THE STRUCTURE
AND FUNCTION OF
NERVOUS TISSUE

VOLUME IV
PHYSIOLOGY II AND BIOCHEMISTRY II

Contributors to This Volume

MARY A. B. BRAZIER

B. G. CRAGG

HUGH DAVSON

EDWARD KOENIG

MARGARET R. MATTHEWS

MASANORI OTSUKA

LINCOLN T. POTTER

GEOFFREY RAISMAN

SYDNEY S. SCHOCHET, JR.

GEORGES UNGAR

A. VAN HARREVELD

THE STRUCTURE
AND FUNCTION OF
NERVOUS TISSUE

Edited by

GEOFFREY H. BOURNE

Yerkes Regional Primate Research Center
Emory University
Atlanta, Georgia

Volume IV
Physiology II and Biochemistry II

1972

ACADEMIC PRESS   New York and London

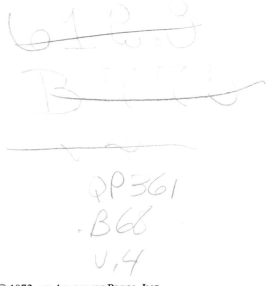

ACADEMIC PRESS, INC.
111 Fifth Avenue, New York, New York 10003

United Kingdom Edition published by
ACADEMIC PRESS, INC. (LONDON) LTD.
24/28 Oval Road, London NW1 7DD

LIBRARY OF CONGRESS CATALOG CARD NUMBER: 68-18660

PRINTED IN THE UNITED STATES OF AMERICA

Contents

Contributors   ix

Preface   xi

Contents of Other Volumes   xiii

1. Plasticity of Synapses

B. G. Cragg

I.	Introduction	2
II.	Short-Term Functional Studies	4
III.	Short-Term Structural Studies	14
IV.	Trophic Effects at Synapses	23
V.	Long-Term Functional Studies	37
VI.	Long-Term Structural Studies	40
VII.	Conclusions	53
	References	55

2. Degeneration and Regeneration of Synapses

Geoffrey Raisman and Margaret R. Matthews

I.	Introduction	61
II.	Degeneration of Synapses	63
III.	Regeneration of Synapses	95
IV.	Summary	99
	References	101

3. Synthesis, Storage, and Release of Acetylcholine from Nerve Terminals

Lincoln T. Potter

I.	Acetylcholine Synthesis	106
II.	Acetylcholine Storage	114
III.	Transmitter Release	120
	References	127

4. Neuronal Inclusions

SYDNEY S. SCHOCHET, JR.

I.	Introduction	129
II.	Inclusions Associated with Viral Infections	132
III.	Nonviral Nuclear Inclusions	135
IV.	Nonviral Cytoplasmic Inclusions	139
V.	Inclusions Derived from Neuronal Fibrous Proteins	159
	References	170

5. Ribonucleic Acid of Nervous Tissue

EDWARD KOENIG

I.	General Aspects of RNA in Nervous Tissue	179
II.	RNA Metabolism	191
III.	Induced Changes in RNA	200
IV.	Special Considerations	208
	References	211

6. Molecular Organization of Neural Information Processing

GEORGES UNGAR

I.	Introduction	215
II.	Chemical Correlates of Information Processing	217
III.	Bioassays for the Molecular Code	220
IV.	Molecular Basis of Neural Coding	231
V.	Concluding Remarks	241
	References	243

7. γ-Aminobutyric Acid in the Nervous System

MASANORI OTSUKA

I.	Introduction	250
II.	Early History	250
III.	Crustacean Neuromuscular Junction	251
IV.	Other Invertebrate Inhibitory Synapses	266
V.	Inhibitory Action of GABA in Nonmammalian Vertebrates	268
VI.	Inhibitory Synapses in Deiters Nucleus	268
VII.	Other Inhibitory Synapses in Mammalian CNS	272
VIII.	Metabolism of GABA in Mammalian CNS	274
IX.	Other Amino Acids Related to GABA	277
X.	General Comments and Conclusion	280
	References	283

8. The Electrical Activity of the Normal Brain

MARY A. B. BRAZIER

I.	Introduction—The Phenomenon as Observed	292
II.	The EEG of Normal Man	293
III.	Neuronal Mechanisms Underlying the EEG	300
IV.	The Effect of Peripheral Stimulation on the Electrical Activity of the Brain	306
V.	Neuronal Mechanisms Underlying the Evoked Potential	316
VI.	Summary	317
	References	317

9. The Blood–Brain Barrier

HUGH DAVSON

I.	Introduction	323
II.	Drainage of the Cerebrospinal Fluid—Arachnoid Villi	330
III.	The Secretion of the Cerebrospinal Fluid—Choroid Plexuses	332
IV.	Chemistry of the Cerebrospinal Fluid	336
V.	Rate of Secretion of Cerebrospinal Fluid	341
VI.	Passage of Infused Material from Blood to Cerebrospinal Fluid	344
VII.	Penetration into Brain	350
VIII.	Permeability of the Choroid Plexus	356
IX.	Slowly Equilibrating Substances	358
X.	Extracellular Space of Brain	358
XI.	Brain–Cerebrospinal Fluid Exchanges	362
XII.	Active Transport Outwards	366
XIII.	Morphology of the Blood–Brain Barrier	369
XIV.	Significance of the Blood–Brain Barrier	376
XV.	Mechanism of Homeostasis	384
XVI.	The Cerebrospinal Fluid and Brain Potentials	387
XVII.	Acid–Base Parameters	391
XVIII.	Some Special Features of the Blood–Brain Barrier System	398
XIX.	Modifications of the Barriers	410
XX.	Ontogeny of the Blood–Brain Barrier	420
XXI.	Special Regions of the Brain	429
XXII.	Peripheral Nerve	431
	Appendix	435
	References	437

10. The Extracellular Space in the Vertebrate Central Nervous System

A. VAN HARREVELD

I.	Space Determinations with Extracellular Markers	449
II.	Electrical Impedance of Central Nervous Tissue	463

III. Chloride and Water Movements in Central Nervous Tissue 474
IV. Electron Microscopy of Central Nervous Tissue 479
V. Mechanisms Involved in the Electrolyte and Water Transport in Central Nervous Tissue 499
 References 506

Author Index 513
Subject Index 539

List of Contributors

Numers in parentheses indicate the pages on which the authors' contributions begin.

Mary A. B. Brazier (291), *Brain Research Institute, School of Medicine, University of California, Los Angeles, California*

B. G. Cragg (1), *Department of Physiology, Monash University, Victoria, Australia*

Hugh Davson (321), *Department of Physiology, University College London, London, England*

Edward Koenig (179), *Department of Physiology, Neurosensory Laboratory, School of Medicine, State University of New York at Buffalo, Buffalo, New York*

Margaret R. Matthews (61), *Department of Human Anatomy, University of Oxford, Oxford, England*

Masanori Otsuka (249), *Department of Pharmacology, Faculty of Medicine, Tokyo Medical and Dental University, Tokyo, Japan*

Lincoln T. Potter (105), *Department of Biophysics, University College London, London, England*

Geoffrey Raisman (61), *Department of Human Anatomy, University of Oxford, Oxford, England*

Sydney S. Schochet, Jr. (129), *Division of Neuropathology, Department of Pathology, University of Iowa, Iowa City, Iowa*

Georges Ungar (215), *Departments of Anesthesiology and Pharmacology, Baylor College of Medicine, Houston, Texas*

A. Van Harreveld (447), *California Institute of Technology, Division of Biology, Pasadena, California*

Preface

Slowly in the course of evolution the generalized irritability of ancient protoplasm became transformed into a nerve impulse. This became possible because of the differentiation of a cell capable of transferring its reaction to stimulation without decrement along extensions of itself to other cells situated a considerable distance away, and even to cells which can store the stimulation and then produce it at will—a process known as "memory." Such cells are known as neurons. These cells and their processes together with supporting cells (neuroglia), investing cells (Schwann cells), various connective tissue, and ectodermal elements form "nervous tissue."

This open-end treatise will deal with nervous tissue as seen through the eyes of anatomists, embryologists, biochemists, pathologists, clinicians, and molecular biologists. So complex is this nervous tissue that all these disciplines have something to contribute to the understanding of its structure and function. The three volumes already published do not of course cover all the aspects of this tissue; subsequent volumes will fill the gap. This synthesis of knowledge is intended as a reference work for graduate students in a variety of disciplines and for those specializing in particular aspects of nervous tissue study who must keep informed of developments in areas other than their own. It is also intended as a general reference work.

The first three volumes were published in rapid succession. Successive volumes will be added from time to time.

Geoffrey H. Bourne

Contents of Other Volumes

Volume I

1. The Origins of the Nervous System
   G. A. Horridge

2. Histogenesis of the Central Nervous System
   Jan Langman

3. Nervous Tissue in Culture
   C. E. Lumsden

4. The Morphology of Axons of the Central Nervous System
   Alan Peters

5. Fine Structural Changes of Myelin Sheaths in the Central Nervous System
   Peter W. Lampert

6. The Morphology of Dendrites
   E. Ramón-Moliner

7. Retrograde Degeneration of Axon and Soma in the Nervous System
   Monroe Cole

8. Morphology of Neuroglia
   P. Glees and K. Meller

9. The Structure and Composition of Motor, Sensory, and Autonomic Nerves and Nerve Fibers
   Lars-G. Elfvin

10. The Perineural Epithelium—A New Concept
    T. R. Shantha and G. H. Bourne

11. The Phenomenon of Neurosecretion
    Helmut O. Hofer

AUTHOR INDEX—SUBJECT INDEX

Volume II

1. The Morphology and Cytology of Neurons
   Totada R. Shantha, Sohan L. Manocha, Geoffrey H. Bourne, and J. Ariëns Kappers

2. The Fine Structure of Brain in Edema
   Asao Hirano

3. Enzyme Histochemistry of the Nervous System
   S. L. Manocha and T. R. Shantha

4. The Nature of Neurokeratin
   M. Wolman

5. The Ultrastructural and Cytochemical Bases of the Mechanism of Function of the Sense Organ Receptors
   Ya A. Vinnikov

6. Part I: Electrical Activity of the Nerve Cell
   Mary A. B. Brazier

6. Part II: Electrical Activity of the Nerve Fiber and Propagation of the Nerve Impulse
   Mary A. B. Brazier

7. Adrenergic Neuroeffector Transmission
   U. S. von Euler

8. Synaptic and Ephaptic Transmission
   Harry Grundfest

9. Macromolecules and Learning
   John Gaito

AUTHOR INDEX—SUBJECT INDEX

Volume III

1. The Subcellular Fractionation of Nervous Tissue
   V. P. Whittaker

2. Identification of Acetylcholine and Its Metabolism in Nervous Tissue
   Catherine Hebb and David Morris

3. Carbohydrate Metabolism in the Nervous System
   J. H. Quastel

4. Key Enzyme Systems in Nervous Tissue
   E. Schoffeniels

5. Phospholipid Metabolism and Functional Activity of Nerve Cells
   Lowell E. Hokin

6. Lipids of Nervous Tissue
   J. Eichberg, G. Hauser, and Manfred L. Karnovsky

7. Serotonin and the Brain
   Irvine H. Page

8. The General Pathology of Demyelinating Diseases
   C. W. M. Adams and S. Leibowitz

9. Metabolic Diseases of the Central Nervous System
   Gian-Carlo Guazzi and Ludo van Bogaert

10. Effects of Ionizing Radiation on Nervous Tissue
    Webb Haymaker

11. Effects of Viruses on Nerves
    George M. Baer

12. Vascular Disorders of Nervous Tissue: Anomalies, Malformations, and Aneurysms
    William F. McCormick

AUTHOR INDEX—SUBJECT INDEX

Volume V

1. The Nerve Growth Factor
   Rita Levi-Montalcini, Ruth H. Angeletti, and Pietro U. Angeletti

2. Neuroglia in Experimentally Altered Central Nervous Systems
   James E. Vaughn and Robert P. Skoff

3. The Pathology of Central Myelinated Axon
   Asao Hirano

4. The Adrenal Medulla
   Norman Kirshner

5. Sites of Steroid Binding and Action in the Brain
   Bruce S. McEwen, Richard E. Zigmond, and John L. Gerlach

6. The Saccus Vasculosus
   H. Altner and H. Zimmermann

7. Representation in the Cerebral Cortex and its Areal Lamination Patterns
   Friedrich Sanides

8. Split-Brain Studies. Funtional Interaction between Bilateral Central Nervous Structures
   Michel Cuénod

9. Electrophysiological Studies of Learning in Simplified Nervous System Preparations
   C. Galeano

AUTHOR INDEX—SUBJECT INDEX

Volume VI

1. Ependyma and Subependymal Layer
   Kurt Fleischhauer

2. Filaments and Tubules in the Nervous System
   Michael L. Shelanski and Howard Feit

3. On the Ultrastructure of the Synapse: The Synaptosome as a Morphological Tool
   D. G. Jones

4. Nonspecific Changes of the Central Nervous System in Normal and Experimental Material
   Jan Cammermeyer

5. The Epiphysis Cerebri
   G. C. T. Kenny

6. Molecular Biology of Developing Mammalian Brain
   Donald A. Rappoport and Richard R. Fritz

7. Excitation and Macromolecules. The Squid Giant Axon
   F. C. Huneeus

8. Macromolecules and Excitation
   Akira Watanabe

9. Dopamine and Its Physiological Significance in Brain Function
   Oleh Hornykiewicz

10. Brain Slices
    G. Frank

AUTHOR INDEX—SUBJECT INDEX

I

Plasticity of Synapses[1]

B.G. Cragg

I.	Introduction	2
II.	Short-Term Functional Studies	4
	A. Recent Experiments	4
	B. Mechanisms of Short-Term Synaptic Modification	8
	C. Summary	14
III.	Short-Term Structural Studies	14
	A. Retina	14
	B. The Neuromuscular Junction	18
	C. Summary and Comments	23
IV.	Trophic Effects at Synapses	23
	A. Growth of Connectivity	24
	B. Experimental Evidence for Inoperative Synapses	25
	C. Synapses on Chromatolytic Neurons	28
	D. Synapses in Degeneration	32
	E. Trans-Synaptic Atrophy	34
	F. Sprouting of Axons and Growth of New Synapses	35
	G. Summary and Comments	36
V.	Long-Term Functional Studies	37
	Summary and Comments	40
VI.	Long-Term Structural Studies	40
	A. Enriched and Impoverished Environments	42
	B. Visual Experience	43
	C. Hormonal and Nutritional Effects on Growth of Synapses	47
	D. Partial Denervations	52
	E. Summary and Comments	53
VII.	Conclusions	53
	References	55

[1] Aided by N.H. and M.R.C. of Australia.

1

I. Introduction

Plasticity of synapses will be taken, in this review, to cover changes in both the efficacy of individual synapses and the numbers of synapses made by axons upon neurons. The subject is in an early stage of development, and most workers have been concerned merely to find situations in which some kind of plastic effect can be shown to occur. This work has produced a small number of relatively clear examples of synaptic modification and a larger number of suggestive results in more difficult situations. The structural effects are often near the limit of reliable measurement, requiring immense labor to produce a significant result, while the demonstration of some of the functional effects requires the use of computers. The next stage will be to determine the mechanisms of synaptic modification in favorable situations, and some evidence has been found that a residuum of active calcium and, possibly also, hyperpolarization can produce facilitation, while depletion of readily releasable transmitter can produce depression.

Progress has been made in thinking about the question of what kind of modification of synapses is required to account for the phenomena of short-term memory and its consolidation into a less frangible long-term form. It appeared from the work of Brindley (1967) that (a) classical conditioning with the possibility of extinction required synapses that would be modified by the activity of the post-synaptic cell and (b) synapses modified by pre-synaptic activity alone were inadequate. This result would exclude the usual form of post-tetanic potentiation, which does not depend on firing of the post-synaptic cell. However, Brindley's analysis was confined to single impulse inputs, and Gardner-Medwin (1969) has shown that, if bursts of impulses are considered to be the essential currency of the nervous system, then simple circuits of neurons with synapses modifiable by pre-synaptic activity alone make possible manipulations of any logical complexity. In this important paper, Gardner-Medwin (1969) also suggests how synapses of short-lasting modifiability could be recycled to provide a long-lasting memory which could be gradually consolidated into a less disruptable form by residual effects in these same active synapses. Figure 1 uses the conventions of Brindley (1967) in which an axon ending in a minimum of two excitatory (unfilled) knobs on a neuron is able to fire that neuron. Thus, a burst of impulses in the pathway of the unconditional stimulus US will fire neuron A and produce a response R. The first spike of a burst of impulses in the conditional stimulus pathway CS will fire neurons B, A, R, and I, and

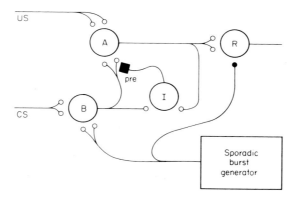

Fig. 1. The neuronal circuit proposed by Gardner-Medwin (1969) in which a short-lived synaptic modification is consolidated to a long-term memory by the activity of a sporadic burst generator. The convention of this diagram is that impulses in two excitatory (unfilled) synapses are needed to fire a cell, while impulses in an inhibitory (filled) synapse stop this firing. The filled square represents an inhibitory synapse that weakens with use. For further explanation, see text.

activation of the inhibitory neuron I prevents further firing of A or R during the rest of the burst, provided that the inhibitory effect of I is of sufficient duration. Activation of US and CS together fires I repeatedly, and the inhibitory synapse made by I is the only modifiable synapse that is postulated. Weakening of this inhibitory synapse with use during the presentation of bursts of impulses at CS and US enables subsequent presentation of CS alone to activate B, A, and R. This conditioning would decay as the inhibitory synapse recovered its potency, but it could be maintained by impulses from a sporadic burst generator which would keep the I synapse depressed, but only if first weakened by CS and US together. Outputs from R during this recycling are prevented by a non-modifiable inhibitory synapse on R represented by the filled knob. This last postulate is analogous to the inhibition of postural motor neurons during paradoxical sleep that coexists with sporadic bursts of impulses in sensory relay nuclei. Gardner-Medwin suggests that, if the time course of weakening of the modifiable I synapse becomes longer with each re-cycling of the conditions for modification, then consolidation will occur. Such a lengthening of time course has been found for post-tetanic po-tentiation by Lloyd (1949) (see Fig. 4), and the modifiable I synapse in Fig. 1 can be replaced by an excitatory synapse exhibiting post-tetanic potentiation with the addition of a few more neurons. In the same way, other particular features of the model can be replaced by logically equivalent arrangements involving a greater number of neuronal elements. In this way, the axo-axonal nature of the modifiable synapse can be avoided.

This approach of drawing simple circuits of neurons and synapses, like all circuits that are drawable, assumes that the number of neurons involved is small and that neuronal connectivity is low. But since learning is not obliterated by small lesions anywhere, there must be many neurons involved in devious circuits in parallel. The more serious objection is to the very concept of a circuit, not because of a lack of connections but because of a lack of structural evidence that connections are not formed between all neighboring neurons within an area of cortex, providing an all-embracing network of connections that is not what is usually meant by a circuit. Structural studies show that connectivity is high, and it has to be supposed that most of the structurally intact synapses, even if modifiable, are in fact turned off at any one time. This dilemma makes urgent some means of identifying inoperative synapses structurally or of obtaining quantitative functional evidence of their prevalence.

II. Short-Term Functional Studies

Electrophysiologists have found a variety of preparations that show some sort of modifiability of input–outptut relations that is presumably due to synaptic plasticity. This work has been reviewed by Morrell (1961a), Sharpless (1964), Bullock (1966), and Kandel and Spencer (1968), and only more recent additions will be mentioned here. These experiments have shown that modification of synaptic action can occur in certain situations, but four related problems need to be discussed: (a) exactly which aspect of the synaptic mechanisms is modified (b) what factors can cause modification (c) what proportion of synapses is modifiable, and (d) the meaning of the various crucial times associated with the process of modification in different preparations.

A. Recent Experiments

Bliss *et al.* (1968) have detected changes in the conductivity of pathways in the cerebral cortex of the unanesthetized cat. A slab of cortex in the suprasylvian gyrus was isolated from all surrounding neuronal connections, leaving the pial blood supply intact. The conductivity was defined as the number of action potentials recorded from a single neuron within an appropriate time slot in the post stimulus histogram divided by the number of electrical stimuli applied to cortex or to white matter nearby. Weak stimuli were used so that the conductivity was less than unity. The time slot contained a peak in the post stimulus histogram some 2–6 msec after the stimulus. The conductivity was tested with a standard stimulus applied at regular intervals, and conditioning stimuli were applied for several minutes.

Most of the pathways tested showed a depression of conductivity with increased frequency of stimulation of the pathway tested, a facilitation with increased neuronal firing caused by stimuli delivered to a different pathway from that used for testing conductivity, and a depression with increased neuronal response to increased stimulation in the test pathway (Fig. 2). The sign of these effects was constant in 19 out of 26 pathways tested, but the sizes of the effects varied from pathway to pathway. The time of conditioning stimulation required to produce an aftereffect was more than 6 minutes and often about 17 minutes, during which time about 2000 stimuli were delivered. The duration of the effect sometimes exceeded 30 minutes and looked as though it would last indefinitely,

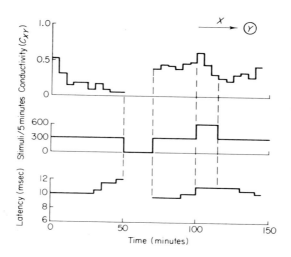

Fig. 2. Changes of cortical conductivity found by Bliss *et al.* (1968) during stimulation of the cortex. The conductivity is the proportion of electrical stimuli that elicit a response in the single neuron whose activity is recorded. Single test stimuli were given at 1/second. During the first conditioning period, this stimulus was turned off, and the conductivity is subsequently increased, while the latency was reduced. During the second period of conditioning the same stimulus was given at 2/second, and the conductivity fell, while the latency increased. Note that the changes last for 20–30 minutes after the conditioning periods.

though in other recordings it passed off with a time constant of about 10 minutes. Although the time slot 2–6 msec after the stimulus limits the number of synapses that can be involved seriatim, some thousands of synapses could be involved in parallel circuits. Single cortical neurons receive an average of 5000–60,000 synaptic connections (Cragg, 1967a) and their axons must make a similar average number of connections. The stimulating electrode is likely to stimulate several axons, for some 100,000 axons cross 1 mm^2 of gray-white boundary in the cat (Sholl, 1955). It is thus not possible to say that the effects are purely homosynaptic or that any particular synapses were modified in the same way as was the behavior of the system as a whole.

The more recent work of Bliss and Lømo (1970) on field potentials in the hippocampus of the rabbit anesthetized with urethane has detected potentiation in a monosynaptic pathway that lasted for several hours after tetanization for only 10–15 seconds. This effect occurred even with stimulus frequencies that were too high to discharge the post-synaptic cell. This simpler situation should make possible an analysis of the mechanism of cortical synaptic modification. It is noted that facilitation occurred at this hippocampal synapse, as in PTP at the neuromuscular junction and at endings of Group I afferents in the spinal cord. It is not yet clear whether the depression which followed afferent stimulation in the work of Bliss *et al.* (1968) is a peculiarity of single synapses in the neocortex or whether it is collective property of the many neurons and synapses activated.

A series of papers has described modifications of neuronal firing in intact cerebral cortex of rats under urethane anesthesia. When the rate of spontaneous firing of single neurons was increased for 10 minutes or more by applying a steady polarizing current, the neuron continued to fire after cessation of the polarizing current at a rate above that found before polarization. This aftereffect might persist for 1–5 hours or as long as the neuron could be held. The polarizing current could be 0.5 μA/mm^2 applied across the cortex (surface positive) or 0.25 μA applied through the extracellular recording electrode (Bindman *et al.*, 1964). It has subsequently been shown that neuronal firing rather than electrical polarization is the essential factor, for similar effects are obtained if the neuronal firing rate is enhanced by cooling of the cortex (Gartside and Lippold, 1967) or prolonged stimulation of the skin (Bindman, 1965; Bindman and Boisacq-Schepens, 1967). The number of action potentials involved in the conditioning period is on the order of 2000–7000. Since the origin of the "spontaneous" neuronal firing that provides the test of conditioning is unknown, it is difficult to say which of the three kinds of contingency of Bliss *et al.* (1968) is involved in these experiments. Both sets of experiments involve abnormal conditions, i.e., neuronally isolated cortex or anesthesia. It remains to be shown that such conditions do not eliminate feedback mechanisms that might oppose such modifiability of the behavior of single units under normal physiological conditions. Boisacq-Schepens (1968) found that the proportion of cortical cells showing prolonged increase in firing rate in unanesthetized rats was only one in four, compared with two in three under urethane. Melzack *et al.* (1969) also described an anesthetic-dependent plasticity of neuronal firing that could be demonstrated by natural stimulation of skin.

A somewhat similar, but longer term, winding-up effect on neuronal firing has been described in unanesthetized rats by Goddard *et al.* (1969). Indwelling bipolar electrodes were implanted in parts of the limbic system, and after recovery electrical stimulation was applied at 62.5/second for 1 minute with 1-msec pulses of 74 μA current. Such stimulation had no apparent effect at first, but after daily application for 1 minute, clonic convulsions were elicited by the same stimulation current at the end of the second week. Convulsions did not occur without electrical stimulation, and could be prevented by making a small electrolytic lesion around the electrode tip. Stimulation for 1 minute every 8 hours or every 7 days was about equally effective, but continuous stimulation for 2–3 days was not effective. This careful work suggests that a repeated raising of neuronal firing rates could have a cumulative effect and has important implications for the genesis of epileptic foci. No doubt, the affected neurons are partially denervated by damage near the electrode, but in addition, there seems to be modification of neuronal excitability or of synaptic efficiency.

The mechanism of the polarization aftereffect in anesthetized rats has been investigated by Gartside (1968a,b). The possibility that reverberating circuits in the cerebral cortex were storing an increased number of impulses after polarization and that these were responsible for the faster neuronal firing was tested by abolishing cortical neuronal firing for about 15 minutes by the use of spreading depression induced by topical application of KCl. After recovery from spreading depression the rate of neuronal firing returned to the enhanced after-polarization value and not to the pre-polarization control value. The enhanced firing rate after polarization had persisted for at least 30 minutes before application of KCl, so some form of consolidation must have occurred in this time. A similar result was found after abolishing neuronal firing throughout the brain by cooling the body below 20°C.

Local applications to the cortex of solutions of drugs known to block protein or RNA synthesis were able to abolish the after-polarization effect without interfering with neuronal firing before or during polarization. The enhanced rate of firing during polarization fell to the prepolarization control level at the end of polarization and there was no aftereffect in the presence of a sufficient dose of cycloheximide, chloramphenicol, neomycin, or 8-azaguanine, while tetracycline and *p*-fluorophenylalanine were relatively ineffective (Fig. 3). The aftereffect is thus dependent on some biochemical reaction that is blocked by the first group of drugs but whether or not this reaction is RNA and protein synthesis has not yet been proved. Dahl (1969) has described a depression of spike and after-potential voltage in the vagus nerve produced by puromycin that is probably not due to inhibition of protein synthesis. However, a promising biochemical approach has been found to the mechanism of the after-polarization effect. We now review some of the other mechanisms that have been proposed for short-term synaptic modifications.

B. Mechanisms of Short-Term Synaptic Modification

In experiments on cerebral cortex where several synapses may be involved seriatim and several thousand synapses in parallel pathways, the overall modification of evoked response could be produced by small changes at many synapses. In contrast to this, the mechanism of synaptic modification is best investigated at single synapses in conditions such that an easily measurable effect occurs. For this reason most work has been done on the neuromuscular junction and on monosynaptic reflexes in the spinal cord, but it is reasonable to regard mechanisms of synaptic modification found to operate in these situations as candidate models for explaining and testing modification mechanisms at other synapses.

The efficacy of the neuromuscular junction is usually investigated by recording the end plate potential intracellularly in the muscle fiber after blocking muscular contraction with curare or magnesium. The agencies causing synaptic modification are then restricted to the number and time distribution of the foregoing pre-synaptic impulses. Three effects occur: a facilitation lasting about 100 msec after a foregoing impulse and decaying in two stages (Mallart and Martin, 1967), a following depression that passes off with a time constant of about 5 seconds, and, after high-frequency tetanic stimulation, a state of post-tetanic potentiation (PTP) that lasts 2–3 minutes. The depression is mainly due to the depletion of the pool of releasable quanta of transmitter by the number of

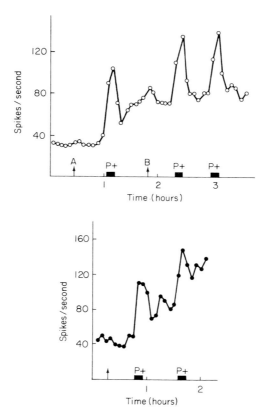

Fig. 3. The effect of inhibitors of protein synthesis on the discharge of cortical neurons after polarization of the cortex (Gartside, 1968b). Top, 0.01 μg of cycloheximide applied topically to the cortex (A) did not prevent electrical polarization (P+) of the cortex raising the firing rate to a higher level that was maintained after the end of polarization. At B, 0.1 μg of cycloheximide did not interfere with the increase in rate of neuronal firing during polarization, but the aftereffect was abolished. Bottom, tetracycline applied at arrow did not prevent the establishment of the aftereffect, and two aftereffects produced a cumulative rise in rate of firing. Thus, the abolition of the aftereffect above was not due to saturation of the firing rate.

quanta released by the foregoing impulses, but there may also be a smaller effect upon the probability of release of quanta (Betz, 1970). When long trains of stimuli are given, recovery from depression is markedly slowed, possible because of depletion of a reserve pool of quanta from which the pool of releasable quanta is refilled. Although the time course of depression and of PTP is short, these mechanisms cannot be rejected as possible explanations for longer-term changes elsewhere because appropriate adaptations of synaptic membranes could prolong the time course and because a small residual effect in the tail of the time course might be effective if it occurred at each of many synapses in a central nervous network.

The possible mechanisms of PTP at the neuromuscular junction have been reviewed by Gage and Hubbard (1966). A pre-synaptic change is involved, for the post-synaptic response to externally applied transmitter is unchanged after repetitive nerve stimulation (Otsuka *et al.*, 1962), while the output of transmitter from the pre-synaptic terminals in response to test stimuli is increased during PTP (Del Castillo and Katz, 1954) and decreased during depression (Elmqvist and Quastel, 1965). In particular, it is the probability of a quantum of transmitter being released by a nerve impulse from among a store of quanta available for release that is increased during PTP. It is not yet known what causes the change in this probability during PTP, but the five suggestions reviewed and rejected by Gage and Hubbard (1966) include hyperpolarization, changes of potassium and sodium gradients, movement of water, and mobilization of transmitter.

Katz and Miledi (1965) suggested that facilitation might be due to a residue of calcium at some pre-synaptic membrane site where it increased the release of transmitter during later nerve impulses. In particular, calcium is thought to be involved in the reaction between the inner side of the axon terminal membrane and the surfaces of the synaptic vesicles which leads to release of transmitter. An experiment with model phospholipid membranes which demonstrates increased adhesion in the presence of an increased concentration of calcium has been described by Blioch *et al.* (1968). This reaction takes place during the action potential and lasts about one-hundredth as long as the subsequent phase of facilitation. In a later paper Katz and Miledi (1968) make two proposals which together could account for a prolonged effect of a residue of calcium at an active site and, thus perhaps, explain PTP as well as facilitation. First, they propose that transmitter release depends on a power (perhaps the fourth power) of the calcium concentration at the active site. A small residue of calcium from one action potential could then have an appreciable facilitating effect on the release of transmitter during a subsequent action potential. In testing this hypothesis, Katz and Miledi (1968) showed that the size of this facilitating effect depended on the external calcium concentration during the first action potential and, thus, on the amount of calcium that entered the terminal, in a manner compatible with the hypothesis. In the giant synapse of the squid, transmitter release is dependent on some power of the external calcium concentration as at the neuromuscular junction (Katz and Miledi, 1970). Second, they proposed that the decline of calcium concentration at the active site after the action potential did not follow an exponential curve but a power law that would leave an effective residuum over a time comparable with that of facilitation. It has not yet been possible to test this second proposal directly, but it is an attractive explanation of the duration of facilitation. In skeletal muscle, also, a persistence of active calcium is responsible in part for the force of contraction increasing with successive closely spaced twitches until it attains the larger value associated with the plateau of a fused tetanus (Jobsis and O'Connor, 1966). In cardiac muscle a form of "memory" can be demonstrated that is probably dependant on a residue of active calcium. Gibbs (1964) showed that the voltage–time integral (area) of the action potential decreases with increased rate of stimulation and that about 3 minutes is required for the area to reach a steady value if the rate of stimulation is changed. This time of adaptation is decreased when the external calcium concentration is reduced. A memory of the previous rate of stimulation can be retained in a inactive cardiac preparation for at least 3 minutes (Gibbs *et al.* 1964) and is probably mediated by the concentration of active calcium.

It is not known whether calcium plays a similar role in the genesis of PTP at synapse in the central nervous system. In the latter, externally applied calcium has a depressant action on the excitability of post-synapse membrane at a lower concentration than that needed to affect the presynaptic membranes of the neuromuscular junction (Kelly *et al.*, 1969), but the significance of this finding is uncertain. A most interesting property of PTP in monosynaptic reflexes of the spinal cord was discovered by Lloyd (1949). As shown in Fig. 4, the time course of decay of PTP is increased markedly after tetanic stimulations of long duration. This finding is confirmed by the results of Beswick and Conroy (1965), but the mechanism has not been investigated. It is compatible with the second postulate of Katz and Miledi (1968) discussed above.

In order to function at a range of frequencies, synapses need to adapt the net rate of production of transmitter to the rate of usage. In the cholinergic neuromuscular junction, Potter (1969) has shown that the rate of formation of acetylcholine is increased by nerve stimulation. In sympathetic nerve endings the concentration of norepinephrine exerts a negative feedback action on the activity of the synthesizing enzyme, tyrosine hydroxylase. Thus, the production of transmitter is derepressed during

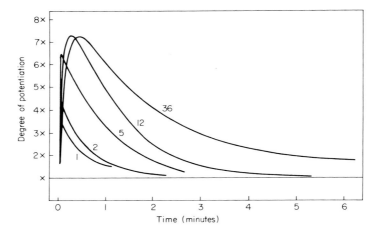

Fig. 4.   The increased duration of post-tetanic potentiation found by Lloyd (1949) after longer periods of repetitive stimulation (1, 2, 5, 12, and 36 seconds) at a constant frequency ($\approx$ 500/second). The electrical stimuli were applied to the central cut end of a muscle nerve, and the reflex response was recorded from the central cut end of an appropriate ventral root.

stimulation. Other mechanisms result in an aftereffect because after 1 hour of stimulation the production of transmitter remains elevated and after 12 hours of increased activity induced by insulin the enzyme tyrosine hydroxylase is increased in activity. Both these aftereffects are blocked by inhibitors of protein synthesis (Weiner, 1970). It is not yet clear whether these mechanisms merely stabilize the store of transmitter or whether there is any overshoot after long periods of increased activity resulting in a strengthening of more active synapses.

An outstanding gap in our knowledge about PTP at central synapses in that almost nothing is known about the behavior of inhibitory synapses after tetanic stimulation. Lloyd (1949) found that the inhibitory effect afferent impulses from stretch receptors in flexor muscles exert on extensor motor neurons showed PTP, but this effect may have been localized at an excitatory ending on an inhibitory interneuron without involving PTP at an inhibitory junction. Inhibitory synapses are prominent on the cell bodies of pyramidal cells in the hippocampus, and Andersen and Lømo (1968) have recorded the intracellular inhibitory post-synaptic potentials (IPSP) produced by electrical stimulation of the fimbria. After tetanic stimulation at 50/second for 10 seconds, the membrane potential takes nearly 10 seconds to recover from hyperpolarization, and during this time test IPSP's are reduced in voltage but lengthened in time.

Excitatory test shocks were not given, and it is not known whether a post-tetanic enhancement or fatigue of inhibition occurs. The latter could be functionally equivalent to PTP, as shown in the circuits of Brindley (1967) and Gardner-Medwin (1969).

Andersen and Lømo (1968) suggest that there are two kinds of excitatory synapses on these pyramidal cells, i.e., those near the cell body that produce an excitatory post-synaptic potential (EPSP) which they call detonator synapses and those far out on the dendrites which need potentiation by repetitive stimulation before they can effectively depolarize the cell. The second group they called intensifying synapses, and these would integrate the pre-synaptic input of impulses over short periods. A somewhat similar distinction between weak and powerful synapses has been made previously by McIntyre (1953) in relation to the dorsal root fibers ending on motor neurons and on neurons of Clarke's column respectively. A sharp distinction between modifiable and unmodifiable synapses has also been found by Morell et al. (1967) in relation to neurons in the third visual area of the cortex in cats (area 19). Single cells in this area respond optimally to light-dark edges or bars moved in certain directions, and Morell et al. (1967) determined the optimum stimulus for each cell studied and recorded the post-stimulus histogram (PSH) of cell firing. Some of these cells also responded to tactile and auditory stimulation, but the PSH was then of a different shape. Combination of the visual stimulus with an auditory or tactile stimulus led to yet another shape of PSH. Morell et al. found than in 102 out of 871 cells studied repeated pairing of the visual and nonvisual stimuli led to a subsequent modification in the shape of the PSH in response to purely visual stimuli. This modification lasted about ½ hour, and could be extinguished by repeated nonpaired visual stimuli or recalled by further pairing. An important point is that cortical neurons showed either clear modifiability of the PSH or no modifiability. There was a suggestion that cells of these two types were grouped in columns. This would follow if the modifiability resided at the terminals of the afferent axons in the columns or at an earlier stage such as the lateral geniculate nucleus. This technique of Morrell et al. of focusing attention on the shape of the PSH is a more subtle method of looking for modifiability than attention to gross rates of firing, but it is more difficult to interpret. There is also the question of whether the neurons can detect the information that resides in the shape of the averaged PSH.

Each of the cortical studies reviewed above has thus detected a proportion of modifiable units and a proportion not modifiable. If this finding were extended throughout the central nervous system, it would be compatible with the neurological failure to localize memory storage to any one structure in the brain. More efficient processing of incoming information could be carried out at all levels in the central nervous system if each were provided with its own modifiable synapses.

C. SUMMARY

Unit and population spike recordings in central nervous system have shown modifiability of input–output relations, but the behavior of individual synapses is still uncertain. At the neuromuscular junction, the retention of a pre-synaptic residue of active calcium is the most likely mechanism of facilitation. In the central nervous system, other possibilities such as post-tetanic hyperpolarization have not been excluded. More elaborate possibilities involving a longer time course and protein synthesis are beginning to be investigated by the use of blocking agents. The agencies producing modification may include post-synaptic cell firing as well as axonal terminal firing, but this effect has not yet been seen in monosynaptic pathways. Almost nothing is known about the modifiability of inhibitory synapses. Only a proportion of single units shows modifiability, and this may be true of synapses also. But there is no reason expect modifiable synapses to be concentrated in any one region of the central nervous system.

III. Short-Term Structural Studies

A. RETINA

The retinal receptors make an unusual form of synapse with bipolar cell dendrites and processes of horizontal cells which are invaginated together into the base of the receptor cell. The bipolar cell dendrite is often flanked on both sides by a horizontal cell process so that a triad of post-synaptic elements is formed (Dowling and Boycott, 1966). In the pre-synaptic terminal of the receptor cell, a prominent synaptic ribbon (Fig. 5) surrounded by vesicles is closely associated with the invaginated post-synaptic processes. This ribbon is also found in receptor cells in the cochlea, vestibular apparatus, pineal eye of amphibia, and electric field detectors of fish. But it is not specific for receptors for it occurs in the axon terminal of the bipolar neuron in the retina. In the rod receptors of the rat, this ribbon can be resolved into a trilaminate structure (Cragg, 1969b) and in the electric field detectors of fish more than three laminae are present (Mullinger, 1969). The retinal receptor synapse has an unusual physiological mechanism since it responds to light by a hyperpolarization associated with a decreased ionic permeability of the membrane (Baylor and Fuortes, 1970). This is a graded rather than an all-or-nothing response, and this is also true of the bipolar neuron, at least in the mudpuppy (Werblin and Dowling, 1969). It can be suggested that the synaptic ribbon is required for vesicle movement toward the post-synaptic membrane in synapses that work without all-or-nothing action potentials. It would be interesting to know whether the ribbons are dissolved in the presence of colchicine, which causes neurotubules to disappear with consequent block of axonal transport (Dahlstrom, 1968; Kreutzberg, 1969).

In spite of these physiological peculiarities, the retinal receptor is an attractive situation for experiments on use and disuse of synapses because there is no neural feedback mechanism on the receptor terminals such as is used to stabilize neuronal firing rates over a wide range of light intensities at higher levels in the visual system. There is every reason to expect that the activity of the receptor synapse is changed by incident light, which is easily controlled.

In the first experiments on this preparation, De Robertis (1958) claimed without statistical tests that when rabbits were kept in darkness for 9 days the synaptic vesicles became smaller, while after shorter periods in darkness the vesicles were congregated close to the synaptic ribbon and region of apposition with the post-synaptic elements. Mountford (1963) performed similar but statistically controlled experiments in guinea pigs and found no significant change in vesicle size. In rats born and reared in complete darkness, I found no significant difference in vesicle size from littermate rats exposed to light for various times from 30 seconds to 4 weeks. There was, however, a significant difference in size between vesicles adjacent to the synaptic ribbon and those in the rest of the synaptic terminal, the former being 9% smaller in diameter than the latter (Cragg, 1969b).

The major difference between the retinal receptors of dark-reared rats and of their light-exposed littermates is in the size of the pre-synaptic receptor terminal itself (Fig. 5). Rearing in darkness or exposure to darkness for 93 days increased the diameter of the receptor terminals by up to 29%, and light exposure as brief as 3 minutes then produced a detectable decrease in terminal diameter. Brief light exposure after dark-rearing also

B. G. Cragg

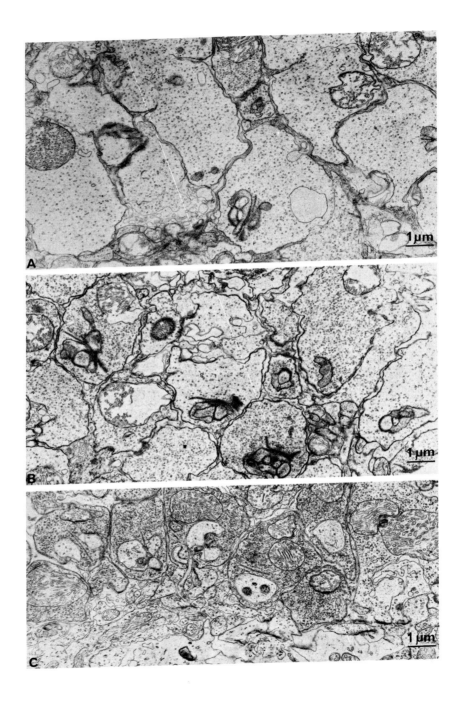

caused an increased electron density of some amorphous substance in the post-synaptic elements (Fig. 5B), and more vesicles were seen post-synaptically. Counting of the synaptic vesicles in unit area of the pre-synaptic receptor terminal showed that the density of vesicles was reduced in darkness and increased after exposure to daylight. Taking the change of terminal diameter into account, the estimated number of vesicles in each terminal (average 18,000) was the same in dark-reared and in light-exposed littermate rats (Cragg, 1969b). Thus, the two main changes on light exposure would be consistent with a change of terminal volume such as would result from a loss of water from the receptor terminals during activity. This is the opposite of the swelling of giant axons during activity found by Hill (1950). Until the ionic basis of the hyperpolarization of the receptor terminals during light exposure is understood, it is impossible to predict what movement of water is to be expected.

It seems surprising that structural changes in synapses should be found in a tissue, such as a retina, that is not usually considered capable of plastic behavior. However, the variations of light exposure involved are extreme, and there is some physiological evidence of changes in the electroretinogram (ERG) under similar conditions. Thus, Zetterstrom (1956) found that in cats reared from birth in darkness the ERG could be elicited reliably by about 4 weeks of age. In the week before this, however, exposure to test flashes (which did not elicit an ERG response) led to the premature appearance of the response when the cat was next tested. It is not clear which component of the ERG was involved in these experiments, and it is possible that more prolonged testing on a single day in the third week would gradually cause a response to develop.

Cornwell and Sharpless (1968) have found a reduction in the b-wave of the ERG of normally reared adult cats after 1 week in darkness that was restored after 3–5 days of room illumination. There is thus evidence that even the retina is capable of fairly long-lasting plasticity of behavior.

Fig. 5. The effect of light and darkness on the synapses made by the rod receptors with bipolar and horizontal cell processes. A litter of rats was reared in diurnal lighting conditions for 97 days. Part of the litter was then kept in complete darkness for 93 days. These rats had wide receptor terminals with a low density of synaptic vesicles (A). Two of these rats were exposed to bright daylight for 2 minutes and 45 seconds immediately before perfusion, the receptor terminals were slightly narrower, and the synaptic vesicles more concentrated (B). The rest of the litter was perfused at the same time after 190 days in diurnal lighting and found to have the usual narrow terminals with a high density of vesicles (C).

B. The Neuromuscular Junction

In the first quantitative work on the neuromuscular junction, Hubbard and Kwanbunbumpen (1968) used exposure to 20 mM KCl solutions to increase the frequency of miniature endplate potentials (mepps). At the phrenic–diaphragm junctions in the rat, 2 hours of this form of stimulation reduced the number of synaptic vesicles found per unit area in electron micrographs, particularly in the part of the terminal near the synaptic cleft. This reduction could have been due to the increased stimulation of the mepps, or it could have been an osmotic effect of the KCl solution. Evidence against the latter possibility was that addition of MgCl$_2$ to the KCl to depress the frequency of mepps prevented the reduction in number of vesicles. More recently, however, hypertonic (360 mM) sucrose solutions have been found to increase the frequency of mepps and to deplete the terminal of vesicles at the frog neuromuscular junction (Clark *et al.*, 1970). These authors found a similar action of black widow spider venom, which was independent of the presence of calcium in the external fluid.

Electrical stimulation is thus preferable to KCl for looking for an effect of excessive use on the neuromuscular junction, and S. F. Jones and Kwanbunbumpen (1970) have stimulated the phrenic nerve at 11.3/second for 90 minutes (61,000 impulses). The diaphragm was maintained *in vitro* at room temperature. In tissue fixed in glutaraldehyde 3 minutes after the end of stimulation there was a reduction of diameter of synaptic vesicles of about 5%. The number of vesicles within 1800 Å of the postsynaptic membrane was also counted. This area is a strip parallel to the synaptic cleft, about 7% of the total width of the terminal, from which vesicles could be expected to be easily released during stimulation. In this area, vesicle numbers were increased by about 17% in tissue fixed 5 minutes after the end of stimulation. S. F. Jones and Kwanbunbumpen (1970) suggest that during stimulation the number of vesicles may be depleted and that this hypothetical deficit is made up with a rebound in the minutes after the end of stimulation.

In all endplates examined after stimulation, the mitochondria were swollen and the cristae disorganized, an appearance not seen in any of the endplates fixed before stimulation. Jones and Kwanbunbumpen suggest that synaptic vesicles are derived from the broken mitochondria. Profiles of the right size are certainly seen in mitochondria (e.g., Fig. 5), but it is difficult to deduce a dynamic process from static micrographs. A striking rearrangement of mitochondria in the axon terminal was also found. Instead of forming a central clump as in control endplates, mitochondria were distributed in a ring adjacent to the inner side of the terminal membrane. This appearance was seen in 7 out of 12 terminals examined 3 minutes after the end of stimulation but was less marked at 5 minutes.

More dramatic reductions in vesicle numbers and diameters were obtained by nerve stimulation in the presence of hemicholinium, which blocks uptake of choline for synthesis of acetylcholine. S. F. Jones and Kwanbunbumpen (1970) suggest that the size of the vesicles is related to their content of acetylcholine, which may swell the vesicle by an osmotic effect. The number of quanta of transmitter released by each nerve impulse fell during stimulation in the presence of hemicholinium, and there was also a fall in the amount of transmitter released in each quantum. The structural and functional findings thus support the hypothesis that the synaptic vesicles carry the transmitter and release it in quanta. As a by-product of this work, S. F. Jones and Kwanbunbumpen (1970) sought an explanation of the slightly elliptical shape of the profiles of synaptic vesicles, whose major and minor axes had an average ratio of 1.3. This profile shape could have been produced by a slight flattening of the vesicles by compression during sectioning, or it could be due to the vesicles themselves having a sausage or disc shape or to random variations around a spherical shape. The histogram of observed vesicle flattening was fitted best by the last hypothesis, with a small effect due to compression in sectioning. The vesicles are thus basically of spherical shape.

A similar technique of counting vesicles close to the synaptic apposition has been applied to the superior cervical ganglion *in vitro* by Quilliam and Tamarind (1969, 1970). These authors found that this local population of vesicles was decreased in number by incubation for 1 hour *in vitro* but increased by nerve stimulation (10 minutes at 10/second or 50/second) and by incubation with drugs that block ganglionic transmission. Incubation with hexamethonium, chlorpromazine, or sucrose also increased the number of vesicles. It is not easy at present to account for these observations, and *in vitro* experiments evidently need careful controls for osmotic effects of drugs.

The possibility that synaptic vesicles and mitochondria carry positive charges on their outer surfaces that determine movements of these particles in the electric fields produced by action potentials has been tested by Landau and Kwanbunbumpen (1969). A steady current of 900 μA was passed through the phrenic nerve to the diaphragm *in vitro* for 3 minutes, and the tissue was then fixed for electron microscopy. It was

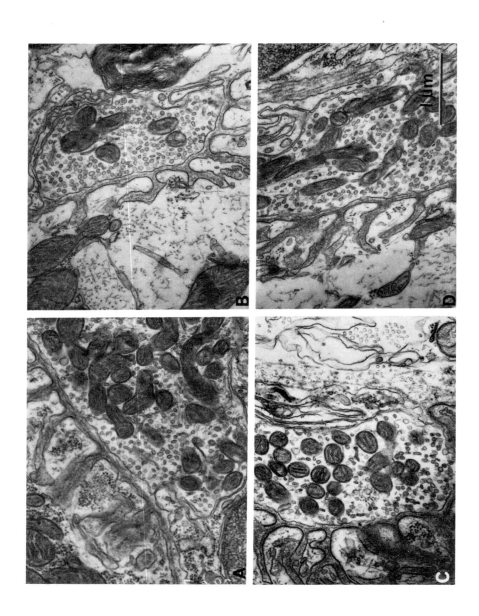

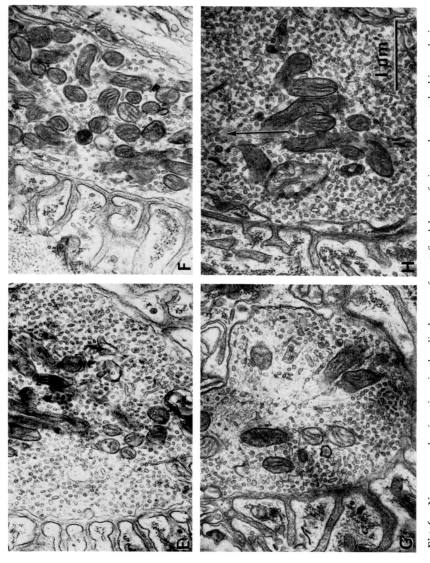

Fig. 6. Neuromuscular junctions in the diaphragm of a rat fixed by perfusion under pentobarbitone during stimulation of one phrenic nerve at 11.5/second A–F stimulated side, G–H opposite, nonstimulated side. The distribution and form of the mitochondria and vesicles is unchanged.

found that depolarizing currents produced a high density of vesicles and mitochondria, while hyperpolarizing currents had the reverse effect and led to a sparse distribution of these particles. It does not necessarily follow that these changes were due to the particles migrating under the imposed electric field, for a change in volume of the terminal containing the particles similar to that found in retinal receptors (Cragg, 1969b) would produce the same result. The same possible explanation applies to the finding of Siegesmund *et al.* (1969) that profiles of synaptic terminals in monkey cerebral cortex contained more vesicles following the passage of electric currents through the brain at a strength that rendered the animal unresponsive to painful stimuli. An early claim by De Robertis and Vaz Ferriera (1957) to have found an increase in the number of synaptic vesicles in the splanchnic nerve endings in the adrenal medulla after stimulation at 100/second for 10 minutes and a depletion after stimulation at 400/second for the same time does not appear to have been tested in the ensuing 13 years, and it would be helpful if negative results were published as readily as new findings. D'Anzi (1969) produced a reflex stimulation of the splanchnic endings in the adrenal medulla by giving rats insulin and found that the number of epinephrine storage vesicles in the cells of the medulla, and the epinephrine content, were greatly depleted after 3–4 hours, but he did not report on the pre-synaptic terminals.

The work of Hubbard, Jones, and Kwanbunbumpen on the neuro-muscular junction represents an advance in showing what structural changes could be produced in axon terminals by excess use. It is, however, an *in vitro* result that might be due to the metabolites produced by the muscle during stimulation in the absence of a vascular circulation; a depletion of vesicle numbers by stimulation was not observed (except in the presence of hemicholinium) but inferred from the rise in vesicle numbers 5 minutes after the end of stimulation. For these reasons I have repeated the experiments *in vivo* in rats anesthetized with pentobarbitone and have fixed the tissue by vascular perfusion with aldehydes during stimulation. The phrenic nerve was cut and stimulated at 11.5/second for 90 minutes at a point 1 cm above the diaphragm on the left side. Maximal contractions of the hemi-diaphragm were still occurring at perfusion, but examination of 10 endplates did not show any with disorganized mitochondria nor with mitochondria aligned around the periphery of the terminal (Fig. 6). Counts of numbers of vesicles within 1800 Å of the synaptic membrane gave an average areal density (per square micron) of 108.5 (SE 5.1) on the stimulated side, and 119.8 (SE 5.4) in 10 terminals on the contralateral control side. These values are not significantly different for the small numbers of terminals found, and of course, the unknown section thickness enters into the vesicle counts as a first-order variable. There is a case for repeating the *in vitro* experiments with curare to block any extraneous effects of muscle contraction upon the neuromuscular junction. An alternative explanation, i.e., that the ultrastructural changes *in vitro* are due to a lack of choline, has been put forward by Parducz and Feher (1970). These authors examined the superior cervical sympathetic ganglion after 90 minutes of nerve stimulation and found no change when the experiment was done *in vivo* but a gross loss of vesicles and damage to mitochondria in nerve terminals when the experiment was done in Locke's solution. Addition of choline to the latter prevented the ultrastructural changes.

C. SUMMARY AND COMMENTS

There is no good reason to expect structural changes in synapses in short-term experiments except in abnormal conditions. The first exposure of dark-reared animals to light, and the prolonged stimulation of the phrenic nerve/diaphragm preparation *in vitro* are abnormal situations for the synapses concerned. Structural changes caused by excess use are of limited value for the interpretation of normal structure because excess use will usually be prevented by neuronal feedback mechanisms. More useful would be a way of recognizing unused synapses if there are any, but the effects of prolonged cooling or anesthesia have not yet been examined. In any case, inoperative synapses in central nervous tissue may be produced by a failure of post-synaptic receptivity rather than a lack of pre-synaptic impulse activity. This topic is reviewed in Section IV.

IV. Trophic Effects at Synapses

In this section we discuss the rise in the number of synapses during development, the significance of the large number of synapses found in the adult central nervous system, and the question of whether or not these synapses are all active. There is a possibility that formed synapses might be rendered inactive by substances derived from the post-synaptic cell, and several pieces of experimental evidence suggest that inactive synapses may occur. It would be of great interest to be able to recognize inactive synapses from their structure as seen by electron microscopy, so the structural changes in synapses during degeneration, trans-synaptic atrophy, and retrograde cell reaction are discussed. Some kind of trophic chemical signal is probably also involved in the sprouting of nerve fibers and production of new synapses that occurs in several situations in response to partial denervation.

A. GROWTH OF CONNECTIVITY

The postnatal increase in number of synapses in the superficial cerebral cortex of the cat was examined qualitatively by Voeller *et al.* (1963). They found axodendritic synapses similar to those in adult cortex present at birth, whereas axosomatic synapses were rarely seen until the end of the first week of postnatal life. Counts of synaptic membrane appositions stained specifically by alcoholic phosphotungstic acid were made by Aghajanian and Bloom (1967) in the parietal cortex of the rat. Between 12 and 26 days after birth, they found a rise from 2×10^8 to 14×10^8 synapses/mm³. There was also some indication of a development and separation of the pre-synaptic projections from the synaptic appositions. Axon terminals were examined in developing rat motor cortex by Armstrong-James and Johnson (1969) and were found to have fewer synaptic vesicles in each terminal profile than the adult rat. There was a rise from 1.1×10^{11} to 12.6×10^{11} in the number of axon terminals per cubic centimeter from 1-day-old to mature rats. The latter figure of 12.6×10^{11} terminals/cm³ is close to the estimate of Aghajanian and Bloom (1967), which was 14×10^8/mm³ or 14×10^{11}/cm³. It is also close to my own estimate of 14×10^{11}/cm³ for rat visual cortex (Cragg, 1968).

Little is yet known about the time of development of synapses at other levels in the nervous system, though Karlsson (1967) found the major rise in the number of axon terminals in the lateral geniculate nucleus of the rat to be in the second week of postnatal life. Bodian (1968) has found that the number of synapses in monkey spinal cord rises steadily from 50 days of gestation to term. Degenerating nerve fibers can be found during prenatal development of the spinal cord in the monkey (Bodian, 1966). Degenerating synapses do not seem to have been described, but this question is relevant to whether synapses can persist structurally in a nonfunctional condition. It is not yet known whether synapses decrease significantly in numbers in aged animals. In 2-year-old senile rats, very few spontaneously degenerating nerve fibers can be detected with the Nauta method although axonal degeneration due to experimental lesions is stainable by the Nauta method for several months (Cragg, 1967a). In other species old age may be associated with a loss of neurons (Brody, 1955), but it has not been shown that this can occur spontaneously and independently of deterioration of the local blood supply.

The number of axonal terminals found in 1 cm³ of adult cerebral cortex is on the order of 10^{12}, while the number of cortical neurons found in the same volume varies from 10^8 in close-packed areas such as monkey visual cortex to 10^7 of the much larger neurons in human motor cortex (Cragg, 1967a). Thus, the average number of synapses associated with one neuron is 10^4–10^5. This does not necessarily imply that each neuron is connected to this number of other neurons, because any one connection between two neurons may be made by many synapses. The highest estimate for this redundancy in cerebral cortex is 60 (Marin-Padilla, 1968). Higher redundancy presumably occurs in the connection between the climbing fiber and the Purkinje cell in the cerebellum, but nothing like this system of coordinated branching of closely approximated axon and dendrite has been seen in cerebral cortex. When all reasonable allowance is made for redundancy and other factors, it is difficult to escape the conclusion that neurons are more highly interconnected than anything else of which we have experience (Cragg, 1967a, 1968). Are all those synapses working, or is a large reserve turned off in some way? Inoperative synapses could represent structurally the behavior learned during development or the potential for future modification of behavior. Some experimental evidence can be interpreted to support the concept of functionally inoperative (modifiable) but structurally intact synapses.

B. EXPERIMENTAL EVIDENCE FOR INOPERATIVE SYNAPSES

The are five examples of experiments which show a loss of effectiveness in previously effective synapses, but in only two of these is there evidence that the ineffective synapses persist structurally. Two further experiments appear to show a sudden gain of effectiveness in previously ineffective synapses, and we shall review these first. Aserinsky (1961) reinvestigated the crossed phrenic phenomenon: When the cord is hemisected above the phrenic motor neurons, the ipsilateral diaphragm becomes inactive, but if the contralateral phrenic nerve is now blocked with local anesthetic, the ipsilateral diaphragm becomes active within 10 minutes. This result is thought to be due to descending impulses crossing below the hemisection to excite the contralateral phrenic motor neurons. If the synapses made by the crossing fibers were normally inoperative but were activated during the experiment, the result would follow. Presumably, hypercapnia and hypoxia would cause an increased frequency of impulses in the inoperative terminals of the crossing fibers. This seems to be an example of preformed but ineffective axon terminals rapidly aquiring control of the post-synaptic cell as a result of enhanced pre-synaptic impulse traffic in the crossing fibers. The effect persists after the local anaesthetic block has worn off (in about 4–12 hours) for 1–2 days in the dog. Little work has been done to establish the structural and functional mechanisms of the effect, however, and Rosenblueth *et al.* (1938) reached the improbable conclusion that some previously unknown form of neural message was transmitted when the phrenic nerve was blocked.

Wall showed that certain rootlets in a dorsal root could be cut without altering the response of a dorsal horn cell to natural stimulation of the skin, yet electrical stimulation of the same rootlets caused monosynaptic responses in the dorsal horn cell (see Cragg, 1967a, p. 651). This suggested that synapses made by fibers in these rootlets onto some dorsal horn cells might be inoperative under natural conditions yet excitable by synchronized electrical stimulation. The evidence that fibers in such rootlets contributed nothing to the dorsal horn cell response under natural conditions is weak, however.

An example of a synapse that persists structurally in an inactive state is the neuromuscular junction paralyzed with botulinum toxin (Thesleff, 1960). Here the failure of transmission is due to inhibition of release of acetylcholine in the nerve terminal, and electron micrographs show no qualitative structural abnormality. These nontransmitting synapses are still able to protect the post-synaptic membrane from the fall in acetylcholine esterase activity that occurs after denervation (Stromblad, 1960; Duchen, 1970).

A denervated external eye muscle in a fish is able to attract innervation from the nerve destined for a neighboring but antagonistic eye muscle after removal of the latter. Marotte and Mark (1970a) have shown that this inappropriate nerve supply loses its function in contracting the muscle when the correct nerve regenerates. The loss of function of the inappropriate nerve occurred at the same time that the function of the appropriate nerve recovered. Electron microscopy has not detected any degeneration or any other qualitative abnormality in the neuromuscular junctions (Marotte and Mark, 1970b). They suggest that synapses may compete for control of the post-synaptic cell and that inappropriate connections may suffer a reduction in transmitter release, a diffusion barrier, or a failure of receptivity in the post-synaptic membrane. Mark (1970) has made this idea the basis of a possible mechanism for memory.

In the remaining examples, synapses are switched off, but there is as yet no evidence as to whether the synapses persist structurally. Jacobson and Baker (1969) transposed large pieces of skin between the back and belly of tadpoles. At larval stage 20 reflex wiping movements of the legs could be elicited by local irritation of the skin. Immediately after metamorphosis into frogs the reflex wiping was correctly directed toward the origin of the irritation. In half the frogs, however, there were also misdirected reflex movements toward the place where the stimulated skin had been taken from, the other half of the frogs developed such misdirected reflexes 3–8 days after metamorphosis. In the latter animals, the reflex response changed apparently spontaneously from a correctly directed to a misdirected wiping movement. This inversion did not occur if grafts were made after larval stage 15. Jacobson and Baker (1969) showed that the inversion was not due to some specific pattern of nerve impulses determined by the skin. The misdirected reflexes were permanent unless the skin graft was returned to its correct orientation (when correctly directed reflexes returned in some frogs), while misdirected reflexes persisted in others. These results suggest that substances derived from the skin may be ingested into the primary sensory neurons and may determine the effectiveness of the central connections made by these neurons. The suddenness of the change is unexplained and brings to mind the sudden specification of ganglion cells in *Xenopus* retina over a period of 10 hours at embryonic stage 30 (Jacobson, 1968a). However, this specification is the first known feature differentiated in these cells after their replication of DNA has ceased (Jacobson, 1968b). The central neurons responsible for the wiping reflex, as well as the skin, are presumably already fully differentiated before the switching of connections takes place. It is possible that some lytic agent appears after metamorphosis and inactivates ill-matched connections that were previously tolerated.

An appearance and disappearance of new connections was seen in the superior cervical sympathetic ganglion by Murray and Thompson (1957) and Guth and Bernstein (1961). The preganglionic pupillo-dilator fibers to this ganglion are derived from roots T1–3, while T4–7 supply vasoconstrictive fibers. Roots T1–3 were crushed, and 1 month later roots T4–7 were found to have acquired a new ability to produce pupillo-dilatation. After 6 months, however, when T1–3 had regenerated back to the ganglion, T4–7 had lost their ability to cause pupillo-dilatation in most instances. This result seems to imply that T4–7 sprouted and formed new synapses in the ganglion and that these synapses became inoperative when T1–3 reestablished their ganglionic connections. It is not known whether the synapses made by T4–7 axons finally degenerated or whether they persisted structurally. A second crush of T1–3 and measurement of the time till T4–7 aquired pupillo-dilator properties a second time might indicate the answer to this question.

Hubel and Wiesel (1970) have published further evidence that cortical visual cells fail to respond to appropriate visual stimulation through an eye that had been closed during a critical period after eye opening. Since fairly normal responses were present in the small number of single cells examined in newborn cats (Hubel and Wiesel, 1963), this suggested that some previously formed synapses had become inoperative. Competition between neurons connected to the two eyes was required for this result, for closure of both eyes produced much less abnormality of cortical cell response.

An experimental approach to the question of whether nonfunctioning synapses can persist structurally is to ask what happens to axon terminals synapsing on cells when the latter degenerate after section of their axons. Do axon terminals degenerate or dedifferentiate and retract, or do they persist for long periods without post-synaptic contacts?

C. Synapses on Chromatolytic Neurons

Blinzinger and Kreutzberg (1968) found that some axon terminals making synapses on facial motor neurons appeared to be displaced from the cell body by glial cells 4 days after section of the facial nerve. Barron *et al.* (1969) and Bodian (1964) did not see this effect in motor neurons of the spinal cord. Hamori (1968) studied the lateral geniculate nucleus in cats 2 months after section of the optic tract combined with ablation of the visual cortex. Axon terminals were still present in the lateral geniculate nucleus but formed into clumps without dendritic elements. There were numerous synaptic thickenings between one axon terminal and another.

There is a strong suggestion that in some situations axon terminals do not remain intact after the cell bodies on which they ended have degenerated. Ablation of the cingulate cortex leads to retrograde degeneration of the neurons in the anterior thalamic nuclei that project to this cortex. In young rabbits, cingulate cortex ablation also leads to degeneration of the medial mammillary neurons that project to the anterior thalamic nuclei (Bleier, 1969). This suggests that the thalamic terminals of these mammillary neurons are not viable in the absence of their post-synaptic elements. A similar situation occurs in the visual system because Van Buren (1963) has found degeneration in retinal ganglion cells in monkeys 4 years after ablation of the visual cortex. However, since the lateral geniculate neurons degenerate within a few weeks of cortical ablation, and retinal ganglion cells in the monkey degenerate within a few months of section of their axons, this result implies that optic nerve terminals are able to persist in the lateral geniculate nucleus for some years (but not 4 years) after the neurons on which they ended have degenerated.

I have started to look at axon terminals in the lateral geniculate nucleus and anterior thalamic nuclei after removal of visual and cingulate cortex in young rats. When the lateral geniculate nucleus (pars dorsalis) was examined 4 months after removal of visual cortex at 11 days of age, light microscopy showed the presence of only one or two neurons in any 30-μ thick cross section of the nucleus, which was grossly shrunken. Electron microscopy showed clusters of persisting axon terminals without post-synaptic elements (Fig. 7A). On the normal contralateral side, such a cluster of terminals had several post-synaptic dendrites (Fig. 7B).

Qualitatively, the surviving axon terminals were not obviously abnormal though there is a strong suggestion that they are larger and fewer than on the normal side. Further work is needed to count and measure these terminals, to determine whether they are of optic or intrinsic origin, and to compare the fate of terminals in the antero-ventral thalamic nucleus after decortication. There is nevertheless an indication that axon terminals may persist independently of their post-synaptic structures in some situations. One such situation might be that the cell body of origin should possess other terminals on intact post-synaptic structures, as the retinal ganglion cells do on the superior colliculus neurons after degeneration of the lateral geniculate nucleus. This does not apply to the intrinsic neurons whose cell bodies are in the lateral geniculate nucleus and whose axon terminals are thought to lie wholly within the nucleus. The identification of the origin of the persisting terminals is thus an important issue.

Electrophysiological experiments have found remarkable changes in synaptic transmission onto neurons undergoing chromatolysis as a result of axonal section. An extreme case is the total block of synaptic transmission that occurred in the stellate ganglion of the cat examined *in vitro* (Brown and Pascoe, 1954). There was normal conduction in the preganglionic axons and in the postganglionic axons up to the point of section.

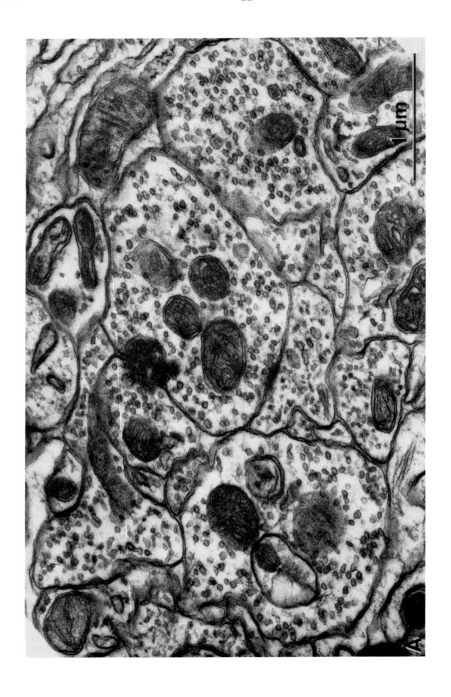

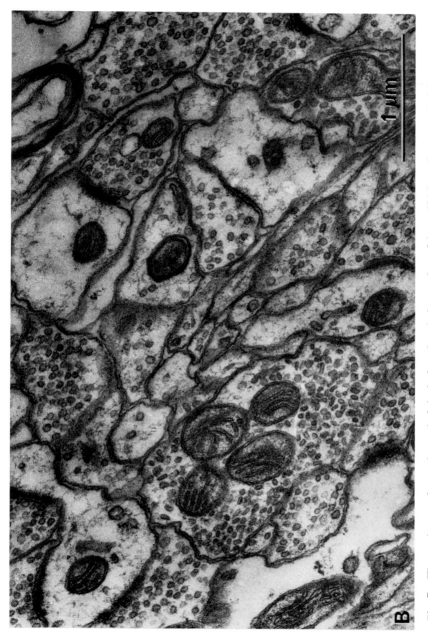

Fig. 7. The persistence of synaptic terminals in the lateral geniculate nucleus of the rat 134 days after removal of the visual cortex at 11 days of age. After decortication the post-synaptic dendrites degenerate but groups of axons terminals persist without post-synaptic elements (A). In a comparable group of synaptic terminals on the contralateral normal side (B) there are numerous post-synaptic dendrites.

The output of acetylcholine from the axon terminals seems to be normal, but the response of the chromatolytic neuron to exogenous acetylcholine is deficient. The monosynaptic responses in spinal motor neurons with cut axons to dorsal root stimulation are not blocked but show striking abnormalities (McIntyre *et al.*, 1959; J. C. Eccles *et al.*, 1958). The latency is increased and is variable, while the threshold to stimulation by some afferents is decreased and to others increased. This does not necessarily mean that the synapses have changed differentially, for antidromic stimulation of the motor axon shows a lowered threshold for invasion of the cell body but a raised threshold in the more distal dendrites. Thus, there is no strong indication that any of the abnormalities that have been described involve changes in any structure other than the post-synaptic neuron, which exhibits chromatolysis.

D. Synapses in Degeneration

Degeneration is the extreme case, for aspects of synaptic structure that are not modified by degeneration are probably not candidates for modification under milder conditions. The topic has been reviewed recently by E. G. Jones and Powell (1970). Section of an axon leads to one of two patterns of structural change at the axon terminal. In one, there is a proliferation of neurofilaments in the axon and an extension of neurofilaments into the terminal. Recently, a correlation of failure of synaptic transmission in the lateral geniculate nucleus in cats has been found with proliferation of neurofilaments and decrease in the number of synaptic vesicles (Pecci-Saavedra *et al.*, 1970). The synaptic vesicles have also been found to increase in diameter in the optic nerve terminals in the pigeon tectum (Cuenod *et al.*, 1970). In the other pattern, the terminal shrinks and the vesicles and mitochondria form a dark fragmenting clump. The times at which these changes appear and the time during which the remains of degenerating synapses can be recognized vary in different situations, extremes being 1–3 days in substantia gelatinosa (Heimer and Wall, 1968) and 1 day to 3 months in pyriform cortex (Westrum, 1969), though in the latter case some slow process of trans-synaptic atrophy may be continuing. An interesting feature of degeneration is that the thickened membrane specialization on the post-synaptic cell or dendrite may persist after the axon terminal has been removed and replaced by a glial cell (Westrum and Black, 1968; Pinching, 1969). This is illustrated in Fig. 8. Thus, structural changes are not likely to be seen in this part of the synapse during any physiological process of synaptic modification.

What then is left for structural modification on the post-synaptic side? There seems to be only the width of the synaptic cleft, and the disposition of the wisps of dark amorphous material that project from the membranes of the synaptic cleft and are particularly well shown by staining with phosphotungstic acid. The synaptic cleft has been found to change in width with strong polarizing currents (Landau and Kwanbunbumpen, 1969) but has not been measured systematically in other physiological conditions that might induce synaptic modification. The projections from the

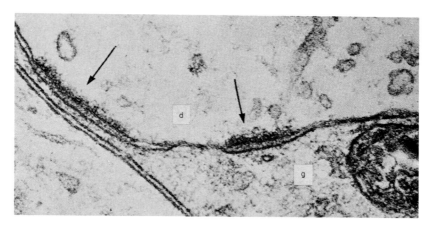

Fig. 8. The post-synaptic membrane specializations (arrows) in the olfactory bulb may remain intact 84 days after cutting the presynaptic axons (Pinching, 1969). These membrane thickenings on a dendrite (d) are now apposed by a glial cell (g) but are apparently unaltered.

terminal membranes have been found to change slightly during postnatal development (Aghajanian and Bloom, 1967) but have not been examined systematically in physiological experiments. There is some not very convincing evidence that these dark projections may contain sialic acid that can be liberated by incubation with neuraminidase (Bondareff and Sjostrand, 1969). Much speculation on the possible role of an outer cell coat of glycoprotein in controlling membrane properties (Schmitt and Samson, 1969) has yet to bear fruit in appropriate experiments. Some substance produced by the post-synaptic cell might pass across the cleft to render the pre-synaptic terminal inoperative by interfering with the liberation of transmitter. In this case there might well be no structural alteration at the level of electron microscopy, as in the botulinum poisoned neuromuscular junction (Thesleff, 1960). There is some experimental evidence against a movement of substances across the synaptic cleft at a squid giant synapse under the conditions studied by Heuser and Miledi (1970). Altogether, it seems unlikely that inoperative synapses would be structurally recognizable unless some physiological stimulus can be applied that alters the structure of functioning synapses but leaves inoperative synapses unaffected, or vice versa. An example from another field of such a stimulus is the action of cortisone which causes greater atrophy in little-used muscles than in posturally active muscles (Goldberg and Goodman, 1969).

E. TRANS-SYNAPTIC ATROPHY

In some situations neurons shrink and stain less brightly with Nissl dyes after axons afferent to them have been sectioned. In the lateral geniculate nucleus of the monkey there are recognizable effects as soon as 4 days after section of the optic nerve (Matthews *et al.*, 1960). It is not known whether this atrophy is due to loss of nerve impulses or to loss of trophic chemical provided by the presynaptic neuron. Now that nerves can be blocked for 2 weeks with local anaesthetic (Robert and Oester, 1970), apparently without causing degeneration, it should be possible to test the first possibility.

What happens to the axon terminals of the neurons that undergo trans-synaptic atrophy? A direct physiological experiment requires electrical stimulation of the optic radiation and electrical recording from visual cortex, and Sakakura and Doty (1969) found abnormally large responses in these circumstances. I have compared the primary visual cortical areas on the two sides in two monkeys 4 months after unilateral optic tract section (Cragg, 1968). No axon terminals of abnormal structure were recognized, but some of unusually large size (1.5 μm diameter) were present on the deafferented side. The average size of the axon terminals throughout the depth of the cortex was 13.5% larger on the deafferented side, while the number of terminals in a unit volume was 23% less. When lesions are made in the lateral geniculate nucleus the terminals which blacken and show degeneration in the visual cortex form a small proportion of the terminals present, even in lamina 4 where the termination is densest. Thus, the change in average size and density of terminals in visual cortex must be largely a secondary effect on terminals whose cell bodies are intracortical. In repeating this work on cats, I have found only small changes in the same direction after 4–10 months survival. This may be related to the long period (2–10 months) required for trans-synaptic atrophy to become conspicuous in the cat's lateral geniculate nucleus (Cook *et al.*, 1951). Very large axon terminals (up to 15-μ diameter) have been found in a condition of psychomotor retardation in man for which there is at present no experimental model (Gonatas *et al.*, 1967).

F. Sprouting of Axons and Growth of New Synapses

Evidence that partial denervation may cause surviving axons to sprout and form new synapses in central nervous tissue continues to increase following the discovery of the phenomenon in muscle (reviewed by Edds, 1953). Liu and Chambers (1958) sectioned the cortico-spinal tract on one side in cats and waited about 300 days for sprouting to occur and for the debris of damaged neurons to be removed (i.e., for Nauta stained sections to become negative). They then cut one dorsal root on each side and studied the distribution of these degenerated root fibers with the Nauta method 4–5 days later. A larger distribution was found on the hemisected side of the cord. McCouch *et al.* (1958) question how much of this was due to sprouting and how much to a fattening of dorsal root axons making the degenerating fibers more prominent in light microscope preparations. These authors found an increased amplitude of pre-synaptic spike potential but no significant increase in "internuncial potentials," suggesting an absence of new functioning terminals. Similarly, J. C. Eccles *et al.* (1962) found no evidence that a section of two-thirds of the dorsal root filaments on one side in young kittens led to the remaining dorsal root filaments aquiring functioning synapses on motor neurons not normally innervated by these roots.

Better structural evidence for sprouting axons has been found by D. C. Goodman and Horel (1966) in the visual system of rats. At 3 months of age, the occipital cortex was removed unilaterally, and 16 months later both eyes were removed. The brains were fixed a few days later, and the extent of fiber degeneration due to the eye removal compared on the two sides of the brain with the Nauta method. On the side of the cortical lesion the dorsal lateral geniculate nucleus was degenerated, and new connections seemed to have been formed by the optic axons in the caudal half of the ventral lateral geniculate nucleus, and also in the caudal part of the lateral nucleus of the optic tract and the subjacent medial quarter of the pretectal nucleus. A similar detection technique was applied by Schneider and Nauta (1969) 14–25 weeks after removal of superficial layers of the superior colliculus in newborn hamsters. In this case, some retinal axons were found to have crossed the tectal midline to end in the normal superior colliculus, and there was an increased retinal projection to the ventra part of the lateral geniculate nucleus. Most surprisingly, there was dense terminal degeneration in the thalamic nucleus lateralis posterior which does not normally receive direct retinal projections.

These light microscopic demonstrations of axonal sprouting have recently been supplemented by electron microscopical evidence of formation of new synapses. Raisman (1969) studied the medial septal nucleus in rats and showed that afferent fibers coming from the fimbria ended mainly on dendrites, with very few axo-somatic endings. Hypothalamic afferents ended on both dendrites and cell bodies. Raisman, then made a lesion in one of these systems of afferents and after 3–6 months studied the distribution of the other system. Destruction of the hypothalamic fibers led to fimbrial fibers occupying abnormally numerous sites on cell bodies, while fimbrial lesions resulted in an unusually high proportion of the hypothalamic terminals being found on dendrites.

In view of the findings of J. C. Eccles *et al.* (1962), functional studies of these sprouting situations are needed to determine whether neurons are really so adaptable in their connections or whether these experiments are recipes for making inoperative synapses.

G. Summary and Comments

During development, the structural connectivity of neurons rises to a uniquely high level by the time that the animal achieves an independent life. There is no functional estimate of neuronal connectivity, but several experiments suggest that synapses may be able to persist structurally in an inoperative, but possibly modifiable, mode. If this is so, effective neuronal connectivity may not exceed the levels that have been considered in simulation of the nervous system. So important a conclusion still needs much more convincing evidence, however. Inoperative synapses have not been recognized by electron microscopy. The lack of change at the post-synaptic membrane during degeneration of the pre-synaptic terminal makes it unlikely that a change could be recognized post-synaptically in inoperative synapses. On the pre-synaptic side, the lack of structural change in motor–axon terminals inactivated chronically with botulinum toxin is not encouraging. The possibilities that remain are that cleft width or glycoprotein attachments to the synaptic membrane could be abnormal in inoperative synapses. It seems more likely, however, that some reaction to a physiological stimulus will be needed to differentiate normal from inoperative synapses structurally.

V. Long-Term Functional Studies

McIntyre (1953) distinguished between weak and powerful synapses made in the spinal cord by dorsal root fibers innervating stretch receptors. In the ventral horn these fibers form weak synapses on motor neurons that show a high degree of post-tetanic potentiation (PTP). If the afferent fibers are cut distal to the dorsal root ganglion, the cell bodies in the ganglion show prominent chromatolysis, and some weeks later electrical stimulation of the afferent fibers shows a change in the monosynaptic reflex response from the ventral horn. Single volleys fail to fire the ventral horn cells, but tetanic stimulation produces an unusually powerful and prolonged PTP (J. C. Eccles and McIntyre, 1953; J. C. Eccles et al., 1959). It would be interesting to know whether the axon terminals show a structural change. A reduction in size of the fibers in the dorsal funiculus has been found recently after section distal to the dorsal root ganglion in rats on the day of birth (Kingsley et al., 1970). In the ventral horn the affected terminals constitute a low proportion of all the terminals present, and this situation is thus unfavorable for electron microscopy. The more concentrated central terminations of the vagus nerve offer a more favorable situation, and one of the reflexes induced by central vagal stimulation changes in a similar way to the monosynaptic cord reflex after distal section of the nerve (Cragg, 1965).

The more powerful synapses made by the primary stretch afferents are on the cells in Clarke's column which relay impulses to the cerebellum. These endings fire the post-synaptic cells with a high safety factor and little sign of PTP (McIntyre, 1953; McIntyre and Mark, 1960). If the afferent fibers are cut distal to the dorsal root ganglia, the endings are weakened but are still able to fire a considerable proportion of the post-synaptic cells some weeks later. A different form of disuse has, however, shown an increase in synaptic efficacy at this termination of stretch afferents on cells of Clarke's column. Sectioning of the tendon of a muscle leads to muscle atrophy, for stretch is an important trophic factor for muscle (Schiaffino and Hanzlikova, 1970). Loss of stretch was expected to reduce the input to the cord of impulses in stretch afferent fibers. It was subsequently shown that afferent activity from unidentified receptors in the atrophying muscle was increased after tenotomy, though the activity in the stretch receptors was not (see reviews by Kozak and Westerman, 1966; Kandel and Spencer, 1968). Thus, the effects of tenotomy could be due to reduced afferent input from the stretch receptors.

In a further attempt to eliminate afferent activity in stretch receptors, April and Spencer (1969) cut ventral roots to deefferent the muscle spindles, as well as cutting the tendon. They studied the post-synaptic responses of Clarke's column neurons with a midline surface electrode positioned on the dorsum of the spinal cord. The afferent volleys on the two sides of the cord produced equal voltage changes at this electrode, but the post-synaptic reflex response was larger on the tenotomized and deefferented side 4–10 weeks after operation. The discharge frequencies in Group I and II afferent fibers from the operated muscle were if anything less than those of the contralateral control muscles during rest and during passive rotation of the ankle. It seemed unlikely that if any increased activity in higher threshold nonstretch afferents produced changes in synaptic efficacy, those changes would be confined to the reflexes of the operated muscles. It was therefore concluded that reduced activity in stretch afferents over a period of weeks had led to an enduring increase in efficacy of the synapses made by the stretch afferents on the neurons of Clarke's column.

More recent work on the monosynaptic reflex in the ventral horn after tenotomy has shown that the maximum size that the reflex response can reach during PTP is unchanged, so the increased response to single test volleys is unlikely to be due to growth of new synapses (Robbins and Nelson, 1970). Moreover, the reflex depression produced by low-frequency stimulation is unchanged, so there is unlikely to be a change in in the fraction of available transmitter released by the test impulses. Robbins and Nelson suggest that the enhanced reflex response on the tenotomized side is due to an increase in size of the total transmitter pool, and might be associated with an increase in size of the afferent axon terminals.

A long-term study has also been made on the optic nerve terminals in the lateral geniculate nucleus. Inhibition is very prominent here, for tetanic electrical stimulation of the optic nerve leads to a delayed depression of synaptic transmission that can last for hours (Hughes *et al.*, 1956). Morlock *et al.* (1965) showed that this depression does not affect on-going cell firing and, so, is probably due to a pre-synaptic change in the optic nerve terminals and is a depression of excitatory terminals rather than a facilitation of inhibitory terminals. Burke and Hayhow (1968) studied transmission through the lateral geniculate nucleus of cats that had been kept in darkness for up to 3 years, and cats in which the retinal receptors had been destroyed by administration of a specific toxin. No significant change was caused by the years in darkness. Most of the retinal ganglion cells continue to discharge in darkness for as long as their activity has been followed (24 hours, Rodieck and Smith, 1966), and it is possible that this discharge continues indefinitely. After destruction of the visual receptors, however, the ganglion cell discharge was silenced. It was found that after only 7 days there was a slight decrease in conduction velocity in the optic nerve and a major decrease in post-tetanic depression. Stimulation at 500/second for 1 hour did not cause any recovery of post-tetanic depression. Burke and Hayhow (1968) interpret this result as due to a strengthening of excitatory syanpses, rather than a weakening of inhibitory synapses, but for this interpretation there appears to be no decisive evidence. It would be useful to show by electron microscopy that the toxin does not cause degeneration in any of the inhibitory synapses in the lateral geniculate nucleus.

A long-term plasticity of response of a different kind was described by R. M. Eccles *et al.* (1962). When the nerves to all except one of a group of synergic antigravity muscles are cut, the afferent fibers in the remaining nerve aquire the ability to elicit stronger monosynaptic reflexes in the weeks after operation. This is so even if the leg is immobilized in plaster or if the spinal cord is cut and, so, is unlikely to depend on increased activity in the stretch afferents of the remaining innervated muscle. At least two possible mechanisms for this effect can be proposed. The remaining muscle will hypertrophy and there may even be muscle fiber division (Hall-Craggs and Lawrence, 1969). If motor neurons derive a trophic substance from muscle, as is suggested by the dependence of the maturation of nerve fibers on contact with muscle (Aitkin *et al.*, 1947), then an increased supply of this substance from a hypertrophying muscle might alter the receptive properties of the motor neuron to the synapses made upon it. It is unlikely, however, that this would work during immobilization, when muscle atrophy would be expected, unless the muscles were strongly stretched (Schiaffino and Hanzlikova, 1970). An alternative possibility is that there could be a partial retraction of synapses made by stretch afferent fibers on motor neurons that became chromatolytic as a result of cutting the other motor nerves. If axons commonly make so many synapses that the maintaining ability of the neuronal cell body is fully extended, then a retraction of synapses affecting part of the axonal ramification could result in enlargement and strengthening of the remaining synapses made by the same axon. This could result in brisker reflex responses when the afferent fibers from the still innervated muscle are stimulated. This possible mechanism could be tested in the visual system where the optic axons to the superior colliculus are collaterals of the optic axons going to the lateral geniculate nucleus (Sefton, 1968). There is evidence that damage to one branch of the optic axon can lead to hypertrophy of the other (see Section IV,F above), and it would be useful to know whether the remaining synapses are correspondingly strengthened.

SUMMARY AND COMMENTS

The fact that tenotomy strengthens dorsal root reflexes suggests that the weakening of reflex responses found after peripheral section of sensory nerves is related to the ensuing chromatolysis of the cell bodies rather than to lack of impulse traffic alone. It may be possible to check this by long-term application of local anaesthetic to the dorsal root without causing degeneration. The strengthening of reflex responses following denervation of synergic muscles in immobilized limbs also suggests that trophic effects on synapses may be important in experiments where changes of use are intended. The lack of functional evidence of modifiability at inhibitory synapses is a glaring omission but the increased responsiveness of the lateral geniculate nucleus after destruction of the retinal receptors could be due to modification or even loss of inhibitory terminals. Thus, functional studies may be more effective in short-term experiments where trophic effects are less likely and structural studies less appropriate.

VI. Long-Term Structural Studies

The problem here is: Do functioning and other conditions of development affect the growth of synapses? Local anaesthetic added to nervous tissue in culture to block conduction did not interfere with the development of the characteristic morphology of the tissue or with the appearance of bioelectric responses after removal of the anesthetic (Crain *et al.*, 1968). These authors review earlier work on the successful development of amphibian embryos under anaesthesia. Davis and Montgomery (1969) have recently succeeded in keeping cats anaesthetised for 3 weeks. Synapses have not yet been studied in any of these preparations by electron microscopy, and it cannot be excluded that functioning may play a necessary part in the normal development and maintenance of synapses. There is much evidence, reviewed below, that the growth of neuropil as seen by light microscopy depends on functional conditions, and this awaits investigation by electron microscopy.

Synapses in general are not seen by light microscopy, not because of their small size but because of a lack of any specific structure that can be recognized at a synapse after staining by methods (such as Golgi–Kopsch or Bielschowsky's silver) that could be expected to stain all parts of neurons. The exception to this general rule are the "boutons" seen in silver preparations when neurofilaments form a ring in the presynaptic terminal (Gray and Guillery, 1966), and the "spines" on dendrites in Golgi preparations that represent the post-synaptic part of the largest of the five classes of synapses (synapses on spines, on dendrites, on cell bodies, on axon hillocks, on axon terminals). There is also a difficult method that may stain mitochondria in axon terminals (Armstrong *et al.*, 1956; Rasmussen, 1957). Quantitative studies of synapses by light microscopy have to assume reliable staining by fickle methods, but recent work has detected a loss of Golgi-stained spines in visual cortex after lesions of the lateral geniculate nucleus or enucleation of one eye in newborn rabbits (Globus and Scheibel, 1967a). This work is distinguished by being able to specify that the loss of spines occurred on the central three quartiles of apical shaft of pyramidal neurons and not on the oblique branches or basilar dendrites or apical shaft branches in layer I. However, some stellate neurons are without spines even in normal material, and this illustrates the selective nature of the information obtainable by this method.

Light microscopy is, however, the method of choice for quantifying the growth of the neuropil, that meshwork of dendrites, axons, synapses, and glial cells which separates the neuronal cell bodies further and further apart during development and constitutes the main zone of neuronal interaction and information processing. The average volume of neuropil per neuron has been widely used to look for effects upon brain development of starvation, hypothyroidism, growth hormone, enriched or impoverished environments, and visual experience. However, a certain volume of neuropil per neuron may permit a corresponding level of intricacy of neuronal interconnections but does not guarantee that this level is achieved. Attempts have been made by light microscopy to estimate how many axons might terminate on the dendrites of an average neuron (Eayrs, 1960b, 1966), but this calculation is still permissive rather that indicative of what actually occurs.

Axon terminals can be seen and counted directly by electron microscopy, and the number distributed in a unit volume estimated (Cragg, 1967a). Division of this number by the number of cell bodies in the same volume of tissue gives the average number of synapses associated with one neuron. This then is a more direct structural measure of neuronal interaction, but it is possible that it may greatly overestimate the latter if a large proportion of synapses is inoperative. Moreover, all standard methods of fixation produce a serious distortion of the tissue: it has been shown that extracellular space decreases from 20–30% of brain volume *in vivo* to 0–5% in electron micrographs (Van Harreveld, 1966, and see the Chapter of this volume where the mechanism is discussed).

It might be supposed that this regrettable, but at present incurable, artifact would prejudice the counting of axon terminals. But in fact, the calculation of density of axon terminals per unit volume of tissue is independent of a change of size in the terminals.

The results to be reviewed of light and electron microscopical estimation of neuropil per neuron or synapses per neuron are uniform in showing that the opportunity for neuronal interaction is increased by development in enriched environments or with visual experience and decreased by impoverished environments, rearing in darkness, starvation, or neonatal thyroidectomy.

A. Enriched and Impoverished Environments

The enriched environment provided for rats in the experiments at Berkeley, California, consisted of periods of formal training on mazes for rats housed in groups in cages provided with wooden toys in brightly lit rooms that were not sound proofed. Littermates in impoverished environment were housed individually in cages with solid metal walls in a dimly lit and quiet room and were minimally handled or stimulated. Initial incredulity that such differences in social and psychophysical conditions could give rise to significant differences in brain weight, cortical thickness, and glial cell numbers seems to have been overcome by the continued series of papers from Berkeley reporting consistent results. Some independent confirmation by workers elsewhere has also been obtained, as mentioned below.

The latest of this series of papers (Rosenzweig *et al.*, 1969) shows that the effect on cortical weight and thickness is greatest in the occipital region (about 6%). The effect still occurred in this occipital cortex containing the visual area when rats were blinded or kept in darkness. The effect occurs in rats of age 105 days kept for 80 days in differential conditions, as well as in young animals. It is found in all strains of rats tested, in both sexes, and to a lesser extent in mice and gerbils. The number of glial cells is increased in the enriched conditions, but the number of neurons is unchanged, so more neuropil surrounds each neuron (Diamond *et al.*, 1964). The neuronal cell bodies are about 10% larger in diameter in the enriched conditions (Diamond *et al.*, 1967). Some of the increased neuropil may be occupied by increased dendritic branching (Holloway, 1966). Confirmation of these trophic effects on cortical volume, brain weight, and glial cell numbers has been obtained by Altman (1968) and Ferchmin *et al.* (1970). An increase in thickness of occipital cortex and hippocampus has been found by Walsh *et al.* (1969). The effects are nevertheless small and detectable only by using litters of rats in carefully controlled conditions. It is doubtful whether quantitative electron microscopy is yet accurate enough or able to handle the large numbers of specimens of tissue required to determine the average number of synapses per neuron in these differential conditions.

Although the occipital cortex shows a greater effect than other cortical areas in rats, it has not yet been excluded that the effect could be due to some general hormonal influence on the growth of the brain rather than to a direct neural response to increased stimulation of sensory receptors.

B. VISUAL EXPERIENCE

The effect of visual experience on the structure of the visual system has been examined by several groups of workers, despite the early negative results of L. Goodman (1932), which did not contain adequate quantitative evidence. In the retina, Eakin (1965) showed that the outer segments of rod receptors in frogs raised in darkness appear to develop normally. However, the terminals of the receptors in rats attain an abnormally large diameter after dark-rearing (Cragg, 1969b, see Fig. 5 of this chapter). The inner plexiform layer of the retina is reduced in thickness in cats reared in darkness (Wieskrantz, 1958; Rasch *et al.*, 1961). The latter group of authors also found a reduced RNA content in all three cell layers of the retina in dark-reared cats and rats and an actual loss of ganglion cells in chimpanzees. Winsburg (1968) found in *Xenopus* that retinal neurons incorporate more precursor into RNA in light than in darkness. The optic nerve issuing from the ganglion cells suffers retarded myelination in dark-reared mice (Gyllensten *et al.*, 1966).

At the lateral geniculate nucleus Chow (1955) found no change in the number or size of neurons in monkeys kept in darkness for 8 months compared with control monkeys, but this experiment did not involve dark-rearing from birth, and cage cleaning resulted in 2–5 minutes of daily exposure to light. We have already mentioned the work of Wiesel and Hubel (1963) and Hubel and Wiesel (1970), which found smaller geniculate neurons with less prominent Nissl substance in the laminae of cells connected to an eye that had been closed during development in young cats. This result was confirmed by Kupfer and Palmer (1964), who found a cessation of growth during dark exposure. A reduced rate of incorporation of leucine into protein was found in the lateral geniculate nucleus of rats in which the opposite eye was shielded from light for 4–7 months after eye opening (Maraini *et al.*, 1967). Acetylcholine ester-ase activity was also reduced in the lateral geniculate nucleus of dark-reared rats (Maletta and Timiras, 1967). However, atrophy of the genic-ulate cells does not seem to occur in adult cats kept for years in darkness (Burke and Hayhow, 1968). The volume of neuropil is reduced in the lateral geniculate nucleus and superior colliculus of dark-reared mice (Gyllensten *et al.*, 1965), but this retardation of growth was partly made up during more prolonged exposure to darkness (Gyllensten *et al.*, 1967). A reduction of 5% in volume of the lateral geniculate nucleus opposite a closed eye in developing rats was found by Fifkova and Hassler (1969), who also found a reduction in the number of neurons.

I have counted synapses by electron microscopy in the lateral geniculate nucleus of rats reared in darkness and used littermate rats brought out into diurnal lighting as controls. The density of synapses per unit volume was reduced by about 30%, but the average diameter of the terminals was increased by 15% in the dark-reared rats (Cragg, 1969a). It has not yet been determined which of the three sources (retina, occipital cortex, intrinsic neurons) of axon terminals in the lateral geniculate nucleus is affected. Greater discrimination of this kind would increase the value of the results, but is particularly difficult to achieve in quantitative studies where all axon terminals must be assigned to their appropriate classes if any are to be discriminated.

In the visual cortex of mice reared in darkness, there is less neuropil around each neuron and the neuronal diameters are slightly less than in similar litters reared in daylight (Gyllensten *et al.*, 1967). These effects were found at about 2 months of age and were somewhat reduced at 4 months. Similar effects were found in rats reared in daylight with uni-lateral closure of eyelids (Fifkova and Hassler, 1969). The thickness of the visual cortex opposite the closed eye was reduced by 16%, and the num-ber of cortical neurons unchanged or higher (11% in layer IV). There was thus less neuropil surrounding each neuron.

Some part of this reduction of neuropil may have been due to reduced dendritic growth, for Coleman and Riesen (1968) have found fewer and shorter dendrites on stellate cells in layer IV of visual cortex in two dark-reared cats. In this work, three pairs of littermate kittens were used, and one of the dark-reared cats showed a larger dendrite growth than any of the light-reared kittens. Globus and Scheibel (1967b) point out that this result supports their contention that variability is the factor that is increased by dark-rearing. These authors examined rabbits born and reared in darkness for 30 days and nonlittermate controls reared in daylight. They found no change in dendritic branching of stellate cells in visual cortex and no change in density of spines, although the spines of dark-reared rabbits were more variable in direction, size, and shape. Valverde (1967), 1968), has also looked at dendritic spines in the visual cortex after dark-rearing. His mice were compared with similar but nonlittermate mice reared in daylight, and fewer spines per unit length of dendritic segment were found on the apical dendrites of pyramidal neurons. All this work on dendrites depends on Golgi staining, in which 1–2% of neurons is picked out on an unknown basis of selection and the number of spines and dendritic branches seen undoubtedly depends on the quality of impregnation. The results suggest that there are effects of dark-rearing on dendrites that are close to the limits of detection by present techniques because of the unreliability and laboriousness of the latter. More dramatic regression of dendrites and spines may occur in transneuronal atrophy (W. H. Jones and Thomas, 1962; Matthews and Powell, 1962; White and Westrum, 1964) and in retrograde cell reaction (Cerf and Chacko, 1958).

I have looked at synapses in the visual cortex of dark-reared rats with electron microscopy and compared synaptic counts with littermate rats brought out from the darkroom at 3 weeks of age to live 4 weeks under diurnal lighting conditions. Initial results (Cragg, 1967b) indicated opposite effects in the upper and lower halves of the visual cortex, the axon terminals becoming smaller but more numerous during light exposure in the lower half of the cortex. Further work has confirmed this result, but the effects are small (8% in diameter and 25% in density), and the presence of opposite effects in the upper and lower halves of the cortex makes contamination of one effect by the other a possibility, depending on how the cortex is divided. A biochemical difference between the upper and lower halves of cortex has also been described during development, malate and citrate dehydrogenase activity increasing in the outer cortical layers and decreasing in the inner (Kuhlman and Lowry, 1956). The cause of such differences is unknown, though the optic radiation from the lateral geniculate nucleus ends mainly in the lower half of the cortex.

Biochemical studies have detected an increased rate of incorporation of labeled amino acids into protein during visual experience. Talwar *et al.*

(1966) found this result in the visual cortex of rabbits exposed to a flickering light for 2 hours after 15–21 days spent in darkness, the control rabbits remaining in darkness. S. P. R. Rose (1967) found a more complicated result on bringing dark-reared rats out into daylight, for incorporation of amino acids into proteins was enhanced after 3 hours but subsequently depressed for 24 hours in comparison with littermates remaining in darkness. It is not yet known whether cortex shows a uniform effect at all depths or different effects in the upper and lower layers. Analogous work on birds has shown that unilateral eye enucleation in newly hatched chicks arrests the growth of the contralateral optic tectum and cerebral hemisphere in weight, protein content and cholinesterase activity. A most interesting result was obtained with eyelid closure alone, which prevents pattern vision without abolishing light perception. Unilateral eyelid closure reduced the growth and cholinesterase activity of the contralateral cerebral hemisphere but not of the optic tectum (Bondy and Margolis, 1969). A visual area that is probably concerned with pattern vision has been described recently in the cerebral hemisphere of the pigeon (Revzin, 1969). This appears to be a good situation for attempting to differentiate the effects of deprivation of pattern vision from the effects of darkness. Light and darkness may have trophic effects on the visual neurons, while the patterning of impulses imposed by pattern vision may effect the development of synapses.

Perhaps the most interesting question one can ask of the biochemical studies is whether they relate to protein synthesis to be used for the growth of new axonal sprouts and synapses or whether control substances are synthesized which turn on preformed but inoperative synapses. A first step would be to see whether a wide range of proteins is produced, or just a few substances, when visual cells are stimulated by pattern vision for the first time. The complexity of the problem is well shown by the progressive labeling of successively heavier fractions of RNA over a period of 10 days in the visual and motor cortical areas (Dewar and Reading, 1970). These authors found that congenitally blind rats had a much reduced rate and range of labeling of RNA fractions in visual cortex but were normal in motor cortex. At the single neuron level, Berry (1969) has found a doubling of the rate of incorporation of precursors into RNA in a single neuron in Aplysia when the frequency of presynaptic stimulation was increased from 0–500 spikes/hour. A most interesting result due to Lux *et al.* (1970) is that axonal transport of proteins is increased in bulk but not in velocity in single motor neurons in cat stimulated antidromically.

C. HORMONAL AND NUTRITIONAL EFFECTS ON GROWTH OF SYNAPSES

There is currently much interest in perinatal factors that might influence the development of the brain favorably or unfavorably. Experimentally alterable perinatal factors have been identified in growing rats that appear to determine behavioral deficits or enhanced problem solving ability. Thus, cretinous rats have unusual difficulty with the Hebb–Williams maze (Eayrs, 1966), while rats treated with growth hormone before birth obtained higher than usual scores on some behavioral tests (Clendinnen and Eayrs, 1961). Structural changes in the brain can also be detected in these two and other similar conditions. It would be of great interest to know whether the structural changes are causal to the behavioral effects. There is the discouraging possibility that both are secondary to molecular mechanisms not yet identified. Some part of the structural plasticity of the rat brain is due to the fact that small neurons are still being produced by mitosis after birth in the olfactory bulb, hippocampus, cerebellum, and perhaps elsewhere (Altman and Das, 1966; Altman, 1968). Much experimental work has been done by the relatively easy technique of measuring brain DNA chemically to assess the total number of neurons and glial cells present. Neuronal size and dendritic branching pattern have also been determined in some experiments, but little work has yet been done on synapses by electron microscopy. This is necessary, however, if the structural connectivity of neurons is to be estimated realistically.

In thyroid deficiency, the postnatal growth of the brain is retarded and there are biochemical, electrophysiological, and behavioral abnormalities (Eayrs, 1960b, 1966). In the cerebral cortex, a reduced growth of neuropil results in the neurons being abnormally closely packed (Eayrs and Taylor, 1951). These neurons have less extensive basal dendrites than usual (Eayrs, 1955). The dendritic field of one neuron encompasses fewer cell bodies and axons so that the opportunities for neuronal interaction are reduced (Eayrs, 1960b). I have counted synapses in the neuropil of the visual cortex and found very little difference in density between severely hypothyroid rats and normal littermates of much larger (20–40%) brain weights. The amount of neuropil surrounding each neuron is reduced, however, by about 20% so that the number of synapses associated with each neuron is reduced by about the same amount (Cragg, 1970). Biochemical estimation of glutamate decarboxylase, which is regarded as a marker for synapses, has shown a 15% reduction in activity (Balazs et al., 1968). The only qualitative structural abnormality in the hypothyroid cortex was the presence of abnormal membranous bodies in neuronal perikarya, dendrites, and synapses. It is by no means clear that the rather modest structural changes found in experimental hypothyroidism can account for the severe retardation of cretinism, and it is quite possible that the number of synapses per neuron is not the appropriate parameter to measure, especially if a proportion of formed synapses is inoperative.

Starvation has been shown to lead to a similar reduction in growth of neuropil (Eayrs and Horn, 1955), and there is much current interest in behavioral deficits associated with malnutrition in man (see Scrimshaw and Gordon, 1968; McCance and Widdowson, 1968). Prenatal protein deficiency produced by feeding the mother rat on a diet with only 8% protein resulted in the birth of baby rats with fewer brain cells (as estimated by DNA content) and less protein per brain cell (Zamenhof *et al.*, 1968). Fish and Winick (1969) have shown that the effect of postnatal starvation is localized according to the stage of development of the neurons. Thus, the number of cells is reduced in the cerebellum and hippocampus where mitosis is still going on, whereas in the brain stem mitosis has almost ceased by birth, but growth in the protein content of the neurons is retarded by starvation.

The effects of other hormones on brain growth has received some study, but the results seem to be less dramatic than in the case of thyroxin. Hypophysectomy at 6 day of age in rats led to an 81% reduction in body weight compared with control rats at 27 days of age, but the depth of the cerebral cortex was not reduced (Diamond, 1968). Brain growth in mice can be slowed by treatment with excess corticosterone during infancy, and a reduced content of DNA indicates a reduced number of neurones and glial cells (Howard, 1968). The closeness of packing of neurons has not yet been studied in these conditions. A remarkable illustration of the sensitivity of some neurons to hormones during development is the lasting change in sexual behavior and periodicity in rats produced by the male sex hormone during the first few days of postnatal life (Harris and Levine, 1962). The mechanism for sex cycles is present in male as well as in female rats at birth, and is inactivated forever by exposure to endogenous or exogenous testosterone in either sex. Barraclough and Gorski (1961) found suggestive evidence that testosterone had a deleterious action on certain neurons in the suprachiasmatic part of the hypothalamus that are involved in the cyclic mechanism. Structural changes in these neurons have not yet been found, but acid phosphatase staining would be a promising approach to this problem for the activity of this lysosomal enzyme rises sharply in damaged neurons.

On the positive side, attempts have been made to enhance brain growth in rats by restricting litter size or administering growth hormone during pregnancy. When one uterine horn is tied off before mating, fetal rats develop in small litters and have a higher content of brain DNA (Van Marthens and Zamenhof, 1969). Various preparations of somatotropic hormone have been administered to pregnant rats, and brain development in the resulting litters studied. Clendinnen and Eayrs (1961) found that the offspring were larger at birth but the cerebral cortex had an unchanged number of neurons. The neurons were larger and had a more extensive dendritic branching pattern. Against this, Zamenhof *et al.* (1966) found an unchanged body weight, an increased brain weight and cortical cell density, and an increased ratio of neurons to glia, implying an increased number and density of neurons. These conflicting results may be due to errors in the differential counting of neurons and glial cells. Eayrs (1960a) found that postnatal treatment with growth hormone increased the dendritic branching of cortical neurons. However, Diamond *et al.* (1969) did not detect changes in cortical depth or body weight after postnatal injection of growth hormone for 3 weeks beginning 7 days after birth. There is thus no clear consensus of opinion on the effects of extraneous growth hormone and no logical reason to expect an artificially raised level of the hormone to promote the growth of a better brain. On the other hand, baby rats growing in large litters may well be at a disadvantage compared with those in small litters, and it would be worth while to examine the degree of independence that synaptic development achieves in these conditions.

I have started to look at the development of synapses in rat visual cortex during starvation and have found an effect very similar to that of thyroidectomy. A newborn litter of rats was separated into two groups kept in identical cages in an incubator at 30°C, and the mother rat spent 18 hours, including the night, with one (small) group and six hours with the other (large) group. All the litter was perfused at 24 days of age, when the starved rats had an average body weight of only 15 gm compared with 46 gm for their better fed littermates. The average brain weights were reduced by 20% and counts of cell bodies in Nissl preparations of the visual cortex showed a density increased by about 20% in the starved rats. There was thus a retardation in the development of the neuropil that separated the cell bodies. Measurements of electron micrographs showed that the size and density of the axon terminals in the neuropil was unchanged. No qualitative abnormalities were recognized (see Fig. 9). Thus, the number of axon terminals associated with one neuron is reduced by about 20%,

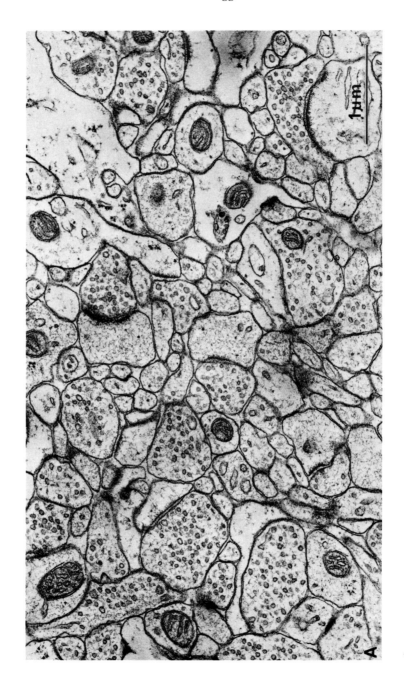

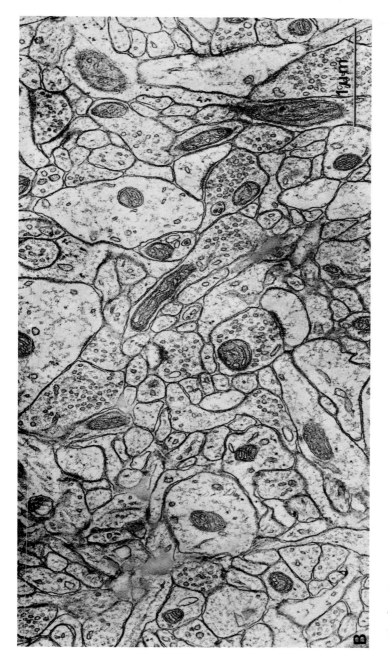

Fig. 9. The development of cortical synapses appears to be normal in rats starved from birth for 24 days and then perfused. In A, the body weight was 15 gm and brain weight 1.05 gm, while in the well-fed littermate B, the body weight was 43 gm and brain weight 1.35 gm. In spite of the huge difference of body weight, the size and density of axon terminals is unchanged.

as with neonatal thyroidectomy (Cragg, 1970). The smallness of this effect compared with the reduction of body weight indicates the priority enjoyed by the brain in development.

D. Partial Denervations

Overactive neurons are produced by partial denervation in experimental models of epilepsy and spasticity. There is some evidence that partially denervated neurons are supersensitive to analeptic drugs (Stavraky, 1961) and, thus perhaps, to any excitatory substances normally present. Synaptic plasticity is also involved, for prolonged bombardment of neurons with impulses arising at the edge of a lesion can, in the presence of partial denervation, lead to the formation of a second autonomous focus of overactive neurons (Morrell, 1961b). Light microscopy has detected a small proportion of dark neurons in the secondary focus. The dark staining is due to an unusually high concentration of RNA in the cell bodies and apical dendrites, possibly because the whole neuron has shrunk. The turnover of RNA in these dark neurons is low (Engel and Morrell, 1970). It is not known whether the condition of these neurons is due to overactivity or to a retrograde reaction to the loss of axons that projected to the area of cortex damaged in the primary epileptic focus. It would be interesting to look for structural changes in the synapses in the secondary focus by electron microscopy, but the situation is heterogeneous because of the combination of increased firing with partial denervation and the presence of the dark neurons. Moreover, individual neurons show a wide range of firing patterns in the secondary epileptic focus, some showing inhibition of firing during paroxysms (Wilder and Morrell, 1967). A loss of synapses on the neurons surrounding the primary focus is shown by the finding of Westrum *et al.* (1964) that in Golgi stained preparations there are fewer spines on the dendrites.

Another form of overactivity resulting from a loss of neurons is the spasticity which can be produced by obstructing the blood supply to the spinal cord for 35–45 minutes. There is a widespread loss of small interneurons, and a permanent extensor rigidity (Gelfan and Tarlov, 1959). Perhaps because of the loss of inhibitory interneurons, ventral root reflex responses to dorsal root electrical stimulation became much more resistant to subsequent anoxia, lasting 13–17 minutes with the animal breathing nitrogen compared with $2\frac{1}{2}$–4 minutes in a normal animal (Van Harreveld, 1964). The loss of synapses has not yet been examined by electron microscopy, but the Rasmussen silver impregnation of axon terminals shows a dramatic reduction in number of synapses on spinal neurons to about 30% of the normal number (Gelfan and Rapisarda, 1964). So great a partial denervation could be expected to lead to much rearrangement of surviving tissue elements including sprouting of axons to form new synapses. The absence of scar tissue to impede regeneration makes this situation rather similar to that produced by heavy particle irradiation, which again destroys neurons without scar formation and seems to lead to regeneration of neuronal processes (J. E. Rose *et al.*, 1960).

E. SUMMARY AND COMMENTS

The density of axon terminals in the neuropil seems strangely constant when the development of neuropil is retarded by thyroidectomy or starvation. If this is a general result, the quantitative studies of neuropil by light microscopy in enriched and deprived environments, in light and darkness, and in abnormal hormone conditions are in effect measuring neuronal connectivity in these conditions. These long-term effects on development of neuropil and synapses are perhaps the most profitable aspect of synaptic plasticity for structural methods of study. There is, however, the possibility that many formed synapses are inoperative but unrecognized, in which case effective connectivity may bear little relation to the structural findings. The correlation of the growth of neuropil with behavioral measures of performance in hypothyroidism, starvation, and treatment with growth hormone suggest nevertheless that neuronal connectivity is a determinant of performance. It is a pity that the same quantitative methods have not yet been applied to human mental deficiency and genius, for which only qualitative statements about the development of gyri and unconvincing histology is available.

VII. Conclusions

New forms of synaptic plasticity are being reported more and more frequently, but it would be particularly helpful to obtain confirmation and agreement on the claims made so far so that work on well-established effects can move on to an analysis of mechanisms. To this end it is necessary that negative results should be published as readily as new positive findings. Failure to confirm a published claim is a significant result that should also be published.

The short-term modifications in synapses detected with electrical methods may offer a limited field for structural correlation because synaptic modification could take place at a molecular level inaccessible to electron microscopy. It is not even certain that the position of synaptic vesicles is frozen at the moment of fixation, for retinal synapses damaged after aldehyde fixation can still show a gross loss of vesicles (Cragg, 1969b). Nevertheless, if changes in the number of vesicles near the synaptic membrane or changes in histochemical staining of calcium could be detected in synapses fixed during depression or PTP, it would be a useful advance.

The more obvious application of structural methods is to longer-term effects on synaptic development. For example, electron microscopy could reasonably hope to distinguish the effects of pattern vision from effects due to unpatterned light exposure at appropriate levels in the visual system, perhaps in the chick cerebral hemisphere. Human mental retardation is accessible to the quantitative methods of studying neuropil, and it should be possible to determine in this way whether the parameters that can be measured are relevant to mental performance. A major uncertainty overhanging the structural approach is the possibility that many inoperative synapses may be present but not recognizable structurally. The evidence for this possibility is at present weak, but it commands attention because neuronal connectivity would otherwise be so extraordinarily high. A method for recognizing inoperative synapses structurally would perhaps be the biggest advance in the field that can be envisaged. Starvation does not greatly decrease the number of synapses in the cortex of developing rats, but it is possible that some other lytic agent such as cortisone might cause a retraction of ineffective synapses. Unfortunately, it is not kuown that retraction of an axon terminal leads to a specific structural picture comparable with the changes that follow axonal degeneration. A counting of synapses may therefore be necessary, and this has not been done in any of the experiments that suggest the existence of inoperative synapses.

In the shorter-term experiments with electrophysiological techniques there is a bewildering variety of effects. Besides facilitation, depression and PTP, depending only on pre-synaptic impulse activity, it is possible that individual synapses may show the dependence on post-synaptic activity which Bliss *et al.* (1968) found in cortical pathways. Some experiments show a strengthening of synapses with use (PTP); others, a strengthening with disuse (the effects of tenotomy on dorsal root afferents). Longer-term aftereffects are often seen if the conditions for synaptic modification are maintained for 10–30 minutes, and this process of consolidation seems to involve protein synthesis (Gartside, 1968b). It would be interesting to know whether the lengthening of the time constant for PTP found by Lloyd (1949) is blocked by inhibitors of protein synthesis. All the above effects are confined to an axonal terminal and a post-synaptic receptor, but there is also evidence that competition between different kinds of axon terminal may be important in determining the efficacy of synapses (Hubel and Wiesel, 1970; Mark, 1970). The modifiability of inhibitory synapses has still to be investigated. The work of Brindley (1967) and Gardner-Medwin (1969) shows that different kinds of modifiable synapses could achieve the same logical manipulations of incoming impulses but at different cost in numbers of neurons and synapses required. The numbers available are remarkably large. A plausible organization of pathways of modifiable conductivity into a scheme that would discriminate patterning in the neural input has been proposed by Uttley (1970).

REFERENCES

Aghajanian, G. K., and Bloom, F. E. (1967). *Brain Res.* **6**, 716.

Aitken, J. T., Sharman, M., and Young, J. Z. (1947). *J. Anat.* **81**, 1.

Altman, J. (1968). *In* "Malnutrition, Learning and Behaviour" (N. S. Scrimshaw and J. E. Gordon, eds.), pp. 332–356. MIT Press, Cambridge, Massachusetts.

Altman, J., and Das, G. D. (1966). *J. Comp. Neurol.* **126**, 337.

Andersen, P., and Lømo, T. (1968). *In* "Structure and Function of Inhibitory Neuronal Mechanisms" (C. von Euler, S. Skoglund, and U. Soderberg, eds.), pp. 335–342. Pergamon, Oxford.

April, R. S., and Spencer, W. A. (1969). *Experientia* **25**, 1272.

Armstrong, J., Richardson, K. C., and Young, J. Z. (1956). *Stain Technol.* **31**, 263.

Armstrong–James, M. A., and Johnson, F. R. (1969). *J. Anat.* **104**, 590.

Aserinsky, E. (1961). *Exp. Neurol.* **3**, 467.

Balazs, R., Kovacs, S., Teichgraber, P., Cocks, W. A., and Eayrs, J. T. (1968). *J. Neurochem.* **15**, 1335.

Barraclough, C. A., and Gorski, R. A. (1961). *Endocrinology* **68**, 68.

Barron, K. D., Chiang, T. Y., and Daniels, A. C. (1969). *Anat. Rec.* **163**, 150.

Baylor, D. A., and Fuortes, M. G. F. (1970). *J. Physiol. (London)* **207**, 77.

Berry, R. W. (1969). *Science* **166**, 1021.

Beswick, F. B., and Conroy, R. T. W. L. (1965). *J. Physiol. (London)* **180**, 134.

Betz, W. J. (1970). *J. Physiol. (London)* **206**, 629.

Bindman, L. J. (1965). *J. Physiol. (London)* **179**, 14P.

Bindman, L. J., and Boisacq–Schepens, N. (1967). *J. Physiol. (London)* **191**, 7P.

Bindman, L. J., Lippold, O. C. J., and Redfearn, J. W. T. (1964). *J. Physiol. (London)* **172**, 369.

Bleier, R. (1969). *Brain Res.* **15**, 365.

Blinzinger, K., and Kreutzberg, G. (1968). *Z. Zellforsch. Mikrosk. Anat.* **85**, 145.
Blioch, Z. L., Glagoleva, I. M., Liberman, E. A., and Nenashev, V. A. (1968). *J. Physiol. (London)* **199**, 11.
Bliss, T. V. P., and Lømo, T. (1970). *J. Physiol. (London)* **207**, 61P.
Bliss, T. V. P., Burns, B. D., and Uttley, A. M. (1968). *J. Physiol. (London)* **195**, 339.
Bodian, D. (1964). *Bull. Johns Hopkins Hosp.* **114**, 13.
Bodian, D. (1966). *Bull. Johns Hopkins Hosp.* **119**, 212.
Bodian, D. (1968). *J. Comp. Neurol.* **133**, 113.
Boisacq-Scheppens, N. (1968). *Arch. Int. Physiol. Biochim.* **76**, 562.
Bondareff, W., and Sjostrand, J. (1969). *Exp. Neurol.* **24**, 450.
Bondy, S. C., and Margolis, F. L. (1969). *Exp. Neurol.* **25**, 447.
Brindley, G. S. (1967). *Proc. Roy. Soc., Ser. B* **168**, 361.
Brody, H. (1955). *J. Comp. Neurol.* **102**, 511.
Brown, G. L., and Pascoe, J. E. (1954). *J. Physiol. (London)* **123**, 565.
Bullock, T. H. (1966). *Neurosc. Res. Program Bull.* **4**, No. 2, 105.
Burke, W., and Hayhow, W. R. (1968). *J. Physiol. (London)* **194**, 495.
Cerf, J. A., and Chacko, L. W. (1958). *J. Comp. Neurol.* **109**, 205.
Chow, K. L. (1955). *J. Comp. Neurol.* **102**, 597.
Clark, A. W., Mauro, A., Longenecker, H. E., and Hurlbut, W. P. (1970). *Nature (London)* **225**, 703.
Clendinnen, B. G., and Eayrs, J. T. (1961). *J. Endocrinol.* **22**, 183.
Coleman, P. D., and Riesen, A. H. (1968). *J. Anat.* **102**, 363.
Cook, W. H., Walker, J. H., and Barr, M. L. (1951). *J. Comp. Neurol.* **94**, 267.
Cornwell, A. C., and Sharpless, S. K. (1968). *Vision Res.* **8**, 1389.
Cragg, B. G. (1965). *Exp. Neurol.* **12**, 190.
Cragg, B. G. (1967a). *J. Anat.* **101**, 639.
Cragg, B. G. (1967b). *Nature (London)* **215**, 251.
Cragg, B. G. (1968). *Proc. Roy. Soc., Ser. B* **171**, 319.
Cragg, B. G. (1969a). *Brain Res.* **13**, 53.
Cragg, B. G. (1969b). *Brain Res.* **15**, 79.
Cragg, B. G. (1970). *Brain Res.* **18**, 297.
Crain, S. M., Bornstein, M. B., and Peterson, E. R. (1968). *Brain Res.* **8**, 363.
Cuenod, M., Sandri, C., and Akert, K. (1970). *J. Cell Sci.* **6**, 605.
Dahl, N. A. (1969). *J. Neurobiol.* **2**, 169.
Dahlstrom, A. (1968). *Eur. J. Pharmacol.* **5**, 111.
D'Anzi, F. A. (1969). *Amer. J. Anat.* **125**, 381.
Davis, C. J. F., and Montgomery, A. (1969). *J. Physiol. (London)* **203**, 13P.
Del Castillo, J., and Katz, B. (1954). *J. Physiol. (London)* **124**, 560.
De Robertis, E. (1958). *Exp. Cell Res., Suppl.* **5**, 347.
De Robertis, E., and Vaz Ferreira, A. (1957). *J. Biophys. Biochem. Cytol.* **3**, 611.
Dewar, A. J., and Reading, H. W. (1970). *Nature (London)* **225**, 869.
Diamond, M. C. (1968). *Brain Res.* **7**, 407.
Diamond, M. C., Krech, D., and Rosenzweig, M. R. (1964). *J. Comp. Neurol.* **123**, 111.
Diamond, M. C., Linder, B., and Raymond, A. (1967). *J. Comp. Neurol.* **131**, 357.
Diamond, M. C., Johnson, R. E., Ingham, C., and Stone, S. (1969). *Exp. Neurol.* **23**, 51.
Dowling, J. E., and Boycott, B. B. (1966). *Proc. Roy. Soc., Ser. B* **166**, 80.
Duchen, L. W. (1970). *J. Neurol.* **33**, 40.

Eakin, R. M. (1965). *J. Cell Biol.* **25**, 162.

Eayrs, J. T. (1955). *Acta Anat.* **25**, 160.

Eayrs, J. T. (1960a). *Anat. Rec.* **136**, 185.

Eayrs, J. T. (1960b). *In* "Structure and Function of the Cerebral Cortex" (D. B. Tower and J. P. Schade, eds.), pp. 43–50. Elsevier, Amsterdam.

Eayrs, J. T. (1966). *Sci. Basis Med.* pp. 317–339.

Eayrs, J. T., and Horn, G. (1955). *Anat. Rec.* **121**, 53.

Eayrs, J. T., and Taylor, S. H. (1951). *J. Anat.* **85**, 350.

Eccles, J. C., and McIntyre, A. K. (1953). *J. Physiol. (London)* **121**, 492.

Eccles, J. C., Libert, B., and Young, R. R. (1958). *J. Physiol. (London)* **143**, 11.

Eccles, J. C., Krnjevic, K., and Miledi, R. (1959). *J. Physiol. (London)* **145**, 204.

Eccles, J. C., Eccles, R. M., and Shealy, C. N. (1962). *J. Neurophysiol.* **25**, 544.

Eccles, R. M., Kozak, W., and Westerman, R. A. (1962). *Exp. Neurol.* **6**, 451.

Edds, M. V. (1953). *Quart. Rev. Biol.* **28**, 260.

Elmqvist, D., and Quastel, D. M. J. (1965). *J. Physiol. (London)* **178**, 505.

Engel, J. P., and Morrell, F. (1970). *Exp. Neurol.* **26**, 221.

Ferchmin, P. A., Eterovic, V. A., and Caputto, R. (1970). *Brain Res.* **20**, 49.

Fifkova, E., and Hassler, R. (1969). *J. Comp. Neurol.* **135**, 167.

Fish, I., and Winick, M. (1969). *Exp. Neurol.* **25**, 534.

Gage, P. W., and Hubbard, J. I. (1966). *J. Physiol. (London)* **184**, 353.

Gardner–Medwin, A. R. (1969). *Nature (London)* **223**, 916.

Gartside, I. B. (1968a). *Nature (London)* **220**, 382.

Gartside, I. B. (1968b). *Nature (London)* **220**, 383.

Gartside, I. B., and Lippold, O. C. J. (1967). *J. Physiol. (London)* **189**, 475.

Gelfan, S., and Rapisarda, A. F. (1964). *J. Comp. Neurol.* **123**, 73.

Gelfan, S., and Tarlov, I. M. (1959). *J. Physiol. (London)* **146**, 594.

Gibbs, C. L. (1964). *Aust. J. Exp. Biol.* **42**, 116.

Gibbs, C. L., Johnson, E. A., and Tille, J. (1964). *Biophys. J.* **4**, 329.

Globus, A., and Scheibel, A. B. (1967a). *Exp. Neurol.* **18**, 116.

Globus, A., and Scheibel, A. B. (1967b). *Exp. Neurol.* **19**, 331.

Goddard, G. V., McIntyre, D. C., and Leech, C. K. (1969). *Exp. Neurol.* **25**, 295.

Goldberg, A. L., and Goodman, H. M. (1969). *J. Physiol. (London)* **200**, 667.

Gonatas, N. K., Evangelista, I., and Walsh, G. O. (1967). *J. Neurophathol.* **26**, 179.

Goodman, D. C., and Horel, J. A. (1966). *J. Comp. Neurol.* **127**, 71.

Goodman, L. (1932). *Amer. J. Physiol.* **100**, 46.

Gray, E. G., and Guillery, R. W. (1966). *Int. Rev. Cytol.* **19**, 111.

Guth, L., and Bernstein, J. J. (1961). *Exp. Neurol.* **4**, 59.

Gyllensten, L., Malmfors, T., and Norrlin, M. L. (1965). *J. Comp. Neurol.* **124**, 149.

Gyllensten, L., Malmfors, T., and Norrlin–Grettve, M. L. (1966). *J. Comp. Neurol.* **128**, 413.

Gyllensten, L., Malmfors, T., and Norrlin–Grettve, M. L. (1967). *J. Comp. Neurol.* **131**, 549.

Hall–Craggs, E. C. B., and Lawrence, C. A. (1969). *J. Physiol.* **202**, 76P.

Hamori, J. (1968). *In* "Structure and Function of Inhibitory Neuronal Mechanisms" (C. von Euler, S. Skoglund, and U. Soderberg, eds.), pp. 71–80. Pergamon, Oxford.

Harris, G. W., and Levine, S. (1962). *J. Physiol. (London)* **163**, 42P.

Heimer, L., and Wall, P. D. (1968). *Exp. Brain Res.* **6**, 89.

Heuser, J., and Miledi, R. (1970). *J. Physiol. (London)* **208**, 55P.

Hill, D. K. (1950). *J. Physiol. (London)* **111**, 304.

Holloway, R. L. (1966). *Brain Res.* **2**, 393.

Howard, E. (1968). *Exp. Neurol.* **22**, 191.

Hubbard, J. I., and Kwanbunbumpen, S. (1968). *J. Physiol. (London)* **194**, 407.

Hubel, D. H., and Wiesel, T. N. (1963). *J. Neurophysiol.* **26**, 994.

Hubel, D. H., and Wiesel, T. N. (1970). *J. Physiol. (London)* **206**, 419.

Hughes, J. R., Evarts, E. V., and Marshall, W. H. (1956). *Amer. J. Physiol.* **186**, 483.

Jacobson, M. (1968a). *Develop, Biol.* **17**, 202.

Jacobson, M. (1968b). *Develop. Biol.* **17**, 219.

Jacobson, M., and Baker, R. E. (1969). *J. Comp. Neurol.* **137**, 121.

Jobsis, F. F., and O'Connor, M. J. (1966). *Biochem. Biophys. Res. Commun.* **25**, 246.

Jones, E. G., and Powell, T. P. S. (1970). *Phil. Trans. Roy. Soc. (London), Ser. B* **257**, 29.

Jones, S. F., and Kwanbunbumpen, S. (1970). *J. Physiol. (London)* **207**, 31.

Jones, W. H., and Thomas, D. B. (1962). *J. Anat.* **96**, 375.

Kandel, E. R., and Spencer, W. A. (1968). *Physiol. Rev.* **48**, 65.

Karlsson, U. (1967). *J. Ultrastruct. Res.* **17**, 158.

Katz, B., and Miledi, R. (1965). *Proc. Roy. Soc., Ser. B,* **161**, 496.

Katz, B., and Miledi, R. (1968). *J. Physiol. (London)* **195**, 481.

Katz, B., and Miledi, R. (1970). *J. Physiol. (London)* **207**, 789.

Kelly, J. S., Krnjevic, K., and Somjen, G. (1969). *J. Neurobiol.* **2**, 197.

Kingsley, J. R., Collins, G. H., and Converse, W. K. (1970). *Exp. Neurol.* **26**, 498.

Kozak, W., and Westerman, R. A. (1966). *Symp. Soc. Exp. Biol.* **20**, 509.

Kreutzberg, G. W. (1969). *Proc. Nat. Acad. Sci. U.S.* **62**, 722.

Kuhlman, R. E., and Lowry, O. H. (1956). *J. Neurochem.* **1**, 173.

Kupfer, C., and Palmer, P. (1964). *Exp. Neurol.* **9**, 400.

Landau, E. M., and Kwanbunbumpen, S. (1969). *Nature (London)* **221**, 271.

Liu, C. N., and Chambers, W. W. (1958). *Arch. Neurol.* **79**, 46.

Lloyd, D. P. C. (1949). *J. Gen. Physiol.* **33**, 147.

Lux, H. D., Schubert, P., Kreutzberg, G. W., and Globus, A. (1970). *Exp. Brain Res.* **10**, 197.

McCance, R. A., and Widdowson, E. M. (1968). "Calorie Deficiencies and Protein Deficiencies." Churchill, London.

McCouch, G. P., Austin, G. M., Liu, C. N., and Liu, C. Y. (1958). *J. Neurophysiol.* **21**, 205.

McIntyre, A. K. (1953). *Abstr. Commun. Int. Physiol. Congr. 19th.* 1953, pp. 107–113.

McIntyre, A. K., and Mark, R. F. (1960). *J. Physiol. (London)* **153**, 306.

McIntyre, A. K., Bradley, K., and Brock, L. G. (1959). *J. Gen. Physiol.* **42**, 931.

Maletta, G. J., and Timiras, P. S. (1967). *Exp. Neurol.* **19**, 513.

Mallart, A., and Martin, A. R. (1967). *J. Physiol. (London)* **193**, 679.

Maraini, G., Carta, F., Franguelli, R., and Santori, M. (1967). *Exp. Eye Res.* **6**, 299.

Marin–Padilla, M. (1968). *Brain. Res.* **8**, 196.

Mark, R. F. (1970). *Nature (London)* **225**, 178.

Marotte, L. R., and Mark, R. F. (1970a). *Brain Res.* **19**, 41.

Marotte, L. R., and Mark, R. F. (1970b). *Brain Res.* **19**, 53.

Matthews, M. R., and Powell, T. P. S. (1962). *J. Anat.* **96**, 89.

Matthews, M. R., Cowan, W. M., and Powell, T. P. S. (1960). *J. Anat.* **94**, 145.

Melzack, R., Konrad, K. W., and Dubrovsky, B. (1969). *Exp. Neurol.* **25**, 416.

Morlock, N. L., Pearlman, A. L., and Marshall, W. H. (1965). *Exp. Neurol.* **11**, 38.

Morrell, F. (1961a). *Physiol. Rev.* **41**, 443.

Morrell, F. (1961b). *In* "C.I.O.M.S. Symposium on Brain Mechanisms and Learning" (J. F. Delafresnaye, A. Fessard, and J. Konorski, eds.), pp. 375–392. Blackwell, Oxford.

Morrell, F., Engel, J. P., and Boeris, W. (1967). *Electroencephalogr. Clin. Neurophysiol.* **23**, 89.

Mountford, S. (1963). *J. Ultrastruct. Res.* **9**, 403.

Mullinger, A. M. (1969). *Tissue Cell.* **1**, 31.

Murray, J. G., and Thompson, J. W. (1957). *J. Physiol. (London)* **135**, 133.

Otsuka, M., Endo, M., and Nonomura, Y. (1962). *Jap. J. Physiol.* **12**, 573.

Parducz, A., and Feher, O. (1970). *Experientia* **26**, 629.

Pecci-Saavedra, J., Vaccarezza, O. L., Reader, T. A., and Pasqualini, E. (1970). *Exp. Neurol.* **26**, 607.

Pinching, A. J. (1969). *Brain Res.* **16**, 277.

Potter, L. T. (1969). *J. Physiol. (London)* **206**, 145.

Quilliam, J. P., and Tamarind, D. L. (1969). *Proc. Int. Congr. Pharmacol., 4th,* 1969 p. 146.

Quilliam, J. P., and Tamarind, D. L. (1970). *Brit. J. Pharmacol.* **39**, 244P.

Raisman, G. (1969). *Brain Res.* **14**, 25.

Rasch, E., Swift, H., Riesen, A. H., and Chow, K. L. (1961). *Exp. Cell Res.* **25**, 348.

Rasmussen, G. L. (1957). *In* "New Research Techniques of Neuroanatomy" (W. F. Windle, ed.), pp. 27–39. Thomas, Springfield, Illinois.

Revzin, A. M. (1969). *Brain Res.* **15**, 246.

Robbins, N., and Nelson, P. G. (1970). *Exp. Neurol.* **27**, 66.

Robert, E. D., and Oester, Y. T. (1970). *Arch. Neurol.* **22**, 57.

Rodieck, R. W., and Smith, P. S. (1966). *J. Neurophysiol.* **29**, 942.

Rose, J. E., Malis, L. I., Kruger, L., and Baker, C. P. (1960). *J. Comp. Neurol.* **115**, 243.

Rose, S. P. R. (1967). *Nature (London)* **215**, 253.

Rosenblueth, A., Klopp, C. T., and Simeone, F. A. (1938). *J. Neurophysiol.* **1**, 508.

Rosenzweig, M. R., Bennett, E. L., Diamond, M. C., Wu, S. Y., Slagle, R. W., and Saffran, E. (1969). *Brain Res.* **14**, 427.

Sakakura, H., and Doty, W. (1969). *Electroencephalogr. Clin. Neurophysiol.* **27**, 687.

Schiaffino, S., and Hanzlikova, V. (1970). *Experientia* **26**, 152.

Schmitt, F. O., and Samson, F. E. (1969). *Neurosci. Res. Program, Bull.* **7**, 281.

Schneider, G. E., and Nauta, W. J. H. (1969). *Anat. Rec.* **163**, 258.

Scrimshaw, N. S., and Gordon, J. E., eds. (1968). "Malnutrition, Learning and Behavior" MIT Press, Cambridge, Massachusetts.

Sefton, A. (1968). *Vision Res.* **8**, 867.

Sharpless, S. K. (1964). *Annu. Rev. Physiol.* **26**, 357.

Sholl, D. A. (1955). *J. Anat.* **89**, 33.

Siegesmund, K. A., Sances, A., and Larson, S. J. (1969). *J. Neurol. Sci.* **9**, 89.

Stavraky, G. W. (1961). "Supersensitivity Following Lesions of the Nervous System." Univ. of Toronto Press, Toronto.

Stromblad, B. C. R. (1960). *Experientia* **16**, 458.

Talwar, G. P., Chopra, S. P., Goel, B. K., and D'Monte, B. (1966). *J. Neurochem.* **13**, 109.

Thesleff, S. (1960). *J. Physiol. (London)* **151**, 598.

Uttley, A. M. (1970). *J. Theor. Biol.* **27**, 31.

Valverde, F. (1967). *Exp. Brain Res.* **3**, 337.

Valverde, F. (1968). *Exp. Brain Res.* **5**, 274.

Van Buren, J. M. (1963). *J. Neurol.* **26**, 402.

Van Harreveld, A. (1964). *In* "Physiology of Spinal Neurons" (J. C. Eccles and J. P. Schade, eds.), pp. 280–304. Elsevier, Amsterdam.

Van Harreveld, A. (1966). "Brain Tissue Electrolytes." Butterworth, London.

Van Marthens, E., and Zamenhof, S. (1969). *Exp. Neurol.* **23**, 214.

Voeller, K., Pappas, G. D., and Purpura, D. P. (1963). *Exp. Neurol.* **7**, 107.

Walsh, R. N., Budtz–Olsen, O. E., Penny, J. E., and Cummins, R. A. (1969). *J. Comp. Neurol.* **137**, 361.

Weiner, N. (1970). *Annu. Rev. Pharmacol.* **10**, 273.

Werblin, F. S., and Dowling, J. E. (1969). *J. Neurophysiol.* **32**, 339.

Westrum, L. E. (1969). *Z. Mikrosk. Anat. Zellforsch. Anat.* **98**, 157.

Westrum, L. E., and Black, R. G. (1968). *Brain Res.* **11**, 706.

Westrum, L. E., White, L., and Ward, A. (1964). *J. Neurosurg.* **21**, 1033.

White, L. E., and Westrum, L. E. (1964). *Anat. Rec.* **148**, 410.

Wiesel, T. N., and Hubel, D. H. (1963). *J. Neurophysiol.* **26**, 978.

Wieskrantz, L. (1958). *Nature (London)* **181**, 1047.

Wilder, B. J., and Morrell, F. (1967). *Neurology* **17**, 1193.

Winsburg, G. R. (1968). *Exp. Cell Res.* **52**, 555.

Zamenhof, S., Mosley, J., and Schuller, E. (1966). *Science* **152**, 1396.

Zamenhof, S., Van Marthens, E., and Margolis, F. L. (1968). *Science* **160**, 322.

Zetterstrom, B. (1956). *Acta Physiol. Scand.* **35**, 272.

2

Degeneration and Regeneration of Synapses[1]

Geoffrey Raisman and Margaret R. Matthews

I. Introduction 61
II. Degeneration of Synapses 63
   A. Practical Steps for the Correlation of Light and Electron Microscopy 66
   B. Ultrastructural Analysis of Normal Neuropil 70
   C. Electron Microscopy of Terminal Degeneration 70
   D. Interpretation of Degeneration 92
   E. Limitations of Degeneration Methods 93
III. Regeneration of Synapses 95
IV. Summary 99
   References 101

I. Introduction

Orthograde or Wallerian degeneration of nerve fibers is a well documented process, and this article will deal particularly with those aspects of orthograde terminal degeneration of synapses which can be seen at the electron microscope level, with only brief references to light microscopic techniques for the study of degeneration. In considering orthograde degeneration of synapses, several recent articles have reviewed or discussed ultrastructural aspects of this field in some detail (Gray and Guillery, 1965; Alksne *et al.*, 1966; McMahan, 1967; Guillery, 1970), and it is not the present intention to review all the published material relevant

[1] To the memory of Sir Wilfrid E. Le Gros Clark.

to this topic. The aim of the section on degeneration of synapses is more to provide a general overview of the applications of orthograde degeneration for the study of nervous connections, its advantages and disadvantages, and the limitations of this type of study. It is hoped that this section may be of help particularly for those who are considering embarking on a course of investigation involving the use of orthograde degeneration at the electron microscope level, and for this purpose an attempt has been made to outline principles relevant to the design of such experiments and also to indicate what supporting light microscopic material will usually have to be prepared.

Regeneration of synapses is, by contrast, a complex and far less understood phenomenon, there being less information available, and little general agreement as to the basic processes involved. The section on regeneration will accordingly take the form of a discussion of possibilities rather than (as in the case of degeneration) a description of established reactions which are sufficiently well understood to be applied routinely as a method for the study of neural connections. It therefore seems appropriate at this stage to define some aspects of the regeneration of synapses. True regeneration may be taken to imply that cut axons re-establish synaptic contacts of the same type with exactly the same postsynaptic elements with which they were formerly in contact; it would result in reconstitution of the precise pattern of connections existing before the lesion. In the peripheral nervous system cut axons do regenerate and may establish their original contacts with some degree of precision. In the central nervous system, however, the reaction is generally far less positive. It is clear that cut axons regenerate and establish effective connections in the central nervous system of cold-blooded vertebrates (Clemente, 1964), and it has been shown in some cases that a striking degree of restoration of point to point relationships may be achieved (Gaze, 1960). In the central nervous system of mammals, effective regeneration in this sense does not occur. However, there is considerable evidence that de-afferented postsynaptic sites may be reinnervated by the formation of new synapses from existing intact axons in the region where the cut axons originally terminated. There is also some suggestion that the cut axons, although not actually regenerating, may form adventitious synapses in the vicinity of the lesion. Both these topics are eminently suited for investigation by electron microscopic techniques; moreover, an understanding of these possibilities is essential to the interpretation of some types of experiments, in particular those involving the use of chronic lesions.

II. Degeneration of Synapses

When a nerve fiber is cut, the portion which is severed from its continuity with the cell body (i.e., the distal segment) is unable to survive, and both the axon and its terminals undergo degeneration, the débris being ultimately removed by phagocytic cells. This is known as Wallerian degeneration. The process of degeneration may be recognized at the light microscopic level by making use of the fact that the axon is fragmented and that the degenerating cytoplasm has a different staining reaction, which may be displayed by the methods of Nauta and Gygax, Glees, Fink and Heimer, and others (for a recent critical appraisal, see Heimer, 1967). These methods are all applicable at the light microscopic level and, thus, obviate the far greater expenditure of time required for electron microscopy. In tracing fiber pathways over large distances through the brain, and in displaying the overall pattern of degeneration within terminal fields (e.g., the laminar pattern of degeneration in structures such as the hippocampus or superior colliculus) light microscopic methods offer considerable advantages over electron microscopy. Paradoxically, despite its lower magnification range, the sensitivity of light microscopy to detect small amounts of degeneration is much greater than that of electron microscopy. This is because the light microscope affords the facility of scanning large volumes of tissue so that it is possible to detect very small numbers of degenerating fibers in a section which may be taken at a thickness of as much as 50 μ and comprise the cross-sectional area of the whole brain. By contrast, an electron microscope section is generally only about 1/800th of this thickness, and usually has an area of not more than one square millimeter. From this it follows that it is nearly always necessary, before commencing an ultrastructural study, to be fully conversant with what the light microscope reveals of the general course and mode of termination of the pathways under study, and also that it is not usually profitable to attempt to use the electron microscope to analyze any but the densest projections found with the light microscope.

There are several advantages which are offered by an electron microscopic study of degeneration and which can rarely or never be achieved by other methods. These include the following.

1. *The identification of degenerating terminals.* It is rarely possible with the light microscope to make a definitive distinction between degenerating axons and degenerating terminals. There are many regions in

which it is uncertain from light microscopy whether a fiber tract gives rise to terminals in addition to axons which continue out of the area to a further terminal region (e.g., Rinvik and Walberg, 1969).

2. *Simultaneous demonstration of normal and degenerating synapses.* In electron micrographs the degenerating terminals are displayed together with all the nondegenerating terminals so that it is possible to assess what proportion of the total number of axon terminals are degenerating. This also means that when terminals are classifiable into different categories, it is possible to see whether the degenerating terminals fall preferentially into particular categories.

3. *Recognition of the postsynaptic structure.* The electron microscope reveals the nature of the postsynaptic elements (dendritic spines, shafts, etc.: Figs. 1, 3, 4, 5) and shows the actual synaptic junctions from which the direction of conduction may be deduced (on the generally accepted hypothesis that the clustering of synaptic vesicles indicates the presynaptic element). By this means complex interactions of processes within regions such as the lateral geniculate nucleus (e.g., Guillery, 1969a,b) or the cerebellar cortex (Eccles *et al.*, 1967) have been worked out. By analogy with recent studies in which electrophysiological and anatomical observations have been correlated, it may be possible to infer something about the possible functions of the synapse. Thus, there is evidence to suggest that in some regions terminals upon cell bodies may be inhibitory (e.g., in the hippocampus and cerebellum, Eccles, 1964; Mugnaini, 1969) and that synapses terminating upon dendritic spines are excitatory (Diamond *et al.*, 1969).

4. *Additional data on the fine structure of the synapse.* Here may be included such information as the types of vesicles in the presynaptic element, the type of synaptic thickening and the contents of the postsynaptic element (spine apparatus, sacs, vesicles etc.) (see Figs. 1–5). These discriminating features are valuable from an anatomical point of view, and may also offer important clues about the functions of the synapses. Under appropriate conditions of fixation, there seems to be a correlation between the presence of flattened or polymorphic synaptic vesicles and symmetrical types of synaptic thickenings (Colonnier, 1968) and, conversely, between spherical synaptic vesicles and asymmetrical thickenings. It has been suggested that the former type of synapse is inhibitory and the latter excitatory (Larramendi *et al.*, 1967; Uchizono, 1968). Similarly, the presence of dense core vesicles, which may be used to distinguish anatomically

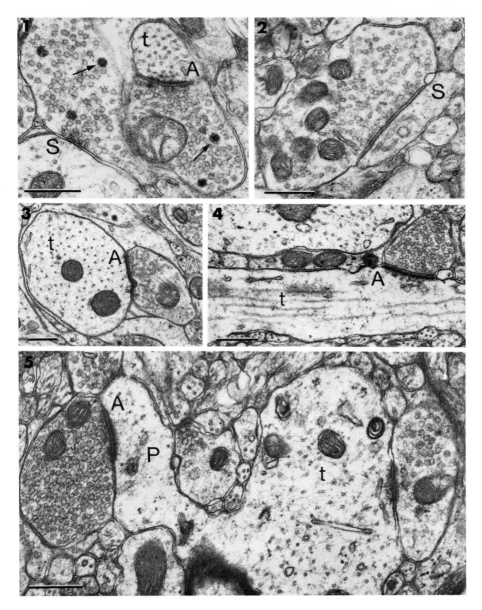

Figs. 1–5. Normal axon terminals making asymmetrical (A) or symmetrical (S) contacts with dendritic shafts (marked by neurotubules, t) or with a dendritic spine (P). Arrows indicate dense core vesicles. Rat, medial septal nucleus. *Except where otherwise stated, the calibration bar in each of the figures represents 0.5 μ. For all tissues except the sympathetic ganglion, primary fixation was by aldehydes, followed by postosmication.*

between the terminals of different pathways (Raisman, 1969a), also seems in some sites to be indicative of the presence of neurohumoral or neurosecretory substances (e.g., the small dense core vesicles in sympathetic postganglionic terminals, Wolfe *et al.*, 1962; the larger neurosecretory vesicles in the axon terminals of the neurohypophysis, Barer *et al.*, 1963).

An example, from our own experience, of an unusual type of synapse whose definition illustrates the use of ultrastructural criteria and which offers interesting correlations with pharmacological and electrophysiological observations is the somatic efferent synapse of the small granule-containing cells of the superior cervical ganglion in the rat (Siegrist *et al.*, 1968; Matthews and Raisman, 1969; T. H. Williams and Palay, 1969). In these synapses (Figs. 6 and 7) the presynaptic vesicle cluster consists largely of dense core vesicles, which closely approach the presynaptic membrane in the intervals of a well-defined series of presynaptic dense projections. In other features these synapses resemble forms common elsewhere in the nervous system, i.e., they have characteristic synaptic thickenings and there is also an increased intermembrane gap containing electron dense material between the pre- and postsynaptic membranes. The dense core vesicles of these cells closely resemble the catecholamine storage vesicles of adrenergic nerves, and evidence from fluorescence microscopy indicates that the cells contain a catecholamine, which is now thought to be dopamine (Björklund *et al.*, 1970). Dopamine most effectively mimics the inhibitory effects on the postganglionic neurons produced by appropriate preganglionic stimulation, and it appears likely that the small cells are involved as inhibitory interneurons (for recent evidence, discussion, and references, sec Libet, 1970; Nishi, 1970). The unusual efferent synapse of the small cells therefore appears to be an inhibitory synapse at which a catecholamine transmitter is released.

A. Practical Steps for the Correlation of Light and Electron Microscopy

Background studies with the light microscope enter into most investigations of the ultrastructure of the nervous system, and it may therefore be helpful to indicate what is most likely to be involved from the technical point of view before embarking on such a line of investigation. First, as has been mentioned above, it is most profitable to apply electron microscopy only to degeneration of pathways in which the terminal degeneration is known to be fairly dense. Second, it is essential to obtain precise

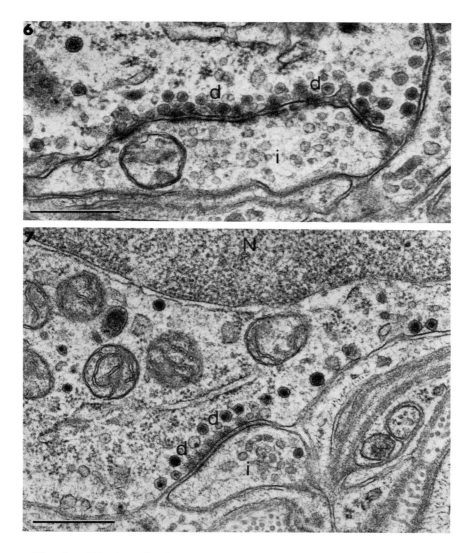

Figs. 6 and 7.   Somatic efferent synapses of the small granule-containing cells of the rat superior cervical ganglion. d, dense core vesicles clustering toward the synaptic contact area; i, irregular vesicular material in the postsynaptic elements; N, nucleus. Osmium fixation.

localization in the ultrathin sections. Unless the terminal field is very well marked by some cytoarchitectonic feature of the tissue, it is frequently necessary to establish appropriate landmarks by a preliminary survey of the degeneration in a series of light microscope sections stained by one of the versions of the reduced silver methods. As the optimal survival times for these methods are about 5–7 days, somewhat longer than those employed for displaying degeneration by electron microscopy, this will usually mean that a separate series of experimental animals must be prepared for light microscopy. However, when the transition is made to the ultrastructural level it may be found that the degeneration is nonetheless too patchy in its fine distribution to be consistently located with the electron microscope. In such cases it is possible to apply the staining methods of Heimer (1969) and Holländer and Vaaland (1968), which show degeneration in semithin (1 or 2 μ) sections from blocks prepared for electron microscopy, so that appropriate areas for ultrathin sections may be selected from the same block face.

Intermediate steps of some kind may be necessary to bridge the gap between the level of organization revealed even by semithin sections and that offered by the electron microscope (see Heimer, 1970). A simple routine which we have found very useful is to make a camera lucida drawing of a stained semithin (light microscope) section from each block face before trimming down for electron microscopy. This gives a view of a wide area of the surrounding tissue, with its landmarks, and facilitates selection of the area for detailed study. After the block has been trimmed down to the desired area for electron microscopy, a further semithin section is taken from this smaller block face, and this is also drawn out in camera lucida and its position matched exactly on the drawing of the original semithin section. Ultrathin sections are now cut from this block face and a drawing of the section is made using the electron microscope. This may be done either by the mapping method described by Alksne *et al.* (1966), which involves using the micrometer scales of the electron microscope stage micromanipulators, or by using a squared electron microscope grid and drawing the relation of the section to the actual grid bars (Fig. 8). The latter method is simpler but of course has the disadvantage that parts of the section are invisible as they lie over the grid bars. However, it does serve to divide the field conveniently into units which can be used for quantitative sampling, and the use of a squared grid of small mesh often avoids the necessity for precoating the grid to support the sections.

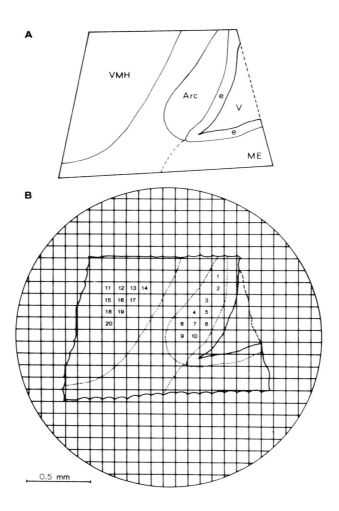

Fig. 8. Method for orientation of ultrathin sections. (A) Camera lucida drawing of a 1 μ thick light microscope section from a trimmed block face (coronal section through the tuberal hypothalamus of the rat) stained with methylene blue and Azur II to show the cytoarchitectonic features. Arc, arcuate nucleus; e, ependyma; ME, median eminence; V, third ventricle; VMH, ventromedial hypothalamic nucleus. (B) A drawing of an adjacent ultrathin section from the same block face lying upon an electron microscope grid. Grid squares 1–10 are from the arcuate nucleus, 11–20 from the ventromedial nucleus.

B. Ultrastructural Analysis of Normal Neuropil

Preparatory to a study of terminal degeneration, the normal population of synapses in the region must be assessed. This analysis involves classification of the synapses by as many features as possible and is most informative when some sort of quantitative estimate of the occurrence of the different types can be obtained. The features which characterize synapses (Figs. 1–5) may differ, often markedly, from one region to another. It may be useful to list examples of the kinds of features in three groups.

1. For the *presynaptic element*, the types of synaptic vesicles (size, shape, contents), other constituents such as mitochondria, which may be distinctive (Szentágothai *et al.*, 1966), size and shape of the axon terminal, the nature of the preterminal segment and parent axon (e.g., the diameter, branching pattern, or presence of myelination), and whether the synapse is of the *en passant* variety.

2. For the *postsynaptic element*, its nature, e.g., dendritic shaft or spine (Figs. 1 and 3–5), cell body (Fig. 32), other axon terminal; its contents, e.g., multivesicular bodies, spine apparatus (Figs. 25 and 26), sacs, tubules, vesicles, etc.

3. For the *contact region*, the type of synaptic thickening, e.g., symmetrical or asymmetrical (Figs. 1–4), continuous or discontinuous (Fig. 9), length, curvature, etc.

C. Electron Microscopy of Terminal Degeneration

Certain criteria have to be satisfied before any specific change in a nerve terminal is interpreted as degeneration. These are (a) that the change appears following a lesion of fibers which enter the area in question, does not occur after lesions of other pathways, and cannot be ascribed to nonspecific effects such as direct vascular or mechanical damage to the terminals; (b) that the change does not occur on the opposite side of the brain (in the case of unilateral pathways), and does not occur in unoperated animals; (c) that after the lesion the changes follow a consistent time course leading ultimately to complete degradation. Several different types of terminal degeneration have so far been recognized, each with its characteristic time course. Since it is not yet possible to predict with certainty what form the degeneration will take in a given pathway, a series of test lesions must be made to ascertain the type of degeneration which occurs in the system, and the optimum time of survival for its

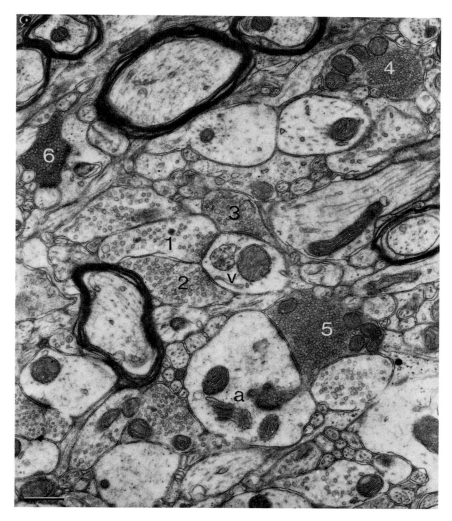

Fig. 9. Neuropil of the rat medial septal nucleus 24 hours after section of the fimbria. Terminals numbered 1 to 6 illustrate a series of intermediate stages varying from normal (1) to definitely degenerating (6). a, spine apparatus; v, multivesicular body.

appearance. The time of onset of degeneration within any given system also appears to depend upon the distance of the lesion from the terminals, i.e., the length of the distal segment. Thus, Miledi and Slater (1970) state that for each additional centimeter of distal stump, the degeneration of the neuromuscular junctions in the rat diaphragm is delayed by a

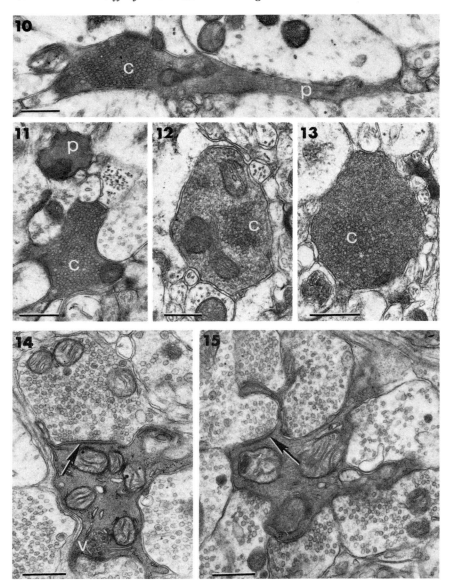

Figs. 10–13.   Early forms of degenerating terminals and presumed preterminal segments (p) showing increased electron density of the matrix and clustering of the synaptic vesicles (c). Rat septum, 48 hours after section of the fimbria.

Figs. 14 and 15.   Darkening and collapse of dendritic profiles attributed to rough handling of the tissue during removal. Arrows, synaptic thickenings; v, multivesicular body. Rat septum, normal material.

further 45 minutes after section of the phrenic nerve. Vaccarezza *et al.*, (1970) estimate a delay of 12 hours for each centimeter of retinogeniculate axons for the onset of degeneration of the retinal terminals in the lateral geniculate nucleus of the Cebus monkey.

The commonest type of degeneration occurring in the *central nervous system* is generally referred to as electron dense degeneration. Detailed descriptions of this type of degeneration have been given for several systems (reviewed in references given on p. 61). The basic morphological features and time course are roughly as follows. In all but the most rapidly degenerating pathways, there is little change during the first 24 hours after axotomy. During the second 24-hour period, changes commence in the terminals. Initially, these changes are slight and equivocal (Fig. 9). There develop a gradual increase in electron density of the background matrix of the terminal and an increasing tendency for the synaptic vesicles to clump together in the center of the terminal, which result in a distinctly abnormal appearance (Figs. 10–13). In identifying this as degeneration, some caution must be exercised in regard to the fixation, as both these effects have been described in normal material in which there have been postulated difficulties in the fixation procedures (see Cohen and Pappas, 1969; V. Williams and Grossman, 1970). The implication of fixation artefacts for degeneration studies has been discussed by numerous authors (e.g., Grofova and Rinvik, 1970; Kruger and Hámori, 1970; J. S. Lund and Lund, 1970; Peters, 1970), and examples are shown in Figs. 14 and 15. At around 2–3 days postoperatively, the degenerating terminals have a considerably increased electron density and the outline of the profile is somewhat collapsed. The collapse and increase in electron density are features common to both the terminals and the axoplasm of the parent axons and preterminal segments (Figs. 10 and 16–18), tending to appear somewhat later in myelinated axons. In the earlier stages of the degeneration the synaptic and other vesicles are still recognizable; the mitochondria usually show characteristic changes such as swelling or shrinkage (Figs. 19–22). It has also been our experience that at this stage of degeneration the unit (trilaminar) structure of the apposed plasma membranes is particularly well seen in the region of the synaptic contact (Figs. 23 and 24). A similar appearance has also been described in relation to degeneration of dendrites induced by irradiation of the cortex (Kruger and Hámori, 1970). Subsequently, the terminal becomes progressively denser and more collapsed, while its organelles (such as synaptic vesicles and mitochondria) become more difficult to distinguish. At this stage the degenerating fragment becomes surrounded by reactive astrocytic pro-

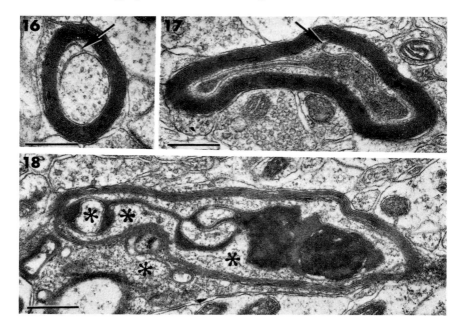

Fig. 16.   Normal myelinated axon. Arrow, mesaxon.

Figs. 17 and 18.   Degenerating myelinated axons in the rat septum 2 days after a lesion of the fimbria. Arrow, mesaxon; *, oligodendrocyte cytoplasm.

cesses (Figs. 25 and 26) which invaginate its surface and may be assumed ultimately to engulf it completely, since at increasing intervals after the lesion degenerating terminals are less and less often found in contact with the postsynaptic element, but continue to be seen as progressively denser, irregular fragments in astrocytes.

The astrocytic reaction in the region in which terminals are degenerating is marked by a general increase in the number and size of the astrocytic processes, as well as an increase in their content of glycogen (Fig. 27) and, somewhat later, of glial filaments. For a further description of possible cell types involved in the reaction to degeneration, reference may be made to Walberg (1963), Bignami and Ralston (1969), Vaughn and Pease (1970), and Vaughn *et al.* (1970). The last part of the terminal to be surrounded by the astrocyte is the region of the synaptic thickening (Figs. 25–27, inset). This fortunate fact means that degenerating terminals can be recognized at a stage when they are still in contact with the postsynaptic element, and thus, the latter may be identified (Figs. 25, 26, 28–33). In most systems, the incidence of degenerating terminals still in

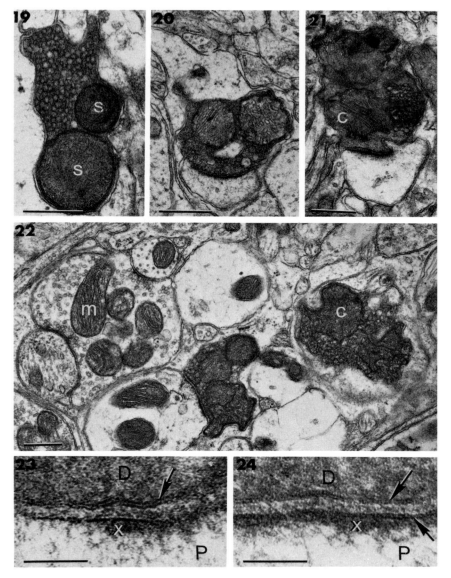

Figs. 19–22. Degenerating axon terminals showing mitochondrial changes—swelling (s) or collapse (c), and deformation of the cristae. m, normal mitochondrion. Rat ventromedial nucleus 2 days after section of the stria terminalis.

Figs. 23 and 24. The region of the synaptic thickening (x) of two degenerating asymmetrical synapses showing the prominent triple layered structure of the unit membranes (arrows). D, degenerating terminal; P, postsynaptic element. Rat septum, 2 days after fimbrial section. Calibration bar = 0.1 μ.

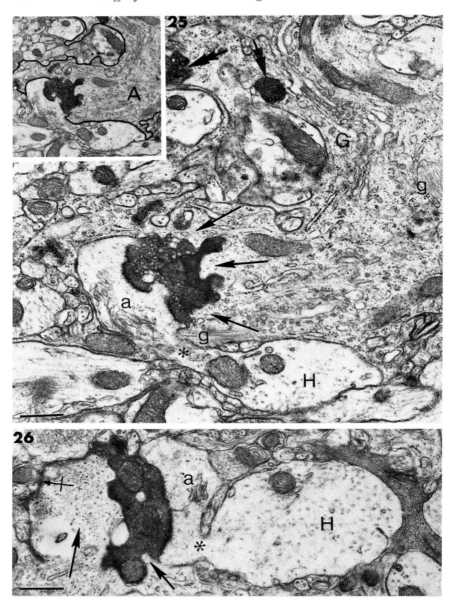

Figs. 25 and 26. Degenerating terminals making contact with dendritic spines. The degenerating terminals are deeply invaginated by astrocytic processes (arrows). a, spine apparatus; *, spine necks; G, Golgi region of astrocyte; g, glial filaments; H, dendritic shafts; double-headed arrows, engulfed degenerating fragments; crossed arrow, attenuated strand of degenerating terminal. Inset shows the astrocytic process (A) of Fig. 25 outlined.

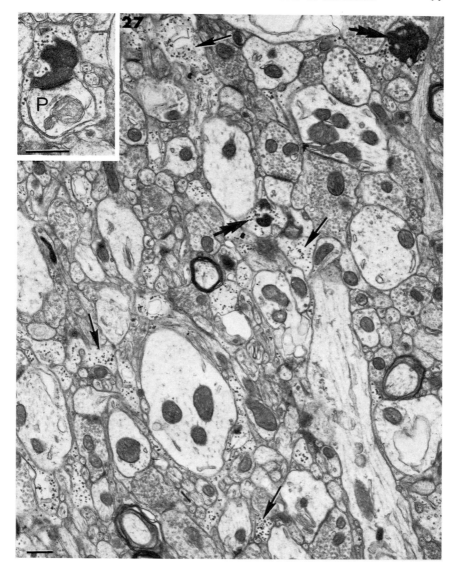

Fig. 27. Field of neuropil showing extensive astrocytic reaction to the presence of terminal degeneration. Arrows, some of the astrocytic processes marked by dense black particulate deposits of glycogen; double-headed arrows, degenerating fragments completely enveloped by astrocytic cytoplasm; inset, a degenerating terminal contacting a dendritic spine (P) and completely surrounded in the plane of section by a reactive, glycogen laden astrocytic process which has not yet penetrated between the degenerating terminal and the synaptic cleft. Rat septum, 5 days after a lesion of the fimbria.

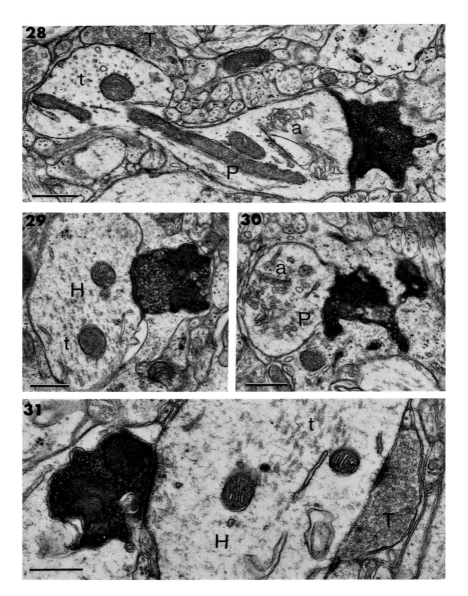

Figs. 28–31. Degenerating axon terminals contacting dendritic shafts (H) or dendritic spines (P). T, normal terminals; t, dendritic tubules; a, spine apparatus. Rat ventromedial nucleus 2 days after a lesion of the stria terminalis.

synaptic contact is at its heaviest between 2 and 7 days postoperatively, and over the second week the process of phagocytosis becomes sufficiently advanced to cause a substantial reduction in the number of profiles still in contact with the postsynaptic element. The majority of degenerating terminals are removed from contact with the postsynaptic elements by 2 or 3 weeks after operation. Although a few degenerating terminals have been described in the inferior olive of the cat after midbrain lesions at as long a survival period as 112 days (Walberg, 1965), this is to be regarded as exceptional. The degree of asynchronism with which degeneration proceeds is such that at any time when terminals are recognizably degenerating but still in contact, a proportion of terminals will not yet show unequivocal signs of degeneration, while others will be completely phagocytosed. This generally does not seriously hinder experimental studies, although it should be realized that the apparent maximum number of degenerating terminals must always be somewhat below the true number and that the choice of survival times is a compromise between the two opposing factors. In some situations, however, (discussed below) the question of asynchronism may be of crucial importance.

Not all features of normal synapses can be equally well distinguished in degenerating synapses. Thus, while the persistence of the synaptic contact with the postsynaptic element resists phagocytosis for sufficiently long for the presynaptic element to be identified as degenerating, the process of collapse and increased electron density may make it difficult to classify degenerating terminals with regard to their true size, contents, or synaptic thickening. In the case of the synaptic thickening, while the asymmetrical types are visible in relation to degenerating terminals even if sectioned somewhat obliquely (Figs. 28, 29, and 31), the symmetrical thickenings may become obscured because the presynaptic element is darkened (e.g., Westman, 1969), and the postsynaptic thickening is generally not sufficiently prominent to be seen with certainty if the section is at all oblique. Under these circumstances it may not even be possible to recognize the existence of a specialized contact area (e.g., Fig. 30). Although this is not an absolute obstacle (Fig. 34; see also, Grofova and Rinvik, 1970) it must be realized that, in a quantitative study, the process of degeneration will tend to give an inflated impression of the number of asymmetrical synapses degenerating in relation to symmetrical synapses.

In the case of the synaptic vesicles, it may be difficult to recognize the difference between spherical and flattened vesicles in degenerating endings (see, however, Walberg, 1966; Holländer *et al.*, 1969; Grofova and Rinvik, 1970). One way of establishing that a pathway may have terminals with

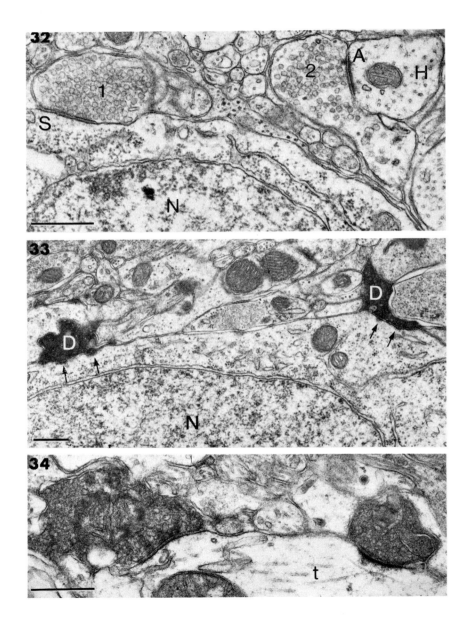

predominantly one or the other type of vesicles is by the use of chronic lesions, leaving a survival time of sufficient length for all the terminals to be removed and then comparing the proportions of terminals of the two types in the residual neuropil with that found in the intact animal. By this method, R. D. Lund (1969) showed that the retino-tectal terminals in the rat contained predominantly spherical synaptic vesicles, i.e., in the optic tectum of the intact animal the proportion of terminals with spherical vesicles to those with flattened vesicles was about 6 to 4, whereas after a chronic lesion of the optic nerve, the proportion was 1 to 4. By contrast with these vesicle types, dense core vesicles are usually easily recognized during the earlier stages of degeneration (cf. Figs. 35 and 36), possibly as they become accentuated by a swelling of the whole vesicle resulting in a wider electron lucent "halo" and a progressive loss of the dense core. Taking advantage of this fact it was shown that in the septal neuropil the terminals of axons from the medial forebrain bundle had a far higher proportion of dense core vesicles than those derived from the hippocampal fibers (Raisman, 1969a).

It now seems fairly certain that the electron dense type of degeneration at the electron microscope level is the equivalent of the dense terminals stained by the Nauta staining methods, and more particularly by the non-suppressive Fink–Heimer type of modifications of light microscopy. This is confirmed by the demonstration of silver particles over electron dense boutons in electron micrographs taken from actual light microscope sections stained by the Nauta technique and then reembedded for electron microscopy (Guillery and Ralston, 1964; Heimer and Peters, 1968).

In some fiber pathways, the section of axons is followed by a different series of changes in the terminals. The axon terminals respond to axotomy by an initial stage which may be described as neurofilamentous hypertrophy (Fig. 37). This type of reaction is less common than the electron dense reaction. It occurs in systems such as the avian retinotectal projection

---

Fig. 32. A normal axosomatic synapse (1) making a symmetrical contact (S) with a cell body (nucleus, N); adjacent normal synapse (2) making an asymmetrical contact (A) with a dendritic shaft (H). Rat ventromedial hypothalamic nucleus.

Fig. 33. Two degenerating axon terminals (D) making axosomatic synapses with a neuronal cell body (nucleus, N) in the medial septal nucleus 2 days after a lesion of the medial forebrain bundle, in the rat. Note discontinuous synaptic thickenings (arrows).

Fig. 34. Two degenerating axon terminals making synaptic contact with the same dendritic shaft. The synapse on the left has a definitely symmetrical thickening, that on the right has an asymmetrical thickening. t, dendritic tubules. Rat medial preoptic area 2 days after a lesion of the stria terminalis.

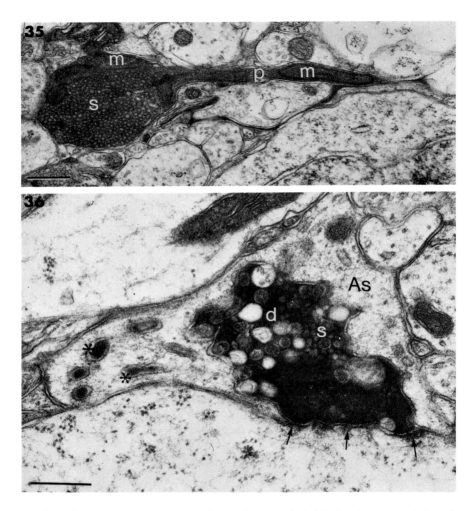

Fig. 35. Degenerating axon terminal and preterminal (p) showing accumulation of predominantly small clear synaptic vesicles (s). m, mitochondria. Rat medial septal nucleus 2 days after a lesion of the fimbria.

Fig. 36. Degenerating axosomatic synapse containing a high proportion of dense core vesicles (d), mixed with the smaller synaptic vesicles (s). The terminal is completely surrounded and invaginated by an astrocytic process (As) except for the contact region. Arrows, discontinuous synaptic thickenings; *, isolated fragments of degenerating terminal. Rat medial septal nucleus 2 days after a lesion of the medial forebrain bundle.

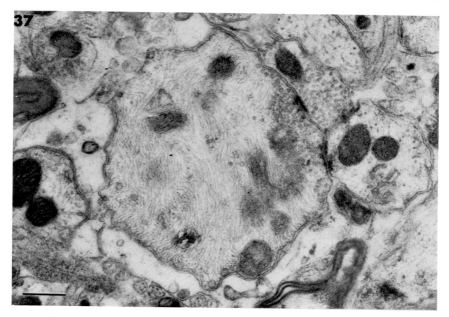

Fig. 37. A synaptic knob from the dorsal lateral geniculate nucleus of the monkey, showing neurofilamentous hypertrophy 11 days after section of the optic nerve. Reproduced with the author's permission from Guillery (1970).

(Gray and Hamlyn, 1962), the retinogeniculate projections of some species (Colonnier and Guillery, 1964; Szentágothai *et al.*, 1966), and the cerebellar corticovestibular system (Mugnaini and Walberg, 1967). During the first few days after the lesion, there is a progressive appearance of neurofilaments in the terminals, and ultimately, the whole terminal becomes filled with a coiled mass of filaments, often with associated mitochondria. At the same time, the synaptic vesicles gradually disappear from the terminals, and this has been circumstantially correlated with a concomitant failure of synaptic transmission (Saavedra *et al.*, 1970). In several systems, the neurofilamentous hypertrophy of the terminals which occurs at short survival periods has been shown to give way to a later stage of electron dense degeneration (R. D. Lund, 1969; Ralston, 1969). In the cerebello-vestibular terminals (Mugnaini and Walberg, 1967) intermediate forms, i.e., electron dense terminals with masses of neurofilaments, have been described at survival times intermediate between those required for the early neurofilamentous reaction and the later times for the electron dense stage. This suggests that the neurofilamentous terminals actually change into electron dense types, although this suggestion must be made with some reserve (for a discussion, see Guillery, 1970). The significance of the neurofilamentous stage is not altogether clear at present, and whether this type of degeneration occurs in any particular system seems to depend upon such factors as the species of the animal. Thus, the retino-geniculate terminals undergo neurofilamentous degeneration in the cat (Szentágothai *et al.*, 1966) and monkey (Colonnier and Guillery, 1964), but electron dense degeneration in the rat (McMahan, 1967). There is, however, an excellent correlation between the ring-like boutons stained by the Glees method of light microscopy and the neurofilamentous rings of electron microscopy which may be seen in degenerating terminals or, in certain sites, in normal terminals or in dendrites (see Guillery, 1970). Furthermore, electron micrographs taken from reembedded light microscope sections stained by the neurofibrillar method of Glees show a silver deposit over areas of neurofilamentous proliferation in degenerating boutons (Walberg and Mugnaini, 1969).

An interesting use of the different types of degeneration was demonstrated by Walberg and Mugnaini (1969). Making use of the fact that the afferents to the lateral vestibular nucleus differ in their mode of degeneration, they were able to produce simultaneously neurofilamentous degeneration of the terminals of the cerebellar cortico-vestibular fibers and electron dense degeneration of the terminals of the primary vestibular afferent fibers at a postoperative survival period of 3 days after a combined lesion of the cerebellum and the vestibular nerve. This study showed that individual postsynaptic elements in the terminal area could receive afferents showing both types of degeneration, and as the neurofilamentous terminals occur only after cerebellar lesions, and had virtually never progressed to the electron dense stage by this time, it was concluded that afferents from both systems converged upon the same postsynaptic element.

Both the processes of degeneration described so far have been used in studies of the central nervous system. A third type of degeneration, comprising swelling and electron lucent changes in the terminals, was described in the cochlear nucleus in earlier material (de Robertis, 1956). It has not subsequently been found to any extent in other sites in the brain and has generally been ascribed to the less perfect preservation of tissue obtained by the earlier methods of fixation and embedding (e.g., see the discussion by McMahan, 1967). However, study of the process of degeneration in the peripheral nervous system, and in several rather atypical sites (such as the neurosecretory axon terminals of the hypothalamo-hypophysial system) suggests the occurrence of at least one other mode of degeneration different from the two types described above. (For what may be yet another type of degeneration, see Cuénod et al., 1970.) In the peripheral nervous system axon terminals fall into three main groups, i.e., preganglionic fibers to autonomic ganglia, postganglionic terminals of ganglion neurons, and the terminals of the somatic moto-neurons in the endplates of striated muscle. While these three systems all show marked similarities in their mode of degeneration (and corres-ponding differences from central nervous degeneration), the present account will be based principally on the degeneration of preganglionic ter-minals in sympathetic ganglia. For accounts of degeneration of postgan-glionic terminals and of motor endplates, there are useful recent articles by Nickel and Waser (1968), Cheng-Minoda et al., (1968), Miledi and Slater (1968, 1970), Roth and Richardson (1969), and Teravainen and Huikuri (1969). Nickel and Waser (1969) have proposed that fixation in a mixture of zinc iodide and osmium tetroxide may produce a selective stain for degenerating motor endplates, and our own observations show that this also applies to degenerating preganglionic terminals. Although this method has great potential use, it will be necessary to establish cri-teria for the specificity of the reaction in individual sites. The main aspects of the degeneration of preganglionic terminals in the sympathetic ganglia are taken from Taxi (1964), Hunt and Nelson (1965), Hámori et al., (1968), Sotelo (1968), and Matthews (1972). Transection of the cervical sympathetic chain below the superior cervical ganglion in the rat results in destruction of the vast majority of the preganglionic fibers to the gan-glion. In comparison with the central nervous system, the reaction of the terminals in this and in most other peripheral sites is extraordinarily rapid. By 2–3 days postoperatively, there are few axon terminals left in-tact; the majority are represented by highly electron dense fragments with little recognizable internal structure and are embedded in the Schwann cell cytoplasm. By a detailed study of the events at closely spaced intervals during the first 6–48 hours after the lesion, it has been possible to see some of the intermediate stages, although the asynchro-nism of the degeneration is such that it is not yet possible to give more than a tentative account of the precise sequence of events.

The normal preganglionic terminal (Fig. 38) contains many synaptic vesicles with a few dense core vesicles and occasional mitochondria. The synaptic thickening is often asymmetrical and may be associated with a row of subjunctional bodies in the cytoplasm of the postsynaptic ele-ment, which in the rat superior cervical ganglion is most often a dendritic shaft or a spine-like profile. The preterminal segment (Fig. 38), like the

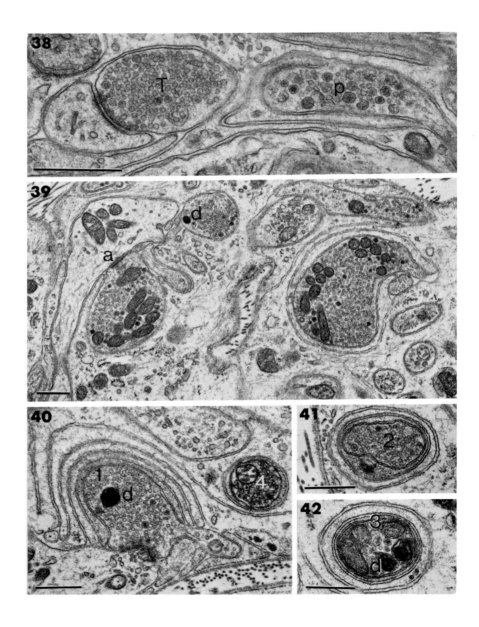

terminal, also contains synaptic vesicles and may have a rather higher proportion of dense core vesicles and mitochondria; it and the terminal profile may form part of a row of varicosities linked by slender connecting segments. Both pre- and postsynaptic elements are enveloped in Schwann cell cytoplasm, which separates the nervous structures from the connective tissue spaces in the ganglion (Figs. 38 and 39). The initial form of the terminal degeneration basically resembles the electron dense degeneration of the central nervous system. The earliest signs are a slight increase in the density of the cytoplasmic matrix and a tendency to clumping of the synaptic vesicles in the center of the terminal, but neither feature appears as clearly as in the central nervous system (Fig. 39). These changes begin to be seen from about 6 hours onward, according to the level of the lesion.

There also appears in a proportion of the terminals a most characteristic organelle not usually found in the electron dense degeneration in the central nervous system, i.e., a type of electron dense, membrane bounded body (Figs. 39, 40, 42, 44) which may contain synaptic or dense core vesicles. These bodies (which are also seen occasionally in unoperated ganglia) are the "axon-cytolysomes" of Hámori *et al.* (1968), and their presence strongly suggests some kind of autophagic process in the terminals. The degeneration is further distinguished from that in the central nervous system by a very early reaction in the enveloping Schwann cells, and this results in the development (at around 12–14 hours postoperatively) of multiple concentric wrappings of satellite lamellae, which are apparently formed by an elaboration of the normal simple mesaxon and which contain lightly granular cytoplasm, poor in organelles (Figs. 39-44). While these multiple wrappings are not incompatible with the persistence of synaptic contact (Fig. 40), the satellite reaction usually leads

---

Figs. 38–42.   Terminals of preganglionic fibers in the rat superior cervical ganglion. Osmium fixation.   Fig. 38. Normal appearance of terminal (T) and preterminal segment (p).   Figs. 39–42. Early and intermediate stages of degeneration, $12\frac{1}{2}$ hours after section of preganglionic nerve fibers (cervical sympathetic chain).   Fig. 39. Early tendency to clustering of vesicles and possible increase of mitochondria in terminal and preterminal profiles; d, cytoplasmic dense bodies; a, attachment plaque.   Figs. 40–42. Slight darkening of terminals and enwrapping in multiple lamellae of satellite cytoplasm; numbering of terminals 1–4 indicates probable progression of changes. From within outward, the satellite lamellae darken and become narrower and more closely spaced. Dense bodies ("axon-cytolysomes," d) appear in some terminals and the matrix undergoes progressive darkening (1, 2) followed by patchy lightening (3) which involves also the intercristal matrix of mitochondria (4).   Fig. 40. Unusual retention of synaptic contact by an enwrapped terminal.

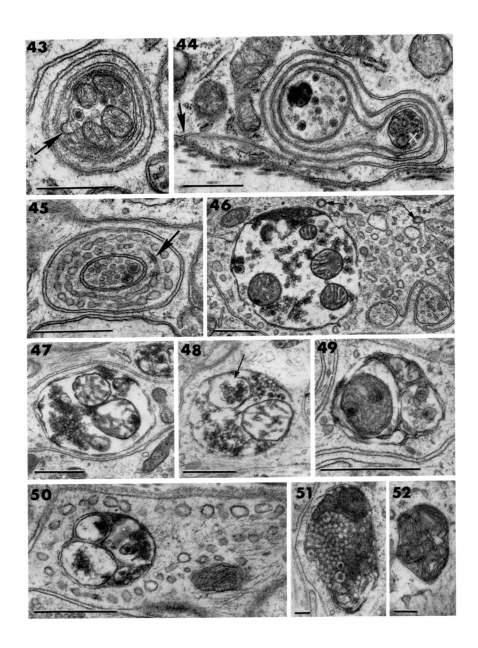

to early detachment of the terminal from the postynaptic site, presumably at a stage when it may not differ significantly in appearance from a normal terminal. Preterminal segments also become enwrapped and from this point onward cannot readily be distinguished from terminals. The satellite lamellae are initially of approximately equal width and of uniform cytoplasmic density, and the intervals between successive lamellae and between the innermost lamella and the terminal profile are approximately equal (Fig. 44). There next develops, from the innermost lamella outward, a progressive darkening of the cytoplasm, and a decrease in the lamellar width and interlamellar intervals (Figs. 40–43). This is most extreme at the interface between the satellite and the terminal, where the membranes may fuse in places (Fig. 42). It is possible that at this stage material derived from the degenerating terminal is taken up into coated vesicles by the innermost satellite lamella (Fig. 43). The degenerating terminal retains a round form even though it may shrink at this stage. Its cytoplasm begins to show a patchy lightening as if empty spaces are appearing (Figs. 42, 43), and the vesicles and mitochondria become sharply outlined by dense material; the mitochondrial cristae and the haloes of the dense core vesicles become similarly enhanced (Fig. 40).

Figs. 43–52.   Intermediate and later stages of degeneration of preganglionic terminals in rat superior cervical ganglion ($12\frac{1}{2}$, $14\frac{1}{2}$, and 18 hours postoperatively).   Figs. 43–45. Aspects of the ensheathment in satellite lamellae: the probable origin of a coated vesicle (arrow, Fig. 43) from the inner face of the innermost satellite lamella surrounding a degenerating profile which shows patchy lightening of the cytoplasmic matrix; and the formation of the satellite lamellae from the mesaxon (Fig. 44; arrow, origin of mesaxon). The enwrapped profile contains a dense body ("axon-cytolysome") which shows a distinct dense core vesicle. Also included in the coils of the mesaxon is a late phagosome (x) resembling that shown in Fig. 52. The membranes separating the satellite lamellae are occasionally replaced, wholly or in part, by rows of irregular vesicles. (Fig. 45; arrow shows point at which appearance as of concentric paired membranes is preserved.) The degenerating terminals undergo expansion and the satellite lamellae disappear, but encircling rings and rows of irregular vesicles are seen in the surrounding satellite cytoplasm (Figs. 46 and 50) together with occasional coated vesicles (arrows). The expanded terminal profile shows apparently empty spaces and the vesicles become aggregated with dense material. The mitochondria swell and the intercristal spaces appear empty (Figs. 47, 48). Some degenerating profiles become subdivided by paired membranes into multilocular forms (Figs. 48–50; arrow in Fig. 48 shows locule containing synaptic vesicles). Others become condensed while remaining apparently unilocular (Fig. 51; this profile was seen to be multilocular in serial sections.) The latest stage recognized is a phagosome containing residues of membranes and barely recognizable structures, bounded by a single membrane (Figs. 44 and 52). Calibration bars in Figs. 51 and 52 = 0.1 μ, others 0.5 μ. Osmium fixation.

Subsequently, the degenerating profile swells and there is a disappearance of satellite lamellae (Fig. 46). In place of lamellae, the profile may now be surrounded by one or more rings of irregular vesicles, which may occasionally be continuous with a remaining part of the mesaxon. Rows of vesicles with occasional coated vesicles may be seen in the vicinity (Figs. 45 and 46). It is probable that the rows and rings of vesicles arise by disruption of the membranes of the satellite lamellae, as described by Rosenbluth (1963) to occur characteristically with osmium as opposed to permanganate fixation. Later, these vesicles appear to move away in the satellite cytoplasm (Figs. 46 and 50). They are selectively impregnated by the zinc-iodide osmium technique of Nickel and Waser (1969; Fig 53), which also acts as a selective stain for degenerating terminals (Fig. 54). The degenerating terminal profile is still approximately spherical and shows extensive clear spaces in which synaptic and dense core vesicles lie in scattered aggregates, clumped together with dense material; the mitochondria are swollen, with dense outer membranes (which show a reduced gap) and clear spaces between the cristae (Figs. 46 and 47). This stage has been likened to the pale swollen terminals described by de Robertis (1956; see Sotelo, 1968). Paired membranes with a narrow interval still separate the profile from the satellite cytoplasm but may fuse in places. The contents of the degenerating terminal next undergo a gradual condensation. In many cases the degenerating terminals are multilocular, being progressively subdivided into compartments by a series of paired membranes (Figs. 48–50). In other cases the terminal seems to remain unilocular as it becomes condensed and darkened (Figs. 51 and 56). These later forms are still more or less rounded, not collapsed and irregular in form like the later degenerating profiles in the central nervous system (compare Figs. 56 and 57), and the synaptic and especially the dense core vesicles are still recognizable. From 18 hours onward most degenerating terminals in the rat superior cervical ganglion have been reduced to dark phagosomes in the Schwann cell cytoplasm (the "Schwann-cytolysomes" of Hámori *et al.*, 1968), surrounded by single membranes and containing residues of membranes but virtually no recognizable organelles (Fig. 52). Over the next few days these phagosomes are gradually transformed into residual bodies in the Schwann cells.

The intraganglionic degeneration, like that in the central nervous system, is markedly asynchronous, but the effect of this asynchronism is even further enhanced by the rapidity with which the degeneration proceeds once it has begun, with the result that at any one survival period only a small proportion of terminals are seen degenerating, even after a lesion which is known to cut virtually all the preganglionic axons. Furthermore, as degenerative changes are not often seen in terminals before they are detached from the synaptic contact, this imposes serious limitations on the use of orthograde degeneration to mark the precise sites of termination of preganglionic fibers (Matthews, 1971).

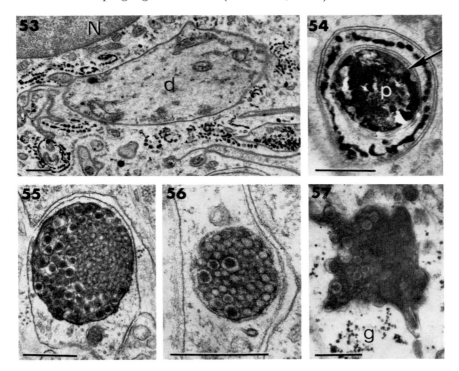

Figs. 53 and 54.   Rat superior cervical ganglion fixed in a mixture of zinc iodide and osmium tetroxide (Nickel and Waser, 1969), 15 hours after section of preganglionic fibers. Figure 53 shows part of a satellite cell (N, nucleus) ensheathing a large dendrite (d) and several smaller profiles; the satellite cytoplasm shows an unusual number of chains of irregular vesicles, many of which are darkly impregnated. Figure 54 shows an impregnated degenerating profile (p). The very narrow innermost satellite lamella (arrow) has darkened cytoplasm; an intermediate turn of the mesaxon is replaced by a row of irregular vesicles, which are heavily impregnated; the innermost and outermost turns of the mesaxon are seen as unimpregnated paired membranes.

Figs. 55–57.   Comparison of terminal degeneration in the median eminence (Fig. 55), the superior cervical ganglion (Fig. 56) and the central nervous system (electron dense type) (Fig. 57). The forms seen in the median eminence and in the ganglion are rounded, whereas the central nervous system shows collapsed, heavily indented forms. g, glycogen granules in reactive astrocytic process. Figures 55 and 57, aldehyde fixation; Fig. 56, osmium fixation.

A type of degeneration intermediate between that described for the preganglionic terminals and the electron dense degeneration typical of the central nervous system occurs in the terminals of the hypothalamo-hypophysial tracts in the neural lobe (Sterba and Brückner, 1967, 1968; Zambrano and de Robertis, 1968; Dellmann and Owsley, 1969; Dellmann and Rodríguez, 1970), and in the terminals of the parvicellular neurosecretory fibers in the median eminence (Budtz, 1970; Réthelyi and Halász, 1970; Raisman, 1971). In both these neurohypophysial sites the degeneration is of an electron dense type but has a rapid mode of onset and is accompanied by a very early phagocytic reaction of the surrounding cells, viz., the tanycytes of the median eminence and the pituicytes. By 24 hours after axotomy, degenerating terminals which may be identified by their synaptic and dense core vesicles are seen totally engulfed in the cytoplasm of the supporting cells (Fig. 55). The degenerating terminals are characteristically rounded, resembling the later forms seen in the sympathetic ganglion and, like these, differing markedly from the collapsed, indented forms seen in the central nervous system (Figs. 55–57).

D. Interpretation of Degeneration

In order to complete the structural interpretation of neuropil patterns it is necessary that both pre- and postsynaptic elements should be identified, and although the placing of a lesion and the subsequent reaction of degeneration serve to mark the origin of the degenerating presynaptic elements, the identification of the remaining (undegenerated) presynaptic elements and of the postsynaptic elements require other means. On some occasions, the electron microscope affords criteria which enable a process to be immediately identified (e.g., the peculiar tubular systems of the axons and axon collaterals of the cerebellar Purkinje cells; Hámori and Szentágothai, 1968). More often, however, it is not possible to identify at once the origin of a particular profile. In these cases it is necessary either to obtain a fortunate plane of section, in which a particular profile can be traced back into continuity with a recognizable element (such as a cell body), or else to reconstruct from serial sections the continuity of such a process. The identification of the nondegenerating elements of the neuropil is often the most difficult part of an electron microscopic study and may require considerable ingenuity, together with a certain felicity of intuition. It is usually at this stage that a series of sections stained by the Golgi technique are useful, as a particular axon or dendrite may be identified by means of the similarity between its branching pattern in electron micrographs and in Golgi sections, or a dendrite may be identified by the presence of spines or varicosities, by its diameter, or even by its predominant orientation. This reliance upon the Golgi technique is rapidly becoming a feature of most electron microscopic studies (Scheibel and Scheibel, 1970). In some cases, however, the inaccessibility of a particular axonal system to selective experimental destruction (e.g., in the retina) may make identification impossible without using a combination of electron microscopy and Golgi staining in the same block. Stell (1967) identified individual horizontal cells in Golgi sections of the retina of the goldfish, cut out areas containing these cells from the section, reembedded them for electron microscopy, and made electron microscope sections, taking advantage of the metallic impregnation effected by the Golgi method to act as a marker at the ultrastructural level for the processes of the cell already identified. By these means he was able to distinguish between the horizontal cell processes and the bipolar cell dendrites in contact with the photoreceptor cells. Details of such techniques may be found in his original article as well as in that of Blackstad (1970).

E. LIMITATIONS OF DEGENERATION METHODS

Basically the application of degeneration methods is limited by the accessibility of fibers to selective experimental destruction. It is therefore inapplicable to regions such as the retina, and to the short fiber systems formed by recurrent axon collaterals and by short axon cells "intrinsic" to particular regions of the central nervous system. For such problems the combined electron microscope–Golgi technique or the laborious methods of reconstruction from serial ultrathin sections are needed. However, a further difficulty in the use of degeneration, even where tracts are accessible to destruction, stems from some of the factors described above, viz., the rapidity of the phagocytic reaction and the asynchronism of degeneration. These factors are seen at their most formidable in the case of the preganglionics to the superior cervical ganglion (but see also Miledi and Slater, 1970). Here, the phagocytic reaction is extremely rapid, leaving very little time before degenerating endings are engulfed. It is not even clear whether many of the endings ever reach a stage of recognizable degeneration before they are detached from the postsynaptic element. The number of degenerating endings seen at any one survival time is relatively small (thus precluding the use of quantitative methods), but as it seems likely that the majority of endings do degenerate over the first day or two, it may be concluded that the process of degeneration is both rapid and asynchronous, so that at any one period of time only a few degenerating endings will be at a recognizable stage. If such conditions were to apply to a tract in the central nervous system, the use of degeneration techniques would be considerably limited. At present there has been no definite instance of this in a central nervous area although our own results with the termination of the medial corticohypothalamic tract do suggest that these may undergo a rapid form of degeneration, possibly analogous to that found in the neurohypophysis after section of the neuro-secretory fibers. It is noteworthy that both the terminal region of the medial corticohypothalamic tract and the neurohypophysis have atypical nonneuronal elements, i.e., the tanycytes of the ependyma of the third ventricle and the pituicytes. This would support the view that the rapid phagocytic reaction is not due solely to a property of the nerve fibers themselves but may be partly a function of the nonnervous elements which engulf them. Thus, in contrast to the tanycytes, pituicytes and Schwann cells, the astrocytes which normally carry out this function in the central nervous system may be slower to react and, therefore, allow the development of a more definite degeneration reaction in the terminals before phagocytosis.

A method which promises to have the same resolution as the electron microscopy of degeneration, but which does not involve placing a lesion, is autoradiography of substances injected at the level of the neuronal perikarya and transported along the nerve fibers to the terminals (Goldberg and Kotani, 1967; Lasek *et al.*, 1968; Hendrickson, 1969; Hendrickson *et al.*, 1970). This method takes advantage of the fact that in the cell bodies amino acids are incorporated into proteins which are then carried down in the axoplasmic flow to the nerve endings. While it suffers from the difficulties associated with diffusion, properly calibrated it may contribute a great deal to the investigation of connections. A particular advantage is that the developed silver grains which constitute the marker need not entirely obscure or distort important features of the terminals, such as size, shape, synaptic vesicles, or synaptic thickenings. Autoradiography would also be of value in analyzing connections in regions of neuropil where degeneration could be used to label one set of connections and autoradiography to label a second set, in the same animal.

Before leaving the subject of identifying terminals by orthograde degeneration, it is worth mentioning the use of chronic survival experiments, in which a sufficient postoperative survival period is left for all degenerating terminals to be removed. At this stage the neuropil is analyzed, the assumption being made that the surviving synapses represent the contacts of undamaged axons present in the tissue at the time of the original lesion. This method of "persisting elements" may be the only way of defining the short axonal systems which are unsuitable for analysis by lesions (e.g., in the cerebral cortex, Szentágothai, 1965a,b), but it does depend upon the assumption that there is no rearrangement in the deafferented terminal areas, an assumption which now seems to require some qualification (see below). An application of the method of persisting elements may also be seen in a recent investigation of the connections of Clarke's column (Réthelyi, 1970). Following a chronic lesion which removed the primary sensory afferents (previously identified by acute lesions as the giant axon terminals), it was possible to identify some of the persisting small axon terminals as belonging to ascending intraspinal fibers by showing that they degenerated after a second (acute) lesion of the spinal cord.

III. Regeneration of Synapses

Up to this point, the discussion has been concerned with the events occurring in the distal stump of the axon after section. These events inevitably lead to degeneration. We must now look at the effects of axon section upon the proximal stump of the axon, upon elements persisting in the denervated area, and also upon the denervated postsynaptic sites. While a comprehensive discussion of retrograde and transneuronal changes is outside the scope of this article, those changes which may lead to the formation of new synapses must be considered, and in this context it is necessary to make a distinction between the central and the peripheral nervous systems (Guth and Windle, 1970).

In the peripheral nervous system section of axons leads to a prompt reaction of both the cut axon and adjacent normal fibers. The cut axon begins to regenerate almost immediately and may, under favorable conditions, reconstitute its original connections. At a very early stage, however, adjacent normal fibers also throw out adventitious collateral sprouts, by means of which the denervated region may be reinnervated. This process has been demonstrated for sensory nerves to skin (Weddell *et al.*, 1941) and also for motor nerves to striated muscle (Edds, 1953). Factors which discourage growth of the original axon or impede its course may well play a part in permitting this heterotypic reinnervation. The existence of collateral sprouting from intact nerve fibers argues strongly that some kind of signal is emitted by the denervated tissue, and that this signal is sufficiently potent to elicit sprouting from undamaged axons (see also Watson, 1970). There is some evidence, based upon selective partial deafferentation of the superior cervical sympathetic ganglion, that when regenerating sprouts from the original cut fibers reach their destination they resume their original connections and functions and, also, that in some way they prevent the functioning of the heterotypic collateral sprouts (Guth and Bernstein, 1961). Rather similar work on heterotypic reinnervation of the eye muscles in the fish also suggests that the endplates formed by the foreign nerves may be rendered ineffectual when the original nerves regenerate (Mark *et al.*, 1970). The factors controlling the growth of the cut fiber are not well understood. Clearly, section of the axon is in itself likely to act as a growth stimulus although the cessation of growth once the axon reaches its target suggests that there is some influence from the denervated sites playing a part.

In the central nervous system in cold blooded vertebrates, cut axons may regenerate and produce effective recovery, but in mammals a far less positive reaction occurs. Despite efforts to encourage regeneration (e.g., Scott and Liu, 1964) the proximal part of the cut axon stump has never been demonstrated to grow back effectively to its original destination. The fate of the proximal stump is to some extent in dispute. Some authors claim that it undergoes retrograde degeneration either as far back as the last branching point of an intact side branch or else all the way back to the cell (for a discussion, see Beresford, 1965). In a recent study the cut axons of the medial lemniscus have been shown not to undergo retrogradely degeneration of a Wallerian type (i.e., fragmentation and dissolution) although they do shrink, and they still retain the potentiality for direct (i.e., orthograde) Wallerian degeneration after a lesion of the dorsal column nuclei (Cole and Nauta, 1970). By analogy with the behavior of axons prevented mechanically from normal regeneration in the fish spinal cord, it has been suggested that cut central axons may satisfy their growth potential by forming adventitious synapses in the region of the lesion (Bernstein and Bernstein, 1969). However, studies on the enzyme histochemistry of the cells of origin of cut central and peripheral fibers suggest that there may be a basic difference in their reaction to axotomy (Barron and Tuncbay, 1964; Barron *et al.*, 1966; Meyer and Cole, 1970). Nevertheless, there is some evidence to suggest that some type of collateral sprouting does occur in the central nervous system. The occurrence of collateral sprouting had already been proposed as a possible cause for the exaggerated reflexes found in human patients with lesions of the spinal cord (McCouch *et al.*, 1958), and in a classical experiment Liu and Chambers (1958) showed that after chronic section of dorsal roots the adjacent intact dorsal root fibers on that side of the spinal cord had a more extensive distribution than normal (i.e., as compared with the opposite intact side). This suggested that the adjacent fibers had extended their distribution to take over part of the denervated territory. In a comparable study, Goodman and Horel (1966) showed that after a chronic lesion of the visual cortical efferent fibers in the rat, the retinal projection became more extensive in two sites (the lateral part of the ventral lateral geniculate nucleus and the lateral part of the nucleus of the optic tract) in both of which the cortical and retinal projections converge to a major extent in the intact animal.

These studies were based upon light microscopy and do not therefore establish that new *synapses* are formed as a result of collateral sprouting. That central deafferentation may indeed lead to the formation of new synaptic contacts was indicated by the finding of Hámori (1968) that when the optic afferents to the lateral geniculate nucleus were chronically destroyed the remaining axon terminals had far more axo-axonic synapses than normal. This conclusion does not imply that entirely new axon terminals had been formed, rather that the existing terminals had acquired more specialized contact areas in order to fill the vacated synaptic sites in their immediate vicinity. Similar evidence has been afforded by work on the septum (Raisman, 1969b). There are two main sources of afferent fibers to the septal nuclei: (a) the medial forebrain bundle, carrying fibers from the hypothalamus and midbrain and (b) the fimbria, carrying fibers from the hippocampus. The fimbrial fibers terminate exclusively upon dendrites (or their spines) where they account for 35% of the dendritic synapses in the medial septal nucleus. After a chronic lesion of the fimbria, examination of the septal neuropil indicates that an abnormally high proportion of the residual axon terminals make more than one synaptic contact and that the axon terminals may be strangely elongated (Figs. 58 and 59), suggesting that they have extended their distribution so as to form new contacts (see also Moore *et al.*, 1971). The afferents from the medial forebrain bundle terminate both upon dendrites and upon cell somata, accounting for some 19% of the dendritic synapses and 24% of the axosomatic synapses in the medial septal nucleus. After a chronic lesion of the medial forebrain bundle, it can be shown by using a second (acute) lesion of the fimbria to elicit terminal degeneration, that the fimbrial fibers have now extended their synaptic distribution so as to occupy sites upon the cell bodies. This transfer of fimbrial fibers to a site which they do not normally occupy seems to indicate that the denervated sites can indeed act as a very powerful stimulus to growth and that the effect

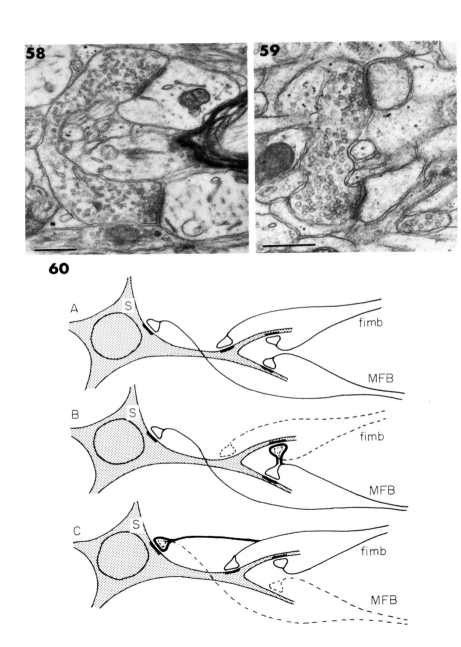

of the adventitious axosomatic synapses formed by the fimbrial fibers is to reoccupy some of the sites which had been denervated by the original lesion of the medial forebrain bundle (Fig. 60).

It is not clear to what extent collateral sprouting is a general phenomenon in the central nervous system (e.g. Westrum, 1969). While it seems possible in the septal nuclei of the rat, it would not be justified to generalize this to all regions, or to all species. The specificity with which synaptic connections are established during normal development of the brain means that there must be many different factors operating over different periods and in different locations to result in the highly ordered and selective network of adult connections (e.g., Gaze, 1970). One must not therefore expect the same rules to apply unreservedly to all systems. Thus experiments in our own laboratory (Field, 1971) show that chronic denervation of the ventromedial hypothalamic nucleus by section of the stria terminalis (a lesion known from acute experiments to cause deafferentation of as many as 50% of the dendritic spines) does not result in multiple synaptic contacts of the type found in the chronically deafferented septum. Ultrastructural studies of the capacity for reconstruction of synapses in the mammalian central nervous system are still in a very preliminary stage, but suggest that the lability of connections may be considerably greater than has often been supposed.

IV. Summary

In this article the degeneration of synapses following axonal injury is considered primarily in relation to its applicability as a tool for the exploration of nervous connections at the ultrastructural level. The design and

---

Figs. 58 and 59. Axon terminals of unusual elongated shapes each making contact with two postsynaptic elements (dendritic shafts in Fig. 58, spines in Fig. 59). Rat medial septal nucleus after a chronic lesion of the fimbria.

Fig. 60. Interpretation of the consequences of chronic deafferentation of the medial septal nucleus. (A) In the normal situation, afferents from the medial forebrain bundle (MFB) terminate on the cell soma (S) and on dendrites, while the fimbrial fibers (fimb) are restricted in termination to the dendrites. (B) Several weeks after a lesion of the fimbria, the medial forebrain bundle fiber terminals extend across from their own sites to occupy the vacated sites, thus forming double synapses (as shown in Figs. 58 and 59). Degenerated connections = discontinuous lines; presumed plastic changes = heavy black lines. (C) Several weeks after a lesion of the medial forebrain bundle, the fimbrial fibers now give rise to terminals occupying somatic sites, which are presumably those vacated as a result of the former lesion.

interpretation of experiments involving the use of degeneration, including ancillary studies, are described from a practical viewpoint as a guide to those who may be taking up such work. The recognition of terminal degeneration is discussed, and contrasts between the various known forms of terminal degeneration are illustrated. The forms of degeneration which are considered are the electron dense degeneration which is the type most commonly seen in the central nervous system, the reaction of neurofilamentous hypertrophy, and the rapid form of degeneration which occurs in the peripheral nervous system, of which the degeneration of preganglionic fibers in a sympathetic ganglion is taken as an example.

Regeneration of synapses is subdivided into true regeneration (defined as restoration of synaptic contact between the two elements of the original synapse) and collateral reinnervation (defined as reoccupation of deafferented postsynaptic sites by neighboring uninjured elements). The section on regeneration is based largely upon the mammalian central nervous system, where, although true regeneration has not been shown, there is evidence for collateral reinnervation in some sites. Too little is yet known about these reactions to enable them to be used as experimental tools, but it is pointed out that they must be borne in mind as factors which may complicate the interpretation of the results of chronic experiments involving degeneration.

A full electron microscopic study of even a simple pathway in the central nervous system may turn out to be extremely complicated. Apart from the laborious nature of electron microscope work at a quantitative level, and the concomitant Nauta and Golgi experiments which are nearly always necessary, it is only with difficulty that we can establish the precise nature of pre- and postsynaptic elements in even a single synaptic relay, let alone in a multisynaptic system. Moreover, the extension of neuropil studies to the chronically deafferented preparation has given a hint that the brain may not be as unresponsive to injury as had previously been supposed. There now seems at least a chance that we have been overlooking quite considerable plastic properties of central nervous circuitry, and the further investigation of these properties promises highly for the study of learning and memory. A knowledge of the factors controlling this plasticity may ultimately yield clues which could help in the positive treatment of injuries of the brain and spinal cord.

ACKNOWLEDGMENTS

The authors wish to thank Dr Pauline M. Field for criticism of the manuscript and for the use of material from an investigation of the distribution of the stria terminalis and Dr Ray W. Guillery for the loan of the micrograph shown in Fig. 37.

Permission to reproduce micrographs and drawings used in previous publications was kindly granted by Elsevier Publishing Company, Amsterdam, The Wistar Institute Press, and by Springer-Verlag, Berlin.

This work was supported by the Medical Research Council and by Grant 70-472 from the Foundations' Fund for Research in Psychiatry.

REFERENCES

Alksne, J. F., Blackstad, T. W., Walberg, F., and White, L. E., Jr. (1966). *Ergeb. Anat. Entwicklungsgesch.* **39**, 3–31.

Barer, R., Heller, H., and Lederis, K. (1963). *Proc. Roy. Soc., Ser. B* **158**, 388–416.

Barron, K. D., and Tuncbay, T. O. (1964). *J. Neuropathol. Exp. Neurol.* **23**, 368–386.

Barron, K. D., Oldershaw, J. B., and Bernsohn, J. (1966). *J. Neuropathol. Exp. Neurol.* **25**, 443–478.

Beresford, W. A. (1965). *Progr. Brain Res.* **14**, 33–56.

Bernstein, J. J., and Bernstein, M. E. (1969). *Exp. Neurol.* **24**, 538–557.

Bignami, A., and Ralston, H. J. (1969). *Brain Res.* **13**, 444–461.

Björklund, A., Cegrell, L., Falck, B., Ritzén, M., and Rosengren, E. (1970). *Acta Physiol. Scand.* **78**, 334–338.

Blackstad, T. W. (1970). *In* "Contemporary Research Methods in Neuroanatomy" (W. J. H. Nauta and S. O. E. Ebbesson, eds.), pp. 186–216. Springer-Verlag, Berlin and New York.

Budtz, P. E. (1970). *Z. Zellforsch. Mikrosk. Anat.* **107**, 210–233.

Cheng–Minoda, K., Ozawa, T., and Breinin, G. M. (1968). *Invest. Ophthalmol.* **7**, 599–616.

Clemente, C. D. (1964). *Int. Rev. Neurobiol.* **6**, 258–301.

Cohen, E. B., and Pappas, G. D. (1969). *J. Comp. Neurol.* **136**, 375–396.

Cole, M., and Nauta, W. J. H. (1970). *J. Neuropathol. Exp. Neurol.* **29**, 354–369.

Colonnier, M. (1968). *Brain Res.* **9**, 268–287.

Colonnier, M., and Guillery, R. W. (1964). *Z. Zellforsch. Mikrosk. Anat.* **62**, 333–355.

Cuénod, M., Sandri, C., and Akert, K. (1970). *J. Cell Sci.* **6**, 605–613.

Dellmann, H.-D., and Owsley, P. A. (1969). *Z. Zellforsch. Mikrosk. Anat.* **94**, 325–336.

Dellmann, H.-D., and Rodríguez, E. M. (1970). *In* "Aspects of Neuroendocrinology" (W. Bargmann and B. Scharrer, eds.), pp. 124–139. Springer-Verlag, Berlin and New York.

de Robertis, E. (1956). *J. Biophys. Biochem. Cytol.* **2**, 503–512.

Diamond, J., Gray, E. G., and Yasargil, G. M. (1969). *In* "Excitatory Synaptic Mechanisms" (J. K. S. Jansen and P. Andersen, eds.), pp. 213–222. Scandinavian University Books, Oslo.

Eccles, J. C. (1964). "The Physiology of Synapses." Springer-Verlag, Berlin and New York.

Eccles, J. C., Ito, M., and Szentágothai, J. (1967). "The Cerebellum as a Neuronal Machine." Springer-Verlag, Berlin and New York.

Edds, M. V., Jr. (1953). *Quart. Rev. Biol.* **28**, 270–276.

Field, P. M., (1971). In preparation.

Gaze, R. M. (1960). *Int. Rev. Neurobiol.* **2**, 1–40.

Gaze, R. M. (1970). "Formation of Nerve Connections." Academic Press, New York.

Goldberg, S., and Kotani, M. (1967). *Anat. Rec.* **158**, 325–332.

Goodman, D. C., and Horel, J. A. (1966). *J. Comp. Neurol.* **127**, 71–88.

Gray, E. G., and Guillery, R. W. (1965). *Int. Rev. Cytol.* **19**, 111–182.

Gray, E. G., and Hamlyn, L. H. (1962). *J. Anat.* **96**, 309–316.

Grofova, I., and Rinvik, E. (1970). *Exp. Brain Res.* **11**, 249–262.

Guillery, R. W. (1969a). *Z. Zellforsch. Mikrosk. Anat.* **96**, 1–38.

Guillery, R. W. (1969b). *Z. Zellforsch. Mikrosk. Anat.* **96**, 39–48.

Guillery, R. W. (1970). In "Contemporary Research Methods in Neuroanatomy" (W. J. H. Nauta and S. O. E. Ebbesson, eds.), pp. 77–105. Springer-Verlag, Berlin and New York.

Guillery, R. W., and Ralston, H. J. (1964). *Science* **143**, 1331–1332.

Guth, L., and Bernstein, J. J. (1961). *Exp. Neurol.* **4**, 59–69.

Guth, L., and Windle, W. F. (1970). *Exp. Neurol., Suppl.* **5**, 1–43.

Hámori, J. (1968). In "Structure and Function of Inhibitory Neuronal Mechanisms" (C. von Euler, S. Skoglund, and U. Söderberg, eds.), pp. 71–80. Pergamon, Oxford.

Hámori, J., and Szentágothai, J. (1968). *Exp. Brain Res.* **5**, 118–128.

Hámori, J., Láng, E., and Simon, L. (1968). *Z. Zellforsch. Mikrosk. Anat.* **90**, 37–52.

Heimer, L. (1967). *Brain Res.* **5**, 86–108.

Heimer, L. (1969). *Brain Res.* **12**, 246–249.

Heimer, L. (1970). In "Contemporary Research Methods in Neuroanatomy" (W. J. H. Nauta and S. O. E. Ebbesson, eds.), pp. 162–172. Springer-Verlag, Berlin and New York.

Heimer, L., and Peters, A. (1968). *Brain Res.* **8**, 337–346.

Hendrickson, A. (1969). *Science* **165**, 194–196.

Hendrickson, A., Wilson, M. E., and Toyne, M. J. (1970). *Brain Res.* **23**, 425–427.

Holländer, H., and Vaaland, J. L. (1968). *Brain Res.* **10**, 120–126.

Holländer, H., Brodal, P., and Walberg, F. (1969). *Exp. Brain Res.* **7**, 95–110.

Hunt, C. C., and Nelson, P. G. (1965). *J. Physiol. (London)* **177**, 1–20.

Kruger, L., and Hámori, J. (1970). *Exp. Brain Res.* **10**, 1–16.

Larramendi, L. M. H., Fickenscher, L., and Lemkey-Johnston, N. (1967). *Science* **156**, 967–969.

Lasek, R., Joseph, B. S., and Whitlock, D. G. (1968). *Brain Res.* **8**, 319–336.

Libet, B. (1970). *Fed. Proc., Fed. Amer. Soc. Exp. Biol.*, **29**, 1945–1956.

Liu, C. N., and Chambers, W. W. (1958). *AMA Arch. Neurol. Psychiat.* **79**, 46–61.

Lund, J. S., and Lund, R. D. (1970). *Brain Res.* **17**, 25–46.

Lund, R. D. (1969). *J. Comp. Neurol.* **135**, 179–208.

McCouch, G. P., Austin, G. M., Liu, C. N., and Liu, C. Y. (1958). *J. Neurophysiol.* **21**, 205–216.

McMahan, U. J. (1967). *Z. Zellforsch. Mikrosk. Anat.* **76**, 116–146.

Mark, R. F., Marotte, L. R., and Johnstone, J. R. (1970). *Science* **170**, 193–194.

Matthews, M. R. (1971). *J. Physiol. (London)* **218**, 95–96.

Matthews, M. R. (1972). In preparation.

Matthews, M. R., and Raisman, G. (1969). *J. Anat.* **105**, 255–282.

Meyer, D. D., and Cole, M. (1970). *Neurology* **20**, 918–924.

Miledi, R., and Slater, C. R. (1968). *Proc. Roy. Soc., Ser. B* **169**, 289–306.

Miledi, R., and Slater, C. R. (1970). *J. Physiol. (London)* **207**, 507–528.

Moore, R. Y., Björklund, A., and Stenevi, U. (1971). *Brain Res.* **33**, 13–35.

Mugnaini, E. (1969). *In* "Excitatory Synaptic Mechanisms" (J. K. S. Jansen and P. Andersen, eds.), pp. 149–169. Scandinavian University Books, Oslo.

Mugnaini, E., and Walberg, F. (1967). *Exp. Brain Res.* **4**, 212–236.

Nickel, E., and Waser, P. G. (1968). *Z. Zellforsch. Mikrosk. Anat.* **88**, 278–296.

Nickel, E., and Waser, P. G. (1969). *Brain Res.* **13**, 168–176.

Nishi, S. (1970). *Fed. Proc., Fed. Amer. Soc. Exp. Biol.* **29**, 1957–1965.

Peters, A. (1970). *In* "Contemporary Research Methods in Neuroanatomy" (W. J. H. Nauta and S. O. E. Ebbesson, eds.), pp. 56–76. Springer-Verlag, Berlin and New York.

Raisman, G. (1969a). *Exp. Brain Res.* **7**, 317–343.

Raisman, G. (1969b). *Brain Res.* **14**, 25–48.

Raisman, G. (1971). In press.

Ralston, H. J. (1969). *Brain Res.* **14**, 99–116.

Réthelyi, M. (1970). *Exp. Brain Res.* **11**, 159–174.

Réthelyi, M., and Halász, B. (1970). *Exp. Brain Res.* **11**, 145–158.

Rinvik, E., and Walberg, F. (1969). *Brain Res.* **14**, 742–744.

Rosenbluth, J. (1963). *J. Cell Biol.* **16**, 143–157.

Roth, C. D., and Richardson, K. C. (1969). *Amer. J. Anat.* **124**, 341–360.

Saavedra, J. P., Vaccarezza, O. L., Reader, T. A., and Pasqualini, E. (1970). *Exp. Neurol.* **26**, 607–620.

Scheibel, M. E., and Scheibel, A. B. (1970). *In* "Contemporary Research Methods in Neuroanatomy" (W. J. H. Nauta and S. O. E. Ebbesson, eds.), pp. 1–11. Springer-Verlag, Berlin and New York.

Scott, D., Jr., and Liu, C. N. (1964). *Progr. Brain Res.* **13**, 127–150.

Siegrist, G., Dolivo, M., Dunant, Y., Foroglou-Karameus, C., de Ribaupierre, F., and Rouiller, C. (1968). *J. Ultrastruct. Res.* **25**, 381–407.

Sotelo, C. (1968). *Exp. Brain Res.* **6**, 294–305.

Stell, W. K. (1967). *Amer. J. Anat.* **121**, 401–423.

Sterba, G., and Brückner, G. (1967). *Z. Zellforsch. Mikrosk. Anat.* **81**, 457–473.

Sterba, G., and Brückner, G. (1968). *Z. Zellforsch. Mikrosk. Anat.* **93**, 74–83.

Szentágothai, J. (1965a). *Progr. Brain Res.* **14**, 1–32.

Szentágothai, J. (1965b). *Symp. Biol. Hung.* **5**, 251–276.

Szentágothai, J., Hámori, J., and Tömböl, T. (1966). *Exp. Brain Res.* **2**, 283–301.

Taxi, J. (1964). *Acta Neuroveg.* **26**, 360–372.

Teravainen, H., and Huikuri, K. (1969). *Z. Zellforsch. Mikrosk. Anat.* **102**, 466–482.

Uchizono, K. (1968). *In* "Structure and Function of Inhibitory Neuronal Mechanisms" (C. von Euler, S. Skoglund, and U. Söderberg, eds.), pp. 33–59. Pergamon, Oxford.

Vaccarezza, O. L., Reader, T. A., Pasqualini, E., and Saavedra, J. P. (1970). *Exp. Neurol.* **28**, 277–285.

Vaughn, J. E., and Pease, D. C. (1970). *J. Comp. Neurol.* **140**, 207–226.

Vaughn, J. E., Hinds, P. L., and Skoff, R. P. (1970). *J. Comp. Neurol.* **140**, 175–206.

Walberg, F. (1963). *Exp. Neurol.* **8**, 112–124.

Walberg, F. (1965). *J. Comp. Neurol.* **125**, 205–221.

Walberg, F. (1966). *Exp. Brain Res.* **2**, 107–128.

Walberg, F., and Mugnaini, E. (1969). *Brain Res.* **14**, 67–76.

Watson, W. E. (1970). *J. Physiol. (London)* **210**, 321–343.

Weddell, G., Gutmann, L., and Gutmann, E. (1941). *J. Neurol. Psychiat.* [N.S.] **4**, 206–225.

Westman, J. (1969). *Exp. Brain Res.* **7**, 51–67.

Westrum, L. E. (1969). *Z. Zellforsch. Mikrosk. Anat.* **98**, 157–187.

Williams, T. H., and Palay, S. L. (1969). *Brain Res.* **15**, 17–34.

Williams, V., and Grossman, R. G. (1970). *Anat. Rec.* **166**, 131–142.

Wolfe, D. E., Potter, L. T., Richardson, K. C., and Axelrod, J. (1962). *Science* **138**, 440–442.

Zambrano, D., and de Robertis, E. (1968). *Z. Zellforsch. Mikrosk. Anat.* **88**, 496–510.

3

Synthesis, Storage, and Release of Acetylcholine from Nerve Terminals

LINCOLN T. POTTER

I. Acetylcholine Synthesis 106
  A. Provision of Choline for Acetylcholine Synthesis 106
  B. Provision of Acetyl-CoA for Acetylcholine Synthesis 110
  C. Choline Acetyltransferase 111
II. Acetylcholine Storage 114
  A. Site of Storage 114
  B. Synaptic Vesicles 115
  C. Turnover of Stores 119
III. Transmitter Release 120
  A. Quantal Release of Acetylcholine 120
  B. Assays of Collected Acetylcholine 122
  C. Possible Release Mechanisms 124
  References 127

The evolution of cholinergic neurotransmission has resulted in the development of several highly specialized processes in cholinergic nerve terminals. These, shown graphically in Fig. 1, include a facilitated transport mechanism for the uptake of choline from the interstitial fluid, an enzymatic step, nearly unique to cholinergic nerve cells, for the synthesis of acetylcholine (ACh), a process for the packaging of ACh in synaptic vesicles in a concentrated state which is physiologically inactive, and a precisely controlled mechanism for the very rapid release of concentrated bursts of ACh toward the post-synaptic membrane.

The intention of this chapter is to summarize current views concerning the above processes, particularly those which have not been discussed in

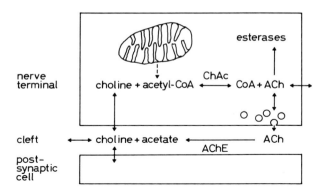

Fig. 1. Acetylcholine metabolism in cholinergic nerve terminals.

detail elsewhere and those which relate to the vesicle hypothesis. The evidence for these views, and detailed references, will be found in the papers cited.

I. Acetylcholine Synthesis

A. Provision of Choline for Acetylcholine Synthesis

Both central and periferal cholinergic neurons require supplies of extraneural choline for maintaining normal tissue levels of ACh and high release rates of the transmitter. In isolated ganglia (Birks and MacIntosh, 1961; Collier and MacIntosh, 1969), diaphragmatic muscles (Potter, 1970), and brain slices (Collier, 1970), added choline is rapidly used for ACh synthesis, and the utilization of either endogenous or exogenous choline is inhibited by a choline analogue, hemicholinium-3 (HC–3), which affects choline uptake but not choline acetyltransferase.

The mechanism of choline uptake by isolated nerve terminals (Marchbanks, 1968a; Potter, 1968; Diamond and Kennedy, 1969), brain slices (Schuberth *et al.*, 1966), squid axons (Hodgkin and Martin, 1965), and red blood cells (Martin, 1968) appears to be the same. In each case choline enters the cellular element by a saturable carrier mechanism and by passive diffusion. In synaptosomes the affinity constant of the carrier for choline is 50–80 μM, and the carrier accounts for most of the total uptake observed at choline levels below 100 μM. Uptake is competitively inhibited by choline analogues, including HC–3 ($K_i = 20$–40 μM) and ACh itself ($K_i = 800$ μM), and is noncompetitively inhibited by eserine

($K_i = 1.3$ mM). As judged by subcellular fractionation, the choline taken up remains in solution within the cells and is largely unmetabolized. [The formation of some phosphorylcholine by synaptosome fractions has been reported, but the possibility that this synthesis took place in cell fragments other than synaptosomes must be considered (Diamond and Kennedy, 1969).] Uptake does not appear to be energy dependent or to require specific ions and is unaffected by ouabain. At low but physiological concentrations (5 μM), choline is concentrated about fourfold by synaptosomes (Marchbanks, 1968a) and twofold by red cells. In the latter, concentration requires extracellular sodium but does not seem to be a function of the sodium electrochemical gradient. Exchange of choline across cell membranes clearly occurs even when there is no net flux (Collier and MacIntosh, 1969; Martin, 1968). These properties of the saturable mechanism may be described as due to facilitated diffusion.

The concentration and amount of free choline in the neuroplasm of cholinergic nerve terminals are of interest because a low and variable level could limit ACh synthesis by the cytoplasmic enzyme choline acetyltransferase. Neither value is known from direct studies since pure cholinergic terminals are not available; they would probably have an altered choline content if they could be isolated. The concentration in cholinergic terminals is probably similar to that in other terminals and cells, however, since the process of choline uptake appears to be the same in different cell types. The amount of free choline in the brain and other tissues has been reported to be in the range 50–500 μmoles/kg (Potter, 1970; Schuberth *et al.*, 1970), of which the lower values are most likely to be accurate, since all tissue-extraction procedures release some lipid-bound choline. From these measurements and from studies of the ability of synaptosomes of mixed-transmitter types to concentrate choline, an internal level of 20–200 μM choline may be estimated. This range is below the affinity constant of choline acetyltransferase for choline [750 μM in brain tissue (Glover and Potter, 1971)], which suggests that the enzyme is not saturated with this substrate under normal conditions in the neuroplasm and that the rate of ACh synthesis is limited by, and will vary with, the choline concentration. The apparent choline level is also far below the estimated concentration of ACh in nerve terminals (50 mM, expressed as if in uniform solution), and other evidence supports the idea that the amount of free choline is much less than the total amount of ACh (Potter, 1970). It is known that HC-3 has a major effect on choline uptake (Birks and MacIntosh, 1961; Potter, 1968; Diamond and Kennedy, 1969), but no effect on the rate of ACh synthesis by soluble choline acetyltransferase (Glover, 1970). During prolonged nerve stimulation, tissues in HC–3 are slowly depleted of their ACh content and resynthesize less than 10% of their original store (Birks and MacIntosh, 1961; Potter, 1970). The amount of choline available for ACh resynthesis thus appears to be less than 10% of the ACh content and at any one time is probably no more than a few percent since choline uptake is not fully arrested by HC–3. It follows from these considerations that the rate of ACh synthesis in nerve terminals is dependent upon the efficiency of choline uptake during nerve stimulation and on the adequacy and stability of the choline supply in the synaptic cleft.

Assuming that the amount of choline in nerves is small, the rate of net transmitter synthesis during the turnover of a large fraction of ACh stores may be used as a rough measure of the rate of net choline uptake by the nerves. The rate of resynthesis during rapid nerve stimulation has been measured in diaphragms during the turnover of 35% of the ACh store in 5 minutes; from the number and size of the nerve terminals the rate of net choline uptake has been estimated as 3–6 pmoles/cm² second (Potter, 1970). At the same external concentration of choline, the net flux rates into squid axons (Hodgkin and Martin, 1965) and red cells (Martin, 1968) are two and four orders of magnitude slower, respectively, indicating that the mechanism for choline uptake in nerve terminals is particularly well developed. From the same experiment with muscles and from similar experiments with ganglia exposed to cat plasma containing about 5 μM choline (Birks and MacIntosh, 1961), it is clear that ACh synthesis can keep pace with its release for long periods, at least at release rates as high as one-quarter those observed during intense nerve stimulation for only 8–18 seconds. An increase in the choline level by a factor of 100 does not affect the relase rate (Birks and MacIntosh, 1961). A stable supply of choline at 5–30 μM is therefore adequate to maintain ACh stores and ACh release.

A decrease in the concentration of choline in the extracellular fluid of peripheral tissues clearly affects the rate of ACh synthesis in their nerves. When ganglia (Birks and MacIntosh, 1961) or muscles (Potter, 1970) are isolated in choline-free media, their content of free choline gradually declines and ACh synthesis slows, with a concomitant decrease in the rate of ACh release during nerve stimulation. These effects indicate that there is little tissue synthesis of choline and that the plasma must ultimately provide most or all of what is required. The plasma of mammals contains 5–50 μM choline, and at least in man this level is held quite constant regardless of food intake, excercise, sex, pregnancy, etc. (Bligh, 1952).

A temporary change of muscle baths to 1 μM choline has little effect on the rate of synthesis because sufficient choline is released from muscle cells to provide that needed by the nerves. In fact, muscles kept in a single small bath release sufficient choline for ACh synthesis for many hours; but ganglia or larger tissues which are perfused or repeatedly washed lose their choline more rapidly. The fact that choline is normally supplied at a stable level which is adequate for ACh synthesis and that other cells tend to maintain that level locally by taking up or releasing choline, indicate that the supply of choline to peripheral tissues does not normally limit ACh synthesis.

Less is known about the adequacy, stability, and source of free choline in the interstitial fluid of the central nervous system (CNS). Choline crosses the blood–brain barrier with difficulty (Potter et al., 1968; Chakrin and Whittaker, 1969; Ansell and Spanner, 1970), and indirect evidence suggests that a phosphocholine compound, most likely phosphatidylcholine (lecithin) or its lyso derivative, may cross instead and be partially degraded to provide choline (Ansell and Spanner, 1970). The amount of free choline in brain tissues is only 1% or so of that in these lipids, so the potential supply is great. The rate of phosphocholine degradation is not likely to be high enough to replace choline as rapidly as it is used for ACh synthesis since ganglia, which have a similar free: bound choline ratio (Friesen et al., 1967), cannot maintain their ACh stores during stimulation in choline-free media. The rate of supply could well match the rate of choline loss from the CNS, however.

When released ACh is hydrolyzed in the synaptic cleft, much of the choline produced is apparently recovered by nerve terminals for ACh resynthesis. The sum of ACh and choline release from stimulated ganglia is roughly halved in the presence of eserine, indicating considerable retention of choline under normal circumstances somewhere in the tissue (Collier and MacIntosh, 1969). In phrenic nerves exposed to labeled choline, endogenous ACh is replaced almost twice as rapidly by labeled ACh when ACh hydrolysis, and thus the reuse of endogenous choline, is prevented (Potter, 1970). This suggests a recapture of about half the choline released as ACh in this tissue; it may be postulated that reuse is yet more important in the CNS where choline ingress and egress are more limited. A probable consequence of the hydrolysis of ACh in the synaptic cleft is a temporary and local increase in the concentration of choline. (The concentration of ACh in vesicles, and presumably in quanta at the moment of release, is estimated below as 150–1000 mM, whereas the cleft choline level is probably closer to 5–50 μM). Given the efficiency of the uptake mechanism and the probability that the level of choline in the neuroplasm is suboptimal for ACh synthesis, the rate of ACh synthesis is probably accelerated during ACh hydrolysis in the cleft.

B. Provision of Acetyl-CoA for Acetylcholine Synthesis

There is general agreement that the acetyl groups of ACh are derived from the intramitochondrial metabolism of glucose (Browning and Schulman, 1968; Sörbo, 1970; Tuček, 1970). The last step in this metabolic chain involves a pyruvate dehydrogenase complex of enzymes which are clearly present in mitochondria of nervous tissues as well as other tissues (pyruvate + NAD + CoA = acetyl-CoA + NADH + CO_2). Brain slices and peripheral nerves which are supplied with large amounts of acetate instead of glucose or pyruvate can synthesize some ACh, but this sequence is not believed to be important, at least in brain tissue, since the metabolic flow of acetate appears to be only a few percent of that of pyruvate and since exogenous acetate is a less effective source of acetyl groups for ACh than exogenous pyruvate. With acetate as the source, acetyl-CoA is produced by an enzyme, acetyl-CoA synthetase, which is found predominantly in mitochondria (acetate + CoA + ATP = acetyl-CoA + AMP + P).

It is much less clear how the acetyl groups of acetyl-CoA in mitochondria reach the enzyme choline acetyltransferase, which is certainly not in mitochondria and is probably free in the neuroplasm. Diffusion of the acetyl-CoA itself would be the simplest explanation and may occur to some extent, but the observed diffusion of acetyl-CoA from brain mitochondria has so far not been sufficient to explain high rates of ACh synthesis. The presumption is, therefore, that intramitochondrial acetyl-CoA is used for the synthesis of citrate (or its metabolites glutamate and *a*-ketoglutarate), acetylcarnitine, or acetate, all of which can pass through mitochondrial membranes and then (in theory) be used by cytoplasmic enzymes for the resynthesis of acetyl-CoA.

The problem with this hypothesis has been to demonstrate that there is a sufficient production of acetyl-CoA by any cytoplasmic enzyme(s) in nerve terminals to account for the known rates of ACh synthesis. The most likely sequence is that intramitochondrial acetyl-CoA is metabolized by the mitochondrial enzyme citrate synthetase to citrate (acetyl-CoA + oxalacetate = citrate + CoA), which diffuses to the cytoplasm and is transformed back to acetyl-CoA by the cytoplasmic enzyme ATP-citrate lyase (citrate + CoA + ATP = acetyl-CoA + oxalacetate + ADP

+ P). Support for this sequence has been obtained from experiments with brain slices, in which glucose 6-^{3}H and glucose 6-^{14}C were provided to give pyruvate doubly labeled in the methyl group: the ^{3}H/^{14}C ratio of the 1- and 2-positions of citrate and of the acetyl group of ACh were found to be the same (Sörbo, 1970). Against this means for the translocation of acetyl-CoA, and still requiring explanation, are observations that exogenous citrate does not readily provide acetyl groups for ACh synthesis and that the measured maximal activity of ATP-citrate lyase in synaptosomes is only 3% of that of choline acetyltransferase.

Less likely means for the provision of cytoplasmic acetyl-CoA include (a) the formation of acetylcarnitine by carnitine acetyltransferase in mitochondria (acetyl-CoA + carnitine = acetylcarnitine + CoA), diffusion of the acetylcarnitine into the cytoplasm, and reversal of this enzymatic reaction there and (b) degradation of acetyl-CoA to CoA by a deacylase, diffusion of the acetate, and resynthesis of acetyl-CoA by "cytoplasmic" acetyl-CoA synthetase. To date, the bulk of the evidence is that carnitine acetyltransferase is an exclusively mitochondrial enzyme which subserves acetyl group transfer within these particles, and measurements of the small fraction of brain acetyl-CoA synthetase which is recovered in soluble subcellular fractions (most remains in mitochondria) show only a few percent of the activity required for ACh synthesis. Clearly, more work is necessary with nervous tissues to establish the means of providing extramitochondrial acetyl-CoA.

The cytoplasmic concentration of acetyl-CoA is not known for any cell. In brain tissues the total content has been reported as 5–8 μmoles/kg (Sollenberg, 1970), of which a considerable part is presumably present in mitochondria. Approximately 20 times as much CoA is present. It may be noted that each of the enzymatic steps which produces acetyl-CoA requires ATP or NAD; as a consequence, it might be expected that ACh synthesis in nerve terminals would be quite dependent upon oxidative metabolism, as indeed it is. It may be postulated as well that the level of acetyl-CoA in the neuroplasm and the ratio of acetyl-CoA to CoA will be highest and, therefore, most nearly optimal for ACh synthesis at times of minimal nerve stimulation.

C. Choline Acetyltransferase

The known properties of choline acetyltransferase from different neural sources, vertebrate and invertebrate, are very similar (cf. Glover and Potter, 1971). The enzyme is a stable, relatively basic protein having a molecular weight of approximately 65,000; to date there is no evidence for different aggregation states. It requires an ionic environment of physiological tonicity for full activity but does not require specific ions and is unaffected by small changes in the concentration of Ca^{++}. In the catalyzed reactions,

$$\text{choline} + \text{acetyl–CoA} \underset{k_2}{\overset{k_1}{\rightleftharpoons}} \text{ACh} + \text{CoA}$$

k_1 is approximately four times k_2, and the equilibrium constant is about 40. The forward reaction is neither activated nor inhibited by either of its substrates over a wide range of concentrations, and the Michaelis constants (determined at pH 7.2 and in 150 mM KCl so as to approximate intracellular conditions) are 750 μM for choline and 10 μM for acetyl-CoA. CoA causes marked product inhibition by competing with acetyl-CoA ($K_i = 16$ μM), but ACh has little effect on its own synthesis at concentrations likely to occur in the neuroplasm, and its maximal effect, at 200 mM, is to cause less than 50% inhibition. Both ACh and bromo-acetylcholine, which is a much more potent inhibitor, i.e., $K_i = 0.2$ μM (Glover, 1970), inhibit synthesis without competing significantly with either choline or acetyl-CoA. In the back reaction, each substrate increases the affinity of the enzyme for the other: the Michaelis constants are 0.75–5 mM for ACh, and 25–250 μM for CoA. These observations show that the reaction mechanism is ordered; it is probable that acetyl-CoA always combines with the enzyme before choline.

From subcellular fractionation studies it is clear that choline acetyltransferase is not present *in* mitochondria or vesicles; in ionic media of isotonic strength it is recovered instead in soluble fractions, whereas in the sucrose solutions usually used for subcellular studies, it reversibly absorbs to membranes, including small vesicles (Potter *et al.*, 1968; Fonnum, 1970). As far as can be determined by these methods, the enzyme should be freely distributed in the neuroplasm of cholinergic nerves, a conclusion in keeping with the presence of large amounts of demonstrably active enzyme in parts of cholinergic axons (e.g., spinal roots) which have few synaptic vesicles (Saunders, 1965). Some calculations suggest, however, that the concentration of the enzyme in nerve terminals is higher than elsewhere in these axons (Hebb *et al.*, 1964), a situation which could arise if there were bulk axoplasmic flow along axons with resorption of fluids near the terminals or if the enzyme adsorbs to vesicles or other structures within the terminals. Any such factor which tended to maintain a high level of the enzyme in nerve terminals, and particularly near the pre-synaptic membrane where the turnover of ACh appears to be maximal, would contribute to the rapid replacement of quanta.

The capacity of peripheral nerve terminals to synthesize ACh is sufficient to maintain ACh stores and, therefore, to match ACh release, during nerve stimulation at 20 Hz for periods of 5–60 minutes. Net synthesis under these conditions replaces an average of 0.12–0.18% of the original store each second (Birks and MacIntosh, 1961; Potter, 1970). The rate of release, however, declines during the first few minutes of such stimulation (Birks and MacIntosh, 1961), and the question arises as to whether the rate of formation of quanta is limited by a lack of active enzyme near the pre-synaptic membrane. It may be argued that this is not the case since the rate of release does not increase in the presence of 700 μM choline (Birks and MacIntosh, 1961), which should considerably accelerate synthesis, and since the rate remains low even when the level of cytoplasmic ACh is increased (see Section II). Synthesis may or may not also keep pace with the higher release rates seen during brief bursts of rapid nerve stimulation, i.e., release of 0.43–0.87% of stores/second (Birks and Mac Intosh, 1961; Potter, 1970). Replacement at this rate would presumably be close to the maximum capacity for synthesis, e.g., the amount of enzyme in the whole diaphragm can synthesize 8% of normal ACh stores/second under optimal test-tube conditions, but less than the total is present in nerve terminals, and the enzyme is probably not saturated with choline.

The net rate of ACh synthesis in nerve terminals varies in relation to the rate of ACh release. When resting diaphragms are placed in eserine, their ACh stores increase by 17% in 5 minutes; this is apparently the result of inhibition of intraneural esterases (not necessarily acetylcholinesterase) since it occurs only slowly with neostigmine (Potter, 1970). The result suggests that transmitter synthesis *at rest* may be more rapid than required to maintain stores and to balance spontaneous release. During nerve stimulation much of the ACh which would have become "surplus" is released and the turnover is increased to at least 35% in 5 minutes. When resting diaphragms or ganglia (Birks and Mac Intosh, 1961) are left in eserine, their ACh content eventually doubles and the rate of synthesis drops to match spontaneous release, which amounts to a turnover of about 6% of the store in diaphragms in 5 minutes. Thus, nerve stimulation can at least double the resting rate of synthesis, and the presence of surplus ACh can decrease it to one-third. Comparison of these figures probably underestimates the acceleration of net synthesis which occurs near the pre-synaptic membrane during nerve stimulation, since this should occur more locally than the synthesis which replaces ACh lost spontaneously, and the synthesis which occurs in the volume of axoplasm affected by eserine.

The most plausible mechanism for the regulation of ACh synthesis will be one which depends upon the level of ACh in the vicinity of choline acetyltransferase. It is perhaps surprising, therefore, that ACh causes so little product inhibition of the enzyme and does not fully inhibit synthesis at any level. Given that the enzyme is present in the neuroplasm, however, the fact that ACh does not compete significantly with either choline or acetyl-CoA can be seen to be of advantage in that it permits rapid ACh synthesis to millimolar levels in the presence of only micromolar concentrations of these substrates. The actual rate of ACh synthesis must depend upon the availability of active enzyme, the concentration of choline and acetyl-CoA, and the ratio of CoA to acetyl-CoA. A reasonable case can be made that none of these factors is responsible for regulating net synthesis since in resting nerves these factors should be at least as optimal for synthesis as during stimulation, when net synthesis increases. Although part of the observed increase may be attributed to a driving of synthesis by increased supplies of choline (from hydrolyzed ACh), this explanation does not account for the decreased synthesis seen when ACh stores are doubled. In the search for a more sensitive control mechanism, it seems more plausible that net synthesis (and the concentration of ACh in the axoplasm) are dependent upon the equilibrium position of choline acetyltransferase with its substrates and products; this mechanism has the merit of responding to the neuroplasmic level of ACh, which is in some kind of equilibrium with the content of vesicles (see Section II,C). Given an equilibrium constant of 40 for the enzyme, if the internal concentration of choline is 20–200 μM and the ratio CoA/acetyl-CoA is anywhere between 1 and 100, the limiting concentration of ACh would be in the reasonable range of 8 μM–8 mM.

II. Acetylcholine Storage

A. Site of Storage

With rare exceptions in normal vertebrate tissues, e.g., the placenta of higher primates (Morris, 1966) and corneal epithelium (Williams and Cooper, 1965), ACh is known to be present only in cholinergic nerves.

The proportion of the total ACh content of the cells which is in their terminals apparently varies with the length of the axons: about two-thirds of the ACh of the cerebral cortex can be isolated in nerve terminals, whereas the proportion is higher in the caudate nucleus and lower in the spinal cord (Whittaker, 1965). When synaptosomes are lysed in distilled water, about half of their ACh can be recovered in association with vesicles the size of synaptic vesicles (De Robertis et al., 1963; Whittaker et al., 1964). A greater fraction of the ACh in terminals is probably in vesicles since vesicles lose ACh with time (Whittaker, 1969) and are clearly sensitive to hypotonic conditions (Marchbanks, 1968b). The cholinergic nerve terminals of *Torpedo* electric tissue can be broken open by mechanical means under isotonic conditions, and in this case about half of the total ACh in the tissue can be recovered in vesicles. With suitable corrections for recovery, the estimated vesicular content is more than 80% of the total in the nerves (Israël et al., 1968; Israël and Gautron, 1969).

In the presence of an esterase inhibitor like eserine, which can enter nerve terminals, the ACh content of isolated tissues slowly increases by a factor of 2 or more, but the amount of ACh which can be recovered in vesicles after subcellular fractionation remains the same (Collier, 1970; Potter, 1970). It is believed that part of the excess ACh is in the terminal neuroplasm rather than elsewhere in the axons because (a) the ratio of surplus to normal stores is higher in ganglia than in their preganglionic nerves (Birks and MacIntosh, 1961), (b) the surplus helps to maintain ACh release during nerve stimulation when synthesis is arrested and ACh stores are declining, and (c) much of the ACh which would become surplus during short periods at rest appears to contribute to release during nerve stimulation (Potter, 1970). (Surplus ACh could accumulate more rapidly in terminals if eserine enters them more rapidly than preterminal axons, if there is more enzyme in the terminals, or more likely, if the conditions for ACh synthesis with regard to choline uptake and the provision of acetyl-CoA from mitochondria are most suitable in the terminals.) Since surplus ACh does not appear to increase the ACh level in vesicles it may be argued that their content is already at a maximum.

B. SYNAPTIC VESICLES

Very little information is available as to the source and turnover of synaptic vesicles. The presence of a few of the right size in preterminal axons (Zelená, 1969) suggests that some or all may be manufactured in the cell body and moved towards terminals, in the same manner as some adrenergic vesicles are transported (Dählstrom and Häggendal, 1970). A precise lineup of vesicles along neurotubules in preterminal and terminal axons has been observed in the nerves of some lower vertebrates (Smith *et al.*, 1970), and this again suggests a form of vesicle transport. It is doubtful, however, that axonal transport of vesicles can supply a sufficient number of new vesicles to match the number of quanta released, e.g., at a stimulation frequency of 20 Hz, and conservatively estimating 25 quanta/impulse/per ending, the release would be 330,000 in 11 minutes; this is a reasonable approximation of the number of vesicles in the phrenic nerve terminals of an endplate in the rat diaphragm [average terminal diameter $= 1.67$ μm, length $= 150$ μm (Potter, 1970); 2000 vesicles/μ^3 located in roughly half the terminal facing the post-synaptic membrane (Jones and Kwanbunbumpen, 1970a,b; see also Elmqvist and Quastel, 1965)]. Moreover, the total membrane surface of this number of vesicles (assuming an average diameter of 50 nm) is more than three times that of the terminals in an endplate. Thus, if release takes place by exocytosis, as is probable (see ACh release), the vesicle membrane must be recovered; this could occur if each vesicle fuses only momentarily with the pre-synaptic membrane and then reforms within the terminal or if vesicles are remade after their total fusion with the membrane. On one hand, the fact that vesicles have a higher lipid and lower ganglioside content than other synaptosomal membranes and no Na^+–K^+–activated ATPase (Whittaker, 1969) suggests that the vesicular and pre-synaptic membranes are different and may remain so. On the other hand, there is no *a priori* reason why the pre-synaptic membrane should not be a mosaic with pieces of vesicle-type membrane which can "flow" to sites of new vesicle formation. Some electron micrographs of nerve terminals suggest that total vesicle fusion may occur (Nickel and Potter, 1970); others of coated vesicles have been interpreted as evidence for vesicle reformation by pinocytosis (Kadota and Kaneseki, 1969); and there is morphological evidence that the number of vesicles near the pre-synaptic membrane changes during nerve stimulation (Hubbard and Kwanbunbumpen, 1968; Jones and Kwanbunbumpen, 1970a,b).

The amount of ACh held in each synaptic vesicle has been estimated by a variety of direct and indirect means. In general, these indicate that the amount corresponds to a solution isotonic or hypertonic to that of the surrounding neuroplasm, i.e., 0.15–1 M, which for mammalian vesicles is 1400–9400 molecules. Recent estimates of quantal size (see ACh release) are of the same order. (1) An upper limit for the average content may be estimated from the amount of ACh which could exist in a crystal which filled the vesicle core (about 310 Å in diameter in mammals). Given crystals of AChCl, which have the lowest volume per molecule, i.e., 249 Å^3 (Herdklotz and Sass, 1970), of any salt likely to exist in vesicles, 63,000 molecules could be accomodated. It is unlikely that this is the case since the equilibrium density of cholinergic vesicles (Whittaker *et al.*, 1964), including those obtained under conditions of high ACh recovery from electric tissue (Israël *et al.*, 1968; p = 1.049, Potter and Nickel, 1970), is considerably lower than that of AChCl crystals [S. G. over 1.2 (Allen, 1962)] or of the known density of lipid-rich membranes, e.g., myelin [p is roughly 1.09 (Cotman *et al.*, 1968)]. (2) Direct measurements of the ACh recovered in isolated vesicles from mammalian brain cortices, coupled with counts of the vesicles, indicate about 300 molecules/vesicle, or 2000 for those obtained from cholinergic nerves (Whittaker, 1965). The latter figure corresponds to an internal concentration of 0.2 *M*. (3) Similar measurements with the larger vesicles obtained from *Torpedo* electric tissue indicate an internal ACh level of about 0.39 *M* (Sheridan *et al.*, 1966), which is close to isotonic for this saltwater fish. Vesicle pellets obtained from this tissue represent about 0.5% of the tissue weight and retain up to 30 mmoles of ACh/kg of pellet; with corrections for recovery and the fractional volume of the pellets occupied by vesicle cores, the internal concentration again appears close to isotonic (Potter, 1971). Values of this order may also be obtained by calculations based on the fractional volume of the tissue occupied by terminals, i.e., 5% (Nickel and Potter, 1970), the volume of terminals occupied by vesicle cores (say 5%), and the recovery of the ACh of the tissue in vesicles (80% of 200–600 μmoles/kg). (4) Measurements of the ACh in diaphragms and of the size of phrenic nerve terminals indicate that the concentration of ACh in the whole terminals is of the order of 50 m*M* (Potter, 1970). Given 50–100% of the ACh in vesicle cores occupying 5% of the terminals yields an estimate of 0.5–1 *M* ACh in the vesicles. Given 50–100% in 330,000 vesicles/terminal gives about 15,000–30,000 molecules/vesicle.

An essential feature of current thinking about cholinergic mechanisms is that ACh must be concentrated from the neuroplasm into synaptic vesicles. As yet it is not known how this is accomplished or how ACh is held within vesicles. What is clear is that ACh is held best at low temperatures (Barker *et al.*, 1967), that it is not rapidly exchanged for external cations (Matsuda *et al.*, 1968; Takeno *et al.*, 1969), including ACh (Marchbanks, 1968b), and that it is labile under hypotonic conditions (Marchbanks, 1968b). These findings indicate that vesicular ACh is protected by a semipermeable membrane. Two possible mechanisms for uptake may be considered. (1) The first, which is consistent with available information, is that neuroplasmic ACh is exchanged for intravesicular Na^+ by a non-energy-requiring carrier in the vesicle membrane. At the time when vesicles are made, whether by pinocytosis or by recovery after momentary fusion with the pre-synaptic membrane, they will be full of extracellular fluid. A sufficent means for filling them with isotonic ACh would then be a carrier which operated according to the outward-directed gradient of sodium ions. Concentration of ACh could occur if the carrier affinities on the two sides of the membrane were such as to make transport of each ion effectively unidirectional (and if Na^+ can leak back inside) or if sodium is, in addition, pumped from the neuroplasm into vesicles by an energy-requiring pump like that in external cell membranes (and similarly directed, considering the orientation of membrane surfaces after vesicle formation). The only enzyme known to occur in vesicle preparations, a Mg^{++}-activated ATPase (Whittaker, 1969), is not like the Na^+-K^+-activated ATPase thought to subserve Na^+ transport, but conceivably, it could function at some stage in a transport process. The strength of vesicle membranes is probably sufficient to maintain a moderate hypertonicity of fluids inside relative to outside, without a binding process for ACh. Some swelling of vesicles as they refill with ACh would account for the changes in vesicle size near the pre-synaptic membrane which are observed between the time of ACh release during nerve stimulation and full recovery (Jones and Kwanbunbumpen, 1970a,b). Unfortunately, attempts in several laboratories to demonstrate concentration of ACh by isolated vesicles in isoionic media have not been successful so far. Ingenious experiments have demonstrated ACh uptake by vesicle preparations in nonionic media, but in each case adsorption of the transmitter could explain the uptake observed (cf. Guth, 1969). (2) ACh could also be taken up and concentrated in vesicles if it is bound by some constituent within them. The obvious precedent for this is the binding of catecholamines by ATP in vesicles (Pletscher *et al.*, 1970) which also contain considerable quantities of proteins which may assist in the binding process. Preparations of cholinergic vesicles which are exposed to water release small amounts of nucleotides and soluble protein (Potter, 1971); and recent studies of the protein suggest that it is sufficiently acidic to neutralize a large fraction of the ACh of vesicles (Whittaker *et al.*, 1971). However, the formation of complexes between ACh and nucleotides or vesicle proteins remains to be demonstrated.

C. TURNOVER OF STORES

The available evidence indicates that the turnover of cytoplasmic ACh in resting nerve terminals is moderately rapid, whereas that in vesicles is slow. When extraneural choline is replaced by radioactive choline, there is rapid exchange labeling of intraneural choline, as expected from the properties of the choline uptake mechanism (Collier and MacIntosh, 1969; Collier, 1970; Potter, 1970). From knowledge of the site and properties of choline acetyltransferase, it would be further expected that cytoplasmic ACh should be rapidly labeled. This is most obvious in nerves treated with eserine where there is a very rapid accumulation of labeled, surplus ACh, without much change in the original store of endogenous ACh (Collier and MacIntosh, 1969; Collier, 1970; Potter, 1970). If eserine is then removed, the labeled ACh disappears, and after short periods, the original store is found to be largely unlabeled. Without eserine, nerves exposed to labeled choline accumulate labeled ACh slowly, the replacement rate being about one-third of the original store each hour in intact tissues. Evidence that the turnover of cytoplasmic ACh occurs even under such conditions is provided by the demonstration that the specific activity of ACh recovered in soluble subcellular fractions is considerably higher than that in vesicles (Chakrin and Whittaker, 1969; Marchbanks, 1969). Even when synaptosomes are exposed to labeled ACh and some enters their cytoplasm, the vesicular content of ACh remains predominantly unlabeled (Marchbanks, 1968b).

In contrast, the turnover of ACh in vesicles during nerve stimulation is rapid. Most of the total store becomes labeled during exposure to radioactive choline, and the specific activity of ACh in vesicles must approach that of the choline used (Collier and MacIntosh, 1969; Potter, 1970). The rate of turnover of ACh in vesicles under such conditions is presumably comparable to the rate of release, the highest measured rate being 0.87% of stores/second (Birks and MacIntosh, 1961). Higher rates of ACh synthesis and release may occur during depolarization of nerves with elevated levels of K^+, but these values may not equal the turnover of ACh in vesicles since there is some recent evidence that K^+ causes a considerably greater release of surplus ACh than occurs during nerve stimulation.

There is reason to believe that a small part of the total store of ACh in nerve terminals, perhaps that contained in vesicles nearest the presynaptic membrane, turns over more rapidly than the rest. This subject is discussed in Section III.

From what has been said so far it would appear that ACh in the majority of vesicles is relatively inert metabolically whenever it is inert physiologically. Nevertheless, there is probably some sort of equilibrium between intra- and extravesicular ACh. Even if the normal situation is one in which the content of vesicles is kept topped-up without much exchange, there is direct evidence that isolated vesicles leak ACh slowly when placed in a medium deficient in ACh (Barker *et al.*, 1967) and indirect evidence that a similar process can occur in stimulated nerve terminals. When choline uptake is inhibited by HC–3, and ACh synthesis is negligible, ACh release declines in proportion to decreasing stores of ACh (Birks and Mac Intosh, 1961; Potter, 1970). In this special circumstance neurophysiological recordings show that the number of quanta remains largely unchanged but that the size of miniature endplate potentials, and thus the number of molecules of ACh/quantum, gradually declines (Elmqvist and Quastel, 1965; Jones and Kwanbunbumpen, 1970b). In terms of the vesicle hypothesis, the interpretation is that full vesicles must slowly give up ACh to empty ones, because of a new equilibrium between intra- and extravesicular ACh.

III. Transmitter Release

A. QUANTAL RELEASE OF ACETYLCHOLINE

This subject is discussed fully in two recent reviews (Katz, 1966, 1969).

The success of the neurophysiological approach to studying ACh release depends on the fact that the post-synaptic membrane at chemical synapses serves as an excellent amplifier for the effects of the transmitter concerned. At vertebrate neuromuscular junctions each molecule of ACh causes a permeability change in the post-synaptic membrane which permits the net flow of (roughly) several thousand ions into the muscle cell. Measurements of potential changes across an endplate membrane thus serve to detect the release of ACh from the associated nerve terminal.

Shortly after microelectrodes were first used to measure endplate potentials, it became clear that these synapses were not silent even in the absence of nerve impulses. Instead, there were spontaneous and random discharges of the post-synaptic membrane about once a second, amounting to a depolarization of 0.5 mV and lasting about 20 msec. These miniature endplate potentials (mepps) were shown to be produced by ACh in that they, like applied ACh, were blocked by curare, and potentiated by esterase inhibitors. The ACh producing mepps must come from nerve terminals since mepps are seen only at endplates and disappear when ACh release is abolished by denervation, by botulinum and several other toxins, or by HC–3. [A very low level of release after denervation may come from Schwann cells (Miledi and Slater, 1968)] Mepps cannot be attributed to single or a few molecules of ACh since the effect of applying graded doses of ACh at endplates is graded levels of depolarization. Thus, each mepp must be produced by the arrival of many ACh molecules at nearly the same time, and these must have been released from a nerve terminal as a burst or "quantum" package. It has been amply demonstrated that the effect of depolarizing nerve terminals, either directly or by nerve impulses, is to greatly increase the frequency but not the size of these quantal bursts up to a few hundred or more in less than a millisecond. ACh release is thus a finely poised and electrically controlled form of secretion.

The release of quanta depends upon the presence of calcium ions in the synaptic cleft at the moment of depolarization of the nerve terminal membrane and on the ability of Ca^{++} to move down a concentration and electrical gradient into the nerve terminal. The number of quanta released generally varies in a graded (nonthreshold) way with the degree of depolarization of the pre-synaptic membrane and as a power function of the extracellular calcium concentration, e.g., as $[Ca^{++}]^4$ at endplates in the frog sartorius muscle (Dodge and Rahamimoff, 1967). Release is facilitated for short periods after one or more depolarizations of the nerve membrane apparently because calcium accumulates within the terminals. Sodium ions compete with calcium ions on the outside, and probably on the inside, of the pre-synaptic membrane. Release does not depend upon the entry of Na^+ during depolarization, which can be blocked by tetrodotoxin, or upon the egress of K^+, which can be blocked with tetraethylammonium ions.

ACh release clearly lags behind the time of depolarization of the pre-synaptic membrane and is particularly delayed at low temperatures. The time course of release is such that most of the interval between depolarization of the pre- and post-synaptic membranes can be attributed to those events which occur after the entry of calcium begins and before the appearance of ACh in the synaptic cleft; the actual rate at which ACh appears in the cleft, as measured by the rise-time of a mepp (less than a millisecond), is nearly constant at different temperatures. The average size of quanta (mepps) at a given junction is unaffected by the resting potential of the pre-synaptic membrane or its degree of depolarization and is only slightly reduced by previous impulses, which cause a temporary decrease in the number of quanta released, apparently due in part to depletion of ACh stores near the membrane (Brooks and Thies, 1962;

Jones and Kwanbunbumpen, 1970b; Christensen and Martin, 1970). Depolarization of the pre-synaptic membrane does not cause detectable nonquantal release of ACh.

Neurophysiological measurements have established upper and lower limits for the number of molecules of ACh in an average quantum. The upper limit of about 10^5 molecules is the amount of ACh which must be discharged from a micropipette at an endplate to give a depolarization whose potential x time area is comparable to a natural mepp (Miledi, 1961). Since the tip of a micropipette cannot be placed opposite the post-synaptic membrane as optimally as the nerve terminal is situated, this method must give an overestimate. A lower limit for the molecular content of a quantum, which may prove to be close to the actual value, has been calculated from analyses of the post-synaptic "noise" produced by the statistical variation in collisions between ACh molecules and endplate receptors (Katz and Miledi, 1970). The smallest calculated effect of ACh represents a potential change which is one or a few thousand times less than an average mepp. Since at least one molecule of ACh must react with one or more receptors to produce each of these elementary effects, the number of molecules in a quantum must be at least a thousand.

B. Assays of Collected Acetylcholine

A number of groups of investigators have collected the ACh which appears in baths surrounding isolated muscles, or in perfusates of ganglia, for assays of the amounts released with and without nerve stimulation and from denervated preparations. Measurement methods have included bioassays on several test muscles (Straughan, 1960; Birks and MacIntosh, 1961; Krnjević and Mitchell, 1961; Mitchell and Silver, 1963; Krnjević and Straughan, 1964; Bowman and Hemsworth, 1965), radiometric analyses after specific isolation procedures for ACh (Collier and MacIntosh, 1969; Potter, 1970), and gas chromatographic determinations (Alkon *et al.*, 1970). In every case it has been necessary to use an esterase inhibitor to prevent ACh hydrolysis during collections; an inhibitor which does not readily enter nerve terminals (neostigmine) has been used as well as eserine and di-isopropylfluorophosphate.

The results obtained by different methods and by different groups are nearly the same. In the case of rat hemidiaphragms (cf. Potter, 1970), which have about 10,000 endplates, the spontaneous release rate is about 2×10^{10} molecules/second, which amounts to less than 1% of the total ACh store of the tissue per minute. This is too high a rate to be accounted for by known rates of spontaneous quantal release from nerve terminals since, even if each quantum represented 40,000 molecules of ACh, 50/second would be required. The supposition is, therefore, that most of the ACh collected at rest comes from preterminal axons, which are known to have a considerable turnover of ACh under resting conditions (Saunders, 1965). Spontaneous release is somewhat greater in eserine, which permits the rapid accumulation of surplus ACh, than in neostigmine, which does not; and the former release rate is reduced by HC–3. These results suggest that much of the spontaneous release may come from the cytoplasm rather than from vesicles. Spontaneous release from ganglia appears to be somewhat less in proportion to the amount of ACh present (Birks and MacIntosh, 1961). In denervated diaphragms the spontaneous release rate is only slightly less than normal and appears to result from the rapid turnover of a store of ACh about 1% of normal size, which may be present in Schwann cells.

At high rates of nerve stimulation the release of ACh increases by a factor of at least 30 over spontaneous release (Potter, 1970) and has been shown to amount to as much as 0.87% of ACh stores/second (Birks and MacIntosh, 1961). Although the amount collected increases with the frequency of stimulation, release per impulse declines, in accord with neurophysiological findings (cf. Brooks and Thies, 1962). With low rates of stimulation of the diaphragm and collection periods of a few minutes, the increase corresponds to about $7–15 \times 10^{-18}$ moles of ACh for each nerve impulse given and per muscle fiber innervated (Krnjević and Mitchell, 1961; Bowman and Hemsworth, 1965; Potter, 1970). A considerable and unknown part of this ACh may come from preterminal axons, and the use of esterase inhibitors is known to increase the rate of depolarization of nerve terminals by backfiring. Because of these uncertainties and the lack of information about the number of quanta/impulse under collection conditions, estimates of the molecular content of quanta based on these data leave much to be improved upon. Assuming 50% release from terminals, no backfiring, and 100 quanta/impulse gives 20,000 molecules/quantum (Potter, 1970).

The presence of surplus ACh in the nerves to diaphragms and ganglia does not change the rate of release of ACh during nerve stimulation (Birks and MacIntosh, 1961), but it does help to maintain release when new synthesis of the transmitter is inhibited through the effects of HC–3 (Potter, 1970). The first result indicates that the level of cytoplasmic ACh does not determine the release rate, which could occur if the release mechanism were already "saturated" with ACh or if surplus ACh were not immediately available for release by impulses. The second result shows that surplus ACh does eventually contribute to the transmitter pool released by impulses. In terms of the vesicle hypothesis, surplus ACh is released only when it is used to refill vesicles.

The rate of release of ACh from ganglia which are stimulated in the presence of HC–3 declines rapidly until roughly a fifth of the total ACh store is depleted, and then more slowly at a rate proportional to the amount of ACh remaining (Birks and MacIntosh, 1961). With the same treatment, the quantal release of ACh from phrenic nerve terminals shows a delayed decrease in the size of quanta (Elmqvist and Quastel, 1965; Jones and Kwanbunbumpen, 1970a). These results show that part of the total store is more readily released than the rest. The evidence is consistent with the interpretation that ACh is released first from full vesicles near the membrane at a rate proportional to the occurrence of vesicle–membrane fusion, and that release then slows according to the rate at which ACh diffuses from full vesicles into those nearest the membrane. Given that that synthesis can match high release rates in the absence of HC–3, it would be expected that ACh nearest the membrane should turn over at a higher rate than the total store. Recent data provide evidence for the preferential release of newly synthesized ACh, which is consistent with this idea. Muscles (Potter, 1970) and ganglia (Collier, 1969) whose stores of ACh have been replaced with labeled ACh release transmitter of the same specific activity as that in the tissue. But when the same tissues are stimulated in the presence of unlabeled choline, the specific activity of released ACh averages about half that found in the tissue, indicating that newly synthesized transmitter is as important for maintaining release as are preformed stores. Similar results have been obtained with potassium-evoked ACh efflux from brain slices (Molenaar *et al.*, 1971) and with norepinephrine in noradrenergic nerves (Kopin *et al.*, 1968). The results obtained with nerve stimulation may be attributed partly to unequal rates of turnover of ACh in different nerve fibers, but direct morphological evidence for the unequal distribution of labeled norepinephrine in single nerve terminals (Budd and Salpeter, 1969) supports the stated interpretation as well.

C. Possible Release Mechanisms

Three mechanisms for the quantal release of ACh may be considered.

1. The possibility that ACh is released in bursts by outward diffusion through calcium-activated "pores" in the pre-synaptic membrane must

be considered unlikely. Such a mechanism should be dependent upon the concentration of ACh in the neuroplasm near the pre-synaptic membrane, whereas the rate of release does not increase with surplus ACh and quanta decrease in size only slightly during rapid nerve stimulation, when there is believed to be considerable depletion of transmitter near the membrane. In addition, one might expect this mechanism to be more dependent upon membrane potential changes, and less temperature dependent, than observed release; and it requires channels for the selection of ACh for release rather than smaller hydrated ions like potassium.

2. Suppose that ACh is released by calcium-activated carrier molecules in the pre-synaptic membrane. These would have to be fully saturated with ACh at normal ACh levels in the neuroplasm in order to carry a fixed number of molecules out of the terminal whenever activated and to thereby account for quanta; small quanta would be released at normal frequency if the level of cytoplasmic ACh fell markedly, as with nerve stimulation in the presence of HC–3. Such carriers could operate independently of changes in membrane potential or permeability (other than those for Ca^{++}) and could show a reasonable Q_{10}.

While this hypothesis is credible, it is less attractive than the vesicle hypothesis. It provides no explanation for the evolution of vesicles as stores for ACh. It would be expected that a carrier-mediated process should show temperature dependence, but the actual rate of output of the ACh in one quantum, as indicated by the rise-time of a mepp, does not change significantly at low temperatures, when the lag between depolarization of the nerve membrane and release does increase considerably. It might be expected that with rapid nerve stimulation there would be a substantial fall in the size of quanta or a slower mepp rise-time; instead, the primary effect is a decrease in mepp frequency. Finally, the available information about transport processes suggests that a large number of carrier molecules would have to act in coordination to account for the release of at least 1000 molecules of ACh in less than a millisecond. While a single carrier might, in theory, move at the rate of molecular relaxation times and therefore carry as many as 10^5 ions/msec, the known rates of carrier-mediated processes are less than 1 ion/msec/site (Baker and Willis, 1969); even the most rapid enzymatic reactions known involve only about 15 molecules/msec/active site.

Some recent evidence obtained by partial labeling of ACh stores (by administration of radiocholine) can be interpreted in favor of a mechanism which releases cytoplasmic ACh. The findings are that the specific activity of released ACh is closer to that which can be recovered in soluble subcellular fractions than to that in vesicles, which show a low specific activity (Marchbanks, 1969). This evidence is still consistent with the vesicle hypothesis. When tissues are exposed to radiocholine, particularly in the presence of eserine and at rest, the specific activity of neuroplasmic ACh rises much faster than that in vesicles (see Section II, C). Depolarization of nerve terminals with elevated levels of potassium may release considerable amounts of this cytoplasmic ACh. Depolarization with nerve impulses is believed to cause rapid turnover of ACh near the pre-synaptic membrane, including that in vesicles, and this region is supplied with choline of the highest specific activity. In addition, isolated vesicles most readily lose newly synthesized ACh (Marchbanks and Israël, 1971). Thus, vesicles near the membrane could contain and release ACh of much higher specific activity than that which can be recovered in vesicles as a whole.

3. The vesicle hypothesis is that the ACh of quanta comes from vesicles. It is generally assumed that the ACh which produces one mepp comes from only one synaptic vesicle although it is conceivable that the coordinated and simultaneous release of the contents of several vesicles is necessary. It is further assumed that the mechanism of release is by exocytosis since release of the contents of a vesicle into the axoplasm near the pre-synaptic membrane, or extrusion of vesicles from a terminal, are much less likely.

The essential requirements for this hypothesis, that ACh be present in vesicles and that vesicle fusion with the pre-synaptic membrane occurs, have been met. It is clear that at least half of the ACh in nerve terminals is present in vesicles, and the amount in each appears to be within an order of magnitude (say 2000 to 20,000 molecules) of the amount which probably produces a mepp. Uncoated vesicles of the same size as other synaptic vesicles have been seen to fuse with the pre-synaptic membrane at cholinergic synapses and to open to the synaptic cleft (Nickel and Potter, 1970). It remains to be demonstrated that the average ACh content of a quantum and a vesicle are the same and that the entry of calcium through the pre-synaptic membrane increases the frequency of vesicle–membrane fusion.

This hypothesis provides a reasonable explanation for all the available information about ACh storage and release, as already indicated elsewhere in this chapter. It is supported further by analogy, by evidence that norepinephrine kept out of vesicles by the action of reserpine is not readily released by nerve impulses, whereas that in vesicles is released (Potter, 1967; Häggendal and Malmfors, 1969).

REFERENCES

Alkon, D. L., Schmidt, D. E., Green, J. P., and Szilagyi, P. I. A. (1970). *J. Pharmacol. Exp. Ther.* **174**, 346.

Allen, K. W. (1962). *Acta Cryst.* **15**, 1052.

Ansell, G. B., and Spanner, S. (1970). In "Drugs and Cholinergic Mechanisms in the CNS" (E. Heilbronn and A. Winter, eds.), p. 143. Försvarets Forskningsanstalt, Stockholm.

Baker, P. F., and Willis, J. S. (1969). *Biochim. Biophys. Acta* **183**, 646.

Barker, L. A., Amaro, J., and Guth, P. S. (1967). *Biochem. Pharmacol.* **16**, 2181.

Birks, R., and MacIntosh, F. C. (1961). *Can. J. Biochem. Physiol.* **39**, 787.

Bligh, J. (1952). *J. Physiol. (London)*, **117**, 234.

Bowman, W. C., and Hemsworth, B. A. (1965). *Brit. J. Pharmacol. Chemother.* **24**, 110.

Brooks, V. B., and Thies, R. E. (1962). *J. Physiol. (London)* **162**, 298.

Browning, E. T., and Schulman, M. P. (1968). *J. Neurochem.* **15**, 1391.

Budd, G. C., and Salpeter, M. M. (1969). *J. Cell Biol.* **41**, 21.

Chakrin, L. W., and Whittaker, V. P. (1969). *Biochem. J.* **113**, 97.

Christensen, B. N., and Martin, R. (1970). *J. Physiol. (London)* **210**, 933.

Collier, B. (1969). *J. Physiol. (London)* **205**, 341.

Collier, B. (1970). In "Drugs and Cholinergic Mechanisms in the CNS" (E. Heilbronn and A. Winter, eds.), p. 163. Försvarets Forskningsanstalt, Stockholm.

Collier, B., and MacIntosh, F. C. (1969). *Can. J. Physiol. Pharmacol.* **47**, 127.

Cotman, C., Mahler, H. R., and Anderson, N. G. (1968). *Biochim. Biophys. Acta* **163**, 272.

Dählstrom, A., and Häggendal, J. (1970). *Advan. Biochem. Psychopharmacol.* **2**, 65.

De Robertis, E., Arnaiz, J. R. de L., Salganicoff, L., Iraldi, A. P., and Zieher, L. (1963). *J. Neurochem.* **10**, 225.

Diamond, I., and Kennedy, E. P. (1969). *J. Biol. Chem.* **244**, 3258.

Dodge, F. A., Jr., and Rahamimoff, R. (1967). *J. Physiol. (London)* **193**, 419.

Elmqvist, D., and Quastel, D. M. J. (1965). *J. Physiol. (London)* **177**, 463.

Fonnum, F. (1970). In "Drugs and Cholinergic Mechanisms in the CNS" (E. Heilbronn and A. Winter, eds.), p. 83. Försvarets Forskningsanstalt, Stockholm.

Friesen, A. J. D., Ling, G. M., and Nagai, M. (1967). *Nature (London)* **214**, 722.

Glover, V. A. S. (1970). Personal communication.

Glover, V. A. S., and Potter, L. T. (1971). *J. Neurochem.* **18**, 571.

Guth, P. S. (1969). *Nature (London)* **224**, 384.

Häggendal, J., and Malmfors, T. (1969). *Acta Physiol Scand.* **75**, 33.

Hebb, C. O., Krnjević, K., and Silver, A. (1964). *J. Physiol. (London)* **171**, 504.

Herdklotz, J. H., and Sass, R. L. (1970). *Biochem. Biophys. Res. Commun.* **40**, 583.

Hodgkin, A. L., and Martin, K. (1965). *J. Physiol. (London)* **179**, 26P.

Hubbard, J. I., and Kwanbunbumpen, S. (1968). *J. Physiol. (London)* **194**, 407.

Israël, M., and Gautron, J. (1969). *Symp. Int. Soc. Cell Biol.* **8**, 137–152.

Israël, M., Gautron, J., and Lesbats, B. (1968). *C. R. Acad. Sci., Ser. D* **266**, 273.

Jones, S. F., and Kwanbunbumpen, S. (1970a). *J. Physiol. (London)* **207**, 31.

Jones, S. F., and Kwanbunbumpen, S. (1970b). *J. Physiol. (London)* **207**, 51.

Kadota, K., and Kanaseki, T. (1969). *J. Cell Biol.* **42**, 202.

Katz, B. (1966). "Nerve, Muscle and Synapse." McGraw-Hill, New York.

Katz, B. (1969). "The Sherrington Lectures X: The Release of Neural Transmitter Substances." Liverpool Univ. Press, Liverpool.

Katz, B., and Miledi, R. (1970). *Nature (London)* **226**, 962.

Kopin, I. J., Breese, G. R., Krauss, K. R., and Weise, V. K. (1968). *J. Pharmacol. Exp. Ther.* **161**, 271.

Krnjević, K., and Mitchell, J. F. (1961). *J. Physiol. (London)* **155**, 246.

Krnjević, K., and Straughan, D. W. (1964). *J. Physiol. (London)* **170**, 371.

Marchbanks, R. M. (1968a). *Biochem. J.* **110**, 533.

Marchbanks, R. M. (1968b). *Biochem. J.* **106**, 87.

Marchbanks, R. M. (1969). *Symp. Int. Soc. Cell Biol.* **8**, 115–135.

Marchbanks, R. M., and Israël, M. (1971). *J. Neurochem.* **18**, 439.

Martin, K. (1968). *J. Gen. Physiol.* **51**, 497.

Matsuda, T., Hata, F., and Yoshida, H. (1968). *Biochim. Biophys. Acta* **150**, 739.

Miledi, R. (1961). *Discovery* **22**, 442.

Miledi, R., and Slater, C. R. (1968). *Proc. Roy. Soc. Ser. B* **169**, 289.

Mitchell, J. F., and Silver, A. (1963). *J. Physiol. (London)* **165**, 117.

Molenaar, P. C., Nickolson, V. J., and Polak, R. L. (1971). *J. Physiol. (London)* **213**, 64P.

Morris, D. (1966). *Biochem. J.* **98**, 754.

Nickel, E., and Potter, L. T. (1970). *Brain Res.* **23**, 95.

Pletscher, A., Berneis, K. H., and Da Prada, M. (1970). *Advan. Biochem. Psychopharmacol.* **2**, 205.

Potter, L. T. (1967). *Circ. Res.* **20**, Suppl. 3, 13.

Potter, L. T. (1968). *In* "The Interaction of Drugs and Subcellular Components on Animal Cells" (P. N. Campbell, ed.), pp. 293–304. Churchill, London.

Potter, L. T. (1970). *J. Physiol. (London)* **206**, 145.

Potter, L. T. (1971). Quoted in *Neurosci. Res. Program, Bull.* **8**, No. 4, 382.

Potter, L. T., and Nickel, E. (1970). *Pharmacologist* **12**, 295.

Potter, L. T., Glover, V. A. S., and Saelens, J. K. (1968). *J. Biol. Chem.* **243**, 3864.

Saunders, N. R. (1965). Ph. D. Thesis, University of London.

Schuberth, J., Sundwall, A., Sörbo, B., and Lindell, J.-O. (1966). *J. Neurochem.* **13**, 347.

Schuberth, J., Sparf, B., and Sundwall, A. (1970). *In* "Drugs and Cholinergic Mechanisms in the CNS" (E. Heilbronn and A. Winter, eds.), p. 15. Försvarets Forskningsanstalt, Stockholm.

Sheridan, M. N., Whittaker, V. P., and Israël, M. (1966). *Z. Zellforsch. Mikrosk. Anat.* **74**, 291.

Smith, D. S., Järlfors, U., and Beránek, R. (1970). *J. Cell Biol.* **46**, 199.

Sollenberg, J. (1970). *In* "Drugs and Cholinergic Mechanisms in the CNS" (E. Heilbronn and A. Winter, eds.), p. 27. Försvarets Forskeningsanstalt, Stockholm.

Sörbo, B. (1970). *In* "Drugs and Cholinergic Mechanisms in the CNS" (E. Heilbronn and A. Winter, eds.), p. 133. Försvarets Forskningsanstalt, Stockholm.

Straughan, D. W. (1960). *Brit. J. Pharmacol. Chemother.* **15**, 417.

Takeno, K., Hishio, A., and Yanagiya, I. (1969). *J. Neurochem.* **16**, 47.

Tuček, S. (1970). *In* "Drugs and Cholinergic Mechanisms in the CNS" (E. Heilbronn and A. Winter, eds.), p. 117. Försvarets Forskningsanstalt, Stockholm.

Whittaker, V. P. (1965). *Prog. Biophys.* **15**, 39.

Whittaker, V. P. (1969). *In* "Handbook of Neurochemistry" (A. Lajtha, ed.), Vol. 2, pp. 327–364. Plenum Press, New York.

Whittaker, V. P., Dowe, G., and Scotto, J. (1971). Proc. 3rd Int. Conf. Neurochem. p. 266.

Whittaker, V. P., Michaelson, I. A., and Kirkland, J. A., (1964). *Biochem. J.* **90**, 293.

Williams, J. D., and Cooper, J. R. (1965). *Biochem. Pharmacol.* **14**, 1286.

Zelená, J. (1969). *Symp. Int. Soc. Cell Biol.* **8**, 73–94.

4

Neuronal Inclusions

SYDNEY S. SCHOCHET, JR.

I. Introduction	129
II. Inclusions Associated with Viral Infections	132
III. Nonviral Nuclear Inclusions	135
A. Marinesco Bodies	135
B. Nuclear Bodies	136
C. Intranuclear Filamentous Inclusions	139
IV. Nonviral Cytoplasmic Inclusions	139
A. Laminated Cytoplasmic Bodies	139
B. Colloid Inclusions and Bunina Bodies	140
C. Acidophilic Granules in Pigmented Neurons and Lattice-Work Inclusions	143
D. Hirano Bodies	145
E. Lewy Bodies	148
F. Lafora Bodies	150
G. Lipofuscin and Its Derivatives	153
V. Inclusions Derived from Neuronal Fibrous Proteins	159
A. Neurofibrillary Tangles Composed of Twisted Tubules	159
B. Neurofibrillary Tangles and Aggregates Composed of Filaments	162
C. Pick Bodies	165
References	170

I. Introduction

The topic of neuronal inclusions obviously encompasses a heterogeneous group of entities. For the purpose of this chapter, they are defined
simply as conspicuous, discrete structures demonstrable by light and
electron microscopy in the nucleus or cytoplasm of neurons. Diffuse

storage deposits found in various metabolic diseases and structures that cannot be resolved by the light microscope generally have been omitted.

Neuronal inclusions can be classified in three categories according to their histopathological significance (Table I). Some of the inclusions are probably normal cellular components; many reflect nonspecific neuronal dysfunction while a few are virtually pathognomonic for specific diseases. Many of the neuronal inclusions are assigned to more than one category, and when encountered in a specimen, their significance must be assessed in relation to other data. For some of the inclusions, current information is inadequate to make more than a tentative or even speculative assignment.

TABLE I

PATHOLOGICAL SIGNIFICANCE

Inclusion	Normal cellular component	Nonspecific neuronal dysfunction	Evidence of specific diseases
Cowdry A inclusions		+	+
Cowdry B inclusions	+	+	
Negri and lyssa bodies			+
Marinesco bodies	+	+ [a]	
Nuclear bodies	+		
Laminated cytoplasmic bodies	+		
Colloid inclusions	+	+ [a]	
Bunina bodies	+	+ [a]	
Acidophilic granules in pigmented neurons (lattice-work inclusions)	+		
Hirano bodies		+	
Lewy bodies			+
Lafora bodies			+
Lipofuscin	+	+	
Granulovacuolar bodies		+	
Neuromelanin	+		
Neurofibrillary tangles composed of twisted tubules		+	
Fibrillary inclusion of Sotelo and Palay	+		
Neurofibrillary tangles composed of filaments		+	
Pick bodies		+	+
Kuru bodies		+	+

[a] Evidence for assignment is tentative or speculative.

There are important differences in the topographic distribution of the various neuronal inclusions (Table II). Some are widely distributed throughout gray matter. However, for many of these, there are still preferred areas where they can be demonstrated more readily. Other inclusions have been found only in certain specific regions. This apparent

TABLE II

PRACTICAL TOPOGRAPHY OF NEURONAL INCLUSIONS

Inclusion	Favorable area for demonstration
Cowdry A inclusions	No area of predilection
Cowdry B inclusions	No area of predilection
Negri and lyssa bodies	Purkinje cells of cerebellum and pyramidal cell layer of hippocampus
Marinesco bodies	Pigmented nuclei
Nuclear bodies	Pigmented nuclei
Laminated cytoplasmic bodies	Lateral geniculate nucleus of cat
Colloid inclusions	Hypoglossal nucleus
Bunina bodies	Anterior horn neurons
Acidophilic cytoplasmic bodies (lattice-work inclusions)	Pigmented nuclei, thalamus of mouse
Hirano bodies	Pyramidal cell layer of hippocampus
Lewy bodies	Pigmented nuclei
Lafora bodies	Cortex and substantia nigra
Lipofuscin	Inferior olivary nuclei, spinal and cranial motor neurons
Granulovacuolar bodies	Pyramidal cell layer of hippocampus
Neuromelanin	Pigmented nuclei
Neurofibrillary tangles composed of twisted tubules	Pyramidal cell layer of hippocampus
Fibrillary inclusions of Sotelo and Palay	Lateral vestibular nucleus of the rat
Neurofibrillary tangles composed of filaments	Anterior horns in sporadic motor neuron disease, variable in experimental models
Pick bodies	Pyramidal cell layer of hippocampus

selective involvement must be interpreted with caution. Some of the inclusions have not been sought with equal thoroughness in locations other than where initially described. Still others, described as distinct entities in different regions of the nervous system and occasionally in different species, may be basically the same structures. These problems are especially significant with the smaller inclusions that are best demonstrated by electron microscopy. Finally, the distribution of some of the experimentally induced lesions is determined by choice of species and route of administration of the toxic or infectious agent rather than by innate characteristics of the affected neuronal population.

The staining characteristics of the various neuronal inclusions are briefly mentioned under their individual descriptions. Virtually all of the inclusions are recognizable when stained with ordinary hematoxylin–eosin. It is desirable to be familiar with the appearance of the inclusions stained in this manner since it is one of the most commonly employed and reliable techniques. Silver stains are the traditional procedures for more dramatically demonstrating the various inclusions derived from neuronal fibrous proteins (the various neurofibrillary tangles and Pick bodies), but these stains are notoriously capricious. Furthermore, they are often not performed unless the lesions are suspected from their appearance in sections stained with hematoxylin–eosin. Other special stains are useful for elucidating the histochemical characteristics of the various inclusions.

Ultrastructural studies have been invaluable in distinguishing and characterizing many of these inclusions, e.g., viral induced inclusions and the various neurofibrillary tangles. Often useful information can be derived from tissue routinely fixed and not originally processed for electron microscopy. This is especially important in the study of human diseases that were unsuspected clinically or involve regions of the nervous system inaccessible for biopsy.

II. Inclusions Associated with Viral Infections

Neuronal inclusions are encountered in a wide variety of naturally occurring and experimentally produced viral infections. Depending on the nature of the infective agent and host, the inclusions can be found in the cytoplasm, the nuclei, or both locations. Nuclear inclusions in neurons, as in other cells, are commonly designated as Cowdry type A or type B (Cowdry, 1934). The type A inclusions are rounded masses of amorphous or particulate material surrounded by a clear halo resulting from margination of the chromatin. This type of nuclear inclusion is characteristic, but not pathognomonic, of virus infection (Pinkerton, 1950). Neurons harboring type A inclusions can be found in patients afflicted with herpes simplex, herpes simiae, varicella-zoster, cytomegalic inclusion disease, and subacute sclerosing panencephalitis (Fig. 1) and in animals with a wide variety of viral diseases. In many viral infections of the nervous system, nuclear inclusions are more abundant in glia and Schwann cells than in neurons. It is often difficult to identify the involved cells with certainity, especially in cytomegalic inclusion disease. Generally, immunofluorescent studies and electron microscopy demonstrate far more extensive involvement by virus than is reflected by inclusion bodies or inflammatory reaction, both of which may be absent. It has been suggested that nuclear inclusions are rendered more conspicuous by the use of acidic fixatives (Reissig and Melnick, 1955; Swanson *et al.*, 1966), but we do not regard this as a significant factor. Histochemical studies of viral induced intranuclear inclusions have revealed mixtures of nucleic acids, proteins, lipids, and carbohydrates (Bozsik *et al.*, 1963; Love and Wildy, 1963; Rosan *et al.*, 1964).

Electron microscopic studies demonstrating the actual viral particles have been especially useful in distinguishing between the type A inclusions due to the herpes viruses and the myxo-paramyxoviruses (Hashida and Yunis, 1970). However, a more specific diagnosis, as with any viral infection, depends on further virologic and serologic procedures.

Type A intranuclear inclusions can also occur in certain nonviral conditions. Occasionally prominent eosinophilic inclusions in both neuronal and glial nuclei have been observed in various forms of hepatocerebral disease (Shiraki and Yamamoto, 1962; Shiraki, 1968). Although morphologically similar to viral induced inclusions, these type A inclusions can be distinguished histochemically by their slightly more intense reactions for polysaccharides and lipids (Shiraki and Yamamoto, 1962). We are unaware of any ultrastructural studies on these structures. Intoxication with lead or bismuth compounds regularly produces Cowdry type A inclusions in the nuclei of renal tubular cells and, to a lesser extent, hepatocytes. However, neurons are not involved in this manner.

The type B intranuclear inclusions are characteristically small and often multiple. In contrast to the type A inclusions, they do not produce displacement or margination of the chromatin. They are generally regarded as less suggestive of viral infection than type A inclusions and, in the nervous system, are most commonly observed in the pigmented neurons of the substantia nigra and locus coeruleus where they are termed Marinesco bodies (*vide infra*). In some cases of subacute sclerosing panencephalitis, the majority of the viral induced inclusions are quite small and have the appearance of type B inclusions. Ultrastructurally, these small inclusions contain the same tubular virus particles as the larger type A inclusion bodies (Périer *et al.*, 1967). The type B inclusions observed in some cases of poliomyelitis (Bodian and Horstmann, 1965) and equine encephalomyelitis (Hurst, 1934) are probably nuclear bodies (*vide infra*) rather than viral induced inclusions.

The Negri (Fig. 2) and lyssa bodies found in many cases of rabies are the best known examples of cytoplasmic inclusions produced by a viral infection. The more common lyssa bodies are distinguished from the Negri bodies by the lack of internal structures, but in human material the distinction is of little significance. These cytoplasmic inclusions were found in 71% of a series of 49 cases of fatal human rabies (Dupont and

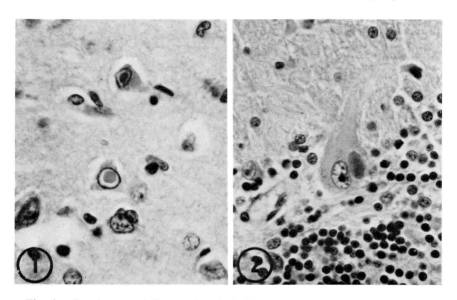

Fig. 1. Cowdry type A intranuclear inclusions in cortical neurons from a patient with subacute sclerosing panencephalitis. Hematoxylin–eosin, ×560.

Fig. 2. Negri body in the cytoplasm of a Purkinje cell from a patient with rabies. Hematoxylin–eosin, ×400.

Earle, 1965; Earle and Dupont, 1966) and were most often encountered in the Purkinje cells of the cerebellum and the pyramidal cells of the hippocampus. The distribution of the neuronal inclusions and the topography of the inflammatory reaction, including the so-called "Babes nodules," were often incongruent and in 30% of the cases; no inclusions were detected. Ultrastructural studies of both human and animal brain tissue have shown that the Negri bodies contain large numbers of bullet-shaped viral particles embedded in a granular matrix (Miyamoto and Matsumoto, 1965; Morecki and Zimmerman, 1969; González-Angulo *et al.*,

1970). The viral particles in the Negri bodies have the same distinctive shape as the rabies virions in extraneural locations (Dierks *et al.*, 1969). Based primarily on morphology, these bullet-shaped viruses are currently classified as rhabdoviruses (Melnick and McCombs, 1966).

In certain species of animals there are various nonviral cytoplasmic inclusions, such as the eosinophilic bodies in the lateral geniculate nucleus of the cat (Szlachta and Habel, 1953) and the eosinophilic bodies in the thalamus of the mouse (Fraser, 1969), that closely resemble Negri bodies. Although these bodies have diagnostic ultrastructures (*vide infra*), they may be confused with Negri bodies when observed by conventional light microscopy, even with the aid of special stains. Particularly, the inclusions in the lateral geniculate nucleus of the cat are virtually indistinguishable from Negri bodies (Innes and Saunders, 1962). Because of the absence of inclusions in many cases of human rabies and the presence of misleading inclusions in certain animals, the diagnosis of rabies should not depend entirely on the recognition of Negri bodies.

Subacute sclerosing panencephalitis is another viral disease of man in which inclusions are commonly encountered in the cytoplasm of neurons and glial cells. By light microscopy, the cytoplasmic inclusions appear as various sized ovoid or irregular elongated eosinophilic masses. Occasionally, these are sufficiently large to almost fill the perikaryon. Neurons containing the cytoplasmic bodies usually harbor type A or B inclusion in their nuclei. Ultrastructurally, the cytoplasmic inclusions contain the same tubular virus particles that are seen in the nuclei (Herndon and Rubinstein, 1968; Parker *et al.*, 1970).

Cytomegalovirus produces conspicuous type A nuclear and granular cytoplasmic inclusions. Although neurons may be involved, the severely affected cells are often difficult to identify with certainty. Ultrastructural studies on infected cell cultures have demonstrated that the granular cytoplasmic bodies consist of aggregates of lysosomes which have engulfed viral particles as they are released from the nucleus (McGavran and Smith, 1965).

III. Nonviral Nuclear Inclusions

A. MARINESCO BODIES

Marinesco (1902) reported the presence of acidophilic intranuclear inclusions in the pigmented neurons of the locus coeruleus and the substantia nigra. The prevalence, morphology, and histochemical reactions of these intranuclear inclusions were studied by Yuen and Baxter (1963) in the brain stems from 160 randomly selected autopsies. The inclusions, which they termed "Marinesco bodies," were present in the majority of patients over 21 years old and increased in number with advancing age. The presence of these inclusions could not be correlated with any particular neurological disorder. From one to six bodies were present in a single nucleus. The diameter of the spherical inclusions ranged from 2 to 10 μ and was not proportional to the patients age. They are red with hematoxylin–eosin (Fig. 3) and van Gieson's, and pink with Masson's trichrome stain. They do not stain with periodic acid-Schiff or Feulgen techniques. The ultrastructure of Marinesco bodies was first reported by Leestma and Andrews (1969), who found them to consist of unbounded ovoid aggregates of granular osmophilic material (Fig. 5). Some were associated with a lattice-like array of fine filaments (Fig. 4). The Marinesco bodies may be variants of nuclear bodies.

B. Nuclear Bodies

Small spherical nuclear inclusions were described ultrastructurally in the cells of a tumor derived from the Shope papilloma (de Thé et al., 1960). Similar inclusions, later designated as "nuclear bodies" (Weber and Frommes, 1963; Weber et al., 1964), have been observed in the nuclei of a wide variety of normal and abnormal cells (Bouteille et al., 1967; Popoff and Stewart, 1968; Dahl, 1970), including neurons (Ishikawa, 1964; Périer et al., 1967; Masurovsky et al., 1970; Dixon, 1970; Dahl, 1970; Seïte, 1970). The bodies (Fig. 6) generally range from 0.2 to 1.5 μ in diameter and may be multiple. Ultrastructurally, they display varying arrangements and proportions of three components: fine granules, fibrils, and coarse granules. When present, the coarse granules are usually located in the center and the fibrils often form a cortex about the other components (Fig. 7). Some authors (Bouteille et al., 1967; Popoff and Stewart, 1968; Seïte, 1970) have regarded the presence of nuclear bodies as a reflection of nuclear or cellular hyperactivity. Others (Dixon, 1970; Dahl, 1970) regarded these inclusions as normal nuclear organelles. In support of the latter interpretation, Dixon (1970) demonstrated that the increased protein synthesis following axon section did not affect the prevalence or morphology of the nuclear bodies in sympathetic neurons. Generally, these inclusions are not readily recognized by light microscopy, but in some tissues, such as the epithelium of the dog epididymis (Nicander, 1964) and in a rhabdomyoma (Wyatt et al., 1970), they are quite conspic-

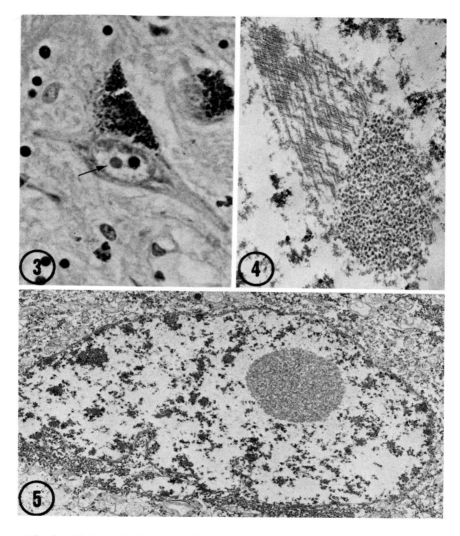

Fig. 3.   Marinesco body (arrow) in the nucleus of a pigmented neuron from the substantia nigra. Hematoxylin–eosin, × 1000.

   Fig. 4.   Electron micrograph of a Marinesco body associated with a lattice-like array of filaments. Uranyl acetate–lead citrate, × 27,500.

   Fig. 5.   Electron micrograph of a Marinesco body in the nucleus of a pigmented neuron from the substantia nigra. Uranyl acetate–lead citrate, × 4500.

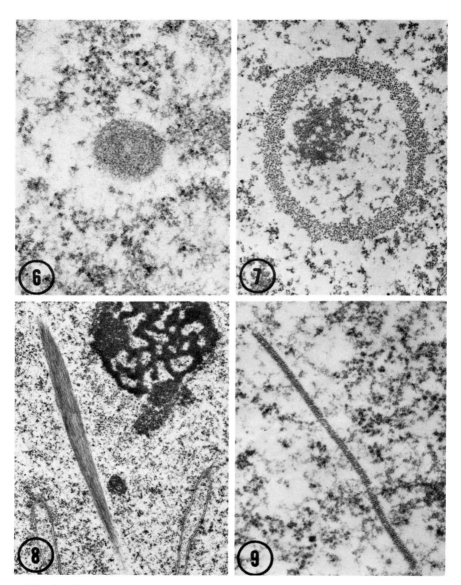

Fig. 6. Electron micrograph of a spherical nuclear body in a neuron from the brain stem of a rat. Uranyl acetate–lead citrate, ×30,000.

Fig. 7. Electron micrograph of a complex sparsely granular and fibrillary nuclear body in a pigmented neuron from the substantia nigra. Uranyl acetate–lead citrate, ×16,500.

Fig. 8. Electron micrograph of a rodlet of Roncoroni in the nucleus of a neuron from the brain stem of a rabbit. Uranyl acetate–lead citrate, ×10,500.

Fig. 9. Electron micrograph of a lattice-like filamentous array in the nucleus of a neuron from the brain stem of a rat. Uranyl acetate–lead citrate, ×30,000.

uous. The small acidophilic nuclear inclusions described in various neurons of the human brain (Wolf and Orton, 1932) and the type B inclusions observed in equine encephalomyelitis (Hurst, 1934) and poliomyelitis (Bodian and Horstmann, 1965) may be further examples of prominent nuclear bodies.

C. INTRANUCLEAR FILAMENTOUS INCLUSIONS

Various forms of intranuclear filamentous inclusions have been described in the neurons of man and animals. The rod-shaped intranuclear inclusions commonly known as the "rodlets of Roncoroni" have long been recognized by light microscopists in a wide variety of neurons (Mann, 1894; Roncoroni, 1895; Prenant, 1897; Holmgren, 1899; Ramón y Cajal, 1909, 1911; Shantha et al., 1969). Siegesmund et al., 1964 provided the first ultrastructural study of the "rodlets of Roncoroni" (Fig. 8) and showed that they are bundles of thin parallel filaments measuring 50–70 Å in diameter. Subsequent electron microscopic studies have demonstrated these filamentous fascicles in many neuronal nuclei even when they are not apparent by light microscopy (Gambetti and Gonatas, 1967; Magalhães, 1967; Sotelo and Palay, 1968; Raine and Field, 1968; Popoff and Stewart, 1968; Andrews and Sekhon, 1969; Masurovsky et al., 1970; Dahl, 1970; Dixon, 1970; Seïte, 1970). Masurovsky et al. (1970) suggested the possibility that extrusion of these intranuclear rodlets may contribute to filaments found in the cytoplasm.

Lattice-like arrays of intranuclear filaments (Figs. 4 and 9) have also been described in various neurons of man and animals (Chandler, 1966; Chandler and Willis, 1966; Magalhães, 1967; Périer et al., 1967; Gambetti and Gonatas, 1967; Sotelo and Palay, 1968; Brown et al., 1968; Andrews and Sekhon, 1969). The relation of these lattice-like inclusions to the "rodlets of Roncoroni" and the various forms of nuclear bodies and the Marinesco bodies is unclear.

IV. Nonviral Cytoplasmic Inclusions

A. LAMINATED CYTOPLASMIC BODIES

Szlachta and Habel (1953) described small round or ovoid acidophilic inclusions that closely resembled Negri bodies in neurons of the lateral geniculate body of nonrabid cats. These bodies measure from 2 to 5 μ in diameter and stain bright red with hematoxylin–eosin (Fig. 10) and

Masson's trichrome. They are argentophilic with the Holmes silver technique. Doolin *et al.*, (1967) performed a comprehensive histochemical analysis of these inclusions and concluded that they are chemically complex, containing predominantly protein but also some lipid and polysaccharide.

These bodies constitute a prominent ultrastructural feature of the neurons of the cat lateral geniculate body (Fig. 11) and were first illustrated by Morales *et al.* (1964). They described the inclusions as multilaminated cytoplasmic bodies composed of parallel rows of tubules each 250 Å in diameter. The rows of tubules were spaced at 750-Å intervals. Smith *et al.* (1964) noted the presence of these lamellar structures in both the perikarya and major dendrites of the lateral geniculate neurons but regarded the inclusions as composed of layers of membranes rather than arrays of tubules. A. Peters and Palay (1966) reported these structures to be confined to the perikarya of the neurons in lamina A and A_1 of the cat lateral geniculate body. These authors also demonstrated that the "dark lines" were actually sheets of tubules about 200 Å in diameter and showed that the intervening, moderately dense material contained fine filaments oriented parallel to the tubules. Doolin *et al.* (1967) demonstrated that pairs of the tubules were intertwined and often coextensive with the adjacent granular endoplasmic reticulum at the periphery of the inclusion. Barron *et al.*, (1967) observed that these bodies persisted in neurons undergoing retrograde atrophy following enucleation of the eye.

Similar laminated cytoplasmic bodies have been found in other parts of the brain. Morales and Duncan (1966) described somewhat smaller inclusions in the stellate neurons of the cat cerebellum, while Herman and Ralston (1970) described them in dendrites and perikarya of neurons in the ventrobasal and posterior nuclear groups of the cat thalamus. Kruger and Maxwell (1969) have demonstrated small laminated cytoplasmic inclusions in neuronal perikarya from the striate cortex of the monkey.

Currently, the significance of the laminated cytoplasmic bodies is unknown. However, their similarity to the Negri bodies by light microscopy prompted Innes and Saunders (1962) to suggest that "the lateral geniculate body is a good area to avoid when taking material from cats for rabies diagnoses."

B. Colloid Inclusions and Bunina Bodies

Large homogeneous cytoplasmic inclusions (Fig. 12) termed "colloid inclusions" (G. Peters, 1935) are commonly encountered in the neurons

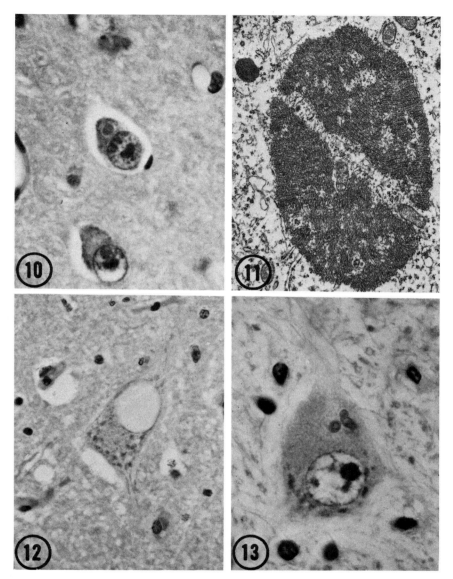

Fig. 10. Eosinophilic spheroid corresponding to a laminated cytoplasmic body in a neuron from the lateral geniculate nucleus of a cat. Hematoxylin–eosin, ×600.

Fig. 11. Electron micrograph of a laminated cytoplasmic body from the lateral geniculate nucleus of a cat. The darker laminae consist of parallel rows of intertwined tubules while the paler laminae consist of finely filamentous material. Uranyl acetate–lead citrate, ×16,000.

Fig. 12. Acidophilic colloid inclusion in a neuron from the hypoglossal nucleus of an elderly patient with no specific neurological disorder. Hematoxylin–eosin, ×600.

Fig. 13. Bunina bodies in an anterior horn cell from a patient with sporadic amyotrophic lateral sclerosis. Hematoxylin–eosin, ×1200.

141

of the hypoglossal nucleus and less commonly in other neurons of the brain stem and spinal cord. G. Peters (1935) described their occurrence in six individuals, including two without neurological disease, ranging in age from 28 to 66 years old. Adams *et al.* (1964) illustrated colloid inclusions in neurons of the hypoglossal nucleus from a patient with striato-nigral degeneration but described the inclusions as resembling Lewy bodies. Forno (1969) briefly mentioned that such inclusions were frequently encountered in the hypoglossal nucleus and indicated that they were different than Lewy bodies. Although their true prevalence and significance is currently unknown, it is our impression that colloid inclusions are quite common, especially in elderly individuals. They are globular in configuration and are stained pink to red in hematoxylin–eosin, red in van Gieson, blue in Nissl, and brown in silver preparations. Neither Best's carmine nor periodic acid-Schiff techniques stain these inclusions strongly.

Recently, three additional studies have been reported. Takei and Mirra (1971) found "intracytoplasmic hyaline inclusion bodies" in the hypoglossal neurons from 150 of 518 consecutive autopsies. They reported the prevalence of the inclusions to increase with age. Mendell and Markesbery (1971) observed these inclusions in 31 of 100 cases but found no consistent pattern relating to age, sex, underlying disease, cause of death, or medications. Wisotzkey and Moossy (1971) noted the inclusions in 82 of 463 autopsy cases and reported the prevalence to increase with age. Based on histochemical findings, all three groups regarded the inclusions as composed of protein or glycoprotein. Mendell and Markesbery (1971) and Wisotzkey and Moossy (1971) studied the ultrastructure of the inclusions and described them as membrane bounded masses of moderately osmophilic granular material.

Biondi (1932) used the term "colloid degeneration" to designate irregular eosinophilic (Alzheimer–Mann stain) inclusions that he observed in a child with "non-encephalitic juvenile Parkinsonism." These inclusions were often multiple and varied widely in size. The larger ones were present in the anterior horn cells of the spinal cord while the smaller ones were found in Clark's column, hypoglossal nucleus, facial nucleus, and substantia innominata. The staining reactions of these inclusions were similar to the "colloid inclusions," from which they were distinguished by G. Peters (1935) on the basis of their distribution, irregular configuration, and more variable size. It is our opinion that these differences are inadequate for regarding "colloid inclusions" and "colloid degeneration" as separate entities.

Bunina (1962) described small eosinophilic, intracytoplasmic inclusions in the anterior horn neurons from certain cases of amyotrophic lateral sclerosis. Although she suggested that they may be evidence of a neurotrophic virus, similar inclusions (Fig. 13) have been seen in cases of Guamanian, familial, and classical amyotrophic lateral sclerosis (Hirano, 1965; Hirano et al., 1969) and even in individuals without recognized neurological disease. Greenfield (1958), in a discussion of lyssa bodies, stated that "acidophilic droplets may be seen in nerve cells in a variety of degenerative conditions which are not related to virus infections." These "droplets" were not illustrated and, thus, cannot be equated with Bunina bodies. Because of their small size and relatively rare occurrence, the histochemical and ultrastructural data necessary to determine the relation of the Bunina bodies to colloid inclusions, acidophilic granules in pigmented neurons, and other cytoplasmic inclusions are lacking.

C. Acidophilic Granules in Pigmented Neurons and Lattice-Work Inclusions

Small acidophilic granules have been observed within the cytoplasm of pigmented neurons in the substantia nigra and locus coeruleus (Marinesco, 1902; Foley and Baxter, 1958; Lipkin, 1959; Lillie and Yamada, 1960; Earle, 1968; Schochet et al., 1970b). Schochet et al. (1970b) examined the substantia nigra from 100 autopsies chosen to represent all decades and found intracytoplasmic acidophilic granules in 80 of the cases. No correlations could be established between the presence of the granules and age, sex, or cause of death. It seems likely that they would have been found in all cases had serial sections been employed. The individual granules ranged from 1 to 7 μ in maximal size and were often multiple. They were stained red with hematoxylin–eosin (Fig. 14) and Mallory's trichrome technique. They could not be recognized in sections stained with luxol-fast blue-PAS, alcian blue, or Bodian silver techniques. The histochemical studies by Lillie and Yamada (1960) suggested that the inclusions were composed of protein. The ultrastructural study of six cases (Schochet et al., 1970b) demonstrated that the granules consisted of sheaves of parallel osmophilic filaments having a diameter of approximately 85 Å. The parallel filaments were interconnected or traversed by a second set of somewhat thinner filaments producing a lattice-work appearance (Figs. 15 and 16). In transverse section, the inclusions appeared as arrays of punctate densities with a uniform center to center spacing of about 140 Å (Fig. 17). Occasionally, small aggregates of the filamentous

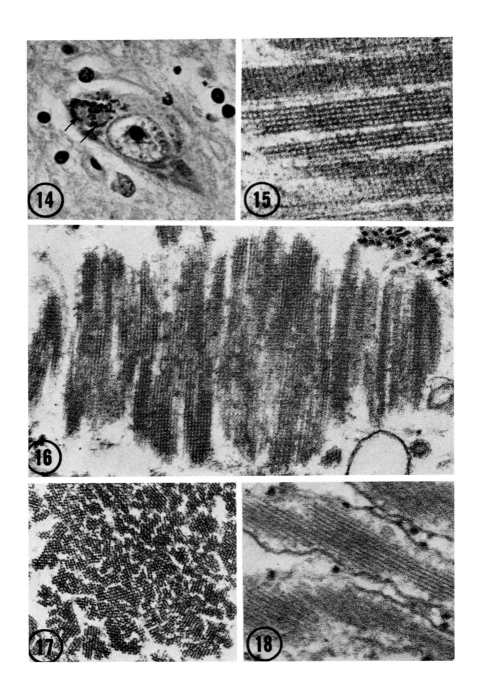

material were observed within dilated cisterns of endoplasmic reticulum and resembled proteinaceous secretory or storage material as found in various nonneural cells (Fig. 18).

These inclusions previously had been observed ultrastructurally and by phase microscopy in the substantia nigra from a case of Batten's disease (Zeman and Donahue, 1968); however, at that time they were not recognized as a ubiquitous component of normal nigral cells. Furthermore, inclusions with this distinctive lattice-work ultrastructure are not limited to pigmented neurons. Virtually identical inclusions have been demostrated in the autonomic ganglia of cats (Elfvin, 1963; Seïte, 1968a,b, 1969a,b) and in the thalamus of mice (Fraser, 1969; Fraser et al., 1970). The significance of the acidophilic granules or lattice-work inclusions is currently unknown. Seïte (1969b) interpreted the inclusions in the sympathetic ganglia of the cats as "a storage form of migrating protein." The presence of these inclusions in both autonomic ganglia and the substantia nigra suggests that they are composed of a protein associated with catecholamine metabolism. Fraser et al. (1970) considered the inclusions in the thalamus of mice to be protein but felt they were related to the aging process. No correlation with age was evident in the studies of human substantia nigra (Schochet et al., 1970b) or cat autonomic ganglia (Seïte, 1969b).

D. HIRANO BODIES

The eponym "Hirano bodies" has been applied to distinctive spheroidal or spindle-shaped acidophilic structures originally observed in the hippocampi of patients with the amyotrophic lateral sclerosis–Parkinsonism dementia complex (Hirano, 1965; Hirano et al., 1966, 1968a). Subse-

---

Fig. 14. Intracytoplasmic acidophilic granules (arrows) in a pigmented neuron from the substantia nigra. Hematoxylin–eosin, × 850.

Fig. 15. Electron micrograph of the acidophilic granules showing that the individual filaments comprising the lattice-work structure are approximately 85 Å in diameter. Uranyl acetate–lead citrate, × 110,000.

Fig. 16. Electron micrograph of the acidophilic granules showing the lattice-work configuration produced by the sheaves of intersecting filaments. Uranyl acetate–lead citrate, × 70,000.

Fig. 17. Electron micrograph of the acidophilic granules. In transverse section the lattice-work inclusions appear as arrays of punctate densities with a uniform center to center spacing. Uranyl acetate–lead citrate, × 61,000.

Fig. 18. Occasionally small aggregates of filamentous material are observed within dilated cisterns of the endoplasmic reticulum. Uranyl acetate–lead citrate, × 95,000.

quently, they have been demonstrated in the hippocampi from patients with Pick's disease (Rewcastle and Ball, 1968; Schochet *et al.*, 1968b), Alzheimer's disease and senile dementia (Wisniewski *et al.*, 1970), and in elderly persons without specific neurological disease (Hirano *et al.*, 1968a). Although they have been encountered most often in the hippocampi, they have also been recognized by their distinctive ultrastructure in the anterior horns of the spinal cord in patients with motor neuron disease (Schochet *et al.*, 1969a; Chou *et al.*, 1970) and in the cerebellum of patients with Kuru (Field *et al.*, 1969). Similar structures have been described in the cerebral cortex adjacent to gliomas (Ramsey, 1967). In animals, they have been identified ultrastructurally in mice with experimental scrapie (David-Ferreira *et al.*, 1968), in old chimpanzees, and in chimpanzees with experimental Kuru encephalopathy (Field *et al.*, 1969).

The Hirano bodies usually appear as spheroidal or spindle-shaped juxtaganglionic structures (Fig. 19) but occasionally appear to be located within neuronal perikarya (Hirano *et al.*, 1966, 1968a; Schochet *et al.*, 1968b). They are stained red with hematoxylin–eosin and Masson's trichrome, purple with phosphotungstic acid–hematoxylin, and are variably argentophilic (Hirano *et al.*, 1968a; Rewcastle and Ball, 1968; Schochet *et al.*, 1968b). They can be readily recognized in plastic embedded sections stained with toluidine blue or paraphenylenediamine.

Ultrastructurally, the Hirano bodies appear to be composed of sheaves of parallel beaded filaments and smooth filaments or sheets of less dense material (Fig. 20). The beaded filaments are approximately 100–150 Å in diameter (Fig. 21) while the smooth filaments of sheets are somewhat thinner. The smooth components occasionally appear as a pair of 40-Å-wide lines separated by a 20–40-Å electron lucent area. Usually, the sheaves are closely packed, and where the beaded filaments are in register, they produce a herringbone pattern (Fig. 22). Occasionally, the bodies appear splintered with one or more small bundles separated from the main mass. Rarely, individual beaded filaments appear widely separated from one another. The ultrastructure of these inclusions has been variously interpreted. Hirano *et al.* (1968a) and Wisniewski *et al.* (1970) regarded the beaded appearance as resulting from the transverse section of parallel filaments embedded in sheets of less dense material while Field *et al.* (1969) and Schochet *et al.* (1969a) suggested that the individual filaments are beaded or tightly coiled. Some Hirano bodies are hollow, or at least deeply indented, and contain an admixture of filaments and vesicles in the cavity. Schochet *et al.* (1968b) and David-Ferreira *et al.* (1968)

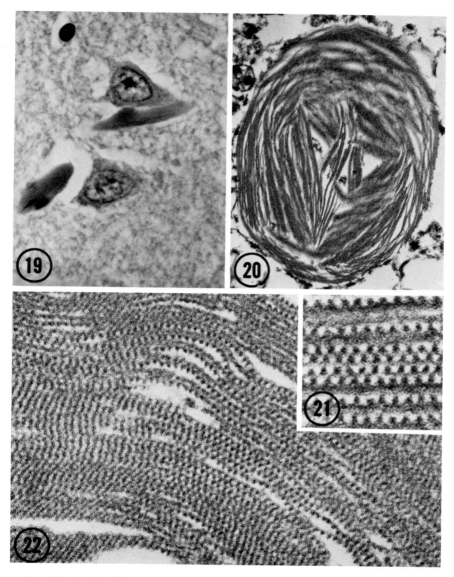

Fig. 19. Acidophilic spindle-shaped Hirano bodies in the hippocampus from a patient with Alzheimer's disease. Hematoxylin–eosin, ×850.

Fig. 20. Electron micrograph of a Hirano body showing the sheaves of beaded and smooth filaments. Uranyl acetate–lead citrate, ×24,000.

Fig. 21. The individual beaded filaments are approximately 100–150 Å in diameter. Uranyl acetate–lead citrate, ×200,000.

Fig. 22. When in register, the parallel beaded filaments produce a herringbone pattern. Uranyl acetate–lead citrate, ×50,000.

described these structures as primarily in neuronal processes, but at least small aggregates of the Hirano body material can be found in the perikaryon (Schochet et al., 1969a). The similar appearing structures described by Ramsey (1967) were within abnormal synapses. Currently, the significance and morphogenesis of these inclusions are unknown.

E. LEWY BODIES

Lewy (1912, 1913) first described spherical bodies in the substantia innominata and in the dorsal motor nucleus of the vagus in brains from patients with idiopathic Parkinsonism. He erroneously equated these bodies to the "corpora amylacea" that had been described in myoclonus epilepsy (Lafora and Glück, 1911). This misinterpretation was corrected by Lafora, who demonstrated that these bodies stained differently than the characteristic neuronal inclusions in myoclonus epilepsy. Trétiakoff (1919) first employed the eponym "Lewy bodies" and focused attention on their frequent occurrence in the substantia nigra and locus coeruleus. Subsequent studies by Hassler (1938), Beheim-Schwarzbach (1952), Greenfield and Bosanquet (1953), Lipkin (1959), Bethlem and den Hartog Jager (1960), and Earle (1968) have established the presence of these inclusions in various brain stem nuclei as a characteristic feature of idiopathic Parkinsonism. In addition to the central nervous system, Lewy bodies have been observed in autonomic ganglia from patients with Parkinsonism (Herzog, 1955; den Hartog Jager and Bethlem, 1960; Vanderhaeghen et al., 1970).

Although mesencephalic neurofibrillary tangles, rather than Lewy bodies, have been regarded as the typical feature of post encephalitic Parkinsonism (Fényes, 1932; Hallervorden, 1933, 1935; von Braunmuhl, 1949; Greenfield and Bosanquet, 1953; Hirano and Zimmerman, 1962; Richardson, 1965; Forno, 1966; Earle, 1968), several studies have recorded the simultaneous occurrence of both Lewy bodies and tangles in this condition (Alvord, 1968; Lipkin, 1959; Earle, 1968). Furthermore, the coexistence of Lewy bodies and neurofibrillary tangles in the mesencephalon has been a characteristic finding in the amyotrophic lateral sclerosis-Parkinsonism dementia complex found on Guam (Hirano, 1965; Hirano et al., 1966). Inclusions resembling Lewy bodies have been observed in the motor neurons of the hypoglossal nucleus and anterior horns of the spinal cord in certain familial cases of amyotrophic lateral sclerosis (Hirano et al., 1967) and in the anterior horns of an apparently sporadic case of amyotrophic lateral sclerosis (Schochet, 1970).

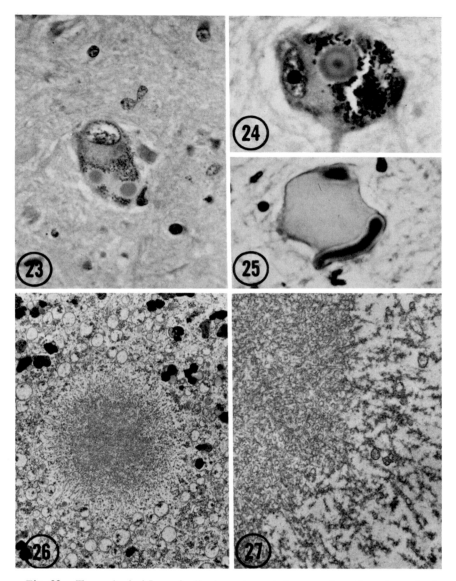

Fig. 23. Two spherical Lewy bodies in a pigmented neuron from the substantia nigra of a patient with Parkinsonism. Hematoxylin–eosin, ×500.

Fig. 24. Spherical Lewy body with multiple laminations in a pigmented neuron from the substantia nigra of a patient with Parkinsonism. Hematoxylin–eosin, ×850.

Fig. 25. Elongated or fusiform Lewy body in dorsal motor nucleus of the vagus. Hematoxylin–eosin, ×800.

Fig. 26. Electron micrograph of a Lewy body showing the central core surrounded by a peripheral zone. Uranyl acetate–lead citrate, ×6000.

Fig. 27. Electron micrograph of a Lewy body showing the linear and circular profiles in the core and the radially oriented irregular filaments in the peripheral zone. Uranyl acetate–lead citrate, ×31,500.

Considerable attention has been given to the possibility that Lewy bodies are a manifestation of senescence (Beheim-Schwarzbach, 1952; Lipkin, 1959; Forno, 1969) or mental illness (Woodard, 1962b). Forno (1969) reconciled these views by concluding that the apparently incidental occurrence of Lewy bodies represents mild early or preclinical cases of Parkinsonism.

Lewy bodies are typically laminated acidophilic spheroids (Figs. 23 and 24), but may be elongated or fusiform (Fig. 25), especially when present in sympathetic ganglia (Herzog, 1955; den Hartog Jager and Bethlem, 1960; Vanderhaegen *et al.*, 1970). Their tinctorial properties with a wide variety of stains have been recorded by Greenfield and Bosanquet (1953). The histochemical studies by Lipkin (1959) suggested that the inclusions were proteinaceous, and the additional studies by Bethlem and den Hartog Jager (1960) indicated that the proteins contained aromatic amino acids. No nucleoproteins, calcium, iron, or heavy metals could be detected. More recently, investigation by den Hartog Jager (1969) has revealed the presence of sphingomyelin.

The original ultrastructural studies by Duffy and Tennyson (1965) and subsequent confirmatory observations (Roy and Wolman, 1969; Forno, 1969) have shown that Lewy bodies are unbounded structures consisting of a central core surrounded by one or more peripheral zones (Fig. 26). The core contains filaments 70–80 Å in width arranged as closely packed linear profiles and/or circular profiles 400–600 Å in diameter. The outer zones are composed of irregular, radially oriented filaments whose diameter varies from 75 to 200 Å (Fig. 27). Although Duffy and Tennyson (1965) suggested that remnants of melanin granules may contribute to the formation of Lewy bodies, den Hartog Jager and Bethlem (1960) have indicated that Lewy bodies may also occur in ganglia that do not contain melanin. Despite the histochemical and ultrastructural studies, the origin and significance of these inclusions in Parkinsonism are currently unknown.

F. Lafora Bodies

These distinctive spheroidal inclusions, now regarded as the hallmark of a familial form of progressive myoclonus epilepsy, were first described in 1911 (Lafora, 1911; Lafora and Glück, 1911). In this disease, large numbers of "Lafora bodies" can be found throughout the gray matter of the central nervous system but are especially abundant in the cerebral cortex, thalamus, pallidum, substantia nigra, and dentate nucleus. By light microscopy, the inclusions appear as homogenous or laminated spheroids, occurring either singly or in small clusters within the neuropil and perikarya of neurons (Fig. 28). Generally, the smaller bodies appear homogenous and are very numerous. Myriads of minute bodies, inconspicuous with hematoxylin–eosin are vividly demonstrated in sections stained with periodic acid-Schiff techniques. The larger bodies are usually laminated and may attain diameters of 20–40 μ. These are composed of dark staining cores surrounded by less intensely staining outer shells that may display radial striations. A common exception is found in the substantia nigra where the inclusions, despite their large size, are often homogenous and may show a Y-shaped crack.

While occasional Lafora bodies can be found in the white matter (van Heycop ten Ham and de Jager, 1963; Schwarz and Yanoff, 1965; van Hoof and Hageman-Bal, 1967), it is usually uninvolved (Seitelberger, 1968). In my material, I have observed only an occasional inclusion in the subcortical white matter. Lafora bodies have also been found in the retina (Yanoff and Schwarz, 1965).

Formerly, Lafora bodies had been reported in extraneuronal locations within the central nervous system (Harriman and Millar, 1955; van Heycop ten Ham and de Jager, 1963; Schwarz and Yanoff, 1965), but these observations have not been substantiated by more recent studies. Many cases of progressive myoclonus epilepsy have deposits of stored material in the myocardium, skeletal muscle, liver, and other visceral organs (Harriman and Millar, 1955; van Heycop ten Ham and de Jager, 1963; Seitelberger et al., 1964; Schwarz and Yanoff, 1965; Sakai et al., 1970) which are similar, but not identical, to the Lafora bodies. The inclusions are not restricted to man. Recently, Lafora bodies have been reported in brain and retina from two purebred dogs (Holland et al., 1970).

Numerous histochemical studies of the Lafora bodies (Harriman and Millar, 1955; Seitelberger et al., 1964; Allegranza et al., 1966; Schwarz and Yanoff, 1965; van Heycop ten Ham, 1965; Janeway et al., 1967; van Hoof and Hageman-Bal, 1967; Collins et al., 1968; Schnabel and Seitelberger, 1968, 1969; Yokoi et al., 1968; Dubois-Dalcq, 1969; Sakai et al., 1970) have been reported, with various results and interpretations. In general, most investigators regard the Lafora bodies to be composed predominantly of polysaccharides. Lafora (1911) referred to the inclusions as "amyloid," meaning starchlike. Subsequent authors have referred to the constituents of the Lafora bodies as acid mucopolysaccharide (Harriman and Millar, 1955), atypical basophilic polysaccharide with an outer shell of mucoprotein (Seitelberger et al., 1964), glycogenlike polysaccharide (van Heycop ten Ham, 1965), a glycoprotein–acid mycopolysaccharide complex (Schwarz and Yanoff, 1965), neutral and acid polysaccharides (Allegranza *et al.*, 1966), sulfated mucopolysaccharide and a neutral saccharide containing moiety (Janeway *et al.*, 1967), mucopolysaccharide (van Hoof and Hageman-Bal, 1967), complex carbohydrate in combination with a tyrosine containing protein (Collins *et al.*, 1968), hexose and protein containing moieties (Dubois-Dalcq, 1969), and polyglucosan–protein complex (Schnabel and Seitelberger, 1969). Enzyme digestion studies (Harriman and Millar, 1955; Edgar, 1963; Seitelberger *et al.*, 1964; Schwarz and Yanoff, 1965; Allegranza *et al.*, 1966; Janeway *et al.*, 1967; van Hoof and Hageman-Bal, 1967; Yokoi *et al.*, 1968; Schnabel and Seitelberger, 1969; Jenis *et al.*, 1970) have also given varying results, but the types of tissue, enzymes, and digestion conditions have rarely been comparable. However, the studies by Yokoi *et al.* (1968) and Schnabel and Seitelberger (1969) have shown that Lafora bodies can be digested by α-amylase and, to a lesser extent, by β-amylase if appropriate tissue, enzyme, and incubation conditions are employed. The acidic properties of the inclusions have been a persistent enigma and have been variously attributed to nonspecific adsorption (Seitelberger *et al.*, 1964) carboxyl groups, sulfate groups (Schwarz and Yanoff, 1965; Allegranza *et al.*, 1966; Janeway *et al.*, 1967), or phosphate groups (van Heycop ten Ham, 1965; Dubois-Dalcq, 1969; Schnabel and Seitelberger, 1969; Sakai *et al.*, 1970).

Recently, Lafora bodies have been isolated from brain tissue and chemically analyzed. Seitelberger (1966) reported them to contain 39% glucose and 45% reducing sugar along with 0.1% sulfur and 0.07% phosphorous. However, the details of the isolation procedures and the determinations were not recorded. Following isolation and acid hydrolysis, Yokoi *et al.* (1968) found Lafora bodies to contain 80–93% glucose and a minimum of 6% protein. Based on their comprehensive study employing histochemical techniques, enzymatic digestions, isolation procedures, infrared spectroscopy, and chemical analyses, Yokoi *et al.* (1968) concluded that the Lafora bodies were composed of an unusual polyglucosan belonging to the same family of compounds as glycogen and amylopectin. Electron probe and histochemical techniques have revealed the presence of phosphorous, suggested to be in phosphate groups, esterified onto the glucose units (Sakai *et al.*, 1970).

A number of electron microscopic studies have been reported (Seitelberger *et al.*, 1964; Seitelberger, 1966; Allegranza, *et al.*, 1966; Namba and Ota, 1966; Sluga and Stockinger, 1967; Odor *et al.*, 1967; van Hoof and Hageman-Bal, 1967; Toga *et al.*, 1968; Collins *et al.*, 1968; Jenis *et al.*, 1970; Vanderhaeghen, 1971), and all have revealed similar ultrastructural features. The Lafora bodies are unbounded structures composed of varying proportions of granular and fibrillar material and have been found only in the perikarya (Fig. 29) and processes (Fig. 30) of neurons. Central cores, when present, are composed predominantly of fine osmophilic granules. The homogeneous inclusions and the peripheral zone of laminated inclusions are composed predominantly of branched fibrils measuring approximately 50–100 Å in diameter. Usually these branched fibrils radiate outward from the center or central core of the inclusion. In some instances, the fibrils appear randomly disposed, but such an appearance may result from nonequatorial sections. Collins *et al.*, 1968 reported the individual fibril to have a granular substructure with a tubular orientation of the subunits while Toga *et al.* (1968) referred to a helicoid orientation. Namba and Ota (1966) spoke of bifilal lamellae rather than fibrils. Randomly interspersed among the fibrils are coarse and fine osmophilic granules. Since the inclusions have no circumferential boundary, cytoplasmic organelles including vesicles, dense bodies, and cisterns of endoplasmic reticulum are entrapped among the peripheral arborizing fibrils (Fig. 31).

Several authors have commented on the histochemical and ultrastructural similarity between Lafora bodies and corpora amylacea (Namba and Ota, 1966; Odor *et al.*, 1967; Toga *et al.*, 1968; Collins *et al.* 1968; Yokoi *et al.*, 1968; Jenis *et al.*, 1970) and between Lafora bodies and the central nervous system deposits in type IV glycogenosis (Jenis *et al.*, 1970; Schochet *et al.*, 1970a). These observations are consistent with the chemical studies indicating that Lafora bodies (Yokoi *et al.*, 1968), visceral deposits in myoclonus epilepsy (Sakai *et al.*, 1970), corpora amylacea (Sakai *et al.*, 1969), and the stored material in type IV glycogenosis (Illingworth and Cori, 1952; Mercier and Whelan, 1970) are all predominantly an amylopectinlike polyglycosan. The histochemical differences among these deposits and the difference from a pure polysaccharide can be attributed to the associated anionic groups. At present, we do not know why various cells in apparently unrelated conditions accumulate this abnormal polysaccharide.

G. LIPOFUSCIN AND ITS DERIVATIVES

Lipofuscin is a yellow to brown pigment that is found in many types of cells including neurons. Although it is commonly referred to as "wear

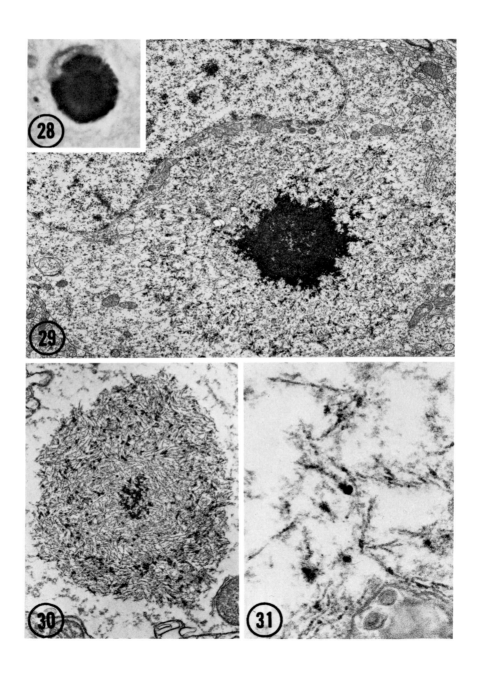

and tear" pigment, its presence does not necessarily indicate cellular senescence for it can be found in neonatal human liver cells (Goldfischer and Bernstein, 1969). In the nervous system, this pigment is reported to be absent at birth but becomes more abundant with advancing age in man (Sulkin, 1953; Brody, 1960; Issidorides and Shanklin, 1961; Samorajski *et al.*, 1964) and in various animals (Few and Getty, 1967; Samorajski *et al.*, 1965, 1968; Reichel *et al.*, 1968; Barden, 1970). Within the adult brain, however, there is considerable regional variation in the distribution of lipofuscin (Friede, 1966). Abnormal deposits of lipofuscin appear as discrete neuronal inclusions in children with Chediak–Higashi disease (Sung *et al.*, 1969).

The histochemical reactions of lipofuscin (Lillie, 1954; Pearse, 1960; Strehler, 1964; Friede, 1966; Porta and Hartroft, 1969) suggest that it is a heterogenous material containing lipids, proteins, and carbohydrates. Among the more readily demonstrated characteristics are autofluorescence, affinity for lipid stains, acid-fastness, and staining with periodic acid-Schiff techniques.

The ultrastructure of neuronal lipofuscin has been extensively studied (Bondareff, 1957; Duncan *et al.*, 1960; Gonatas *et al.*, 1963; Samorajski *et al.*, 1964, 1965, 1968; Sulkin and Sulkin, 1967; Few and Getty, 1967; Miyagishi *et al.*, 1967; Pallis *et al.*, 1967). The pigment granules are membrane bounded conglomerates of lipid globules, osmophilic granules and lamellar material. When present, the lamellae may be arranged as either asymmetric curved bands or in highly organized paracrystalline arrays (Samorajski *et al.*, 1965). Current histochemical and ultrastructural evidence suggests that the pigment granules are derived from the residua of lysosomes (Essner and Novikoff, 1960; Samorajski *et al.*, 1964; Miyagishi *et al.*, 1967; Barden, 1970). The sequestered material accumulates because of limitations in the hydrolytic capacity of the lysosomal enzymes and modifications of the residua through lipid peroxidation or polymerization and cross linkage of lipoproteins (Barden, 1970).

Fig. 28. A Lafora body in the cytoplasm of a neuron from the cerebral cortex of a patient with progressive myoclonus epilepsy. Hematoxylin–eosin, × 950.

Fig. 29. Electron micrograph of a laminated Lafora body in the perikaryon of a neuron. Uranyl acetate–lead citrate, × 5000.

Fig. 30. Electron micrograph of a small laminated Lafora body in a neuronal process. Uranyl acetate–lead citrate, × 21,000.

Fig. 31. Electron micrograph showing the branched filaments and associated cytoplasmic organelles at periphery of a Lafora body. Uranyl acetate–lead citrate, × 70,000.

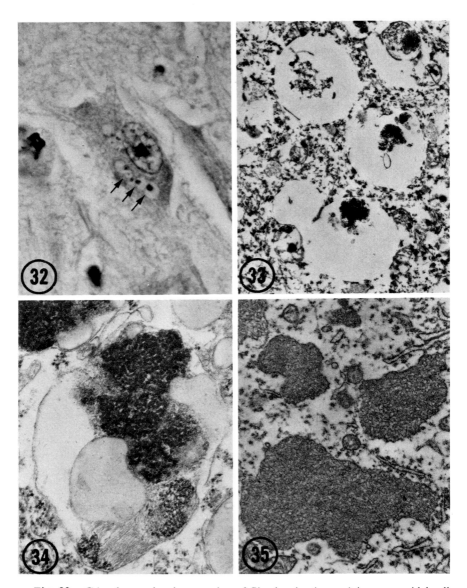

Fig. 32. Granulovacuolar degeneration of Simchowicz (arrows) in a pyramidal cell from the hippocampus of a patient with Alzheimer's disease. Hematoxylin–eosin, ×1000.

Fig. 33. Electron micrograph showing that the granulovacuolar degeneration consists of membrane bounded vacuoles containing a central mass of amorphous material. Uranyl acetate–lead citrate, ×10,500.

Fig. 34. Electron micrograph of neuromelanin showing the lipid, finely granular and coarsely granular components. A portion of the pigment granule is distinctly laminated. Uranyl acetate–lead citrate, ×36,000.

Fig. 35. Electron micrograph of neuronal cytosomes from a case of Batten's disease showing the "finger print" arrays of curved membranes. Uranyl acetate–lead citrate, ×16,500.

It has been suggested that the granulovacuolar change of Simchowicz is an intracellular degenerative process involving lipofuscin (Moossy, 1962) or at least material resembling lipofuscin (Hirano *et al.*, 1968a). The cells actually harboring these inclusions usually contain less lipofuscin than the adjacent cells (Margolis, 1959). They occur predominantly in the pyramidal cell layer of the hippocampus and have been seen in cases of senile dementia, Alzheimer's disease (McMenemey, 1963; Woodard, 1962a), Pick's disease (McMenemey, 1963; Rewcastle and Ball, 1968; Schochet *et al.*, 1968b; Seitelberger, 1969b), amyotrophic lateral sclerosis (van Bogaert and Bertrand, 1926), amyotrophic lateral sclerosis-Parkinsonism dementia complex (Hirano *et al.*, 1961, 1966), mongolism (Haberland, 1969), and in elderly individuals with no specific neurological disorder. Granulovacuolar degeneration also has been described in various brain stem nuclei in cases of progressive supranuclear palsy (Steele *et al.*, 1964) and in the parietal cortex along with neurofibrillary tangles and argentophilic globules in a child with tuberous sclerosis (Hirano *et al.*, 1968b).

The inclusions are often multiple, and consist of small vacuoles 2 to 8 μ in diameter that contain a smaller dense granule (Fig. 32). The central cores are stained intensely by hematoxylin and silver techniques, weakly with luxol-fast blue, and variably with Congo red and periodic acid-Schiff stains. The surrounding vacuoles remain unstained with any of the usual histological procedures.

Ultrastructurally, the inclusions appear as membrane bounded (Schochet *et al.*, 1968b; Hirano *et al.*, 1968a) or unbounded (Rewcastle and Ball, 1968) vacuoles containing a central mass of amorphous osmophilic material (Fig. 33). Occasionally, they are incorporated within a neurofibrillary tangle (Hirano *et al.*, 1968a) or Pick body (Schochet *et al.*, 1968b).

The significance of these inclusions is unknown. Woodard (1962a) emphasized a correlation between the number of granulovacuolar inclusions and the diagnosis of Alzheimer's disease. Rewcastle and Ball (1968) noted a frequent association with Pick bodies, while Hirano (1968a) pointed out parallels in the distribution of the granulovacuolar inclusions, neurofibrillary tangles, and Hirano bodies.

Neuromelanin may be another derivative of lipofuscin. In man, it is most abundant in the substantia nigra, locus coeruleus, and dorsal motor nucleus of the vagus; however, serial sections have shown that the pigmented neurons occur in columns extending from the mesencephalon to the nucleus retroambigualis (Bazelon *et al.*, 1967). Similar deposits are present in primates and, to a lesser extent, in carnivores but are absent in lower mammals (Marsden, 1969). Fenichal and Bazelon (1968) studied 44 children and found neuromelanin accumulation beginning during the first 5 years of life and increasing steadily throughout childhood. During adult life, the intensity of the pigmentation normally remains constant (Foley and Baxter, 1958; Moses *et al.*, 1966) and is even present in albinos.

The histochemistry of neuromelanin has been studied extensively (Lillie, 1955, 1957; Lillie and Yamada, 1960; Barden, 1969). While many of the reactions are common to all melanins, differences in basophilia and metal reduction properties distinguish neuromelanin from the other melanins. Barden (1969) was able to experimentally interconvert the histochemical properties of neuromelanin and lipofuscin and provided evidence that neuromelanin can be derived from metal catalyzed pseudo-peroxidation of catechol derivatives in association with lipofuscin. Neuromelanin in contrast with lipofuscin, accumulates especially in those neurons with a histochemically intact Golgi apparatus (Barden, 1970).

A number of electron microscopic studies (Duffy and Tennyson, 1965; Moses *et al.*, 1966; Schochet *et al.*, 1970b; and others) have shown that the neuromelanin granules morphologically resemble lipofuscin more closely than the melanosomes of the skin and eyes. Moses *et al.*, (1966) attributes the characteristic argentophilic properties of neuromelanin to a coarsely granular electron-dense material that is present in addition to the usual components of lipofuscin (Fig. 34).

The material accumulating in the neurons of patients with the nonganglioside variants of "amaurotic familial idiocy" or Batten's disease has been regarded by some authors to be ceroid or lipofuscin (Zeman and Hoffman, 1962; Zeman and Alpert, 1963; Donahue *et al.*, 1967; Zeman and Dyken, 1969). The term "ceroid," originally used by Lillie *et al.*, (1941) to designate a pigment in the livers of cirrhotic rats, has also been applied to pigments occurring in man and in vitamin E deficient animals (Papenheimer and Victor, 1946; Einarson, 1953; Sulkin and Srivanij, 1960; Miyagishi *et al.*, 1967; Nishioka *et al.*, 1968). Most authors now regard ceroid and lipofuscin as essentially the same material (Friede, 1966; Miyagishi *et al.*, 1967; Nishioka *et al.*, 1968; Porta and Hartroft, 1969). The ultrastructure of the neuronal cytosomes from patients with Batten's disease vary from that of typical lipofuscin to predominantly "finger print" arrays of curved membranes (Herman *et al.*, 1971) (Fig. 35).

V. Inclusions Derived from Neuronal Fibrous Proteins

A. NEUROFIBRILLARY TANGLES COMPOSED OF TWISTED TUBULES

Alzheimer (1907) described argentophilic fibrillary structures in the cortical neurons of a patient with a progressive presenile dementia. These fibrillary inclusions have since been called Alzheimer's neurofibrillary tangles and are regularly found in cases of Alzheimer's disease and senile dementia (Alzheimer, 1907; Morel and Wildi, 1952; von Braunmühl, 1957; Hirano and Zimmerman, 1962; McMenemey, 1963, 1968; Ishii, 1966), amyotrophic lateral sclerosis–Parkinsonism dementia complex (Malamud et al., 1961; Hirano et al., 1961, 1966, 1969; Hirano and Zimmerman, 1962; Hirano, 1965), postencephalitic Parkinsonism (Fényes, 1932; Hallervorden, 1933, 1935; von Braunmühl, 1949; Greenfield and Bosanquet, 1953; Hirano and Zimmerman, 1962; Richardson, 1965; Forno, 1966; Earle, 1968) and progressive supranuclear palsy (Steele et al., 1964; Weinmann, 1967; Blumenthal and Miller, 1969; Seitelberger, 1969a). They can also be found in elderly individuals without specific neurological disease (Hirano and Zimmerman, 1962; McMenemey, 1963), in cases of apparently nonencephalitic Parkinsonism (Hirano and Zimmermann, 1962), and in cases of mongolism (Bertrand and Koffas, 1946; Jervis, 1948; Solitare and Lamarche, 1966; Haberland, 1969). Rarely they have been described in cases of Pick's disease (Berlin, 1949; McMenemey, 1963; Schochet et al., 1968b), "inclusion" encephalitis (Malamud et al., 1950; Corsellis, 1951; Krücke, 1957; Noyan, 1966), Kufs' disease (Hallervorden, 1938; Norman, 1963; Chou and Thompson, 1970), amyotrophic lateral sclerosis (van Bogaert and Bertrand, 1926; Schaffer, 1926; Hirano and Zimmerman, 1962), and tuberous sclerosis (Hirano et al, 1968b).

The topographic distribution of neurofibrillary tangles varies among the different conditions (Hirano, 1970). Neurofibrillary changes can be found throughout the cerebral cortex in patients with Alzheimer's disease, senile dementia, or old age. They are especially abundant in the hippocampus, where they may be found even when absent elsewhere (von Braunmühl, 1957; Margolis, 1959; Hirano and Zimmerman, 1962; McMenemey, 1963). In postencephalitic Parkinsonism the basal ganglia and brain stem are maximally affected. Among the basal ganglia, the amygdalae are the most frequently involved (Hirano and Zimmerman, 1962), while in the brain stem, the pigmented and periaqueductal nuclei are the most commonly involved. The spinal cord may contain neurofibrillary tangles, especially in the amyotrophic lateral sclerosis–Parkinsonism dementia complex and in familial Alzheimer's disease (Feldman *et al.*, 1963). The cerebellar cortex remains strikingly uninvolved regardless of the disease process.

The neurofibrillary tangles in the cortex are usually triangular or flame-shaped (Fig. 36), while those in subcortical neurons are more commonly globose (Fig. 37) (Hirano *et al.*, 1961). The tangles stain variably with hematoxylin–eosin and periodic acid-Schiff techniques but are intensely argentophilic. They are congophilic and birefringent in polarized light. These properties are dependent upon the orientation of the fibrillary components and do not indicate the presence of amyloid. Krigman *et al.* (1965) reported the neurofibrillary tangles to have no enzyme activity, but a more recent study (Johnson and Blum, 1970) revealed high activity of two nucleoside phosphatases.

Electron microscopic studies of cerebral tissue from patients with Alzheimer's disease (Terry, 1963, 1968; Kidd, 1963, 1964; Terry *et al.*, 1964; Luse and Smith, 1964; Krigman *et al.*, 1965; Gonatas *et al.*, 1967; Wisniewski *et al.*, 1970), amyotrophic lateral sclerosis–Parkinsonism dementia complex (Hirano, 1965; Hirano *et al.*, 1968a, 1969; Wisniewski *et al.*, 1970), and postencephalitic Parkinsonism (Wisniewski *et al.*, 1970; Schochet *et al.*, 1970b) have shown the neurofibrillary tangles to consist of bundles of abnormal fibrillary material (Figs. 38 and 39). Although all of these authors have illustrated the same structures, the interpretation and terminology have varied somewhat. Kidd (1963, 1964) interpreted the fibrillary structures as double stranded helices. Terry initially employed the terms "hollow fibrils" (1963) and "neurofilaments" (Terry *et al.*, 1964) while Luse and Smith (1964) spoke of "thick neurofilaments." Krigman *et al.* (1965) and Hirano (1965; Hirano *et al.*, 1968a) referred to "hollow filaments," and Gonatas *et al.* (1967) used the term "fibrils." More recently, the components of the Alzheimer neurofibrillary tangles have been interpreted as twisted hollow tubules (Terry, 1968; Wisniewski *et al.*, 1970; Terry and Wisniewski, 1970; Hirano, 1970). These abnormal twisted tubules have a maximal diameter of about 200 Å and, at intervals of 800 Å, appear to narrow to a diameter of about 100 Å (Fig. 39). In transverse section they display a circular or arciform configuration and occasionally contain a central dot. These distinctive tubular elements are morphologically unlike either the normal neurofilaments (100 Å in diameter) or the normal neurotubules (220–240 Å in diameter) and are currently considered unique to the human species (Wisniewski *et al.*, 1970). The morphogenesis of the twisted tubules and their relation to the normal neuronal fibrous proteins is as yet unknown.

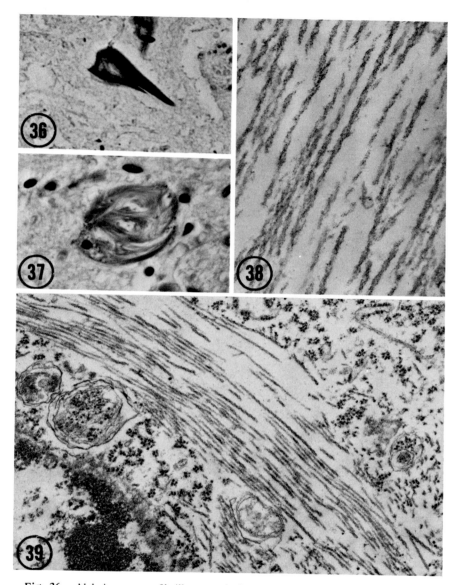

Fig. 36. Alzheimer neurofibrillary tangle in a neuron from the hippocampus of a patient with Alzheimer's disease. Bodian silver stain, ×800.

Fig. 37. Globose neurofibrillary tangle in a neuron from the brain stem of a patient with postencephalitic Parkinsonism. Hematoxylin–eosin, ×700.

Fig. 38. Electron micrograph of an Alzheimer neurofibrillary tangle showing periodic constrictions along the length of the abnormal twisted tubules. Uranyl acetate–lead citrate, ×57,000.

Fig. 39. Electron micrograph of an Alzheimer neurofibrillary tangle showing the skeins of abnormal twisted microtubules. Uranyl acetate–lead citrate, ×31,500.

B. Neurofibrillary Tangles and Aggregates Composed of Filaments

In addition to the Alzheimer neurofibrillary tangles that are composed of abnormal twisted tubules, there are various fibrillary aggregates composed of either normal neurofilaments or abnormal filamentous material that resembles neurofilaments. Sotelo and Palay (1968) described sharply circumscribed aggregates of neurofilaments within neurons of the lateral vestibular nucleus of normal rats. Subsequently, these so-called "fibrillary bodies" were encountered in the ventral cochlear nucleus, posterior colliculus, and spinal cord of rats. The spheroidal or lobulated masses are clearly separated from the surrounding cytoplasm by a limiting envelope that varies from a single membrane to a complicated honeycomb structure (Fig. 40). Other types of filamentous aggregates and tangles are unbounded. Schochet *et al.* (1969a) reported a case of sporadic motor neuron disease characterized by large hyaline conglomerates (Fig. 41) in the anterior horn neurons of the spinal cord and occasional motor neurons of the brain stem. These hyaline conglomerates stained pale blue with hematoxylin–eosin and were moderately argentophilic. Ultrastructurally, they were composed of interwoven skeins of filaments averaging 100 Å in diameter (Fig. 42). At the periphery of some of the masses were beaded strands identical to the components of the Hirano bodies. Similar accumulations of filaments, but within enlargements of the proximal portion of axons, have been described in the anterior horns of the spinal cords from patients with rapidly progressive or subacute amyotrophic lateral sclerosis (Carpenter, 1968; Chou *et al.*, 1970) and in rats and mice intoxicated with iminodipropionitrile (Chou and Hartmann, 1964, 1965).

The subarachnoid or intracerebral injection of aluminum compounds in rabbits, cats, and monkeys has produced neurofibrillary tangles, particularly in the anterior horn neurons of the spinal cord and large neurons of the brain stem (Klatzo *et al.*, 1965; Terry and Peña, 1965; Wisniewski *et al.*, 1966, 1967, 1970; Klatzo, 1968; Wisniewski and Terry, 1970). These tangles resemble the conglomerates observed in the case of sporadic motor neuron disease but are more intensely argentophilic and congophilic (Fig. 43). Ultrastructurally, they consist of compact bundles of filaments averaging 100 Å in diameter (Fig. 44). The application of aluminum phosphate to cultures of fetal rabbit dorsal root ganglia also produced aggregates of filaments, but these tended to be more spheroidal than the tangles produced *in vivo* (Seil *et al.*, 1969).

Mitotic spindle inhibitors have been reported to produce prolifera-

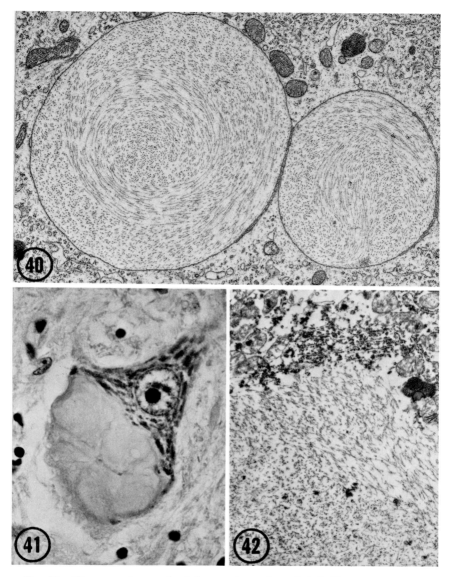

Fig. 40. Electron micrograph of the membrane bounded fibrillary bodies of Sotelo and Palay in a neuron from the anterior horn of a rat spinal cord. Uranyl acetate–lead citrate, ×10,500.

Fig. 41. Hyaline conglomerate in a neuron from the anterior horn of the spinal cord of a patient with sporadic motor neuron disease. Hematoxylin–eosin, ×830.

Fig. 42. Electron micrograph of a hyaline conglomerate showing the component filaments that are 100 Å in diameter. Uranyl acetate–lead citrate, ×10,000.

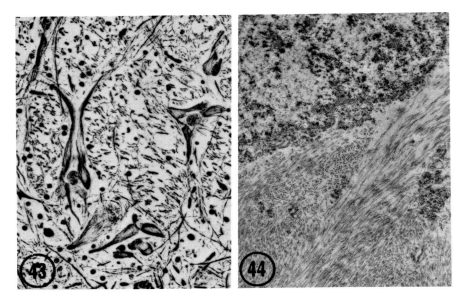

Fig. 43. Experimental neurofibrillary tangles induced by intracisternal injection of aluminium hydroxide in a rabbit. Bodian silver, ×370.

Fig. 44. Electron micrograph showing the 100 Å filaments comprising the neurofibrillary tangles induced by the intracisternal injection of aluminum hydroxide. Uranyl acetate–lead citrate, ×6000.

tions of filaments in various neurons of both man and animals. Schochet *et al.* (1968a) reported prominent acidophilic crystals and fibrillary tangles ultrastructurally composed of 100-Å filaments (Figs. 45 and 46) in the anterior horn neurons of a child with lymphocytic leukemia who had been given intrathecal vincristine. Shelanski and Wisniewski (1969) described an increase in argentophilic fibrillar material, especially in the spinal ganglia, in three patients with leukemia who had been treated with intravenous vincristine. Experimentally, tangles composed of 100-Å filaments have been produced in several species of animals by the intrathecal administration of low doses of colchicine, vincristine, vinblastine, or podophyllotoxin (Wisniewski and Terry, 1967; Wisniewski *et al.*, 1968, 1970) and by the intraperitoneal administration of vincristine (Journey *et al.*, 1969). Filamentous tangles have also been produced by *in vitro* the application of mitotic spindle inhibitors to cultures of nerve tissue (Burdman, 1966; Peterson and Bornstein, 1968; Seil and Lampert, 1968; Bunge and Bunge, 1969; Peterson, 1969). Intracisternal administration of relatively high doses of vincristine to rabbits produced both filamentous tangles and acidophilic crystals in neurons (Schochet *et al.*, 1968a) and acidophilic crystals alone in oligodendroglia (Schochet *et al.*, 1969b). In longitudinal section the crystals appear as parallel rows of punctate osmophilic densities (Fig. 47), while in transverse section the crystals appear as compact arrays of circular profiles approximately 300 Å in diameter (Fig. 48). Some of the circular profiles contain a central density. Schochet *et al.* (1968a) suggested that the crystals were in continuity with the filaments from which they were derived by a helical orientation of the filamentous material. By implanting vinblastine in the forebrain of rats, Hirano and Zimmerman (1970) induced the rapid development of crystals in oligodendroglia and neurons prior to the proliferation of filaments. Furthermore, the filaments were more numerous in the astrocytes and ependyma than in the neurons. Similar crystalline aggregates also have been produced by the Vinca alkaloids in leukocytes, platelets, and fibroblasts (Bensch and Malawista, 1968, 1969; White, 1968; Krishan and Hsu, 1969) and in solutions of purified microtubule protein (Marantz and Shelanski, 1970). These crystalline arrays have been variously regarded as derived from the normal microtubules, from helical assembly of the microtubule protein subunits, or from the associated filaments which may be polymers of microtubule protein rather than normal neurofilaments (Shelanski and Taylor, 1970).

C. Pick Bodies

Alzheimer (1911) provided the first microscopic study of Pick's disease, a progressive nonarteriosclerotic dementia histologically characterized by the presence of large numbers of enlarged neurons containing globular argentophilic inclusions—the so-called "Pick bodies." Neurons containing these inclusions can be found in any area of the cortex undergoing the earlier stages of degeneration, but are most readily demonstrated in Ammon's horn and the hippocampal gyrus. In some cases of Pick's disease, they are especially numerous in the dentate fascia. Although these globular inclusions are typically found in cases of Pick's disease, they have been reported in Lissauer's paralytic dementia and an assortment of other conditions (Williams, 1935). Hirano *et al.* (1968b) even described them, along with neurofibrillary tangles and granulovacuolar bodies, in an unusual case of tuberous sclerosis.

The Pick bodies are usually described as intensely argentophilic intracytoplasmic globules (Fig. 49). Although not generally emphasized, the inclusion bodies can be recognized in sections stained with hematoxylin–

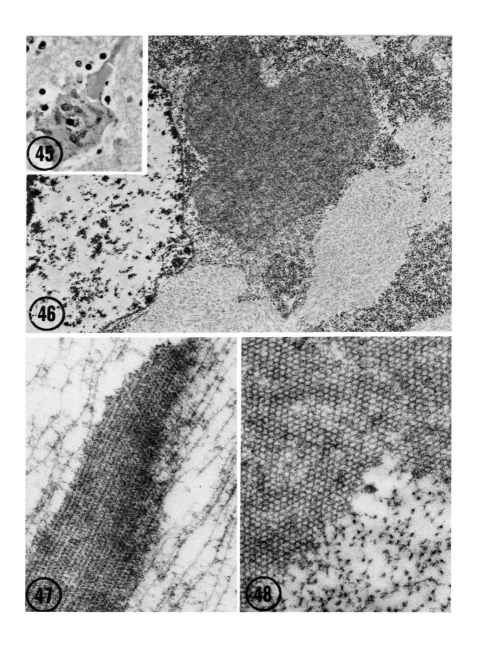

eosin where they appear as basophilic spheroids. They are commonly homogeneous but may contain minute lacunes or even granulovacuolar bodies. In an unusual case reported by Schochet and Earle (1970), some of the hematoxylinophilic Pick bodies contained small eosinophilic cores (see Fig. 53). These central spheroids were not stained by trichrome, phosphotungstic acid–hematoxylin or periodic acid-Schiff techniques, but the entire inclusion was typically argentophilic.

Ultrastructurally, the Pick bodies appear as unbounded, but circumscribed, conglomerates of granular and randomly arranged fibrillar material (Fig. 50) (Rewcastle and Ball, 1968; Schochet et al., 1968b). Rewcastle and Ball (1968) reported the fibrillar material in their case to consist of thin, straight tubules with a diameter of 75–120 Å, while Schochet et al. (1968b) illustrated fibrillar material consisting of periodically constricted tubules with a maximal diameter of 200 Å (Fig. 51). Further study of the latter case has demonstrated other Pick bodies containing an admixture of both neurofilaments and periodically constricted or twisted tubules (Fig. 52). It is probably significant that rare Alzheimer neurofibrillary tangles were present in the case reported by Schochet et al (1968b) whereas none were present in the case reported by Rewcastle and Ball (1968). The random arrangement of the fibrillar components of the Pick bodies contrasts with the orderly arrangement in the neurofibrillary tangles and accounts for the absence of congophilia and birefringence. Occasional lipofuscin particles and granulovacuolar bodies are incorporated within the Pick bodies.

The similarity of the Pick cells to neurons undergoing reactive changes secondary to axonal injury had been emphasized by Onari and Spatz (1926), who suggested that Pick's disease may primarily affect axons. Furthermore, Williams (1935) demonstrated Pick bodies in a wide variety

---

Fig. 45. Neurofibrillary tangles and an acidophilic crystal in a neuron from the anterior horn of the spinal cord of a child who had been given intrathecal vincristine. Hematoxylin–eosin, × 240.

Fig. 46. Electron micrograph showing the skeins of filaments and crystal that resulted from the intrathecal administration of vincristine. Uranyl acetate–lead citrate, × 8000.

Fig. 47. Electron micrograph of a portion of an acidophilic crystal. In longitudinal section they appear as parallel rows of punctate osmophilic densities. Uranyl acetate–lead citrate, × 45,000.

Fig. 48. Electron micrograph showing that in transverse section the acidophilic crystals appear as closely packed arrays of circular profiles. Uranyl acetate–lead citrate, × 42,000.

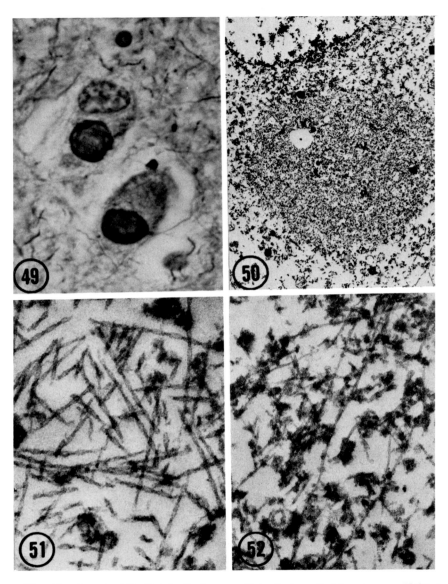

Fig. 49. Argentophilic Pick bodies in pyramidal cells from the hippocampus. Holmes stain, ×900.

Fig. 50. Electron micrograph of a Pick body showing the poorly demarcated mass of granular and fibrillar material. Uranyl acetate–lead citrate, ×4000.

Fig. 51. Electron micrograph of a Pick body in which the fibrillar material consists of randomly arranged twisted tubules with a maximum diameter of 200 Å. Uranyl acetate–lead citrate, ×60,000.

Fig. 52. Electron micrograph of a Pick body in which the fibrillar material consists predominantly of filaments 100 Å in diameter. Uranyl acetate–lead citrate, ×50,000.

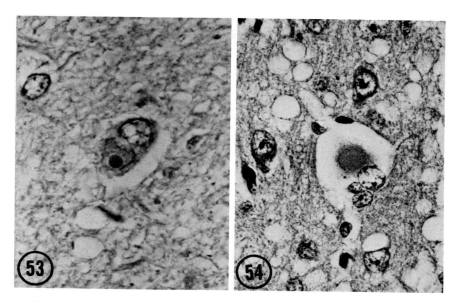

Fig. 53.   Unusual Pick body with an acidophilic core in the center of the basophilic spheroid. Hematoxylin–eosin, × 500.

Fig. 54.   Spheroidal intracytoplasmic inclusion in a cortical neuron from a chimpanzee with experimental Kuru encephalopathy. Holmes stain, × 500.

of diseases, all of which presumably affect the proximal portion of the axon. Nevertheless, large numbers of these inclusions are the most characteristic histological feature of Pick's disease.

Argentophilic spheroids (Fig. 54), very similar by light microscopy to Pick bodies, have been observed in the deeper layers of the cerebral cortex of chimpanzees afflicted with experimental Kuru encephalopathy (Lampert *et al.*, 1969). Ultrastructurally, these spheroids were composed predominantly of randomly arranged tubules about 200 Å in diameter admixed with a few filaments 100 Å in diameter. If the twisted neurotubules are indeed unique to man (Wisniewski *et al.* 1970), one would expect any animal counterpart of the Pick body to be composed of neurotubules and/or neurofilaments.

ACKNOWLEDGMENTS

My appreciation is extended to Dr. William F. McCormick for encouragement and review of the manuscript and to Mrs. Virginia Reighard for typing the manuscript. The preparation of this chapter was supported in part by funds from the Department of Neurology, University of Iowa.

REFERENCES

Adams, R. D., van Bogaert, L., and Vander Eecken, H. (1964). *J. Neuropathol. Exp. Neurol.* **23**, 584–608.

Allegranza, A., Canevini, P., and Strada, G. P. (1966). *Proc. Int. Congr. Neuropathol.,* *5th,* 1965, pp. 999–1003.

Alvord, E. C., Jr. (1968). *In* "Pathology of the Nervous System" (J. Minckler, ed.), Vol. I, pp. 1152-1161. McGraw-Hill, New York.

Alzheimer, A. (1907). *Zentralbl. Nervenheilk. Psychiat.* **30**, 177–179.

Alzheimer, A. (1911). *Z. Gesamte Neurol. Psychiat.* **4**, 356–385.

Andrews, J. M., and Sekhon, S. S. (1969). *Bull. Los Angeles Neurol. Soc.* **34**, 163–174.

Barden, H. (1969). *J. Neuropathol. Exp. Neurol.* **28**, 419–441.

Barden, H. (1970). *J. Neuropathol. Exp. Neurol.* **29**, 225–240.

Barron, K. D., Doolin, P. F., and Oldershaw, J. B. (1967). *J. Neuropathol. Exp. Neurol.* **26**, 300–326.

Bazelon, M., Fenichel, G. M., and Randall, J. (1967). *Neurology* **17**, 512–519.

Beheim–Schwarzbach, D. (1952). *J. Nerv. Ment. Dis.* **116**, 619–631.

Bensch, K. G., and Malawista, S. E. (1968). *Nature (London)* **218**, 1176–1177.

Bensch, K. G., and Malawista, S. E. (1969). *J. Cell Biol.* **40**, 95–107.

Berlin, L. (1949). *Arch. Neurol. Psychiat.* **61**, 369–384.

Bertrand, I., and Koffas, D. (1946). *Rev. Neurol.* **78**, 338–345.

Bethlem, J., and den Hartog Jager, W. A. (1960). *J. Neurol., Neurosurg. Psychiat.* **23**, 74–80.

Biondi, G. (1932). *Z. Gesammte Neurol. Psychiat.* **140**, 226–251.

Blumenthal, H., and Miller, C. (1969). *Arch. Neurol. (Chicago)* **20**, 362–367.

Bodian, D., and Horstmann, D. M. (1965). *In* "Viral and Rickettsial Infections of Man" (F. L. Horsfall, Jr. and I. Tamm, eds.), 4th ed., Chapter 18, p. 430. Lippincott, Philadelphia, Pennsylvania.

Bondareff, W. (1957). *J. Gerontol.* **12**, 364–369.

Bouteille, M., Kalifat, S. R., and Delarue, J. (1967). *J. Ultrastruct. Res.* **19**, 474–486.

Bozsik, G., Horányi, B., and Papp, M. (1963). *Acta Neuropathol.* **2**, 362–370.

Brody, H. (1960). *J. Gerontol.* **15**, 258–261.

Brown, W. J., Kotorii, K., and Riehl, J.-L. (1968). *Neurology* **18**, 427–438.

Bunge, R. P., and Bunge, M. B. (1969). *J. Neuropathol. Exp. Neurol.* **28**, 169.

Bunina, T. L. (1962). *Korsakov J. Neuropathol. Psychiat. (USSR)* **62**, 1293–1299.

Burdman, J. A. (1966). *J. Nat. Cancer Inst.* **37**, 331–335.

Carpenter, S. (1968). *Neurology* **18**, 841–851.

Chandel, R. L. (1966). *Nature (London),* **209**, 1260–1261.

Chandler, R. L., and Willis, R. (1966). *J. Cell Sci.* **1**, 283–286.

Chou, S-M., and Hartmann, H. A. (1964). *Acta Neuropathol.* **3**, 428–450.

Chou, S-M., and Hartmann, H. A. (1965). *Acta Neuropathol.* **4**, 590–603.

Chou, S-M., and Thompson, H. G. (1970). *Arch. Neurol. (Chicago)* **23**, 489–501.

Chou, S-M., Martin, J. D., Gutrecht, J. A., and Thompson, H. G. (1970). *J. Neuropathol. Exp. Neurol.* **29**, 141–142.

Collins, G. H., Cowden, R. R., and Nevis, A. H. (1968). *Arch. Pathol.* **86**, 239–254.

Corsellis, J. A. N. (1951). *J. Ment. Sci.* **97**, 570–583.

Cowdry, E. V. (1934). *Arch. Pathol.* **18**, 527–542.

Dahl, E. (1970). *J. Anat.* **106**, 255–262.

David-Ferreira, J. F., David-Ferreira, K. L., Gibbs, C. J., Jr., and Morris, J. A. (1968). *Proc. Soc. Exp. Biol. Med.* **127**, 313–320.

den Hartog Jager, W. A. (1969). *Arch. Neurol.* **21**, 615–519.

den Hartog Jager, W. A., and Bethlem, J. (1960). *J. Neurol., Neurosurg. Psychiat.* **23**, 283–290.

de Thé, G., Rivière, M., and Bernhard, W. (1960). *Bull. Cancer* **47**, 570–584.

Dierks, R. E., Murphy, F. A., and Harrison, A. K. (1969). *Amer. J. Pathol.* **54**, 251–273.

Dixon, J. S. (1970). *Anat. Rec.* **168**, 179–186.

Donahue, S., Zeman, W., and Watanabe, I. (1967). *In* "Inborn Disorders of Sphingolipid Metabolism" (S. M. Aronson and B. W. Volk, eds.), pp. 3–22. Pergamon, Oxford.

Doolin, P. F., Barron, K. D., and Kwak, S. (1967). *Amer. J. Anat.* **121**, 601–622.

Dubois–Dalcq, M. (1969). *Acta Neuropathol.* **12**, 205–217.

Duffy, P. E., and Tennyson, V. M. (1965). *J. Neuropathol. Exp. Neurol.* **24**, 398–414.

Duncan, D., Nall, D., and Morales, R. (1960). *J. Gerontol.* **15**, 366–372.

Dupont, J. R., and Earle, K. M. (1965). *Neurology* **15**, 1023–1034.

Earle, K. M. (1968). *J. Neuropathol. Exp. Neurol.* **27**, 1–14.

Earle, K. M., and Dupont, J. R. (1966). *Tex. Rep. Biol. Med.* **24**, 317–325.

Edgar, G. W. F. (1963). *Epilepsia* **4**, 120–137.

Einarson, L. (1953). *J. Neurol., Neurosurg. Psychiat.* **16**, 98–109.

Elfvin, L.-G. (1963). *J. Ultrastruct. Res.* **8**, 403–440.

Essner, E., and Novikoff, A. B. (1960). *J. Ultrastruct. Res.* **3**, 374–391.

Feldman, R. G., Chandler, K. A., Levy, L. L., and Glaser, G. H. (1963). *Neurology* **13**, 811–824.

Fenichel, G. M., and Bazelon, M. (1968). *Neurology* **18**, 817–820.

Fényes, I. (1932). *Arch. Psychiat. Nervenkr.* **96**, 700–717.

Few, A., and Getty, R. (1967). *J. Gerontol.* **22**, 357–368.

Field, E. J., Mathews, J. D., and Raine, C. S. (1969). *J. Neurol. Sci.* **8**, 209–224.

Foley, J. M., and Baxter, D. (1958). *J. Neuropathol. Exp. Neurol.* **17**, 586–598.

Forno, L. S. (1966). *J. Neurosurg. Suppl.* **24**, 266–271.

Forno, L. S. (1969). *J. Amer. Geriat. Soc.* **17**, 557–575.

Fraser, H. (1969). *J. Pathol.* **98**, 201–204.

Fraser, H., Smith, W., and Gray, E. W. (1970). *J. Neurol. Sci.* **11**, 123–127.

Friede, R. L. (1966). "Topographic Brain Chemistry," pp. 425–430. Academic Press, New York.

Gambetti, P., and Gonatas, N. K. (1967). *Riv. Patol. Nerv. Ment.* **88**, 188–196.

Goldfischer, S., and Bernstein, J. (1969). *J. Cell Biol.* **42**, 253–261.

Gonatas, N. K., Terry, R. D., Winkler, R., Korey, S. R., Gomez, C. J., and Stein, A. (1963). *J. Neuropathol. Exp. Neurol.* **22**, 557–580.

Gonatas, N. K., Anderson, W., and Evangelista, I. (1967). *J. Neuropathol. Exp. Neurol.* **26**, 25–39.

González-Angulo, A., Márquez-Monter, H., Feria-Velasco, A., and Zavala, B. J. (1970). *Neurology* **20**, 323–328.

Greenfield, J. G. (1958). *In* "Neuropathology" (J. G. Greenfield *et al.*, eds.), pp. 132–229. Arnold, London.

Greenfield, J. G., and Bosanquet, F. D. (1953). *J. Neurol., Neurosurg. Psychiat.* **16**, 213–226.

Haberland, C. (1969). *Acta Neurol. Psychiat. Belg.* **69**, 369–380.

Hallervorden, J. (1933). *Klin. Wochenschr.* **12**, 692–695.

Hallervorden, J. (1935). *Deut. Z. Nervenheilk.* **136**, 68–77.

Hallervorden, J. (1938). *Monatsschr. Psychiat. Neurol.* **99**, 74–80.

Harriman,. D. G. F., and Millar, J. H. D. (1955). *Brain* **78**, 325–349.

Hashida, Y., and Yunis, E. J. (1970). *Amer. J. Clin. Pathol.* **53**, 537–543.

Hassler, R. (1938). *J. Psychol. Neurol.* **48**, 387–476.

Herman, M. M., and Ralston, H. J. (1970). *Anat. Rec.* **167**, 183–196.

Herman, M. M., Rubinstein, L. J., and McKhawn, G. M. (1971). *Acta Neuropathol.* **17**, 85–102.

Herndon, R. M., and Rubinstein, L. J. (1968). *Neurology* **18**, 8–20.

Herzog, E. (1955). *In* "Handbuch der speziellen pathologischen Anatomie und Histologie" (O. Lubarsch, F. Henke, and R. Rössle, eds.) Vol. 13, Part 5, pp. 357–542. Springer-Verlag, Berlin and New York.

Hirano, A. (1965). *In* "Slow, Latent and Temperate Virus Infections" (D. C. Gajdusek, C. J. Gibbs, and M. Alpers, eds.), NINDB Monogr. No. 2, pp. 23–37. Nat. Inst. Health, Washington, D.C.

Hirano, A. (1970). *Alzheimer's Dis. Related Conditions, Ciba Found. Symp.* pp. 185–207.

Hirano, A., and Zimmerman, H. M. (1962). *Arch. Neurol. (Chicago)* **7**, 227–242.

Hirano, A., and Zimmerman, H. M. (1970). *Lab. Invest.* **23**, 358–367.

Hirano, A., Malamud, N., and Kurland, L. T. (1961). *Brain* **84**, 662–679.

Hirano, A., Malamud, N., Elizan, T. S., and Kurland, L. T. (1966). *Arch. Neurol. (Chicago)*, **15**, 35–51.

Hirano, A., Kurland, L. T., and Sayre, G. P. (1967). *Arch. Neurol. (Chicago)* **16**, 232–243.

Hirano, A., Dembitzer, H. M., Kurland, L. T., and Zimmerman, H. M. (1968a). *J. Neuropathol. Exp. Neurol.* **27**, 167–182.

Hirano, A., Tuazon, R., and Zimmerman, H. M. (1968b). *Acta Neuropathol.* **11**, 257–261.

Hirano, A., Malamud, N., Kurland, L. T., and Zimmerman, H. M. (1969). *In* "Motor Neuron Diseases" (F. H. Norris, Jr. and L. T. Kurland, eds.), Vol. 2, pp. 51–60. Grune & Stratton, New York.

Holland, J. M., Davis, W. C., Prieur, D. J., and Collins, G. H. (1970). *Amer. J. Pathol.* **58**, 509–529.

Holmgren, E. (1899). *Anat. Anz.* **16**, 388–397.

Hurst, E. W. (1934). *J. Exp. Med.* **59**, 529–542.

Illingworth, B., and Cori, G. T. (1952). *J. Biol. Chem.* **199**, 653–660.

Innes, J. R. M., and Saunders, L. Z. (1962). "Comparative Neuropathology," p. 393. Academic Press, New York.

Ishii, T. (1966). *Acta Neuropathol.* **6**, 181–187.

Ishikawa, H. (1964). *Z. Zellforsch. Mikrosk. Anat.* **62**, 822–828.

Issidorides, M., and Shanklin, W. M. (1961). *J. Anat.* **95**, 151–159.

Janeway, R., Ravens, J. R., Pearce, L. A., Odor, D. L., and Suzuki, K. (1967). *Arch. Neurol. (Chicago)* **16**, 565–582.

Jenis, E. H., Schochet, S. S., Jr., and Earle, K. M. (1970). *Mil. Med.* **135**, 116–119.

Jervis, G. A. (1948). *Amer. J. Psychiat.* **105**, 102–106.

Johnson, A. B., and Blum, N. R. (1970). *J. Neuropathol. Exp. Neurol.* **29**, 463–478.

Journey, L. J., Burdman, J., and Whaley, A. (1969). *J. Nat. Cancer Inst.* **43**, 603–619.

Kidd, M. (1963). *Nature (London)*, **197**, 192–193.

Kidd, M. (1964). *Brain* **87**, 307–320.

Klatzo, I. (1968). *In* "International Academy of Pathology Monograph, The Central Nervous System" (O. T. Bailey and D. E. Smith, eds.), pp. 209–212. Williams & Wilkins, Baltimore, Maryland.

Klatzo, I., Wisniewski, H., and Streicher, E. (1965). *J. Neuropathol. Exp. Neurol.* **24,** 187–199.

Krigman, M. R., Feldman, R. G., and Bensch, K. (1965). *Lab. Invest.* **14,** 381–396.

Krishan, A., and Hsu, D. (1969). *J. Cell Biol.* **43,** 553–563.

Krücke, W. (1957). *Nervenarzt* **28,** 289-301.

Kruger, L., and Maxwell, D. S. (1969). *J. Ultrastruct. Res.* **26,** 387–390.

Lafora, G. R. (1911). *Virchows Arch. Pathol. Anat. Physiol.* **205,** 295–303.

Lafora, G. R., and Glück, B. (1911). *Z. Gesammte Neurol. Psychiat.* **6,** 1–14.

Lampert, P. W., Earle, K. M., Gibbs, C. J., Jr., and Gajdusek, D. C. (1969). *J. Neuropathol. Exp. Neurol.* **28,** 353–370.

Leestma, J. E., and Andrews, J. M. (1969). *Arch. Pathol.* **88,** 431–436.

Lewy, F. H. (1912). *In* "Handbuch der Neurologie" (M. Lewandowsky, ed.), pp. 920–933. Springer-Verlag, Berlin and New York.

Lewy, F. H. (1913). *Deut. Z. Nervenheilk.* **50,** 50–55.

Lillie, R. D. (1954). "Histopathological Technic and Practical Histochemistry," 2nd ed., pp. 248-254. McGraw-Hill (Blakiston), New York.

Lillie, R. D. (1955). *J. Histochem. Cytochem.* **3,** 453–454.

Lillie, R. D. (1957). *J. Histochem. Cytochem.* **5,** 325–333.

Lillie, R. D., and Yamada, H. (1960). *Okajimas Folia Anat. Jap.* **36,** 155–163.

Lillie, R. D., Daft, F. S., and Sebrell, W. H., Jr. (1941). *Publ. Health Rep.* **56,** 1255–1258.

Lipkin, L. E. (1959). *Amer. J. Pathol.* **35,** 1117–1133.

Love, R., and Wildy, P. (1963). *J. Cell Biol.* **17,** 237–254.

Luse, S. A., and Smith, K. R., Jr. (1964). *Amer. J. Pathol.* **44,** 553–563.

McGavran, M. H., and Smith, M. G. (1965). *Exp. Mol. Pathol.* **4,** 1–10.

McMenemey, W. H. (1963). *In* "Greenfield's Neuropathology" (W. Blackwood *et al.* eds.), pp. 520–580. Williams & Wilkins, Baltimore, Maryland.

McMenemey, W. H. (1968). *In* "International Academy of Pathology Monograph, The Central Nervous System" (O. T. Bailey and D. E. Smith, eds.), pp. 201–208. Williams & Wilkins, Baltimore, Maryland.

Magalhães, M. M. (1967). *Exp. Cell Res.* **47,** 628–632.

Malamud, N., Haymaker, W., and Pinkerton, H. (1950). *Amer. J. Pathol.* **26,** 133–153.

Malamud, N., Hirano, A., and Kurland, L. T. (1961). *Arch. Neurol. (Chicago)* **5,** 401–415.

Mann, G. (1894). *J. Anat.* **29,** 100–108.

Marantz, R., and Shelanski, M. L. (1970). *J. Cell Biol.* **44,** 234–238.

Margolis, G. (1959). *Lab. Invest.* **8,** 335–370.

Marinesco, G. (1902). *C. R. Acad. Sci.* **135,** 1000–1002.

Marsden, C. D., (1969). *In* "Pigments in Pathology" (M. Wolman, ed.), pp. 395–420. Academic Press, New York.

Masurovsky, E. B., Benitez, H. A., Kim, S. U., and Murray, M. R. (1970). *J. Cell Biol.* **44,** 172–191.

Melnick, J. L., and McCombs, R. M. (1966). *Progr. Med. Virol.* **8,** 400–409.

Mendell, J., and Markesbery, W. R. (1971). *J. Neuropathol. Exp. Neurol.* **30,** 233–239.

Mercier, C., and Whelan, W. J. (1970). *Eur. J. Biochem.* **16,** 579–583.

Miyagishi, T., Takayata, N., and Iizuka, R. (1967). *Acta Neuropathol.* **9**, 7–17.

Miyamato, K., and Matsumoto, S. (1965). *J. Cell Biol.* **27**, 677–682.

Moossy, J. (1962). Personal communication.

Morales, R., and Duncan, D. (1966). *J. Ultrastruct. Res.* **15**, 480–489.

Morales, R., Duncan, D., and Rehmet, R. (1964). *J. Ultrastruct. Res.* **10**, 116–123.

Morecki, R., and Zimmerman, H. M. (1969). *Arch. Neurol. (Chicago)* **20**, 599–604.

Morel, F., and Wildi, E. (1952). *Proc. Int. Congr. Neuropathol.,* 1st. 1952. Vol. 2, pp. 347–374.

Moses, H. L., Ganote, C. E., Beaver, D. L., and Schuffman, S. S. (1966). *Anat. Rec.* **155**, 167–183.

Namba, M., and Ota, T. (1966). *Bull. Yamaguchi Med. Sch.* **13**, 233–250.

Nicander, L. (1964). *Exp. Cell Res.* **34**, 533–541.

Nishioka, N., Takahata, N., and Iizuka, R. (1968). *Acta Neuropathol.* **11**, 174–181.

Norman, R. M. (1963). *In* "Greenfield's Neuropathology" (W. Blackwood *et al.*, eds.), pp. 324–440. Williams & Wilkins, Baltimore, Maryland.

Noyan, B. (1966). *Proc. Int. Congr. Neuropathol.,* 5th, 1965, pp. 486–489.

Odor, D. L., Janeway, R., Pearce, L. A., and Ravens, J. R. (1967). *Arch. Neurol. (Chicago)* **16**, 583–594.

Onari, K., and Spatz, H. (1926). *Z. Gesammte Neurol. Psychiat.* **101**, 470–511.

Pallis, C. A., Duckett, S., and Pearse, A. G. E. (1967). *Neurology* **17**, 381–394.

Pappenheimer, A. M., and Victor, J. (1946). *Amer. J. Pathol.* **22**, 395–413.

Parker, J. C., Jr., Klintworth, G. K., Graham, D. G., and Griffith, J. F. (1970). *Amer. J. Pathol.* **61**, 275–291.

Pearse, A.G.E. (1960). "Histochemistry, Theoretical and Applied," 2nd ed., pp. 661–680. Little, Brown, Boston, Massachusetts.

Périer, O., Vanderhaeghen, J.-J., and Pelc, S. (1967). *Acta Neuropathol.* **8**, 362–380.

Peters, A., and Palay, S. L. (1966). *J. Anat.* **100**, 451–486.

Peters, G. (1935). *Z. Gesammte Neurol. Psychiat.* **153**, 779–783.

Peterson, E. R. (1969). *J. Neuropathol. Exp. Neurol.* **28**, 168.

Peterson, E. R., and Bornstein, M. B. (1968). *J. Neuropathol. Exp. Neurol.* **27**, 121–122.

Pinkerton, H. (1950). *Amer. J. Clin. Pathol.* **20**, 201–207.

Popoff, N., and Stewart, S. (1968). *J. Ultrastruct. Res.* **23**, 347–361.

Porta, E. A., and Hartroft, W. S. (1969). *In* "Pigments in Pathology" (M. Wolman, ed.), pp. 191–235. Academic Press, New York.

Prenant, A. (1897). *Arch. Anat. Microsc. Morphol. Exp.* **1**, 366–373.

Raine, C. S., and Field, E. J. (1968). *Brain Res.* **10**, 266–268.

Ramón y Cajal, S. (1909). "Histologie du système nerveux de l'homme et des vertébrés" (Transl. by L. Azoulay), Vol. I, p. 200. Maloine, Paris.

Ramon y Cajal, S. (1911). "Histologie du système nerveux de l'homme et des vertébrés" (Transl. by L. Azoulay), Vol. II, p. 550. Maloine, Paris.

Ramsey, H. J. (1967). *Amer. J. Pathol.* **51**, 1093–1109.

Reichel, W., Hollander, J., Clark, H. J., and Strehler, B. L. (1968). *J. Gerontol.* **23**, 71–78.

Reissig, M., and Melnick, J. L. (1955). *J. Exp. Med.* **101**, 341–352.

Rewcastle, N. B., and Ball, M. J. (1968). *Neurology* **18**, 1205–1213.

Richardson, E. P. (1965). *In* "Parkinson's Disease, Trends in Research and Treatment" (A. Barbeau, L. J. Doshay, and E. A. Spiegel, eds.), pp. 63–68. Grune & Stratton, New York.

Roncoroni, L. (1895). *Arch. Psichiat.* **16**, 447–450.

Rosan, R. C., Nahmias, A. J., Kibrick, S., and Kerrigan, J. A. (1964). *Exp. Cell Res.* **36**, 611–624.

Roy, S., and Wolman, L. (1969). *J. Pathol.* **99**, 39–44.

Sakai, M., Austin, J., Witmer, F., and Trueb, L. (1969). *Arch. Neurol. (Chicago)* **21**, 526–544.

Sakai, M., Austin, J., Witmer, F., and Trueb, L. (1970). *Neurology* **20**, 160–176.

Samorajski, T., Keefe, J. R., and Ordy, J. M. (1964). *J. Gerontol.* **19**, 262–276.

Samorajski, T., Ordy, J. M., and Keefe, J. R. (1965). *J. Cell Biol.* **26**, 779–795.

Samorajski, T., Ordy, J. M., and Rady-Reimer, P. (1968). *Anat. Rec.* **160**, 555–573.

Schaffer, K. (1926). *Arch. Psychiat.* **77**, 675–679.

Schnabel, R., and Seitelberger, F. (1968). *Pathol. Eur.* **3**, 218–226.

Schnabel, R., and Seitelberger, F. (1969). *Acta Neuropathol.* **14**, 19–37.

Schochet, S. S., Jr. (1970). Unpublished observations.

Schochet, S. S., Jr., and Earle, K. M. (1970). *Acta Neuropathol.* **15**, 293–297.

Schochet, S. S., Jr., Lampert, P. W., and Earle, K. M. (1968a). *J. Neuropathol. Exp. Neurol.* **27**, 645–658.

Schochet, S. S., Jr., Lampert, P. W., and Lindenberg, R. (1968b). *Acta Neuropathol.* **11**, 330–337.

Schochet, S. S., Jr., Hardman, J. M., Ladewig, P. P., and Earle, K. M. (1969a). *Arch. Neurol. (Chicago)* **20**, 548–553.

Schochet, S. S., Jr., Lampert, P. W., and Earle, K. M. (1969b). *Exp. Neurol.* **23**, 113–119.

Schochet, S. S., Jr., McCormick, W. F., and Zellweger, H. (1970a). *Arch. Pathol.* **90**, 354–363.

Schochet, S. S., Jr., Wyatt, R. B., and McCormick, W. F. (1970b). *Arch. Neurol. (Chicago)* **22**, 550–555.

Schwarz, G. A., and Yanoff, M. (1965). *Arch. Neurol. (Chicago)* **12**, 172–188.

Seil, F. J., and Lampert, P. W. (1968). *Exp. Neurol.* **21**, 219–230.

Seil, F. J., Lampert, P. W., and Klatzo, I. (1969). *J. Neuropathol. Exp. Neurol.* **28**, 74–85.

Seïte, R. (1968a). *C. R. Acad. Sci.* **266**, 2444–2446.

Seïte, R. (1968b). *C. R. Soc. Biol.* **162**, 1972–1975.

Seïte, R. (1969a). *C. R. Acad. Sci.* **268**, 97–99.

Seïte, R. (1969b). *Z. Zellforsch. Mikrosk. Anat.* **101**, 621–646.

Seïte, R. (1970). *J. Ultrastruct. Res.* **30**, 152–165.

Seitelberger, F. (1966). *Proc. Int. Congr. Neuropathol.*, 5th, 1965, pp. 153–163.

Seitelberger, F. (1968). *In* "Pathology of the Nervous System" (J. Minckler, ed.), Vol. I, pp. 1121–1134. McGraw-Hill, New York.

Seitelberger, F. (1969a). *Acta Neurol.* **24**, 276–284.

Seitelberger, F. (1969b). *In* "Neurosciences Research" (S. Ehrenpreis and O. C. Solnitzky, eds.), Vol. 2, pp. 253–299, Academic Press, New York.

Seitelberger, F., Jacob, H., Peiffer, J., and Colmant, H. J. (1964). *Fortschr. Neurol. Psychiat.* **32**, 305–345.

Shantha, T. R., Manocha, S. L., Bourne, G. H., and Kappers, J. A. (1969). *In* "The Structure and Function of Nervous Tissue" (G. H. Bourne, ed.), Vol. 2, pp. 1–67. Academic Press, New York.

Shelanski, M. L., and Taylor, E. W. (1970). *Alzheimer's Dis. Related Conditions, Ciba Found. Symp.* pp. 249–266.

Shelanski, M. L., and Wisniewski, H. (1969). *Arch. Neurol. (Chicago)*, **20**, 199–206.

Shiraki, H. (1968). *In* "International Academy of Pathology Monograph, The Central Nervous System" (O. T. Bailey and D. E. Smith, eds.), pp. 252–272. Williams & Wilkins, Baltimore, Maryland.

Shiraki, H., and Yamamoto, T. (1962). *Proc. Int. Congr. Neuropathol.*, *4th*, 1961, pp. 173–179.

Siegesmund, K. A., Dutta, C. R., and Fox, C. A. (1964). *J. Anat.* **98**, 93–97.

Sluga, E., and Stockinger, L. (1967). *Acta Neuropathol.* **7**, 201–217.

Smith, J. M., O'Leary, J. L., Harris, A. B., and Gay, A. J. (1964). *J. Comp. Neurol.* **123**, 357–378.

Solitare, G. B., and Lamarche, J. B. (1966). *Amer. J. Ment. Defic.* **70**, 840–848.

Sotelo, C., and Palay, S. L. (1968). *J. Cell Biol.* **36**, 151–179.

Steele, J. C., Richardson, J. C., and Olszewski, J. (1964). *Arch. Neurol. (Chicago)* **10**, 333–359.

Strehler, B. L. (1964). *Advan. Gerontol. Res.* **1**, 343–384.

Sulkin, N. M. (1953). *J. Gerontol.* **8**, 435–445.

Sulkin, N. M., and Srivanij, P. (1960). *J. Gerontol.* **15**, 2–9.

Sulkin, N. M., and Sulkin, D. F. (1967). *J. Gerontol.* **22**, 485–501.

Sung., J. H., Meyers, J. P., Stadlan, E. M., Cowen, D., and Wolf, A. (1969). *J. Neuropathol. Exp. Neurol.* **28**, 86–118.

Swanson, J. L., Craighead, J. E., and Reynolds, E. S. (1966). *Lab. Invest.* **15**, 1966–1981.

Szlachta, H. L., and Habel, R. E. (1953). *Cornell Vet.* **43**, 207–212.

Takei, Y., and Mirra, S. S. (1971). *Acta Neuropathol.* **17**, 14–23.

Terry, R. D. (1963). *J. Neuropathol. Exp. Neurol.* **22**, 629–642.

Terry, R. D., (1968). *In* "International Academy of Pathology Monograph, The Central Nervous System" (O. T. Bailey and D. E. Smith, eds.), pp. 213–224. Williams & Wilkins, Baltimore, Maryland.

Terry, R. D., and Peña, C. (1965). *J. Neuropathol. Exp. Neurol.* **24**, 200–210.

Terry, R. D., and Wisniewski, H. (1970). *Alzheimer's Dis. Related Conditions, Ciba Found. Symp.* pp. 145–168.

Terry, R. D., Gonatas, N. K., and Weiss, M. (1964). *Amer. J. Pathol.* **44**, 269–297.

Toga, M., Dubois, D., and Hassoun, J. (1968). *Acta Neuropathol.* **10**, 132–142.

Trétiakoff, C. (1919). Cited by Greenfield and Bosanquet (1953).

van Bogaert, L., and Bertrand, I. (1926). *Arch. Neurol. Psychiat.* **16**, 263–284.

Vanderhaeghen, J.-J. (1971). *Acta Neuropathol.* **17**, 24–36.

Vanderhaeghen, J.-J., Périer, O., and Sternon, J. E. (1970). *Arch. Neurol. (Chicago)* **22**, 207–214.

van Heycop ten Ham, M. W. (1965). *Arch. Neurobiol.* **28**, 647–666.

van Heycop ten Ham, M. W., and de Jager, H. (1963). *Epilepsia* **4**, 95–119.

van Hoof, F., and Hageman-Bal, M. (1967). *Acta Neuropathol.* **7**, 315–326.

von Braunmühl, A. (1949). *Arch. Psychiat. Nervenkr.* **181**, 543–576.

von Braunmühl, A. (1957). *In* "Handbuch der speziellen pathologischen Anatomie und Histologie" (O. Lubarsch, F. Henke, and R. Rössle, eds.), Vol. 13, Part 1A, pp. 337–539. Springer-Verlag, Berlin and New York.

Weber, A. F., and Frommes, S. P. (1963). *Science* **141**, 912–913.

Weber, A., Whipp, S., Usenik, E., and Frommes, S. (1964). *J. Ultrastruct. Res.* **11**, 564–576.

Weinmann, R. L. (1967). *Neurology* **17**, 597–603.

White, J. G. (1968). *Amer. J. Pathol.* **53**, 447–461.

Williams, H. W. (1935). *Arch. Neurol. Psychiat.* **34**, 508–519.

Wisniewski, H., and Terry, R. D. (1967). *Lab. Invest.* **17**, 577–587.

Wisniewski, H., and Terry, R. D. (1970). *Alzheimer's Dis. Related Conditions, Ciba Found. Symp.* pp. 223–248.

Wisniewski, H., Karczewski, W., and Wisniewska, K. (1966). *Acta Neuropathol.* **6**, 211–219.

Wisniewski, H., Narkiewicz, O., and Wisniewska, K. (1967). *Acta Neuropathol.* **9**, 127–133.

Wisniewski, H., Shelanski, M. L., and Terry, R. D. (1968). *J. Cell Biol.* **38**, 224–229.

Wisniewski, H., Terry, R. D., and Hirano, A. (1970). *J. Neuropathol. Exp. Neurol.* **29**, 163–176.

Wisotzkey, H. M., and Moossy, J. (1971). *Abstr. 47th Annu. Meeting Amer. Ass. Neuropathol.*

Wolf, A., and Orton, S. T. (1932). *Bull. Neurol. Inst. New York* **2**, 194–209.

Woodard, J. S. (1962a). *J. Neuropathol. Exp. Neurol.* **21**, 85–91.

Woodard, J. S. (1962b). *J. Neuropathol. Exp. Neurol.* **21**, 442–449.

Wyatt, R. B., Schochet, S. S., Jr., and McCormick, W. F. (1970). *Arch. Otolaryngol.* **92**, 32–39.

Yanoff, M., and Schwarz, G. A. (1965). *Trans. Amer. Acad. Ophthalmol. Otolaryngol.* **69**, 701–708.

Yokoi, S., Austin, J., Witmer, F., and Sakai, M. (1968). *Arch. Neurol. (Chicago)* **19**, 15–33.

Yuen, P., and Baxter, D. W. (1963). *J. Neurol., Neurosurg. Psychiat.* **26**, 178–183.

Zeman, W., and Alpert, M. (1963). *Ann. Histochim.* **8**, 255–257.

Zeman, W., and Donahue, S. (1968). *Pathol. Eur.* **3**, 332–340.

Zeman, W., and Dyken, P. (1969). *Pediatrics* **44**, 570–583.

Zeman, W., and Hoffman, J. (1962). *J. Neurol., Neurosurg. Psychiat.* **25**. 352–362.

5

Ribonucleic Acid of Nervous Tissue

EDWARD KOENIG[1]

I. General Aspects of RNA in Nervous Tissue 179
   A. Introduction 179
   B. Brain Tissue RNA 180
   C. Cellular RNA 182
   D. RNA Changes during the Life Cycle 189
II. RNA Metabolism 191
   A. Uptake of RNA Precursors 191
   B. Analysis of RNA Classes Synthesized 193
III. Induced Changes in RNA 200
   A. Effects of Functional Activity 201
   B. Effects of Axotomy 205
   C. Other Effects 206
IV. Special Considerations 208
   A. Origin of Axonal RNA 208
   B. Future Prospects 210
   References 211

I. General Aspects of RNA in Nervous Tissue

A. INTRODUCTION

A prominent histological feature of nerve cells stained with basic aniline dyes is the Nissl or tigroid substance. At the turn of the century Barker (1899), in his monumental book on the nervous system, detailed

[1] The author is the recipient of a Research Career Program Award (NB 14254) from the National Institute of Neurological Diseases and Stroke.

the first systematic histochemical analysis of Nissl substance by Held, stating finally "that the Nissl bodies belong to the group of nucleo-albumins." Referring to the subsequent analysis of McCallum and Scott, he notes that these workers also concluded that Nissl's "stainable substance [was] of a nucleoproteid" nature (Barker, 1899). Moreover, Scott (1898), based on his studies of nerve cells in the ventral horn in pig embryos, surmised that Nissl bodies were derived from the nerve cell nucleus, clearly a discerning observation in view of present day knowledge.

Thus, at a time in the history of neuroscience when the acrimony surrounding the neuron doctrine was at its peak, the essential chemical character of Nissl substance had been deduced. However, it is doubtful that an appreciation of the chemical composition of the "nucleins" extended beyond the simple recognition at the time that they were non-dialyzable, multibasic phosphorous-containing acids.

The modern era in nucleic acid neurochemistry may be said to have had its origin with the classic work of Hydén (Landström *et al.*, 1941; Hydén, 1943), utilizing the scanning microspectrophotographic techniques of the Caspersson school. In the tradition of a cytological approach, Jan-Erik Edström (1953, 1958, 1960) later made important contributions to the quantitative and qualitative analyses of nucleic acid at the cellular level. Indeed, much of what is presently known about RNA content and base composition of isolated cellular material derives principally from the methods and techniques he developed in the Göteborg Laboratory.

B. Brain Tissue RNA

The practice of basing tissue nucleic acid concentration on phosphorous content was introduced by Chargaff and Zamenhof (1948) and was predicated by the need to make comparisons among various nucleic acids of different sources and purity. On the basis of such analyses, Logan *et al.* (1952) found that cerebral cortex from dog brain contained 10.3 mg P/100 gm wet weight, while white matter contained about half of that amount, viz., 4.9 mg P/100 gm. The sciatic nerve of the cat was similar to that of brain white matter, containing 4.7 mg P/100 gm. The corresponding grey and white matter values for monkey (Bodian and Dziewiatkowski, 1950) were for caudate nucleus, 11.5 mg P/100 gm and, for corpus callosum, 6.4 mg P/100 gm.

More recent data from May and Grenell (1959) and from Mandel *et al.* (1964), using several methods for analysis, show somewhat higher values but are nonetheless comparable. They range in the rabbit, for example, from 6.5 mg P/100 gm for cerebellar white matter to 19.5 mg P/100 gm for the olfactory bulb; most cell-rich structures, however, fall in the range of 11–15 mg P/100 gm tissue. Estimations of RNA of whole rat brain by Winick and Noble (1966) based simply on RNA mass concentration yields a calculated value from their data of 236 mg RNA/100 gm. This value is higher than the corresponding value converted from published RNA-P concentrations. Data from Bondy (1966) indicates a value

TABLE I

NUCLEIC ACIDS IN WHOLE BRAIN OF VARIOUS VERTEBRATES[a]

	RNA-P (μg/100 mg wet weight)	DNA-P (μg/100 mg wet weight)	PP (μg/100 mg wet weight)	RNA-P / DNA-P	RNA-P / Dipl. DNA-P
Trout	13.4	15.2	7.0	0.88	0.48
Carp	14.6	14.2	—	1.02	0.36
Newt	10.0	34.3	10.0	0.29	—
Frog	7.3	9.4	7.3	0.78	1.17
Turtle	13.1	6.2	6.5	2.11	1.06
Grass snake	13.0	6.3	10.0	2.06	1.03
Chicken	8.8	2.4	9.7	2.00	0.44
Rat	11.1	8.5	10.6	1.30	0.74
Guinea pig	11.5	9.3	14.5	1.35	0.81
Rabbit	10.4	7.5	12.4	1.39	0.74

[a] Mandel et al. (1964).

of about 180 mg RNA/100 gm wet tissue, which represents an average of the sum of RNA concentrations obtained for purified subcellular fractions. The two sets of values probably can be regarded as upper and lower limits, respectively, of brain RNA concentration.

A survey of brain RNA-P from various animals spanning the vertebrate scale by Mandel et al. (1964) shows little difference among the classes analyzed (Table I). The absence of any phylogenetic relationship is self-evident from the data.

C. Cellular RNA

From a classical point of view, RNA was believed to be restricted to the nerve cell nucleus and to the cytoplasm of the perikaryon and basal regions of dendrites. Such a distribution was based mainly on staining of the structural counterpart of RNA, viz., Nissl bodies. In the light microscope, distal reaches of dendrites showed little or no evidence of Nissl substance, but the axonal process was unique in exhibiting a total lack of basophilia, an observation first noted by Schaffer in 1893. Although ribosomes were observed electronmicroscopically throughout the cytoplasm of dendrites and have been used as a criterion of a post-synaptic structure, their absence in axoplasm has been verified repeatedly on the electronmicroscopic level since the initial observations of Palay and Palade (1955). In the motoneuron of the monkey, Bodian (1965) has reported what appeared to be a nonrandom distribution of ribosomes in close apposition to the sub-synaptic membrane of large synapses in the proximal region of dendrites.

Early attempts to ascertain whether the axon contains RNA by ultraviolet (uv) microspectrophotometry resulted in negative findings (Nurnberger *et al.*, 1952). However, evidence suggestive of a local synthesis of acetylcholinesterase in the axon (E. Koenig and Koelle, 1961; Clouet and Waelsch, 1961) prompted J.-E. Edström to examine the giant axon of the Mauthner neuron in goldfish. Direct microanalysis of Carnoy-fixed axons, dissected free of myelin, demonstrated unequivocally the presence of RNA in the axon (J.-E. Edström *et al.*, 1962). Indeed, a comprehensive study of RNA in the Mauthner axon carried out by A. Edström later (1964) showed that the total RNA content of the axon exceeded that of the cell body by a factor of 4 in the specimens analyzed, notwithstanding a RNA concentration (w/v) in the axon that was about $\frac{1}{20}$ of that in the perikaryon. The concentration along the axon was not constant but decreased from 0.05 to 0.03% along the proximal two-thirds and then increased again distally to reach a value of 0.07% at the terminals. Topographical differences in RNA concentration were not observed, however, in the giant axons of the crayfish abdominal nerve cord, which had an average concentration of 0.02% (Andersson *et al.*, 1970). Axons from the stretch receptor neuron of the lobster also had a similar concentration of 0.06% (Grampp and Edström, 1963). In still another axon type, Lasek (1970) demonstrated RNA in the giant axon of the squid. Concentration, calculated on the basis of his data indicate again that it is of the same order of magnitude, viz., 0.02–0.03%. On a unit length basis, he found RNA amounts equal between axoplasm and Schwann sheath; on a protein basis, the sheath contained four times as much as axoplasm.

In mammals, the only axon studied to date has been taken from the spinal accessory nerve of the cat (E. Koenig, 1965) and the rabbit (E. Koenig, 1967a). Axons from this nerve showed an order of magnitude lower concentration (i.e., 0.003–0.006%). It has been suggested (E. Koenig, 1969) that concentration may be an inappropriate parameter as a measure of RNA for mammalian axons, where the surface-to-volume ratio is very high, because there is evidence that RNA is associated with synaptosomal membrane (Austin and Morgan, 1967; Balázs and Cocks, 1967) and the axolemma (E. Koenig, 1968). In the giant axons (Andersson *et al.* 1970) and in the mammalian axon (E. Koenig, 1970a), RNA is primarily extramitochondrial in distribution.

Base composition of the several axonal systems studied is compared in Table II. Points to be made are (a) base composition is very similar between myelin sheath (which contain no glial cell nuclei) and axon of Mauthmer fiber; (b) based on the adenine/guanine ratio, the Mauthner axon and the axon from the cat spinal accessory nerve are quite similar but very different from that of the crayfish axon; and (c) the adenine/guanine ratios of the former two are characteristic of a ribosomal type (see below), whereas the high adenine-uracil content of crayfish axons signifies a DNA-like character. An important distinction to be made between various axons, however, is that the RNA analyses of Mauthner and mammalian axons included the axolemma, while the crayfish axonal analysis was on axoplasm only. Both estimations of concentration and base composition could be influenced by the exclusion of the axolemma if a significant proportion of RNA is associated with it.

Hydén has emphasized repeatedly that the large neuron is richly endowed with RNA, comparing favorably to that of exocrine pancreas cells, whose capacity for synthesizing protein is especially noteworthy. RNA concentration of various neuronal perikarya vary from 1–5.7% w/v (Table III). Some of the reported differences may well be real. However, the wide range of values is also indicative of the difficulties inherent in estimating cell volume accurately, owing to errors introduced by preparative procedures (e.g., fixation, nonisoosmotic conditions) and by imprecise measurements due to geometrical irregularities. Analyses of RNA concentration in freshly isolated cells yield considerably lower values (up to 50% lower) than is often the case with fixed material (Hydén, 1960).

On the basis of his analysis of anterior horn cells from the rabbit, J.-E. Edström (1956) concluded that there was a direct proportionality

TABLE II

COMPARATIVE ASPECTS OF RNA OF DENUDED AXONS AND AXONAL SHEATH

Source	Content (pg/μ)	Concentration (%; w/v)	A	G	C	U	A/G	Refs.[a]
Axon: Mauthner neuron (goldfish)	0.15	0.03–0.07	18.3	38.6	25.5	18.0	0.56	(1)
Myelin sheath: Mauthner axon	0.2		20.9	37.6	23.4	18.0	0.60	(1)
Med. and Lat. axons: abdominal nerve cord (crayfish)	1–2	0.02	30.3	21.7	13.6	34.6		(2)
Schwann sheath: nerve cord	2–2.5	0.22	28.1	27.4	15.5	29.1		(2)
Axon: spinal accessory (cat)	0.002	0.006					0.57	(3)

[a] Key to refs. (1) A. Edström (1964). (2) Andersson *et al.* (1970). (3) Koenig (1965).

between surface area of the nerve cell body and its RNA content. A proportionality was observed also between the volume of the nucleolus and the RNA content of the cells from nucleus supraopticus in the rat (J.-E. Edström and Eichner, 1958). In light of the fact that the bulk of cytoplasmic RNA is ribosomal and what is presently known about the nucleolus as a site of ribosomal synthesis, the relationship between nucleolar volume and RNA content of a cell is readily understandable.

There is a paucity of quantitative data on the RNA content of various glial cell types, owing primarily to the difficulty in obtaining pure, morphologically well-defined samples. On the basis of a modified, selective Nissl staining procedure, H. Koenig (1964) has estimated that oligodendrocytes have RNA concentrations several fold higher than that of nerve cells. Schwann cells and ganglion satellite cells similarly stain intensely, in contrast to astrocytes, which hardly exhibit discernable staining. Ultraviolet cytospectrophotometric studies (Pevzner, 1965) have indicated that satellite cells of the cat superior cervical ganglion do contain a rather high RNA concentration (Table III).

The preponderance of RNA in the nerve cell is generally of the ribosomal type, which is distributed throughout the cytoplasm of the perikaryon and dendrites but not the axons (see above). According to Mahler *et al.* (1966) about 80% of the total RNA of rat brain is ribosomal. In certain neurons, such as the large ones from Deiters nucleus, cytoplasmic RNA can represent more than 95% of the total RNA (Table III).

Purified RNA, extracted from large and small subunits of ribosomes, fall into three classes characterized by their sedimentation coefficients ($s_{20,w}$) (Table IV). The large subunit yields a 28 S component and a 5 S component; the small subunit contains a 17–18 S component. All three classes of RNA have high molar proportions of guanine and cytosine (Table IV), yielding a guanine + cytosine/adenine + uracil that is usually greater than 1.2. Since ribosomal RNA generally predominates in the cell, the average base composition of the cell's RNA would reflect it (Table III). However, there are examples of cells in Table III that do not meet this expectation and depart significantly from the usual 28–37% cytosine or guanine. Assuming that random and/or systematic errors were not operating in those instances, other factors might have to be invoked, such as the relative contributions made by various nonribosomal subcellular fractions. However, considerations of this type do point out the limited usefulness of determining average base composition of a cell's total RNA, except in those instances where induced changes are sufficiently large, quantitatively, or extreme, in a qualitative sense, to reveal themselves.

TABLE III

A Survey of RNA Analysis of Nervous Tissue Cells

Source	Content (pg)	Refs.[a]	Concentration (%; w/v)	Refs.[a]	Molar proportions (%) A	G	C	U	Refs.[a]
Neuronal RNA									
Deiters (rabbit)	700–1550	(2)			18.6	30.1	29.2	22.0	(1)
Deiters (rabbit)			1.3–1.5 (unfixed)	(2)	19.7	33.5	28.8	18.0	(3)
Cell nucleus: Deiters (rabbit)	56	(4)	0.5	(5)	21.3	26.6	30.8	21.3	(4)
Anterior horn (rabbit)	540	(6)	2.5						
Anterior horn (rat)					21.6	30.4	24.9	23.3	(7)
Anterior horn (rat)					19.1	29.5	30.2	21.2	(8)
Hypoglossus (rabbit)	170–235	(9)	1.5 (unfixed)	(10)	21.1	24.8	31.9	22.2	(11)
			3.5 (fixed)		19.7	25.0	34.6	20.8	(12)
Hypoglossus (rat)	160	(7)			20.9	36.2	24.9	18.1	(7)
Purkinje, cerebellum (rabbit)	140–230	(13) (14)	2.1 (fixed)	(13)	20.7	29.6	27.8	21.9	(14)
Pyramidal, hippocampus (rat)	110	(15)			17.7	24.5	37.8	20.0	(15)
Cortex (rat)					18.2	25.5	36.3	20.0	(16)
Supraopticus (rat)	50–70	(17)			18.9	36.0	26.9	18.3	(17)

Sample	RNA content	Ref	RNA content (fixed)	Ref	Base composition				Ref
Paraventricularis (rat)					19.3	34.5	27.3	18.9	(17)
Gasserian gangl. (rat)					18.0	34.9	27.5	18.8	(17)
Stretch receptor (lobster)	2900				26.0	27.7	24.1	22.2	(18)
Abdominal cord gangl. (crayfish)	300–600		5.7 (fixed)		24.4	22.5	26.1	27.0	(19)
Spinal cord (goldfish)					21.1	32.5	26.5	20.0	(20)
Superior cervical gangl. (cat)	160	(21)	3.0 (fixed)	(21)					
Gangl. cell: retina (bovine)	25–100		1.2–2.0	(22)					
Nonneuronal RNA									
Glia: cortex (rat)					25.3	29.0	26.5	19.2	(23)
Glia: Deiters nucleus (rabbit)	15	(24)			20.8	28.8	31.8	18.6	(3)
Glia: anterior horn (rat)					25.8	27.3	25.4	21.6	(7)
Glia: sup. cerv. gangl. (cat)			5.4 (fixed)	(21)					
Rod cell: retina (rabbit)	0.65	(25)	0.36 (unfixed)	(25)	21.4	27.4	28.6	22.6	(25)
Rod cell nucleus (rabbit)	0.39	(25)	0.42 (unfixed)	(25)	24.4	25.8	26.5	23.3	(25)
Rod cell inner segment (rabbit)	0.26	(25)			16.9	29.7	31.7	21.7	(25)

[a] Key to Refs.: (1) E. Koenig (1968). (2) Hydén (1960). (3) Egyházi and Hydén (1961). (4) Hydén and Egyházi (1962a). (5) Hydén (1962). (6) J.-E. Edström (1956). (7) Slagel et al. (1966). (8) Hartman et al. (1968). (9) J.-E. Edström (1957). (10) Brattgard (1957). (11) J.-E. Edström (1957). (12) Daneholt and Brattgard (1966). (13) Jarlstedt (1962). (14) Jarlstedt (1966b). (15) Ringborg (1966). (16) Hydén and Lange (1965). (17) J.-E. Edström et al. (1961). (18) Grampp and Edström (1963). (19) Andersson et al. (1970). (20) J.-E. Edström et al. (1962). (21) Pevzner (1965). (22) J.-E. Edström and Eichner (1957). (23) Hydén and Egyházi (1963). (24) Hydén and Pigon (1960). (25) E. Koenig (1967b).

TABLE IV

CHARACTERISTICS OF RIBOSOMAL RNA FROM BRAIN

Class (s_{20})	Source	Concentration	A	G	C	U	Refs.[a]
17 S + 28 S	guinea pig brain		19.5	32.1	29.0	19.3	(1)
17 S + 28 S	mouse brain		18.7	32.4	27.2	21.8	(2)
4 S (5 S) + 17 S + 28 S	rat cortex	125 mg/100 gm	18.4	32.3	31.2	18.1	(3)
4 S (5 S)	rat cortex		19.8	32.2	28.3	19.7	(3)
17 S	rat cortex		19.0	31.9	30.1	18.0	(3)
28 S	rat cortex		17.4	35.0	30.3	17.3	(3)

[a] Key to Refs.: (1) Yamagami *et al.* (1965). (2) Kimberlin (1967). (3) Mahler *et al.* (1966).

D. RNA CHANGES DURING THE LIFE CYCLE

RNA content increases rapidly during the first few weeks postnatally in most vertebrates analyzed and tends to level off sharply thereafter (Mandel *et al.*, 1964). The increase in RNA from birth to adult levels varies from approximately 1.5- to 5-fold (Fig. 1). Presumably, the degree of neurological maturity at the time of birth may be a factor, as in the case of the guinea pig, for example. Generally, the RNA increase parallels that of DNA. Man, however, is an exception in this respect; brain RNA content increases 25-fold from birth to the adult, while DNA in-

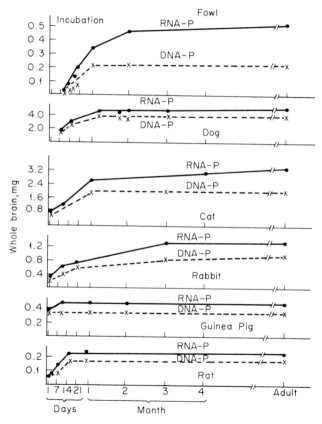

Fig. 1. Increase in RNA and DNA of the whole brain in different species of vertebrates during postnatal growth (rat, guinea pig, rabbit, dog, cat) or during incubation and after hatching (chicken). (From Mandel *et al.*, 1964, with permission of the publisher.)

creases only sevenfold, and at that, most of the DNA ($\approx 75\%$) is present at 10 months (Mandel *et al.*, 1964).

An analysis of pyramidal cells taken from the CA_3-region of the rat hippocampus showed significant differences in RNA content and base composition obtained at different periods of life (Table V). RNA content increased fourfold from the neonatal rat to the adult in this neuron type, only to diminish again in the senescent animal to about half of the maximum value. The overall base composition of the cell also showed definitive changes with age, but remained unchanged during prenatal and neonatal periods (Table V). Quantitative changes in RNA content of motoneurons in the human (Hydén, 1967a) showed a similar pattern to that seen in the rat, with a peak content occurring during adult middle age (Table V).

TABLE V

AGE DEPENDENT ANALYSES OF CELLS FROM HIPPOCAMPUS AND ANTERIOR HORN

Source	Age or period	Content (pg/cell)	A	G	C	U
pyramidal neuron:						
CA_3, hippocampus [a]	fetal rat	19	20.9	26.2	30.8	22.1
	neonatal rat	24	21.0	27.6	31.0	20.8
	adult rat	110	17.7	24.5	37.8	20.0
	senescent rat	53	14.9	29.0	36.9	19.3
motoneuron (man)[b]	0–20 years	402				
	21–40 years	553				
	41–60 years	640				
	61–80 years	504				
	80 years	420				

[a] Ringborg (1966)
[b] Hydén (1967a).

Some studies (Bernsohn and Norgello, 1966; Adams, 1966) indicate that the base composition of brain tissue ribosomal RNA may differ between the neonatal and the adult rat. Although the base ratio differences reported for the two age groups are small but statistically significant in each study, there are discrepancies between the two sets of results. Therefore, it would seem that a much larger series of determinations are necessary in order to establish whether the small differences are indeed real.

Murthy (1970) compared the ability of various ribosomal systems isolated from newborn and adult rat brain to support amino acid incorporation (i.e., synthesize protein). He concluded on the basis of his analysis that there are no inherent differences as regards to ribosome composition (i.e., as determined by its sedimentation characteristics) or amino acid incorporating capacity. The principal difference he noted between the neonatal and adult rats was that there was a higher proportion of membrane-bound polyribosomes (i.e., multiple ribosomes attached to a single messenger RNA strand) in the young brain with correspondingly lower proportions of "free" monomeric ribosomes (i.e., unattached). This was consistent with other findings on the rates of incorporation of labeled precursors into RNA of neonatal and adult rat brain slices; neonatal brain synthesized RNA at rates that were several times greater than adult (Orrego, 1967; Guroff et al., 1968; Itoh and Quastel, 1969).

II. RNA Metabolism

A. UPTAKE OF RNA PRECURSORS

Precursors that have been used to study RNA synthesis include ^{32}P, inorganic phosphorus; ^{3}H- or ^{14}C-orotic acid, a precursor of pyrimidines; ^{3}H- or ^{14}C-pyrimidine nucleosides, such as uridine and cytosine; and ^{3}H- or ^{14}C-purine bases, adenine and guanine and corresponding purine nucleosides. ^{3}H- or ^{14}C-thymidine is commonly used as a specific precursor of DNA. *In vivo* studies generally employ injections of precursor into the subarachnoid space or into a ventricle in order to bypass the blood–brain barrier and to exclude somatic organs that are metabolically active. While the intrathecal route insures high concentrations of precursor in brain tissue, the distribution is nonuniform, falling off significantly in the brain parenchyma with distance from the site of injection (Shimada and Nakamura, 1966; Hogenhuis and Spaulding, 1967). Shimada and Nakamura (1966) obtained labeled RNA throughout the whole neuraxis with subcutaneous injections of ^{3}H-uridine into neonatal mice. Subcutaneous injections into the adult animal (Leblond and Amano, 1962), albeit with ^{3}H-cytidine, resulted in poor uptake in the CNS, suggesting that this particular route is suitable only in the very young animal when the blood–brain barrier is not yet fully developed.

The early studies, utilizing the intrathecal route for injection of precursors (H. Koenig, 1958a,b), made it evident that nervous tissue was actively engaged in RNA turnover, contrary to earlier reports in which there had been a lack of appreciation for the importance of the blood–brain barrier. This was true not only for grey matter, as might have been anticipated, but for white matter as well. Such observations led to the conclusion that interfasicular oligodendrocytes share with neurons the characteristic of an active RNA metabolism (H. Koenig, 1958a,b). Microanalysis of RNA extracted from nerve cells and adjacent glia from the hypoglossal nucleus of the rabbit indicated that the specific radioactivity of bases from glial RNA was much higher than that from nerve cells (Daneholt and Brattgård, 1966). Compared with liver in the rat, brain RNA metabolism is about one-third the rate, according to von Hungen *et al.* (1968), which is undoubtedly due to the more rapid rate of turnover of RNA of all classes. Nonetheless, the rate in nervous tissue is quite high for a tissue lacking a large population of dividing cells.

Autoradiographic studies (H. Koenig, 1958b; Leblond and Amano, 1962; Shimada and Nakamura, 1966) have provided graphic evidence of a fundamental axiom of eucaryotic biology; namely, that RNA precursors are initially incorporated into macromolecular RNA in the nucleus, the principal repository of the cell's DNA. Fractionation studies (see below) have verified this repeatedly. Reduced silver grains appear initially over the nucleoplasm and nucleolus, with the latter structure exhibiting the highest grain density. Subsequently, the grains begin to appear over the cytoplasm, and their number increases with time, while the grain density over the nucleus declines (Fig. 2). Long-term autoradiographic studies indicate that cells retain significant amounts of labeling, even beyond 50 days (H. Koenig, 1958b; Hogenhuis and Spaulding, 1967). This has led to the suggestion that there is a reutilization of degradation products of rapidly turning over RNA for synthesis of more stable RNA (Hogenhuis and Spaulding, 1967) and for DNA synthesis of slowly dividing glial cells (H. Koenig, 1958a,b).

Although reutilization of labeled degraded products very likely occurs, on the basis of theoretical considerations (von Hungen *et al.*, 1968), it is not regarded to be significant enough to invalidate estimations of turnover rates based on radioactive decay of labeled RNA. Two definitive studies bearing on the question of turnover rates of brain RNA have been carried out by Bondy (1966) and von Hungen *et al.* (1968) in rats. Both studies agree that the half-life of cytoplasmic RNA is approximately 12–12.5 days, corresponding to a turnover rate of about $0.17\%/$ hour, a value close to $0.2\%/$hour calculated also by Kimberlin (1967). von Hungen and co-workers (1968) provided evidence that the ribosome, which is composed of about 40% RNA and 60% protein (Palade, 1964),

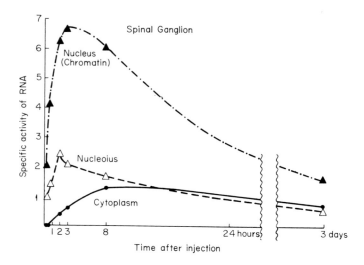

Fig. 2. Specific activity of nuclear RNA (dark triangles), nucleolar RNA (light triangles) and cytoplasmic RNA (dots) in spinal ganglion cells at various time intervals after cytidine-^{3}H injection. Nucleolar RNA behaves as the precursor of cytoplasmic RNA. (From Leblond and Amano, 1962, courtesy of the authors.)

turns over as a unit. This was consistent with findings from nonnervous tissue that newly synthesized ribosomal RNA leaves the nucleus as part of intact subunits (Girard *et al.*, 1964; Perry, 1965) with their complements of associated protein. Both soluble (i.e., 4 S) and mitochondrial RNA fractions showed RNA components that turn over at more rapid rates (Fig. 3). Nuclear RNA showed heterogenous decay rates, containing components with very short and long half-lives. Indeed, von Hungen *et al.* (1968) observed that up to 5 % of the radioactivity was still associated with the nuclear fraction after 84 days, corroborating autoradiographic findings (see above).

B. ANALYSIS OF RNA CLASSES SYNTHESIZED

Fractionation and separation of RNA into different classes, depending on molecular weight and composition, has involved the use of three principal techniques, viz., methylated albumin–kieselghur column chromatography, ultracentrifugation in linear density sucrose gradients, and electrophoresis in porous acrylamide-agarose gels. The relatively recent introduction of the use of gel electrophoresis for the separation of macromolecular RNA by Tsanev (1965), Loening (1967), and Dingman and

Peacock (1968) has already gained wide recognition as having the best resolving powers of any of the methods presently employed.

In brain tissue a number of studies have centered around (a) a characterization of RNA classes synthesized in the nucleus, (b) an analysis of precursor–product transformation in the nucleus, and (c) a study of kinetics of RNA transfer from the nucleus to the cytoplasm (Jacob *et al.*, 1966, 1967; Vesco and Giuditta, 1967; Kimberlin, 1967; Balázs and Cocks 1967; Murthy, 1968; Takahashi *et al.*, 1969; Tencheva and Hadjiolov, 1969; Saborio and Alemán, 1970; Løvtrup-Rein, 1970; Løvtrup-Rein and Grahn, 1970; R. P. Peterson, 1970). Some of the salient findings are summarized below.

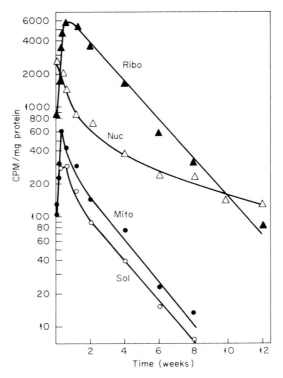

Fig 3. Time course of the RNA label originally injected as 2.5 μCi of 6-¹⁴C-orotic acid in fractions isolated from rat brain cortex: ribosomal (Ribo), nuclear (Nuc), mitochondrial (Mito), and soluble (Sol). Each *time point* is based on pooled homogenate from 10 brains. Note that up to 2 weeks the turnover of RNA from the mitochondrial and soluble fractions is markedly quicker than that from the ribosomal fraction. (From von Hungen *et al.*, 1968, courtesy of the authors and permission of the publisher.)

1. Synthesis of Ribosomal and Transfer RNA

The nucleolus of eucaryotic cells had been shown by several investigators to be the site of ribosomal and transfer RNA synthesis (for review, see Perry, 1967). The 28 S and 18 S ribosomal RNA components of the cytoplasm are synthesized initially in the nucleolus as parts of a high molecular weight precursor, sedimenting at 45 S in the ultracentrifuge (Scherrer and Darnell, 1962; Rake and Graham, 1964; Penman, 1966). The 45 S precursor then undergoes cleavage in the nucleolus to yield short-lived intermediates (i.e., 41 S, 36 S) that ultimately become converted to 32 S, and finally to 28 S (Weinberg et al., 1967). The 18 S ribosomal component is derived from a short-lived 20 S precursor that is split off early in the processing of the 45 S (Weinberg et al., 1967). The 45 S and 32 S ribosomal precursors have been identified in brain tissue (Vesco and Giuditta, 1967; Tencheva and Hadjiolov, 1969; Saborio and Alemán, 1970; Løvtrup-Rein, 1970) in addition to a 38 S (Løvtrup-Rein, 1970). The origin of the 5 S ribosomal component and the 4 S transfer RNA is less well understood, but the synthesis of these classes in the nucleolus are apparently independent of that of the 45 S precursor (Perry and Kelley, 1968).

The appearance of ribosomal RNA components in the cytoplasm is delayed, owing to the sequence of steps involving the synthesis of the 45 S precursor, transformation of the 45 S to 28 S and to 18 S components, and finally, the transfer of the two components to the cytoplasm. The earliest reported indication of labeling in the cytoplasm occurs in the 18 S component 30 minutes after injection (Jacob et al., 1967). Cytoplasmic transfer RNA (tRNA), on the other hand, shows evidence of labeling as early as 20 minutes following intracerebral injection (Saborio and Alemán, 1970). At 1 hour after injection, both 28 S and 18 S show more discernable evidence of labeling, and continue to increase in radioactivity such that at 6 hours the 28 S and 18 S peaks are labeled quite prominantly.

The temporal relationship in the labeling patterns of nuclear and cytoplasmic RNA can be seen in Fig. 4, which is taken from the study of Saborio and Alemán (1970). These investigators used a double labeling technique, utilizing two types of precursors to differentiate the synthesis of ribosomal RNA (rRNA) from that of total RNA. Both rRNA and tRNA classes contain a certain proportion of methylated bases. Methylation occurs during the synthesis of the 45 S precursor (Muramatsu and Fujisawa, 1968). Each rat was injected with ^{14}C-uridine and ^{3}H-methyl-methionine, with the latter serving as a methyl donor for the methylation reaction. On the basis of their analysis, Saborio and Alemán (1970) estimated that the times required for passage of rRNA from the nucleus were 26 minutes for the 18 S and 33 minutes for the 28 S components, respectively. Inspection of Figs. 4 and 2 will show an interesting parallel between the form of the tritium specific radioactivity curves of the two figures, i.e., loss of specific radioactivity over the nucleolus (Fig. 2) and that of the [3H]-methyl labeled rRNA (Fig. 4). Although there are differences in the times to reach peak specific radioactivity, such differences might well exist between spinal ganglion cells and cells of the CNS (see below). The similar shapes of the decay curves are notable and provide complementary morphological and biochemical verification of the nucleolar origin of ribosomal RNA.

On the basis of hybridization experiments, rRNA is complementary to approximately 0.15% of the DNA (Stévenin *et al.*, 1968), corresponding to about 6000 cistrons coding for the 28 S components. The large redundancy led Stévenin *et al.* (1968) to suggest the existence of either many nucleolar organizers or one nucleolar organizer with many cistrons coding for rRNA.

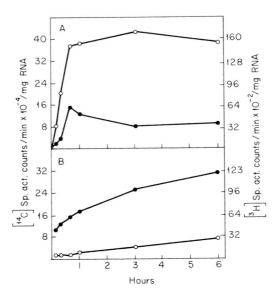

Fig. 4. Specific activity of total RNA from nuclear (A) and cytoplasmic (B) fractions. — ○ —, [14C] specific activity (uridine-14C); — ● —, [3H] specific activity (methyl-methionine-3H). (From Saborio and Alemán, 1970, courtesy of the authors.)

2. Synthesis of Messenger RNA

The synthesis of messenger (mRNA) in brain has received attention by several investigators. However, mRNA is defined operationally by the fact that it specifies particular polypeptides encoded in the genome, a function ordinarily impossible to demonstrate in practice. This causes difficulties in identifying the synthesis of this class with certainty and has led to the use of a number of criteria as a basis of identification. The following are the salient characteristics of mRNA: (1) Its synthesis is dependent on DNA, requiring a chromatin-associated RNA polymerase. (2) Its synthesis is rapid and undelayed. (3) Its base composition is low in guanine-cytosine content, while the proportions of adenine and uracil are high, conferring a DNA-like composition to it (dRNA). (4) Its sedimentation characteristics are broad and poorly defined (i.e., polydisperse in a linear density gradient), reflecting a wide spectrum of molecular weights. (5) It is able to form double stranded hybrids with DNA (i.e., base pairing between corresponding complementary base sequences of RNA and DNA). (6) It is associated with ribosomes, forming polysomal aggregates during the translation process. (7) As part of the polysomes, it exhibits a high degree of susceptibility to low concentrations of ribonuclease, owing to the fact that it is single-stranded and not complexed to protein. (8) It shows a capacity to stimulate amino acid incorporation in an *in vitro* ribosomal system.

At early intervals (< 1 hour) following intrathecal injection, extraction of nuclear RNA yields a radioactivity profile in a linear density gradient that is polydisperse in character (i.e., 8–80 S), with a large proportion sedimenting ahead of 28 S; this RNA is DNA-like in base composition (Jacob et al., 1966; Egyházi and Hydén, 1966; Vesco and Giuditta, 1967; Murthy, 1968). Because of the uncertainty of its messenger function, the designation "dRNA" is regarded as a more acceptable denotation for this nondescript nuclear DNA-like RNA. Hybridization experiments (Stévenin et al., 1968; Bondy and Roberts, 1968) show that a certain proportion of nuclear dRNA apparently never reaches the cytoplasm but remains restricted to the nucleus. According to Stévenin et al. (1969), the nuclear restricted portion amounts to 35% of the total dRNA. The functional significance of this nuclear restricted RNA is unknown at present. The total nuclear dRNA is complementary to approximately 1.2% of the homologus DNA (Stévenin et al., 1968, 1969).

Sedimentation analysis of mRNA in the cytoplasm is generally based upon short pulse-labeling experiments of less than 1 hour to minimize labeling of ribosomal components. Pulse-labeled RNA associated with polysomes shows a polydisperse character, ranging from 4–40 S (Jacob et al., 1967; Takahashi et al., 1969), although sedimentation values of up to 80 S have been reported (Vesco and Giuditta, 1967). On the other hand, there is evidence that dRNA in the cytoplasm is distributed principally in the 4–18 S region of the gradient (Samec et al., 1967; Murthy, 1968). The cytoplasmic dRNA represents 65 % of the total dRNA and will hybridize with about 0.8 % of homologous DNA (Stévenin et al., 1969). Making certain assumptions regarding the size of polypeptide chains synthesized, these authors estimated that 30,000–300,000 cistrons coded for mRNA in rat brain. This estimate was regarded as conservative because only the more redundant DNA sequences would be assayed with the methods employed.

Recent evidence indicates that mRNA may be transferred to the cytoplasm from the nucleus in the form of ribonucleoprotein complexes (dRNP) (Samec et al., 1967, 1968). These dRNP particles are associated with the microsomal fraction and are released with treatment by sodium deoxycholate. They exhibit a higher specific radioactivity than that of the polysomes for up to 2 hours; thus, the possibility exists that they may represent occult mRNA in transit. Subribosomal RNP particles have been found in other tissue microsomal fractions, and mRNA transport function ascribed to them, but the evidence at best is circumstantial (see Samec et al., 1968). The dRNP particles sediment in a polydisperse fashion, ranging from 20–60 S, and the dRNA associated with them exhibits a polydisperse pattern of 8–15 S, characteristic of mRNA that supports amino acid incorporation into ribosomal proteins in vitro (Bondy and Roberts, 1967; Samli and Roberts, 1969).

The half-lives calculated for hybridizable RNA in the adult rat brain range from 2.5 hours to 5 days (Bondy and Roberts, 1968). Based on studies using actinomycin D and labeled amino acid incorporation into brain slices of the rat in vitro, Orrego and Lipmann (1966) found a half-life for mRNA of 2.6 hours. Bondy and Roberts (1968) compared the hybridizability of newly synthesized RNA between adult and neonatal rat, observing (a) that proportions of nuclear and cytoplasmic hybridizable RNA's are similar in the newborn and adult animals; however, (b) that the turnover rate in the former is greater. Therefore, it appeared that mRNA in the adult is relatively more stable than that in the immature. In vivo (see Roberts et al., 1970) and in vitro (Orrego and Lipmann, 1966) studies indicate that incorporation of amino acids into brain protein occurs at a rate in neonatal animals that is 1–2 orders of magnitude greater.

In comparison with liver, brain mRNA apparently constitutes a much greater proportion of the RNA synthesized, which is consistent with the finding that RNA polymerase activity is also higher in brain (Bondy and Waelsch, 1965).

3. *Analysis of RNA Synthesized Based on Cell Type*

Hetereogeneity of cell types in the nervous system has long been widely recognized and appreciated from the earliest days of neurohistology. The microanalytical approaches and cellular fractionation procedures that have been developed in recent years reflect attempts to take cognizance of the fact that metabolic differences very likely exist among the specialized cell types of the nervous system.

A study by R. P. Peterson (1970), using agarose gel electrophoresis to characterize the RNA synthesized in specific cells of the abdominal ganglion of *Aplysia*, a mollusk, reflects a cellular orientation. The *Aplysia* has special advantages insofar as some of the cell bodies are gigantic (e.g., 400–800 μ in diameter) and the function of many specified. However, the neuronal network is based on axo-axonal synapses and the cell bodies are excluded as intervening elements in the transmission of excitation, similar to that of vertebrate spinal ganglion cells. Peterson, analyzing nuclear and cytoplasmic RNA's separately from microdissected cells, was able to resolve several high molecular weight RNA species from the nuclear extracts that were believed to represent precursor rRNA in this invertebrate, i.e., 38 S instead of 45 S (see above). In addition, he observed what appeared to be transition peaks corresponding to 31 S and 21 S precursors to 27 S and 18 S, respectively. After 30 minutes of incubation, there was also a labeled polydisperse cytoplasmic RNA in the range of 6–12 S that was found to turn over very rapidly. Significant differences were also noted in the rates at which the final 27 S and 18 S rRNA products, in addition to a 14 S RNA fraction reached the cytoplasm of two different cell types of the same ganglion. Based on autoradiographic analysis, Watson (1965) also observed significant differences in the ratio of cytoplasmic/nuclear grain counts of various cell types, especially after several hours. The existence of such distinctions between various cell types have been considered already in the context of comparing Figs. 2 and 4 (see above).

Perhaps the most extreme example of a delay in the transfer of RNA from the nucleus to the cytoplasm is that of the rod cell of rat retina. In this cell type the cytoplasm is limited to the inner segment, which is in the form of an appendage, physically removed from the nucleus to varying degrees, depending on the relative position of the cell in the outer nuclear layer. Significant labeling of inner segment RNA was apparent 2–3 hours after intraocular injection, and at that time it was associated with the 4 S region. At 18 hours, the picture remained unchanged; however, at 24 hours the ribosomal peaks were labeled maximally. The levels of labeling (i.e., rRNA) remained unchanged up to 20 days after intraocular injection, indicating an extremely low rate of turnover. The nuclear radioactivity profile also exhibited a stable labeling pattern that was transformed only at a slow rate compared to nervous tissue in general. At no time up to 20 days did the level of labeling in the inner segment exceed that of the nucleus (E. Koenig, 1971b). The metabolic picture is consistent with the absence of a discernible nucleolus and with the results of microanalysis of this cell type (E. Koenig, 1967a) (see Table III).

In a recent study, Løvtrup-Rein and Grahn (1970) fractionated rat nuclei derived from neurons, astrocytes, and "other glial cells," following an intracranial injection of labeled precursor. They observed similarities between neurons and astrocytes with regard to rate of intranuclear transformation of rRNA precursor; i.e., 45 S→38 S→35/32S + 18 S→28 S + 18 S. The nonastroglia (i.e., oligodendroglia and microglia, according to these authors) were significantly out of phase in terms of time of appearance of various species (i.e., the latter showed a much slower rate of appearance). In addition, there was evidence that the nonastrocytic glial population synthesized less RNA. RNA sedimenting at 25 S and 12 S and turning over rapidly was observed in nuclei from all cel types. These species with lower S values were postulated to be mRNA on the basis of analogy to other systems. Assuming no error in identification of cell types, some of these findings with respect to RNA synthesis of various glial cell types are inconsistent with conclusions drawn from cytological studies (see Section I,C.).

III. Induced Changes in RNA

Interests have long centered around changes in RNA associated with functional activity in the nervous system. Indeed, the high concentration of RNA in the nervous system coupled with the role of RNA in biology as a carrier of molecular information has provided circumstantial grounds for postulating that RNA is directly linked in some vague manner to information storage. Whatever the merits of the logic of the arguments put forward for this hypothesis, its greatest shortcoming lies in its failure thus far to accomodate well-established principles of neurophysiology. Until mechanisms can be postulated that are consonant with these established principles and experimental evidence gained to support them, it seems only reasonable that RNA changes associated with electrophysiological activity be interpreted as being due to secondary causes; i.e., altered metabolic demands arising from certain sectors of the metabolic economy whose rates of turnover are affected by functional activity.

A. EFFECTS OF FUNCTIONAL ACTIVITY

In vitro electrical stimulation of rat brain cortex slices produced a 40% decrease in the rate of RNA synthesis (Orrego, 1967). This occurred in the absence of a change in the rate of RNA breakdown. The inhibition of RNA synthesis under these conditions was traced to a diminished rate in the phosphorylation of uridine diphosphate (UDP), presumably because ATP was diverted to other nonsynthetic reactions of higher priority (e.g., ionic transport processes). Itoh and Quastel (1969) have shown that the rate of RNA synthesis in brain slices *in vitro* is directly dependent on endogenous ATP, and the ATP levels will vary depending on type of substrate supporting energy metabolisn. Prolonged electrical stimulation (i.e., 3 hours) of the cervical sympathetic nerve *in situ* in the anaesthetized cat, on the other hand, produced significant increases in RNA content of superior cervical ganglion cells (Pevzner, 1965). The satellite cells, in contrast, showed a reduction in RNA content. This led Pevzner to infer that there might have been a transfer of RNA from satellite cells to nerve cell, an hypothesis advanced by Hydén earlier (1959, 1962) (see below). Although the results of *in vitro* and *in vivo* studies are in apparent contradiction in some respects the experimental conditions are not at all comparable. Depending upon the purpose to be served, the approach of using direct electrical stimulation to increase "functional" activity can provide useful information; however, the unphysiological conditions of stimulation tend to obfuscate any "functional" significance in the latter experiments. The brain slice studies clearly show that RNA synthesis becomes impaired when the availability of ATP becomes limiting; however, little can be inferred from the information at hand as regards to where RNA synthesis stands in the rank order of metabolic priorities of the cells.

Several studies have employed certain forms of physiological stimulation in order to excite selectively certain functional cell types by synaptic activation. These have included cells from the following structures in which adequate stimuli have produced increases in RNA content: supraopticus (rat), NaCl in drinking water (J.-E. Edström and Eichner, 1958), thirst (J.-E. Edström *et al.*, 1961); nucleus Deiters (rabbit), rotation (Hydén and Pigon, 1960); Purkinje cells of the cerebellum (rat), proprioceptive, exterioceptive, and vestibular stimulation (Jarlstedt, 1966a). In the investigation by Jarlstedt, a direct correspondence was observed between the activation of selective pathways and the increase in Purkinje cell RNA of only those regions of the cerebellum to which the pathways were known to distribute anatomically. In all instances, nonspecific stimuli were without effect. Finally, Hydén (1964) observed that forced swimming for 20–30 minutes in barracudas to virtual exhaustion resulted in a progressive increase in RNA content of motoneurons that reached a peak of 30% above control after 4.5 hours.

In an autoradiographic study in mice by Watson (1965), stimulation by NaCl in drinking water caused a transient increase in the ratio of grain counts between cytoplasm and nucleus of supraoptic and paraventricular neurons after intracranial injection of ³H-uridine. Similar transient increases were observed in vestibular nuclei following vestibular stimulation and in spinal ganglia and anterior horn cells after exercise. The increased cytoplasm/nucleus ratio appeared after an initial latent period of one to three days following onset of stimulation and lasted over a period of several days. The increased ratio was believed to signify an increase in the rate of RNA transfer from nucleus to cytoplasm and tended to appear sooner with greater intensity of stimulation. The ratio invariably returned to control levels despite continued stimulation. After periods of rest, subsequent stimulation produced increased ratios, but always lower in magnitude compared with that of the first exposure to stimulation.

Not all instances of stimulation produce increased RNA concentration in nerve cells. For example, sound stimulation failed to increase RNA content of spiral ganglion cells in guinea pig (Hallén *et al.*, 1965). Watson (1965) failed to observe changes in the cytoplasm/nucleus ratio of grain counts (see above) of superior cervical ganglion cells or cells of the hypoglossal nucleus in the rat after electrical stimulation of up to 5 hours (hypoglossal cells were stimulated antidromically). Under well-controlled conditions, sustained stretch stimulation of the slowly adapting stretch receptor neuron of the lobster for up to 6 hours resulted in no alteration in RNA content (Grampp and Edström, 1963).

The work on the stretch receptor neuron of the lobster by J.-E. Edström and Grampp was later extended (1965). Again, under carefully controlled experimental conditions, attempts were made to assess the effects of physiological stimulation on several RNA parameters. Eight hours of continuous stretch stimulation resulted in no significant difference in RNA content compared with unstimulated, control cells, confirming earlier observations. In addition, no significant change in the base composition compared with that of paired control occurred, controverting the very small change in the adenine base ratio found in the earlier study (Grampp and Edström, 1963). Finally, RNA synthesis, as measured by ^{32}P uptake into ribonuclease digestible product, was not affected by stimulation. In these experiments, too, actinomycin D, an inhibitor of DNA dependent RNA synthesis, had no overt effect on the biophysical properties of the excitable membrane or on the ability of the stretch receptor neuron to continue discharging for up to 24 hours. In addition to blocking RNA synthesis completely, actinomycin D promoted the loss of 10–20% of the cell's RNA that was rich in adenine and poor in cytosine. The findings emerging from this investigation are instructive because they indicate that severe impairment of RNA synthesizing capacity of a nerve cell does not affect the functional properties of the cell (i.e., excitability). However, because the preparation was kept in a non-nutritive physiological medium, the results cannot be considered pertinent to the question of RNA synthesizing potential that might be realized during "functional" activity (see below). Nonetheless, the conclusion can hardly be less apparent that there is a notable lack of short-term dependence (i.e., < 24 hours) of the excitable plasmalemma upon the cytoplasmic protein synthesizing machinery (see Section IV).

Very recent studies, using the giant R2 cell of *Aplysia* (see above), have yielded very interesting results relating to the question of RNA metabolism and functional activity. It was demonstrated that incorporation of labeled RNA precursor was significantly enhanced by electrical stimulation of afferent connectives (R. P. Peterson and Kernell, 1970), and a direct proportionality was in fact shown to exist between the rate of "spikes" (i.e., action potentials) generated and the rate of incorporation (Berry, 1969). However, Kernell and Peterson (1970) clearly demonstrated that the increased rate of incorporation was not caused by spike activity per se, but rather to something unspecifiable at present that was related to *synaptic activation.* Thus, trains of spikes, evoked by intracellular current pulses at rates that caused increased uptake with afferent nerve stimulation (Peterson and Kernell, 1970), did not produce a rate of incorporation significantly different from that of unstimulated, control cells. Yet, when the R2 cells were activated synaptically to produce EPSP's (excitatory postsynaptic potentials) but not of sufficient magnitude to generate propagated action potentials, a small but significant increase in RNA labeling occurred. These workers raised the possibility that a trophic substance might be coreleased with transmitter and that the trophic substance might then exert an action upon the metabolic machinery. Such a concept is indeed worthy of serious consideration for future investigation. If true. it would contribute much to an understanding as to reasons for contradictory results among various experiments of this type (see above).

A gel electrophoretic analysis of nuclear and cytoplasmic RNA's labeled in stimulated and unstimulated R2 cells was carried out also by Peterson and Kernell (1970). A consistent observation they made was that stimulation caused an appreciable increase in labeling of high molecular weight RNA (> 27 S) of the cytoplasm after 1.4 hours, incubation. These authors considered the possibility that the same classes of RNA were being synthesized in the unstimulated cells, but at a lower rate.

Based on a number of experimental observations that include assays of certain enzyme systems and on analyses of protein and RNA, Hydén (1959) has put forward the hypothesis that the neuron and its adjacent glia form a functional metabolic unit. In his concept of this unit, the glia are regarded as accessory metabolic centers, capable of providing the neuron with various substrates and metabolic intermediates, especially during increased neuronal activity. In a later extension of this hypothesis, Hydén, postulated that the glia can also provide the nerve cell with macromolecular RNA. The evidence is mainly circumstantial in which increases in enzymic activities or RNA content in the nerve cell are correlated with corresponding decreases in the glia (Hydén and Pigon, 1960). Complementary qualitative changes in RNA base composition have also been noted between nerve cells and surrounding glia, induced by chemical means (Egyházi and Hydén, 1961). Detailed discussion of this hypothesis may be found in reviews by Hydén (1962, 1967b). There is no doubt that the entire question of molecular traffic between nerve cells and glia, particularly that involving macromolecules, is highly deserving of concentrated investigative effort. The answers to many problems in neurobiology, including those concerned with neurogenesis, neurospecificity, and topographic differentiation of the neuronal plasma membrane (see Section IV), may lie with appropriate analysis of intercellular macromolecular transfer.

Induced qualitative changes in cellular RNA, indicated by significant departures from control base proportions, have been observed under various stimulus conditions (Hydén and Egyházi, 1962a, 1963, 1964; Hydén and Lange, 1965; Rappoport and Daginawala, 1968). The frame of reference of these experiments was learning, a subject that has come under review by several authors (Gaito, 1969; Hydén, 1967b, 1969).

B. EFFECTS OF AXOTOMY

Apparently, since the time of Nasse and Valentin in 1839, it was known that the division of an axon could lead to degeneration of the decentralized portion although it was Waller in 1850 and, later, Türck in 1852 who studied the phenomenon systematically in the peripheral and central nervous systems, respectively. After the introduction of Nissl stains, the retrograde reaction developing over the first few days after axotomy in the cell body (i.e., chromotolysis) also became a well-characterized pattern. The classical picture, after a variable time lag, usually involved an initial increase in cell volume, dissolution of Nissl bodies, and an eccentric location of the nucleus. From an ultrastructural standpoint, the dissolution of Nissl substance entails a fragmentation of the granular endoplasmic reticulum (Andres, 1961; Pannese, 1963; Mackey et al., 1964). All apparent signs of chromotolysis, save that of the increase in volume, can be completely blocked by administering actinomycin D at the time of neurotomy (Torvik and Heding, 1967), indicating the likelihood of genetic induction (i.e., derepression) being an essential antecedent to chromotolysis.

A microanalytical study of the changes in RNA content and concentration during the retrograde reaction was carried out on hypoglossal neurons by Brattgård et al. (1957). According to their findings, the RNA content remains constant for the first 9 days after axotomy and then increases to reach a broad peak over 4–7 weeks that is twice that of uninjured control and then returns to about 1.3 times that of control by 11 weeks. The early change in cell volume reduces the RNA concentration to half until increased RNA synthesis raises it, reaching normal values by 11 weeks.

Autoradiographic studies, showing incorporation of labeled nucleosides at varying intervals after axotomy, reveal the following changes. Within 48 hours after division of the axon, there is a striking increase in the incorporation of labeled nucleosides into DNA of perineuronal glial cells and endothelial cells of blood vessels, restricted to the affected nucleus (Watson, 1965; Sjöstrand, 1965). The labeled glial cells are predominantly of the microglial type (Sjöstrand, 1965). The cytoplasm/nucleus ratio of grain counts of labeled RNA increases in the regenerating cell bodies, peaking between the third and fifth days, but showing elevated values from the second to eleventh days (Watson, 1965). Since the increased ratio reflects an increased RNA synthesis and transfer to the cytoplasm, Watson concluded that there must be an increased rate of turnover because the RNA content remains essentially constant over this period (Brattgård *et al.*, 1957).

In a comprehensive autoradiographic study on regeneration of axotomized hypoglossal neurons subsequently, Watson (1968) used ultraviolet spectrophotomicrography to measure changes in RNA of the nucleolus and of the whole cell body. He observed that division of the axon resulted in a 1.5- to 2-fold increase in RNA content of the nucleolus after a variable latent period; the latency in onset of the increase varied directly with the proximity of the nerve injury to the cell bodies (i.e., shorter lag time with closer axotomy). Total cell RNA content began to increase at a time when the nucleolar RNA content had reached its maximum. The elevated levels in the nucleolus extended from about 2–4 weeks, with the shorter duration being directly related to the proximity of the injury. The duration of total cell RNA, in turn, was dependent on the time that the nucleolar content was above control level. Thus, axotomy was found to produce a transient increase in the synthesis of ribosomal RNA in the nucleolus, and a succeeding increase in the number of cytoplasmic ribosomes, the magnitude of which was modulated by the closeness of nerve injury. Other experiments showed that stimulation of nucleolar RNA synthesis was independent of the state of innervation (i.e., end organ innervation was not a prerequisite to stimulation). Intracranial injection of actinomycin D at various intervals after nerve injury allowed determination of the "decay" of the nucleolar RNA. Faster rates of decay were observed during the peak elevation of nucleolar RNA. Finally, labeling with ^{3}H-uridine, indicated that the increase in the cytoplasm/nucleus ratio of grain counts (see above) coincided with the increase in nucleolar RNA content.

C. Other Effects

1. *Nerve Growth Factor*

Nerve growth factor (NGF) is a protein that stimulates cell proliferation in embryonic sensory and sympathetic ganglia *in vivo* and *in vitro* (for review, see Levi-Montalcini and Angeletti, 1968). It can be extracted from a number of tissues, including ganglia, but the best sources are submaxillary glands of male mice or snake venoms. Toschi *et al.* (1964) found that NGF stimulated very significantly the rate of incorporation of ^{3}H-uridine into RNA of explanted spinal ganglia from chick embryos. The effects of puromycin and actinomycin D showed that whatever the mode of action of this trophic substance, it was very likely mediated through a synthesis of RNA. Subsequently, Toschi *et al.* (1966) analyzed the labeled RNA from NGF-treated ganglia and compared it with that from untreated ganglia. Within the limits of resolution achieved by these workers, it was concluded that NGF does not induce qualitative changes in the types of RNA synthesized in the embryonic ganglia.

2. *Actinomycin D*

Actinomycin D has been used very widely as a specific inhibitor of DNA-dependent RNA synthesis (for review, see Reich and Goldberg, 1964). As such, investigators have utilized it to assess the metabolic stability of mRNA, but reports have questioned its specificity of action (Revel *et al.*, 1964; Honig and Rabinovitz, 1965; Laszlo *et al.*, 1966; Pastan and Friedman, 1968). An investigation of its effects on the nervous system from several points of view has been carried out by H. Koenig *et al.* (1970). Intrathecal or intracranial injections of actinomycin D caused marked alterations in the fine structure of nuclear chromatin of neurons and glia, reflected as a clumping of chromatin and a loss of nucleolar RNA. A correlation between binding of ^{3}H-actinomycin D to DNA and the potency of inhibition of RNA synthesis indicated to these investigators that the generally accepted mechanisms of steric hinderance was inadequate to account for the potency of inhibition; i.e., a ratio of $10 : 10^6$ molecules, actinomycin D : DNA, caused 70% inhibition 6 hours after injection). In conjunction with the morphological transformation of chromatin, the high potency indicated another mode of action; therefore, the hypothesis was advanced that actinomycin D acts as a cross-linking agent between segments of DNA, altering the conformational state of DNA and its ability to act as a template. Injections of 1 mg into the lumbar theca of cats and 20 μg into the rat brain resulted 24 hours later in 97% inhibition of ^{14}C-lysine incorporation into protein. Maximum inhibition of RNA synthesis was reached 6–8 hours after injection. Some objections were raised to the use of actinomycin D as a reliable indicator of mRNA stability. Readers interested in the biochemical, morphological, and neurological effects of actinomycin D in addition to those of other antimetabolites of RNA metabolism are referred to a recent review (H. Koenig, 1969).

3. *Nitriles*

The nitriles were known to be neurotoxic substances for some time. Malononitrile was shown to alter the Nissl picture before the turn of the century (Barker, 1899). Recent experiments have shown that injections of tricyanoaminopropene into rabbits can produce dramatic increases of 25% in RNA content of nerve cells of Deiters nucleus in just 1 hour; glia, in contrast, exhibit a loss in RNA content of 44% (Egyházi and Hydén, 1961). Base composition is also affected in both neurons and glia, showing enhancements in the proportions of bases that already dominated for each cell type (i.e., guanine for nerve cells and cytosine for glia) (Egyházi and Hydén, 1961; Hydén and Egyházi, 1962a). Again the induction of RNA changes in nerve cells and surrounding glia that appear to be reciprocal in character has been used to support the hypothesis that the two cell types are intimately linked in a metabolic unit (see Section III).

Apparently, tricyanoaminopropene does not produce outward signs of neurotoxicity, at least in short-term experiments (Egyházi and Hydén, 1961). However, another nitrile, β,β-iminodipropionitrile (IDPN), produces a waltzing syndrome after several weeks of ingestion or by intraperitoneal injection that arises, presumably, because of characteristic axonal lesions that develop in the proximal portions of the axon, called axonal balloons (Hartmann *et al.*, 1958; Chou and Hartmann, 1964; Slagel and Hartmann, 1965). Microanalysis of most affected cells show no significant changes in RNA content, while axonal balloons have appreciable RNA, exhibiting an average concentration of 0.23% (w/v) (Slagel *et al.*, 1966; Hartmann *et al.*, 1968).

IV. Special Considerations

A. Origin of Axonal RNA

In all instances where myelin-free axons have been analyzed with sufficiently sensitive methods, it has been possible to demonstrate the presence of RNA. For reasons discussed elsewhere (E. Koenig, 1970b, 1971a), it is no longer tenable to regard the axon as incapable of autochthonous protein synthesis. The source of axonal RNA has come under examination by several investigators. There are reports indicating that RNA in the axon is derived from the cell nucleus by a mechanism of proximodistal flow (Bray and Austin, 1968; J. A. Peterson *et al.*, 1968). The evidence, however, is very tenuous at best because the results are subject to several interpretations. The various possibilities for the origin of axonal RNA are as follows: (1) RNA can be synthesized in the cell nucleus and transported undegraded into the axon, as already considered. (2) RNA is synthesized locally in the axon from precursors that reach it through intraaxonal, interfasicular, and/or transcellular (i.e., satellite cell) routes. (3) RNA is synthesized in the satellite cell and transferred to the subjacent axon. (4) Axonal RNA originates by any combination or all of the foregoing means.

Some experiments where the satellite cell was excluded from consideration are those that were carried out on explanted NGF-treated sensory ganglia from embryonic chick (Amaldi and Rusca, 1970). Ganglia were pulsed *in vitro* with ^{3}H-uridine and then chased with cold uridine. Autoradiography of the preparation showed progressive increase in grain density over the neurites with increasing pulse intervals. No indication of a moving front of radioactivity was observed by these workers. Since neurites must be regarded as undifferentiated axons, extrapolation to differentiated axons may not be valid. For example, ultraviolet microscopic studies of embryonic neuroblasts (Hughes and Flexner, 1956) showed that outgrowing axons absorbed radiation in the region of 260 nm; however, one of the apparent signs of axonal differentiation was an abrupt loss of ultraviolet absorption. Although the source of absorption was unknown, a reasonable inference is that it could be RNA. Furthermore, the possibility of a local synthesis cannot be excluded by the experiments of Amaldi and Rusca although the tacit assumption is that the labeled RNA must have originated in the cell nucleus.

The evidence for a "local" synthesis of axonal RNA now is more than suggestive. This is not to exclude the cell body as an additional source of RNA, but "local" synthesis would encompass axonal RNA synthesized intraaxonally and/or in its satellite cell (i.e., Schwann cell or oligodendrocyte), which would then be transferred to the axon. The evidence for a local synthesis is based on the findings that labeled RNA precursors are incorporated into axonal RNA *in vitro* in the absence of the cell body (E. Koenig, 1967a, 1970b; A. Edström *et al.*, 1969). Analysis of specific radioactivity of the axon and of purified nerve mitochondria based on protein mass but due to labeled RNA indicated that most of the labeled RNA was extramitochondrial in distribution (E. Koenig, 1970a). In dissected Mauthner axon fibers (i.e., axon with myelin sheath, but lacking sheath nuclei), RNA was labeled *in vitro* in both the sheath and the axon, and this labeled RNA sedimented in the region of 4 S in a sucrose gradient (A. Edström *et al.*, 1969). Although axonal mitochondria could account for this labeling, this explanation could hardly be valid for the myelin sheath. Moreover, when the Mauthner axon was dissected from the spinal cord *after* incubation of the whole cord *in vitro*, analysis of labeled RNA extracted from myelin-free axons showed RNA sedimenting in the 28–30 S and 16 S regions of the gradient. The results can be interpreted to indicate that the higher molecular weight RNA species found in the axon after incubation *in situ*, but not found in axons incubated after their isolation, were derived from satellite cell nuclei. The results of some preliminary pulse-chase experiments on the spinal accessory nerve of the rabbit were consistent also with this possibility of an intercellular transfer of macromolecular RNA (E. Koenig, 1970b). In earlier experiments by A. Edström (1964), transection of the spinal cord in fish, which included the Mauthner axon, produced striking alterations in base composition that reached a maximum after 2–3 days. Of interest in this context were the findings that the changes in the axonal RNA were paralleled by similar changes in the myelin sheath, indicating possibly a type of metabolic interdependence.

The machinery concerned with protein turnover of the excitable membrane is yet to be characterized and mechanisms for membrane renewal elucidated. There is a tacit assumption that the cytoplasmic machinery (i.e., polysomes) probably fulfills this function. However, topographic or regional differentiation of the membrane, in which differences in subunit composition of delimited membrane areas are distinguished from those of contiguous regions, raises the likelihood that a local, intrinsic membrane machinery (i.e., RNA) may exist (E. Koenig, 1970b). The possibility of intercellular macromolecular transfer provides a plausible mechanism for topographic differentiation by specifying and/or regulating the local membrane machinery (see E. Koenig, 1971a).

B. Future Prospects

Attempts to anticipate the direction and the form future research will take are not inappropriate for a review, but changes in the scientific *Zeitgeist* are generally impossible to predict. Certain trends are evident, however, and presumably, they will run their course. For example, there probably will be increased efforts to characterize the various classes of RNA synthesized in specific cell types during a variety of functional states as well as during neurogenesis. Other areas that will receive increasing attention concern factors, particularly extracellular ones, and mechanisms controlling transcription and translation during development, functional differentiation, and functional activity. There are probably few areas other than nucleic acid research that promise to offer more in the way of understanding some of the basic mechanisms underlying the compelling phenomena of neurobiology such as neurodifferentiation, neurotrophism, neurospecificity, and neuroplasticity.

REFERENCES

Adams, D. H. (1966). *Biochem. J.* **98**, 636.

Amaldi, P., and Busca, G. (1970). *J. Neurochem.* **17**, 767.

Andersson, E., Edström, A., and Jarlstedt, J. (1970). *Acta Physiol. Scand.* **78**, 491.

Andres, K. H. (1961). *Z. Zellforsch. Mikrosk. Anat.* **55**, 49.

Austin, L., and Morgan, I. G. (1967). *J. Neurochem.* **14**, 377.

Balázs, R., and Cocks, W. A. (1967). *J. Neurochem.* **14**, 1035.

Barker, L. F. (1899). "The Nervous System." Appleton, New York.

Bernsohn, J., and Norgello, H. (1966). *Proc. Soc. Exp. Biol. Med.* **122**, 22.

Berry, R. W. (1969). *Science* **166**, 1021.

Bodian, D. (1965). *Proc. Nat. Acad. Sci. U.S.* **53**, 418.

Bodian, D., and Dziewiatkouski, D. (1950). *J. Cell. Comp. Physiol.* **35**, 155.

Bondy, S. C. (1966). *J. Neurochem.* **13**, 955.

Bondy, S. C., and Roberts, S. (1967). *Biochem. J.* **105**, 1111.

Bondy, S. C., and Roberts, S. (1968). *Biochem. J.* **109**, 533.

Bondy, S. C., and Waelach, H. (1965). *J. Neurochem.* **12**, 751.

Brattgàrd, S.-O., Edström, J.-E., and Hydén, H. (1957). *J. Neurochem.* **1**, 316.

Bray, J. J., and Austin, L. (1968). *J. Neurochem.* **15**, 731.

Chargaff, E., and Zamenhof, S. (1948). *J. Biol. Chem.* **173**, 327.

Chou, S. M., and Hartmann, H. A. (1964). *Acta Neuropathol.* **3**, 428.

Clouet, D., and Waelsch, H. (1961). *J. Neurochem.* **8**, 201.

Daneholt, B., and Brattgàrd, S.-O. (1966). *J. Neurochem.* **13**, 913.

Dingman, C. W., and Peacock, A. C. (1968). *Biochem. J.* **7**, 659.

Edström, A. (1964). *J. Neurochem.* **11**, 309.

Edström, A., Edström, J.-E., and Hökfelt, T. (1969). *J. Neurochem.* **16**, 53.

Edström, J.-E. (1953). *Biochim. Biophys. Acta* **12**, 361.

Edström, J.-E. (1956). *J. Neurochem.* **1**, 159.

Edström, J.-E. (1957). *In* "Metabolism of the Nervous System" (D. Richter, ed.), p. 429. Academic Press, New York.

Edström, J.-E. (1958). *J. Neurochem.* **3**, 100.

Edström, J.-E. (1960). *J. Bhiophys. Biochem. Cytol.* **8**, 39.

Edström, J.-E., and Eichner, D. (1957). *Z. Zellforsch. Mikrosk. Anat.* **48**, 187.

Edström, J.-E., and Eichner, D. (1958). *Nature (London)* **181**, 619.

Edström, J.-E., and Grampp, W. (1965). *J. Neurochem.* **12**, 735.

Edström, J.-E., Eichner, D., and Schor, N. (1961). *In* "Regional Neurochemistry" (S. S. Kety and J. Elkes, eds.), p. 274. Pergamon, Oxford.

Edström, J.-E., Eichner, D., and Edström, A. (1962). *Biochim. Biophys. Acta* **61**, 178.

Egyházi, E., and Hydén, H. (1961). *J. Biophys. Biochem. Cytol.* **10**, 403.

Egyházi, E., and Hydén, H. (1966). *Life Sci.* **5**, 1215.

Gaito, J. (1969). *In* "The Structure and Function of Nervous Tissue" (G. H. Bourne, ed.) Vol. 2, p. 493. Academic Press, New York.

Girard, M., Latham, H., Penman, S., and Darnell, J. E. (1964). *Proc. Nat. Acad. Sci. U.S.* **51**, 205.

Grampp, W., and Edström, J.-E. (1963). *J. Neurochem.* **10**, 725.

Guroff, G., Hogans, A. F., and Udenfriend, S. (1968). *J. Neurochem.* **15**, 489.

Hallén, O., Edström, J.-E., and Hamberger, A. (1965). *Acta Oto-laryngol.* **60**, 121.

Hartmann, H. A., Lalich, J. J., and Akert, K. (1958). *J. Neuropathol. Exp. Neurol.* **17**, 298.

Hartmann, H. A., Lin, J., and Shively, M. C. (1968). *Acta Neuropathol.* **11**, 275.

Hogenhuis, L. A. H., and Spaulding, S. W. (1967). *Nature (London)* **215**, 287.

Honig, G. R., and Rabinovitz, M. (1965). *Science* **149**, 1504.

Hughes, A., and Flexner, L. B. (1956). *J. Anat.* **90**, 386.

Hydén, H. (1943). *Acta Physiol. Scand.* **6**, Suppl. 17.

Hydén, H. (1959). *Nature (London)* **184**, 433.

Hydén, H. (1960). *In* "The Cell" (J. Brachet and A. E. Mirsky, eds.), Vol. 4, p. 215. Academic Press, New York.

Hydén, H. (1962). *Endeavour* **21**, 144.

Hydén, H. (1964). *Recent Advan. Biol. Psychiat.* **6**, 31.

Hydén, H. (1967a). *In* "The Neurosciences" (G. C. Quarton, T. Melnechuk, and F. O. Schmitt, eds.), p. 265. Rockefeller Univ. Press, New York.

Hydén, H. (1967b). *In* "The Neurosciences" (G. C. Quarton, T. Melnechuk, and F. O. Schmitt, eds.), p. 765. Rockefeller Univ. Press, New York.

Hydén, H. (1969). *In* "On the Biology of Learning" (K. H. Pribram, ed.), p. 97. Harcourt, New York.

Hydén, H., and Egyházi, E. (1962a). *J. Cell Biol.* **15**, 37.

Hydén, H., and Egyházi, E. (1962b). *Proc. Nat. Acad. Sci. U.S.* **48**, 1366.

Hydén, H., and Egyházi, E. (1963). *Proc. Nat. Acad. Sci. U.S.* **49**, 618.

Hydén, H., and Egyházi, E. (1964). *Proc. Nat. Acad. Sci. U.S.* **52**, 1030.

Hydén, H., and Lange, P. W. (1965). *Proc. Nat. Acad. Sci. U.S.* **53**, 946.

Hydén, H., and Pigon, A. (1960). *J. Neurochem.* **6**, 57.

Itoh, T., and Quastel, J. H. (1969). *Science* **164**, 79.

Jacob, M., Stévenin, J., Jund, R., Judes, C., and Mandel, P. (1966). *J. Neurochem.* **13**, 619.

Jacob, M., Samec, J., Stévenin, J., Garel, J. P., and Mandel, P. (1967). *J. Neurochem.* **14**, 169.

Jarlstedt, J. (1962). *Exp. Cell Res.* **28**, 501.

Jarlstedt, J. (1966a). *Acta Physiol. Scand.* **67**, 243.

Jarlstedt, J. (1966b). *Acta Physiol. Scand.* **67**, Suppl. 271.

Kimberlin, R. H. (1967). *J. Neurochem.* **14**, 123.

Kernell, D., and Peterson, R. P. (1970). *J. Neurochem.* **17**, 1087.

Koenig, E. (1965). *J. Neurochem.* **12**, 357.

Koenig, E. (1967a). *J. Neurochem.* **14**, 437.

Koenig, E. (1967b). *J. Cell Biol.* **34**, 265.

Koenig, E. (1968). *J. Cell Biol.* **38**, 562.

Koenig, E. (1969). *In* "Handbook of Neurochemistry" (A. Lajtha, ed.), Vol. 2, p. 423. Plenum Press, New York.

Koenig, E. (1970a). *In* "Protein Metabolism of the Nervous System" (A. Lajtha, ed.), p. 259. Plenum Press, New York.

Koenig, E. (1970b). *Advan. Biochem. Psychopharmacol.* **2**, 303.

Koenig, E. (1971a). *In* "Macromolecules and Behavior" (J. Gaito, ed.), 2nd Appleton, New York (in press).

Koenig, E. (1971b). *Invest. Ophthalmol.* (in press).

Koenig, E., and Koelle, G. B. (1961). *J. Neurochem.* **8**, 169

Koenig, H. (1958a). *Proc. Soc. Exp. Biol. Med.* **97**, 255.

Koenig, H. (1958b). *J. Biophys. Biochem. Cytol.* **4**, 785.

Koenig, H. (1964). *In* "Morphological and Biochemical Correlates of Neural Activity" (M. M. Cohen and R. S. Snider, eds.), p. 39. Harper, New York.

Koenig, H. (1969). *In* "Motor Neuron Disease" (F. H. Norris and L. T. Kurland, eds.), Vol. 2, p. 347. Grune & Stratton, New York.

Koenig, H., Lu, C. Y., Jacobson, S., Sanghavi, P., and Nayyar, R. (1970). *In* "Protein Metabolism of the Nervous System" (A. Lajtha, ed.), p. 491. Plenum Press, New York.

Landström, H., Caspersson, T., and Wolfart, G. (1941) *Z. Mikrosk. Anat. Forsch.* **49**, 534.

Lasek, R. J. (1970). *J. Neurochem.* **17**, 103.

Laszlo, J., Miller, D. S., McCarty, K. S., and Hochstein, P. (1966). *Science* **151**, 1007.

Leblond, C. P., and Amano, M. (1962). *J. Histochem. Cytochem.* **10**, 162.

Levi-Montalcini, R., and Angeletti, P. (1968). *Physiol. Rev.* **48**, 534.

Loening, U. E. (1967). *Biochem. J.* **102**, 251.

Logan, J. E., Mannell, W. A., and Rossiter, R. J. (1952). *Biochem. J.* **51**, 470.

Løvtrup-Rein, H. (1970). *J. Neurochem.* **17**, 853.

Løvtrup-Rein, H., and Grahn, B. (1970). *J. Neurochem.* **17**, 845.

Mackey, E. A., Spiro, D., and Wiener, J. (1964). *J. Neuropathol. Exp. Neurol.* **23**, 508.

Mahler, H. R., Moore, W. J., and Thompson, R. J. (1966). *J. Biol. Chem.* **241**, 1283.

Mandel, P., Rein, H., Harth-Edel, S., and Mardell, R. (1964). *In* "Comparative Neurochemistry" (D. Richter, ed.), p. 149. Macmillan, New York.

May, L., and Grenell, R. G. (1959). *Proc. Soc. Exp. Biol. Med.* **102**, 235.

Muramatsu, M., and Fujisawa, T. (1968). *Biochim. Biophys. Acta* **157**, 476.

Murthy, M. R. V. (1968). *Biochim. Biophys. Acta* **166**, 115.

Murthy, M. R. V. (1970). *In* "Protein Metabolism of the Nervous System" (A. Lajtha, ed.), p. 109. Plenum Press, New York.

Nurnberger, J. A., Engström, A., and Lindström, B. (1952). *J. Cell. Comp. Physiol.* **39**, 215.

Orrego, F. (1967). *J. Neurochem.* **14**, 851.

Orrego, F., and Lipmann, F. (1966). *J. Biol. Chem.* **242**, 665.

Palade, G. E. (1964). *Proc. Nat. Acad. Sci. U.S.* **52**, 613.

Palay, S. L., and Palade, G. E. (1955). *J. Byophys. Biochem. Cytol.* **1**, 69.

Pannese, E. (1963). *Z. Zellforsch. Mikrosk. Anat.* **60**, 711.

Pastan, I., and Friedman, R. M. (1968). *Science* **160**, 316.

Penman, S. (1966). *J. Mol. Biol.* **17**, 117.

Perry, R. P. (1965). *Nat. Cancer Inst., Monogr.* **18**, 325.

Perry, R. P. (1967). *Progr. Nucl. Acid Res. Mol. Biol.* **6**, 220.

Perry, R., and Kelley, D. E. (1968). *J. Cell. Physiol.* **72**, 235.

Peterson, J. A., Bray, J. J., and Austin, L. (1968). *J. Neurochem.* **15**, 741.

Peterson, R. P. (1970). *J. Neurochem.* **17**, 325.

Peterson, R. P., and Kernell, D. (1970). *J. Neurochem.* **17**, 1075.

Pevzner, L. Z. (1965). *J. Neurochem.* **12**, 993.

Rake, A., and Grahm, A. (1964). *Biophys. J.* **4**, 267.

Rappoport, D. A., and Daginawala, H. F. (1968). *J. Neurochem.* **15**, 991.

Reich, E., and Goldberg, L. H. (1964). *Progr. Nucl. Acid Res. Mol. Biol.* **3**, 184.

Revel, M., Hiatt, H. H., and Revel, J.-P. (1964). *Science* **146**, 1311.

Ringborg, U. (1966). *Brain Res.* **2**, 296.

Roberts, S., Zomzely, C. E., and Bondy, S. C. (1970). *In* "Protein Metabolism of the Nervous System" (A. Lajtha, ed.), p. 3. Plenum Press, New York.

Saborio, J. L., and Alemán, V. (1970). *J. Neurochem.* **17**, 91.

Samec, J., Mandel, P., and Jacob, M. (1967). *J. Neurochem.* **14**, 887.

Samec, J., Jacob, M., and Mandel, P. (1968). *Biochem. Biophys. Acta* **161**, 377.

Samli, M. H., and Roberts, S. (1969). *J. Neurochem.* **16**, 1565.

Schaffer, K. (1893). *Neurol. Zentralbl.* **12**, 849.

Scherrer, K., and Darnell, J. (1962). *Biochem. Biophys. Res. Commun.* **7**, 486.

Scott, I. H. (1898). *Trans. Roy. Can. Inst.* **5**.

Shimada, M., and Nakamura, T. (1966). *J. Neurochem.* **13**, 391.

Sjöstrand, J. (1965). *Z. Zellforsch. Mikrosk. Anat.* **68**, 481.

Slagel, D. E. and Hartmann, H. A. (1965). *J. Neuropathol. Exp. Neurol.* **24**, 599.

Slagel, D. E., Hartmann, H. A., and Edström, J.-E. (1966). *J. Neuropathol. Exp. Neurol.* **25**, 244.

Stévenin, J., Samec, J., Jacob, M., and Mandel, P. (1968). *J. Mol. Biol.* **33**, 777.

Stévenin, J., Mandel, P., and Jacob, M. (1969). *Proc. Nat. Acad. Sci. U.S.* **62**, 490.

Takahashi, Y., Hsü, C. S., and Suzuki, Y. (1969). *Brain Res.* **13**, 397.

Tencheva, Z. S., and Hadjiolov, A. A. (1969). *J. Neurochem.* **16**, 769.

Torvik, A., and Heding, A. (1967). *Acta Neuropathol.* **9**, 146.

Toschi, G., Gandini, D. A., and Angeletti, P. U. (1964). *Biochem. Biophys. Res. Commun.* **16**, 111.

Toschi, G., Dore, E., Angeletti, P. U., Levi-Montalcini, R., and Haën, C. (1966). *J. Neurochem.* **13**, 539.

Tsanev, R. G. (1965). *Biochim. Biophys. Acta* **103**, 374.

Vesco, C., and Giuditta, A. (1967). *Biochim. Biophys. Acta* **142**, 385.

von Hungen, K., Mahler, H. R., and Moore, W. J. (1968). *J. Biol. Chem.* **243**, 1415.

Watson, W. E. (1965). *J. Physiol. (London)* **180**, 741.

Watson, W. E. (1968). *J. Physiol. (London)* **196**, 655.

Weinberg, R. A., Loening, U., Willems, M., and Penman, S. (1967). *Proc. Nat. Acad. Sci. U.S.* **58**, 1088.

Winick, M., and Noble, A. (1966). *J. Nutr.* **89**, 300.

Yamagami, S., Kawakita, Y., and Naka, S. (1965). *J. Neurochem.* **12**, 607.

6

Molecular Organization of Neural Information Processing[1]

GEORGES UNGAR

I. Introduction 215
II. Chemical Correlates of Information Processing 217
   A. Chemical Analysis 217
   B. Action of Metabolic Inhibitors 218
III. Bioassays for the Molecular Code 220
   A. Types of Assays 221
   B. Reliability of the Assays 222
   C. Specificity of the Method 227
   D. The Chemical Problem 230
IV. Molecular Basis of Neural Coding 231
   A. Neural Codes 232
   B. Labeled Pathways 234
   C. Molecular Hypotheses 235
V. Concluding Remarks 241
   References 243

I. Introduction

The output of behavior and the coordination of physiological functions in living organisms requires the existence of a communication system. This system receives information from the external and internal environments and is capable of integrating, storing, and retrieving it. This in-

[1] The research work referred to in this chapter is supported by U.S.P.H.S. grant MH–13361.

formation processing in higher organisms is essentially the function of the nervous system in cooperation with some hormonal mechanisms.

The nervous system is composed of discrete units, the neurons, linked together with synapses to form a network of connections whose complexity has been increasing in the course of evolution. In the vertebrate series, at least, the most important feature of the development of the nervous system has been the formation of successive hierarchic levels correcting and controlling each other but capable of autonomy when disconnected.

It has been obvious for a long time that neurons of the central nervous system are not connected randomly, and it is implicit in the so-called "law of specific energies" of Johannes Müller that sensory information is coded in the pathways through which the impulses travel. It is at present generally admitted that the sensory input and the motor output follow well-defined pathways, but the area in between remains controversial because it is largely unknown. The uncertainty concerning the existence of specific localizations in this important and extensive portion of the brain has caused a considerable polarization of opinion, and I shall return to it in Section IV,C,2.

The best known biological information processing, the transmission of hereditary characters, is based on a molecular code. It is understandable, therefore, that attempts have been made to apply the same principle to the mechanism by which acquired information is processed in the nervous system. There have been several allusions in earlier literature to molecular phenomena playing a role in memory (Ribot, 1881; James, 1890), but they probably represented metaphors rather than concrete chemical processes. The term "engram" proposed by Semon (1904) did not originally have the chemical connotation often attributed to it today. Definite molecular hypotheses were not formulated until the late 1940's (von Foerster, 1948; Monné, 1948; Katz and Halstead, 1950), and they were mostly an offshoot of the powerful growth of molecular biology.

The molecular approach really started a little over a decade ago with the first analytical data published by Hydén (1959) followed by the first use of metabolic inhibitors by Dingman and Sporn (1961) and the planarian experiments by McConnell (1962). The literature kept growing at a fast rate in the 1960's, and the number of laboratories working on problems related to molecular neurobiology has been increasing.

The physical, as opposed to chemical, nature of the neural process is so strongly anchored in tradition that intrusion of chemical phenomena into the study of the nervous system has always met with determined opposition. It took over 25 years for the chemical mediation of synaptic transmission to be fully accepted, and as Schmitt and Samson (1969) noted, "The concept that information-bearing macromolecules may condition the storage and retrieval of information...seems likely to encounter as much skepticism as did the neurohumoral concept."

II. Chemical Correlates of Information Processing

Our knowledge of the chemical processes associated with neural activity lags very much behind the wealth of information provided by electrophysiology. The situation was reviewed recently (Ungar and Irwin, 1968), and I shall mention here only the points that are particularly relevant to the problem of information processing.

There have been three main strategies in the study of this problem: (a) direct chemical analysis of the brain, (b) use of metabolic inhibitors, and (c) detection of chemical changes by means of bioassays.

A. CHEMICAL ANALYSIS

Hydén's pioneering work (1959) was based on the hypothesis that the information contained in the electrical pattern of impulses was able to modify somehow the sequence of RNA bases and thus encode the information. What Hydén and his co-workers actually found in a series of experiments (1967, 1969) is a change in the composition of the nuclear RNA in the neurons involved in the acquisition of information. The change in RNA composition was expressed in terms of base ratios which, in the experimental group, shifted towards the "DNA-like" type. This change was absent in the control group subjected to the same amount of stimulation but without acquisition of information. In recent years, the change in base ratios was interpreted as an increase in messenger RNA rather than the synthesis of new RNA species (Hydén, 1967).

There have been no published attempts at replicating these extremely elegant experiments, done in isolated neurons with accurate microtechniques, outside of Hydén's laboratory. There are, however, other experimental data suggesting that acquisition and fixation of information is associated with increased synthesis of RNA. Glassman's group (1969) found increased incorporation of double labeled uridine in a short-term learning situation in mice. Similar results were obtained by Bowman and Strobel (1969) with cytidine. Increased synthesis with base ratio changes was observed by Shashoua (1968) in goldfish trained to acquire a new swimming skill and injected with labeled orotic acid, a precursor of both pyrimidine bases. Studies of amino acid incorporation have also produced some positive results (Hydén and Lange, 1968; Bateson *et al.*, 1969; Beach *et al.*, 1969). Using a different approach, Bogoch (1968) detected changes in a number of brain glycoprotein fractions in pigeons subjected to simple training procedures.

Rappoport and Daginawala (1968) observed quantitative and qualitative changes of RNA in the perfused catfish head submitted to olfactory stimuli, but their results are difficult to interpret in terms of information processing. Increased protein synthesis was also observed in brain areas as a result of sensory stimulation without deliberate training (Rahmann, 1965; Rensch and Rahmann, 1966; Telwar *et al.*, 1966; Rose, 1967).

This brings up the interpretation of this whole approach to the chemical correlates of neural information processing. The results undoubtedly prove that increased neural activity is associated with an elevation of RNA and protein metabolism. They leave, however, some important questions unanswered, e.g.: (a) Are the changes correlated with the acquisition of new information or only with increased neural activity? (b) Are they indispensable for information processing? (c) Do they represent a code? The first question has been the object of several discussions reviewed by Glassman (1969) and Booth (1970) and remains open. Attempts have been made to answer the second question by using inhibitors of RNA and protein synthesis; these experiments will be discussed in the following section. The third, most controversial, question will be considered in Section III with the bioassay approach.

B. Action of Metabolic Inhibitors

The importance of RNA and protein synthesis for information processing has been investigated by the use of inhibitors. If these have an effect on the acquisition of information, it is clear that the metabolic changes are not merely coincidental but are necessary for the adequate operation of the nervous system.

The first attempt at answering this question was made by Dingman and Sporn in 1961, using 8-azaguanine, an inhibitor of RNA synthesis. Although the results of these experiments were inconclusive, they undoubtedly stimulated other similar approaches. Another inhibitor of the DNA–RNA transcription, i.e., actinomycin D, was first unsuccessfully tried (Barondes and Jarvik, 1964) on short-time retrieval in mice, but Agranoff *et al.* (1967) found that it inhibited long-time fixation of memory in gold-fish.

Most of the work in this area was done with inhibitors of the RNA-protein translation such as puromycin and cycloheximide (and its acetoxy derivative). Results were obtained in mice in Flexner's laboratory and in goldfish by Agranoff and his colleagues. Details of this research have been reviewed by Glassman (1969) and Cohen (1970), and only a brief outline will be given here.

Inhibitors of protein synthesis seem to act by interfering with the conversion of short-term memory into long-term fixation of information. Short-term memory does not require protein synthesis, and puromycin treated mice, trained to an avoidance task, performed it perfectly if tested within 15 minutes. Three hours later, however, they showed complete amnesia (Barondes and Cohen, 1966). Puromycin could produce amnesia at later stages, also, if the site of injection was changed: Within the first day or two, bitemporal injections were effective, but more delayed injections had to be given over wider areas of the cortex (Flexner *et al.*, 1964, 1967). Agranoff *et al.* (1965) further specified some critical points. They found that in the goldfish puromycin was effective only if it was given less than an hour after training.

The precise mode of action of puromycin on memory is still in doubt. Flexner and Flexner (1968) believe that the amnesic effect is due to formation of abnormal peptides ("peptidyl-puromycin"). This hypothesis is supported by the observation that the effect can be abolished by injections of saline which "wash out" the toxic metabolites. It is possible that puromycin produces effects other than inhibition of protein synthesis, i.e., swelling of neuronal mitochondria (Gambetti *et al.*, 1968) and abnormal electrical activity (Cohen and Barondes, 1967).

Cycloheximide, a powerful inhibitor of protein synthesis, is free of these side effects. Barondes and Cohen (1967) have shown that this agent also causes amnesia but only in mice that have not been submitted to prolonged training. This effect was not abolished by saline injections. An advantage of cycloheximide is that it can inhibit cerebral protein synthesis even after subcutaneous injection (Barondes and Cohen, 1968a). When mice were trained shortly after such an injection, they remembered the task up to about 3 hours after training but not after 6 hours. Injections given 30 minutes after training were ineffective. Davis and Agranoff made similar observations in goldfish (1966).

It seems, therefore, that the protein necessary for the consolidation of information is synthesized at an early stage. This synthesis may be stimulated by "arousal" produced by pharmacological, electrical, or behavioral manipulations (Barondes and Cohen, 1968b; Davis and Agranoff, 1966).

Probably, the most important information provided by these experiments is the demonstration of a definite sequence of events in the fixation of information (Agranoff, 1965; McGaugh, 1966; Cohen, 1970): During a first phase, extending for a few hours after training, the inhibitors are without effect; during the second phase (lasting for a few days), fixation can be abolished by hippocampal application of the agent; and a final phase requires extensive applications of the drug to produce amnesia.

The use of metabolic inhibitors in the search for the chemical correlates of information processing is beset with difficulties. Some facts, such as the neutralization of the effect of puromycin by cycloheximide (Flexner and Flexner, 1966), the dependence of the amnesic effect on the duration, the extent and difficulty of the training (Barondes and Cohen, 1967), and the "washout" effect, remain obscure. On the whole, the experiments do suggest that protein synthesis is necessary for the consolidation of memory, but they do not answer the question of the role of the protein synthesized.

III. Bioassays for the Molecular Code

The problem of the molecular code of neural information is at the same stage today as the neurohumoral theory was 50 years ago. Confronted with the need to demonstrate that stimulation of nerves releases active substances, the only possible approach was the use of biological assay methods. In the absence of appropriate physical or chemical methods, the substances released could be characterized only by their pharmacological effects as exemplified by the original experiments of Loewi (1921).

Bioassays have always been unpopular with scientists trained in chemical and physical disciplines. They imply the use of biological material with its inherent variability, they have limited reliability and accuracy, and they require considerable patience and equanimity. In spite of these disadvantages, bioassays played an extremely important role at the critical stage of several important advances of the biological sciences. The bioassay is the life blood of pharmacology, but it was also the original and indispensable approach to the study of hormones, vitamins, antibiotics, and of course, neurotransmitters.

Application of bioassays to the problem of molecular coding of neural information has been obscured by the terms "memory transfer," "transfer of learning," and others which emphasized the sensational aspects of these experiments. In my laboratory at least, their purpose has been to test information-carrying molecules in view of their isolation and chemical identification. The principle of the assays is (a) to supply donor animals with information that modifies their behavior in some easily observable and measurable fashion, (b) to prepare an extract of the central nervous system that contains the molecular species in which the information is assumed to be coded, (c) to administer the extract to recipient animals, and (d) to test their behavior and detect changes that can in any way be related to the information given to the donors. By using appropriate controls, one should be able to ascertain whether the extract taken from the donors is specifically responsible for the behavioral changes observed in the recipients.

A. TYPES OF ASSAYS

Since the first experiments, published in 1962 by McConnell, a large variety of techniques have been proposed using a number of different animal species. During a first period (1962–1965) assays were done in planarian worms only; from 1965 on, besides rodents (rats, mice, and hamsters), which were the most widely used animals, chicks (Rosenthal and Sparber, 1968) and goldfish (Zippel and Domagk, 1969; Fjerdingstad, 1969; Braud, 1970) were introduced. The latter promise to be the most useful and convenient experimental animals.

The planarian experiments became the center of a lively controversy, and the reader is referred to the recent reviews by McConnell and Shelby (1970) and Corning and Riccio (1970) for their discussion. The weight of evidence is very much in favor of the basic correctness of the results, but their interpretation, particularly concerning the chemical identity of the active material, still remains in doubt.

The bulk of the experiments was done in rats and mice, beginning with the almost simultaneous publications in 1965 of Reinis, Fjerdingstad *et al.*, Ungar and Oceguera-Navarro, and Babich *et al.* They can be divided into two groups. In the first group the recipients were tested by being trained identically with the donors and the results evaluated in terms of an increased rate of learning of the experimental animals as compared with the controls. In the second group, the recipients were tested without reinforcement so that they did not actually "learn" anything during the test, and if they responded similarly to the donors, this could only be attributed to the information contained in the extracts.

The first type of experiments cannot properly be called bioassays for the molecular code since the animals were supplied information as to the response expected from them. When successful, these assays indicate that the brain of trained animals may contain some material that accelerates the acquisition and fixation of information but do not prove the existence of an actual molecular code in which the information was recorded. This does not mean that these studies are worthless, only that their interpretation should be more restricted. In a number of cases, the original studies done with reinforcement were repeated without training of recipients and their conclusions were validated (Fjerdingstad *et al.*, 1966; Rosenblatt *et al.*, 1966a,b; Dyal *et al.*, 1967; Ungar and Irwin, 1967; Golub *et al.*, 1970).

The bibliography of the bioassay approach has now close to 100 publications and could not be surveyed here in its entirety. The reader is referred to the volumes edited by Byrne (1970) and Fjerdingstad (1971) and to the reviews of Rosenblatt (1970), Ungar (1971), and Ungar and Chapouthier (1971). The behavioral patterns used include simple situations like habituation (Ungar and Oceguera-Navarro, 1965; Ungar, 1967a,b) fixation of postural asymmetry (Giurgea *et al.*, 1969), conditioned approach (Babich *et al.*, 1965) or avoidance (Ungar, 1967a,b; Ádám and Faiszt, 1967), passive avoidance (Gay and Raphelson, 1967; Ungar *et al.*, 1968; Golub *et al.*, 1969; Wolthuis, 1969), brightness discrimination (Fjerdingstad *et al.*, 1965; Gibby *et al.*, 1968; Wolthuis *et al.*, 1969); spatial discrimination (Rosenblatt, 1970; Krylov *et al.*, 1969), color and taste discrimination (Zippel and Domagk, 1969), instrumental conditioning (Rosenblatt and Miller, 1966; Dyal *et al.*, 1967; McConnell *et al.*, 1968), and more complex choices (Rosenblatt, 1969).

B. Reliability of the Assays

By surveying the literature of the last 5 years it has been possible to determine some of the conditions of successful assays (Ungar, 1970a, 1971; Ungar and Chapouthier, 1971). The most important of these conditions can be listed as follows:

a. *Optimal duration of donor training.* In most cases this lasted at least 5 to 6 days, sometimes up to 10 days. The guiding consideration is that the donors should have learned the task to the highest possible criterion and, also, should have been given time to accumulate an excess of the coded material in their brains. Short training has never been successful, but sometimes prolonged overtraining has also resulted in inactive extracts. It is probable that appropriately spaced rest periods during training can improve the results (Golub *et al.*, 1970).

b. *Preparation and dosage of extracts.* A great deal of confusion has resulted from the premature assumption by many workers that the active substance was RNA. Some RNA preparations were active, and I shall return to this point in a moment (Section III,D). Further purification, however, may have resulted in loss of activity. As a general rule, it is recommended to use only crude extracts to begin with and, if they give positive results, purify them under the guidance of the assay. In the absence of information on the stability of the active material, the usual precautions should be observed during extraction and purification.

Almost all successful assays used doses of extracts equivalent to the weight of the recipient's brain, and better results were obtained with two, three, or even four brain equivalents. High dosage is particularly necessary when the extract is introduced by intraperitoneal route.

c. *Interval between injection and testing of recipients.* This seems to have been the most frequent cause of error because in the majority of experiments the effect of the injection is detectable only 24 hours after injection and reaches its maximum 2 or 3 days later. The best procedure is to test the recipients several times for at least 4 to 5 days.

For the other conditions (interval between last training session and removal of the brain, selection and pretesting of recipients, route of injection, and statistical treatment of results) see the reviews mentioned above.

The necessity to fulfill all these conditions has contributed to make the bioassay approach highly controversial. The planarian experiments were criticized on the ground of doubts on the trainability of these flatworms and the exact nature of the behavioral change induced in the recipients. The vertebrate experiments were questioned soon after their publication; those of Babich *et al.* (1965) were attacked more particularly and several failures to replicate them were published (Gross and Carey, 1965; Gordon *et al.*, 1966; Luttges *et al.*, 1966; Kimble and Kimble, 1966). This culminated in the publication of a collective paper signed by 23 authors from seven laboratories (Byrne *et al.*, 1966) in which negative results were mentioned without experimental details. In spite of the cautious conclusions of the authors, this was believed to have put an end to the whole bioassay approach. It is, of course, evident that bioassays are particularly vulnerable to criticism at the early stage of their development when the experimental variables are still unknown.

It is noteworthy that during the intervening years the positive publications have been rapidly increasing while only a few sporadic negative papers appeared, all by workers who did not seem to be informed of the recent developments. An example is the work of Frank *et al.* (1970), who set out to test the validity of "memory transfer" by experiments in which "the entire procedure, from initial test of donor to intraperitoneal injection of recipients, was completed within 5 minutes" and the recipients were tested once 6 hours after injection. The fact that they were obviously dealing with phenomena entirely unrelated to memory, learning, or any form of information processing did not prevent the authors from applying their data to the criticism of the "RNA specific memory hypothesis."

It is obvious, from the facts mentioned earlier in this section, that these bioassays are difficult experiments requiring the collaboration of a team of workers having a reasonable competence in both the biochemical and behavioral aspects of the problem. Their validity cannot be tested in a few animals by inexperienced students. For reasons mentioned earlier, there are occasional negative assays, even in the most experienced hands. This may occur with all bioassay methods, even with those using clear cut physiological responses such as a muscle contraction.

Reliability can be expressed in terms of a replication of an experimental design in the same laboratory or independently in several laboratories. Table I shows the distribution of the results obtained in my laboratory with 115 extracts of brain taken from rats trained for dark avoidance and 34 control extracts (Ungar *et al.*, 1968). Although it includes several extracts that have given negative results, it is obvious that the behavior of the recipients of trained donor brain extract was significantly different from that of the recipients of control extracts.

Table II shows the results obtained with the same assay in four different laboratories using slightly different techniques which probably explains the quantitative differences. Negative results were published from one laboratory (Hutt and Elliott, 1970) in which the donor training was different in one critical respect. Extracts prepared from donors that received the type of training given by these workers had yielded negative results in our hands also. They were satisfied, however, that this does not "appear sufficient to account for the failure to replicate." Besides neglecting to observe the precise conditions of the positive experiments, these "replications" attempt to invalidate with groups of 10 animals the results obtained with almost 1200 experimental and 400 control recipients. Similar features have been characteristic of many of the negative experiments and bring up the question of how much weight should be given

TABLE I

DISTRIBUTION OF DARK-AVOIDANCE TRAINED AND UNTRAINED RAT BRAIN EXTRACTS
PREPARED DURING A 2-YEAR PERIOD ACCORDING TO THEIR EFFECTS ON TIME SPENT
IN THE DARK BOX (DBT) BY THE RECIPIENTS.[a]

DBT (sec)	Experimental		Control	
	No.	%	No.	%
10– 29.5	3	2.6	0	0
30– 49.5	23	20.0	0	0
50– 69.5	49	42.6	1	2.9
70– 89.5	33	28.7	2	5.9
90–109.5	7	6.1	7	20.5
110–129.5	0	0	10	30.6
130–149.5	0	0	14	41.0
Total	115	100	34	100
< 90	108	93.9	3	8.8
≥ 90	7	6.1	31	91.2

$$\chi^2 = 101; \quad P < 0.0001$$

DBT ± SD		DBT ± SD	
62	17.3	120	20

$$t = 16.2; \quad P < 0.0001$$

[a] Statistical analysis by χ^2 and t-tests.

to them. There is a practically infinite number of ways in which negative results can be obtained while positive results require the fulfillment of well-defined conditions.

The quantitative reliability of the bioassays was studied in Rosenblatt's laboratory and in mine. Rosenblatt (1970) published a dose-response curve for his bar-door assay, and I gave quantitative data for a brightness discrimination experiment (Ungar, 1967b). We studied extensively the dose-response relationship in the dark-avoidance extracts (Ungar et al., 1968). Figure 1 presents data obtained with different types of preparations. The presence of aberrant points indicates the possibility of individual assays giving misleading results.

Negative results will be obtained as long as some of the important variables are unknown or deliberately ignored. It is probable that all the

TABLE II

Results of Dark Avoidance Experiments in Four Laboratories [a]

| | Time in dark box (%) | | | | | | | |
| Time of test | Gay and Raphelson (1967) | | Ungar et al. (1968, 1970a,b) | | Wolthuis (1969) | | Golub et al. (1969) | |
	E	C	E	C	E	C	E	C
Preinjection:	—	—	72.6	72.6	73.8	74.0	—	—
Postinjection (hours):								
2–16	17.6	59.3	—	—	—	—	—	—
6	—	—	—	—	55.6	66.7	—	—
24 + 48	—	—	34.6	66.7	—	—	—	—
24	—	—	—	—	45.1	65.7	64	64
30	—	—	—	—	44.9	62.8	—	—
48	—	—	—	—	50.8	59.8	15	38
72	—	—	—	—	—	—	11	40
N	8	8	1140	400	32	32	10	10
Recipient species	Rats		Mice		Mice		Rats	
Type of extract	"RNA"		Peptide		Crude supernatant		"Peptide" and "RNA"	
Dose, gm donor brain/kg recipient	20		40		12		15 and 4	
Route	i. p.		i. p.		i. p.		i. p. and intracranial	
P	< 0.05		< 0.001		< 0.05 (24 and 30 hours)		< 0.01 (48 and 72 hours)	

[a] Percentage values are used because Wolthuis tested for 120 seconds while in the other laboratories 180-second tests were used. Golub et al. tested their recipients with partial reinforcements. There were other minor differences in the training and testing practices of the four laboratories.

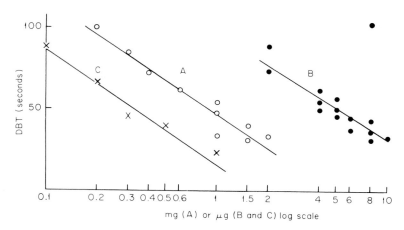

Fig. 1. Dose response curve of dark avoidance inducing substance. Abscissa: dose per 25 gm mouse (log scale). Ordinate: time spent in dark box out of 180 seconds A, dialyzate; B, active fraction after gel filtration; C, pure scotophobin. (For description of these preparations, see Section III,D).

variables will never be controlled, and this is the frustrating aspect of all bioassays and the reason why they are often regarded as a temporary expedient, to be replaced by more reliable methods as soon as these become available.

C. SPECIFICITY OF THE METHOD

It is evident that, if the substances being tested in the bioassays represent a code, the method must have a high degree of specificity. In other words, the material extracted from the brain of animals trained to a given task should induce in the recipients a behavior related to the training received by the donors.

This problem has been discussed by Rosenblatt (1970), Ungar (1970a,b, 1971), and Ungar and Chapouthier (1971), and there is agreement on the existence of an at least limited specificity, particularly in regard to the stimulus received by the donors. It was shown, for example, that extracts of brain taken from donors habituated to a sound induce habituation to sound but not to a sudden change in air pressure (air puff) and vice versa (Ungar, 1967a,b).

In other series of experiments, cross transfers were attempted between donors trained to escape electric shock into the lighted or the unlighted arms of a T or Y maze (Ungar, 1967b; Røigaard-Petersen *et al.*, 1968). These tests of specificity failed because escape into the unlighted arm did not prove transferable (Chapouthier and Ungerer, 1969).

A great deal of work was done with left–right discrimination, especially in Rosenblatt's laboratory (1970). It gave highly inconsistent results because it depended on a number of factors, particularly on the natural bias of the donors and of the recipients for one side or the other. We gave a partial explanation of these results by assuming that the message contained in the extracts and communicated to the recipients was not only to turn left or right but also to overcome their natural bias (Ungar and Irwin, 1967).

We made an attempt at cross-transfer between two passive avoidances, i.e., the dark avoidance mentioned above and the avoidance of step down from a platform. Material from the brain of donors trained to avoid the dark induced only dark avoidance in the recipients and had no effect on the latency of step-down. Conversely, extracts from donors trained to avoid the step-down increased in the recipients the latency of step-down but failed to influence the time spent in the dark (Ungar, 1970a). The recent studies of Rosenblatt (1969), where the donors were trained to respond to the same stimulus either by pressing a bar or pushing a door, also suggest the possibility of response specificity.

The most definite proof of stimulus specificity within the same sensory modality was supplied by Zippel and Domagk (1969). They trained goldfish to switch their preference from red to green by receiving food in the compartment of the tank signaled by a green light. After receiving an injection of the extract of brain taken from these donors, the recipients also switched their preference from red to green. Similar experiments were done with taste discrimination.

We have repeated these experiments (Ungar *et al.*, 1971b) and extended them to several combinations of colors: red (630–> 700 nm) vs blue (370–510 nm); blue vs green (480–629 nm) and orange (580–> 700 nm) vs yellow (560–630 nm). Figure 2 shows the results of the experiments; within the first 3 days after injection the preferences of the recipients changed in the direction predicted by the training of the donors. Our experiments differed in many respects from those of Zippel and Domagk. The natural preferences in the strain of goldfish used by us were green > blue > red, and our donors were trained by negative reinforcement; they received an electric shock in the compartment signaled by the wrong color.

An interesting feature of these assays was the suggestion of a "context specificity." For example, when donors trained to prefer red to blue were tested to choose between red and green they showed no significant red preference and when they were tested with blue and green did not avoid blue. The same effect was observed in the recipients of their brain. It seems, therefore, that the information encoded was a whole context of preferring red to blue and not preference of red against any other color.

There is, of course, need for many more experiments to evaluate the limit of specificity and to define exactly the sort of information that is recorded in the molecular code.

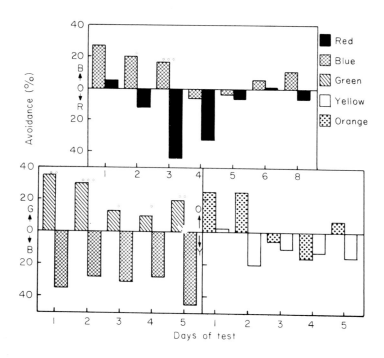

Fig. 2. Avoidance of colors by goldfish injected with brain extracts taken from donor fish trained to avoid those colors. The columns indicate the percentage avoidance of the recipients, corrected by their preinjection performance to account for their natural bias. The markings of the columns show the preference acquired by the donors whose brain extracts were injected. In the first experiment (top) one group of recipients was treated with brain extracts from donors trained to prefer red and avoid blue; the other group received extracts from donors trained to prefer blue and avoid red. In the second experiment (bottom left) the fish were injected with extracts from blue-preferring or green-preferring donors and the subjects of the third experiment (bottom right) received brain extracts from donors that preferred either yellow or orange. The asterisks indicate statistical significance (*, < 0.05; **, < 0.01; ***, < 0.001).

D. The Chemical Problem

The molecular approach to the neural coding problem has been strongly influenced by the advances of molecular genetics which showed that genetic information is stored in a DNA code which, for its expression, has to be transcribed into RNA and translated into the language of proteins. Since DNA cannot be modified by environmental influences, it was assumed that RNA must be involved in the coding of acquired information. This assumption, supported by Hydén's findings (1959), was accepted by McConnell, and many of the later workers using vertebrates (Fjerdingstad *et al.*, 1965; Babich *et al.*, 1965, among the earlier studies). There was something paradoxical in this assumption if we consider that according to the central dogma of molecular genetics RNA cannot contain information that is not already present in DNA and no new RNA sequences can be created by environmental influences. The original hypothesis of Hydén assuming RNA changes to be produced by an "instructional" process has to be changed to a "selectional" hypothesis by which the acquired information utilizes DNA sequences already present but repressed (Morrell, 1961). This would allow the synthesis of a kind of RNA and protein not previously made by that particular cell.

In surveying the bioassay experiments, it seems evident that information transfer was accomplished with brain preparations aimed at isolating RNA (Fjerdingstad *et al.*, 1965; Ádám and Faiszt, 1967; Krylov *et al.*, 1969; Gay and Raphelson, 1967) as well as with extracts made to obtain a peptide-rich fraction (Ungar and Oceguera-Navarro, 1965; Rosenblatt *et al.*, 1966b; Golub *et al.*, 1969; Zippel and Domagk, 1969). We attacked this problem in my laboratory (Ungar and Fjerdingstad, 1971) by preparing, from the same pool of brain taken from dark-avoiding rats, an "RNA-rich" extract and a so-called peptide extract. We found that both extracts were capable of inducing dark avoidance in mice. By submitting these extracts to proteases and to ribonuclease we found that their activity was destroyed by a protease (trypsin) but not by ribonuclease. This result suggested that the active substance was a peptide that could be somehow linked to RNA and extracted with it. This assumption was confirmed when we separated the active peptide by dialysis at low pH and left behind the inactive RNA. Faiszt and Ádám (1968) showed that the active material was associated with ribosomal RNA. This was confirmed in my laboratory by W. J. Hodges, who was also able to separate the dark-avoidance inducing peptide by dialyzing ribosomal RNA at pH 3.7.

Up to date, we have characterized, by their susceptibility to enzymic hydrolysis, three peptides corresponding to three different behavioral patterns: The sound-habituation inducing peptide is destroyed by chymotrypsin; the dark-avoidance inducing peptide is inactivated by trypsin; and the peptide which induces step-down avoidance is destroyed by both proteases (Ungar, 1970a,b).

Two-and-a-half years ago, I decided to isolate one of the active substances and chose dark avoidance as the easiest to test (see Fig. 1). We collected about 5 kg of trained rat brain over a period of 2 years. The best starting method of purification proved to be preparation of RNA and dialysis of the peptide at low pH. This phase of purification yielded about 1 mg of material/gram of fresh weight of brain. After purification by gel filtration on Sephadex G-25 this was reduced to 5 μg/gm. This material was further purified by thin-layer chromatography until we obtained a unique spot containing all the activity in 0.1 μg/gm. This spot was absent from similarly purified extracts of untrained brain.

$$
\begin{array}{ccccccccccccccc}
1 & 2 & 3 & 4 & 5 & 6 & 7 & 8 & 9 & 10 & 11 & 12 & 13 & 14 & 15 \\
\end{array}
$$

Ser-Asp-Asn-Asn-Gln-Gln-Gly-Lys-Ser-Ala-Gln-Gln-Gly-Gly-Tyr-NH$_2$

Fig. 3. Amino acid sequence of scotophobin, as established by mass spectrometry (Ungar *et al.*, 1971a).

After having established the amino acid composition and determined the *N*-terminal group, sequence determinations were made by mass spectrometry of the whole peptide and of the two fragments obtained by tryptic hydrolysis. The name scotophobin (from the Greek skotos, dark, and phobos, fear) was given to this peptide, most probable structure of which is shown in Fig. 3. The structure has now been confirmed by synthesis (Ungar *et al.*, 1971a).

IV. Molecular Basis of Neural Coding

The processing of information by the nervous system implies the existence of a system of signals into which information has to be translated in order to be taken up, integrated, stored, retrieved, and utilized. Such a system of signals came to be called a code. This concept is widely accepted for genetic information, but its validity is still questioned by students of the nervous system (E. Roberts, 1965; Moore *et al.*, 1966). It has been reviewed and discussed, among others, by Perkel and Bullock (1968), Kandel and Spencer (1968), and Uttal (1969).

A. NEURAL CODES

The study of the nervous system has been dominated throughout its history by the electrical activity it exhibits. The bioelectrical phenomena are considered to be the outstanding characteristics of neurons, and it is well established that the pattern of electrical impulses traveling along the axon represents information. Adrian (1928) showed that the intensity of stimuli put into sensory receptors is converted into frequencies, representing a "stimulus code" (Uttal, 1969).

It has been assumed that information, after its integration at the higher centers, is also represented by complex electrical patterns, forming a code. In other words, if this code were known, we should be able to take a pattern and retranslate it into a visual image, a complex perception, a feeling, or a thought. The existence of what Uttal calls a "systemic code" is at present purely hypothetical in spite of the volume of data collected on electrical phenomena picked up by a variety of recording techniques (Adey, 1966). The significance of these electrical signals for information coding has been discussed by John (1967), Adey (1969), and most exhaustively by Perkel and Bullock (1968).

As far as we know at present, a given electrical pattern has meaning only within a specific neural pathway. Picking up signals in the auditory pathway, for example, will tell us something about the intensity of the sound stimulus, and if we could distinguish between the individual neurons and record from them, we might gain information on the quality of the sound received. However, as soon as we reach the higher centers where information of different sensory modalities is combined, the meaning is lost. There are grave doubts on the possibility at higher levels, say in the cortex, of recognizing signals coming from different sensory sources and different levels of integration.

It is likely, therefore, that the most important elements of information are coded by what Perkel and Bullock call "labeled lines" and the electrical signals have meaning only within the context of each line. This idea is not new. As I mentioned earlier, it is implicit in Müller's "law of specific energies" and the concept of "local signs" of Sherrington (1906). Like other information processing machines, the brain seems to have a "program" built into its structure, but unlike the machines, the brain can constantly reprogram itself in terms of incoming information.

Let us examine the inborn structural code and the possible mechanisms of reprogramming. The centers and pathways of the nervous system are organized according to a plan laid down in the genome. The sensory receptors are connected by well-defined pathways to specific centers and the motor centers in turn have their constant connections with the muscles or other effector organs. We also know that certain responses are regularly elicited by a given stimulus without learning. These reflexes, organized into more or less complex behavioral patterns, are called instincts. The network of innate connections is the expression of genetic information and represents a code since it can direct the nerve impulses along specific channels.

A nervous system possessing fixed connections can only produce stereotyped behavior whose adaptive capabilities are limited to whatever situations are anticipated by heredity. To account for the "plasticity" of higher organisms, their ability to learn from experience and to adapt to unforeseen situations, the nervous system must be able to form new connections. The central problem of information processing is the mechanism by which these new connections can be created.

The earlier hypotheses assumed that learning is supported by the growth of new synapses (Ramón y Cajal, 1911; Hebb, 1949; Eccles, 1965). The main objection to this hypothesis is the slowness of the growth process compared with the rapidity of memory fixation. Elul (1966) proposed an explanation based on a more rapid process of deformation of the neural membrane by electrokinetic phenomena, but it still remains conjectural. Kandel and Spencer (1968) discussed the data supporting the various hypotheses on synaptic efficiency as the basic condition in learning, i.e., effect of use and disuse, formation of dominant and mirror foci, fixation of postural asymmetries, and possible "trophic" effects of neural activity.

To have general validity, any explanation must be able to account for the extreme rapidity with which information may be acquired and retained for indefinite periods. The important phenomenon is the one that takes place at the very beginning of the process. The explanation that best fulfills the condition is the "functional validation" (Jacobson, 1969) of synapses that are anatomically present but "are not functionally operative" (Cragg, 1967), by the mechanism known as "concurrent activity," "simultaneous firing," "temporal contiguity," etc. This mechanism can be traced back almost 100 years to Brown-Sequard, Wedensky, Pavlov, and Baer (John, 1967), but its importance was particularly emphasized by Hebb (1949).

I shall have more to say about the creation of new synaptic connections. In the meantime, I should like to state very briefly my belief that information is identified in the nervous system by the pathways through which the appropriate impulses travel; the electrical code contributes only quantitative elements which are probably lost in long time storage.

B. Labeled Pathways

There is good circumstantial evidence that the structural information built into the nervous system is organized on chemical principles. Sperry (1963), Weiss (1965), and Jacobson (1969) believe that the organization of neural pathways can best be explained by a molecular recognition mechanism. "Each individual cell carries a set of distinctive marking proteins on its surface. . . . Effective synapses form between cells which have identical or nearly identical proteins on their surfaces (R. B. Roberts and Flexner, 1966)." Most of the evidence for this view comes from experiments on regeneration of the optic nerve. At a given stage during embryonic life, nerve cells lose their pluripotentiality and can make synapses only with specific neurons.

It is probable that this high differentiation of synaptic connections is only an extreme refinement of the general ability of all cells to recognize each other and form aggregates composed of homologous cells. Moscona and Moscona (1963) showed that adhesion between similar cells is genetically determined and can be abolished by puromycin and, locally, by proteases and by removal of calcium. They characterized the recognition molecules as glycoproteins.

There has been a great deal of speculation recently on the intersynaptic material or "gap substance" (Johnston and Roots, 1965; Kelly, 1967; Bloom and Aghajanian, 1968). The role of calcium in controlling synaptic transmission (as in cell aggregation just mentioned) has been emphasized by Penn and Loewenstein (1966), Miledi and Slater (1966), and Grenell (1969).

Labeling of the neural pathways during embryonic development can explain innate stereotyped responses and may also serve for the coding of acquired information. Sperry admitted the possibility that the innate labeling system may be adapted to facilitate the "plasticity" of the adult brain (1963). In Jacobson's view (1969), "the modifiability of neuronal connections in the adult is regarded as the continuation of developmental processes." A similar opinion was expressed by R. B. Roberts and Flexner (1966): ". . . identity reactions could strengthen frequently used synapses if inducers were transmitted across synapses at simultaneous firings. Such a process would be specific; it would not facilitate other synapses of the same cell."

The most plausible mechanism for the creation of new synaptic connections is the "concurrent activity" mentioned above (Section IV,A). The permeability changes taking place when two contiguous neurons fire simultaneously or at very brief intervals could favor the movement of material across the synaptic gap. This movement is probably directed from the pre-synaptic to the post-synaptic element, in agreement with the usually accepted sequence of events in conditioning. It is possible that the passage of some coded molecules would create new functional connections in some of the hitherto inert synapses. Cragg (1967) estimated that only about 1 % of the average number of 10^4 synapses on each cortical neuron is actually functional.

Exchange of material at synaptic junctions has been discussed by Droz (1969), who has raised the question of the fate of the material transported by axoplasmic flow when it reaches the axonal ending. Korr et al. (1967) saw labeled material leave nerve endings and enter muscle cells. Waxman and Pappas (1969) observed pinocytosis at the post-synaptic membrane and Loewenstein (1966) studied the exchange of substances between cells that "recognize" each other.

The labeled pathways, by undergoing constant switches among themselves, could explain the most intricate processes of information processing. In the words of Sperry (1958), by the "opening and closing of different patterns at different times, the single morphological network can in effect be transformed into many different types of circuits with widely differing properties and capacities."

C. Molecular Hypotheses

The molecular interpretation of neural information processing has often been regarded as the antithesis of the connectionist view. This position has been maintained both by the proponents of the molecular hypothesis (McConnell, 1965) and its opponents (Glassman, 1969). In fact, I believe that not only is there no contradiction between the specific organization of neural connections and the assumption of a molecular code but the two concepts complement each other. The molecular code organizes the innate connections and is capable also of reprogramming them.

The data supplied by the various approaches to the problem of the chemical correlates of information processing (Sections II and III) have been, on the whole, interpreted in three different ways: (a) nonspecific interpretations, (b) "nonneurological" hypotheses based on the existence of "tape recorder" molecules, and (c) hypotheses based on the molecular labeling of pathways.

1. *Nonspecific Interpretations*

The role of protein synthesis associated with information processing is most commonly interpreted as being necessary for increasing the closeness and, perhaps, the number of synaptic contacts, for synthesizing and metabolizing neurotransmitters, or maintaining increased neuronal function. This is the least controversial interpretation since it does not actually represent molecular coding. The newly synthesized molecules do not encode information directly or indirectly; they merely maintain neural function and adjust it to the increased demands presumably created by the acquisition of information. The molecules would be of the same species regardless of the particular piece of information processed.

It is certain that increased function requires increased protein synthesis not only in the nervous system but in all cells. For a discussion of this problem from the point of view of neural function see a review by Ungar and Irwin (1968) and the volume edited by Lajtha (1970). It is probable that some of the newly synthesized protein is used for maintenance of the machinery which keeps the neurons excitable and capable of conducting impulses. Another fraction may adjust the process of synaptic transmission to increased demands. There have been a number of hypotheses involving these basic processes of neural function (Overton, 1969; Sachs, 1961; Briggs and Kitto, 1962; Smith, 1962), but their discussion is not relevant to the coding problem.

A large number of studies indicate that synaptic transmitters play a role in information processing (McGaugh and Petrinovitch, 1965; Deutsch, 1966), but this is not surprising and does not contribute much to our understanding of the coding process, except perhaps by supplying a simplified model for it, as I shall try to show below. In fact, acceptance of the nonspecific interpretations neither contradicts nor supports the molecular hypothesis. Molecular coding, if it exists, is superimposed on the basic processes of neural function whose integrity requires biochemical maintenance.

2. *"Nonneurological" Hypotheses*

Ever since the first experimental demonstration of cerebral localizations by Hitzig and Fritsch exactly 100 years ago, a lively debate has been going on between localizationists and antilocalizationists. Nobody questions today the localization of certain sensory and motor functions in the brain, but opinion is still divided and somewhat confused on the possibility of applying the same principle to higher nervous ("mental") functions. The most influential antilocalizationist of recent times was Lashley, whose concept of "equipotentiality" of different parts of the brain (1950) is still with us. It is being supported by a school of electrophysiology which emphasizes "macropotentials" (John, 1967) at the expense of the unit activity. As I mentioned earlier, the only certainly established electrical code is the pattern and, more particularly, the frequency of firing of the unit.

All the "nonneurological" molecular hypotheses are based on the field theory which, according to Hebb (1949), represents the brain "as having all the finer structure of a bowlful of porridge." These hypotheses tend to replace neural nets with "molecular nets" (Schmitt, 1962), which float in the porridge. Landauer (1964) assumed that an electrical pattern may give rise to the synthesis of a new molecular species of RNA which stores the information contained in the pattern. The synthesis takes place in the glia, but the RNA is transferred to the neurons which become sensitized to future occurrences of the same pattern.

Since neurons stop dividing at a very early age, one could make a case for the nervous system not being ruled by the "central dogma" of molecular biology and synthesizing RNA not specified in DNA. Such an assumption was made first by Hydén in his first hypothesis (1959) and by Hechter and Halkerston (1964). Even the possibility of changing DNA by methylation of its bases was raised by Griffith and Mahler (1969). Others did not go that far; they only postulated conformational changes in RNA molecules under the influence of changes in electrical fields (Katchalsky and Oplatka, 1966; Stanford and Lorey, 1969).

The hypothesis proposed by Robinson (1966) avoids the heresy of requiring new RNA nonspecified in the genome. He believed that a given pattern of firing causes the release of a set of "pattern molecules." These are picked up by glial cells in which they induce the formation of complementary substances ("pattern comolecules"). When the same firing pattern occurs again the pattern molecules will be recognized by their comolecules.

The essential weakness of all these theories is that they have no explanation for the encoding and the decoding process: Even if it were proven that electrical patterns contain all the information, we do not see how this can be converted into a molecular code and how this molecular code is translated into a behavioral response or a retrievable memory trace. These difficulties become even greater in the most extreme of these hypotheses (McConnell, 1965), which postulates that acquired information coded in "tape-recorder" molecules, is stored not only in the nervous system but in all cells of the body, like genetic information.

One should, finally, question the basic assumption of these "non-neurological" interpretations. It seems today that Lashley's "search of the engram" (1950) was probably a wild goose chase. There is probably no such thing as an engram in either the anatomical or chemical sense, and it was therefore somewhat naive to expect the destruction of specific information by removal of parts of the brain. Information is probably distributed in the brain at a number of hierarchic levels so that practically the whole central nervous system is involved in the acquisition of every new set of information. Lashley's experiments prove only that the specificity of neural pathways is much more subtle and much less inflexible than the early localizationists or connectionists imagined and that it is compatible with a diffuse distribution of information. Memory traces are only routing schedules for nerve impulses and are retrieved every time these retrace their original path.

3. *Molecular Code of Labeled Pathways*

A number of hypotheses have been proposed in which the molecular coding is superimposed on the anatomical organization of the pathways: The code is represented by the substances that label the channels. We have seen above (Section IV,B) the evidence for such labeling underlying the development of the nervous system. It may be considered that when "the chemical coding of information is adventitious to an anatomical coding of memory" (Booth, 1970) the former is redundant and therefore unnecessary. This argument loses its validity if one regards the chemical coding as the means by which new connections can be formed and maintained for long periods of time.

Katz and Halstead (1950) believed that information was encoded in "nucleoprotein" molecules which, by their presence in the cell membrane, were able to create new connections. Their hypothesis is now obsolete because it was formulated before the DNA–RNA–protein system of cellular information processing was elucidated, but the basic idea may still be correct.

The most remarkable speculations were published by Szilard in 1964 based on the presence of "specific membrane proteins" in each category or neurons, corresponding to their functional specificity. He believed that some neurons are "congenitally determined" and can produce only stereotyped responses. However, when they make contact with a "memory neuron" and both neurons fire simultaneously, the specific protein of the former penetrates into the latter where it induces the formation of a complementary molecule "just as an antigen induces its antibody." This process called "transprinting" results in the formation of a new synaptic connection. Rosenblatt (1967) further developed these ideas and assumed that, during activity, both pre- and post-synaptic cells released specific, mutually complementary substances, finally located in the synaptic gap.

The hypothesis I have proposed (Ungar, 1968, 1970b,c) emphasizes the continuity of the mechanism by which the nervous system becomes organized and which allows it to process acquired information. The genetically determined labels by which neurons recognize each other will later on serve as "connectors" between neurons brought together by the simultaneous activity induced through experience. When a functional synaptic junction is formed between two pathways hitherto unconnected, the two labels form a complex which becomes the code for that particular synapse. Analogous synapses are formed probably at hundreds of sites each marked by the same coded complex. This can be extracted from the brain, and when it is injected into recipients it will induce the appropriate behavior by recreating in their brain the connection for which it is coded.

Figure 4 and 5 show two examples of the application of the hypothesis. Figure 4 represents the diagram of a Pavlovian conditioning paradigms with the behavioral, the physiological, and the presumed molecular events shown in parallel. In Fig. 5, escape training in a T maze introduces the elements of feedback which contribute to the elaboration of the behavior.

A similar theory was formulated by Best (1968), who calls the pathway-specific substance a "neuron identification code" (NIC). The code words of the pathways involved in a given information form polymers, "poly-NIC" molecules, which stand for the connections and, consequently, represent the record of the experience.

I estimated that the innate labeling of the pathways would require about 10^7 distinct molecular species (Ungar, 1968). If the specificity of these molecules resides in the amino acid sequences, there are theoretically enough hexapeptides to label all the pathways. It is more likely, however, that the neuronal recognition system evolved progressively. In a simple nervous system, individual amino acids could suffice for coding all the pathways and the suspected transmitter function of a few amino acids (Aprison and Werman, 1968) may represent the vestige of this primitive labeling system. The division of neurons according to the transmitters they release and to which they respond also represents a cod-

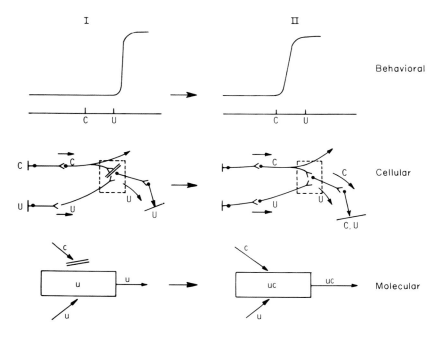

Fig. 4. Diagram of the behavioral, cellular, and molecular events in classical conditioning. I, before training; II, at criterion. At the behavioral level, the response that was elicited only by the unconditioned stimulus (U) si now produced by the conditioned stimulus (C). At the cellular level, the neuronal circuit corresponding to the unconditioned response has, before training, no connection with the pathways of the conditioned stimulus. As a result of training, the junction is achieved between them so that the response is elicited by the conditioned stimulus. At the molecular level, the unconditioned pathway, labeled u during development of the nervous system, becomes connected to the neuronal circuit carrying the conditioned stimulus (c) by the mechanism of "concurrent activity" (precedence of firing in C would favor release of label c and its penetration into U). In this fashion, merging of molecular markers c and u would make a functional synapse, labeled uc, through which the response could be elicited by the conditioned stimulus.

ing system. For example, cholinergic neurons can form effective connections only with cholinoceptive elements. It is unlikely, however, that this system can be endowed with plasticity.

It is tempting to speculate that as, in the course of evolution, the role of acquired information gained in importance for successful survival, the need for increased plasticity of the nervous system created more and more intricate coding processes. The connector complexes coding for the variety of human experience may represent enormously large molecules, unless one assumes that the emergence of language has evolved a new simplified

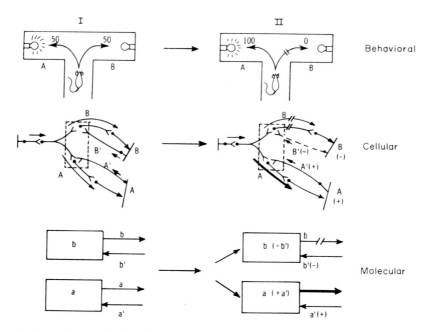

Fig. 5. Diagram of a brightness discrimination paradigm. Before training, the animal runs theoretically half the time into each arm of the T maze. If it is systematically shocked in the unlighted arm, at the end of training it will run 100% into the lighted arm. This behavior is controlled by the feedback the brain receives from the result of each run: unlighted arm, pain; lighted arm, no pain. Run into the lighted arm (*A*) is reinforced by positive feedback (*A'*) and run into the unlighted arm (*B*) is inhibited by negative feedback (*B'*). At the molecular level, this may be accomplished by the formation of molecular complex *bb'* having an inhibitory action and *aa'* having a facilitatory action on some critical synaptic junctions.

code. Perhaps the superiority of the human brain is due to the fact that it handles information in a symbolic code, instead of the cumbersome complexes of pathway markers. If such a symbolic code exists, it must have evolved from other more primitive forms and must also be based on chemical principles.

V. Concluding Remarks

Of all the experimental approaches to the molecular coding of neural information surveyed in this chapter, only the bioassay method can actually help to isolate and identify the code words. Two other promising approaches, one immunological (Janković *et al.*, 1968; Rosenblatt, 1970), the other based on DNA–RNA hybridization (Machlus and Gaito, 1969), have deliberately been left out of the survey because it is too early to assess their value. At some later stage, it may be possible to replace the bioassays by more reliable methods such as those just mentioned or by radioimmunoassays. It is likely, however, that for the next few years we shall have to put up with the uncertainties and frustrations of the biological assays.

To take full advantage of this method, concerted efforts should be made to isolate the greatest possible number of code words. We have started collecting material for identification of the peptide that induces habituation to sound and are making plans for studying some of the substances related to color discrimination in the goldfish. I hope that the identification of scotophobin will break down some of the resistance to this approach.

Objections to a molecular coding stem largely from the ingrained idea that the nervous system is an electronic machine. Generations of neurophysiologists have been exploring it by electrical means, and now the electronic computer has become an extremely useful model for its operations. The important part of the model, however, is the computing principle, not the means by which it is accomplished. Computation can be achieved by mechanical, optical, and many other processes, and living systems seem to use chemical computing, as exemplified by the processing of genetic information. Transcription of DNA sequences into RNA is the result of chemical computation and so is the translation of RNA into protein in which the ribosome plays the role of a computing unit.

The nervous system can be regarded as a chemical computer operating by means of molecular switches. The decision of a neuron to fire or not to fire is the result of computation, accomplished by molecular means. A given behavior is the outcome of computations by many thousands of units organized into complex circuits. Almost 30 years ago, Craik (1943) compared the nervous system to "a calculating machine capable of modeling or paralleling external events." In today's language we can say that the brain "simulates" the universe, more specifically, the interaction of each individual with his own particular universe. Such a mechanism adjusts this interaction continuously to assure the best possible adaptation and, by preserving the memory of past interactions, maintains the continuity of the individual and, in man, the consciousness of personality.

The question remains open whether the mechanisms proposed in this chapter can explain the functioning of such a computer. In a lucid discussion of this problem, Weiss (1965) called the molecular recognition phenomenon "a universal feature of living nature" and underlined its importance in the development of the nervous system as well as in its ability to adapt to new situations. He asserted that "the hierarchical organization of the central nervous system has superimposed upon the rigid base mechanisms of the lower forms systems of greater adaptive flexibility. The newer systems can. . .form new words from the letters of the innate vocabulary." In terms of what we know of the code at present, it would probably be more correct to say that, by acquiring new information and processing it, the nervous system forms new sentences with the words of the innate vocabulary. Discovering the rules of grammar and syntax by which the sentences are formed is the essential aim of future research.

REFERENCES

Adám, G., and Faiszt, J. (1967). *Nature (London)* **216**, 198.

Adey, W. R. (1966). *In* "Progress in Physiological Psychology" (E. Stellar and J. M. Sprague, eds.), Vol. 1, p. 1. Academic Press, New York.

Adey, W. R. (1969). *Neurosci. Res. Program, Bull.* **7**, 75.

Adrian, E. D. (1928). "The Basis of Sensation. The Action of Sense Organs," Christophers, London.

Agranoff, B. W. (1965). *Perspect. Biol. Med.* **9**, 13.

Agranoff, B. W., Davis, R. E., and Brink, J. J. (1965). *Proc. Nat. Acad. Sci. U. S.* **54**, 788.

Agranoff, B. W., Davis, R. E., Casola, L., and Lim, R. (1967). *Science* **158**, 1600.

Aprison, M. H., and Werman, R. (1968). *In* "Neurosciences Research" (S. Ehrenpreis and O. C. Solnitzky, eds.), Vol. 1, p. 143. Academic Press, New York.

Babich, F. R., Jacobson, A. L., Bubash, S., and Jacobson, A. (1965). *Science* **149**, 656.

Barondes, S. H., and Cohen, H. D. (1966). *Science* **151**, 594.

Barondes, S. H., and Cohen, H. D. (1967). *Proc. Nat. Acad. Sci. U. S.* **58**, 157.

Barondes, S. H., and Cohen, H. D. (1968a). *Science* **160**, 556.

Barondes, S. H., and Cohen, H. D. (1968b). *Proc. Nat. Acad. Sci. U. S.* **61**, 923.

Barondes, S. H., and Jarvik, M. E. (1964). *J. Neurochem.* **11**, 187.

Bateson, P. P. G., Horn, G., and Rose, S. P. R. (1969). *Nature (London)* **223**, 535.

Beach, G., Emmens, M., Kimble, D. P., and Lickey, M. (1969). *Proc. Nat. Acad. Sci. U. S.* **62**, 692.

Best, R. M. (1968). *Psychol. Rep.* **22**, 107.

Bloom, F. E., and Aghajanian, G. K. (1968). *J. Ultrastruct. Res.* **22**, 361.

Bogoch, S. (1968). "The Biochemistry of Memory." Oxford Univ. Press, London and New York.

Booth, D. A. (1970). *In* "Molecular Mechanisms in Memory and Learning" (G. Ungar, ed.), p. 1. Plenum Press, New York.

Bowman, R. E., and Strobel, D. A. (1969). *J. Comp. Physiol. Psychol.* **67**, 448.

Braud, W. G. (1970). *Science* **168**, 1234.

Briggs, M. H., and Kitto, G. B. (1962). *Psychol. Rev.* **69**, 537.

Byrne, W. L., ed. (1970). "Molecular Approaches to Learning and Memory." Academic Press, New York.

Byrne, W. L., Samuel, D., Bennett, E. L., Rosenzweig, M. R., Wasserman, E., Wagner, A. R., Gardner, R., Galambos, R., Berger, B. D., Margules, D. L., Fenichel, R. L., Stein, L., Corson, J. A., Enesco, H. E., Chorover, S. L., Holt, C. E., III, Schiller, P. H., Chiappetta, L., Jarvik, M. E., Leaf, R. C., Dutcher, J. D., Horovitz, Z. P., and Carlson, P. L. (1966). *Science* **153**, 658.

Chapouthier, G., and Ungerer, A. (1969). *Rev. Comportement Anim.* **3**, 64.

Cohen, H. D. (1970). *In* "Molecular Mechanisms in Memory and Learning" (G. Ungar, ed.), p. 59. Plenum Press, New York.

Cohen, H. D., and Barondes, S. H. (1967). *Science* **157**, 333.

Corning, W. C., and Riccio, D. (1970). *In* "Molecular Approaches to Learning and Memory" (W. L. Byrne, ed.), p. 107. Academic Press, New York.

Cragg, B. G. (1967). *J. Anat.* **101**, 639.

Craik, K. J. W. (1943). "The Nature of Explanation." Cambridge Univ. Press, London and New York.

Davis, R. E., and Agranoff, B. W. (1966). *Proc. Nat. Acad. Sci. U. S.* **55**, 555.

Deutsch, J. A. (1966). *Dis. Nerv. Syst.* **27**, 20.

Dingman, W., and Sporn, M. B. (1961). *J. Psychiat. Res.* **1**, 1.

Droz, B. (1969). *Int. Rev. Cytol.* **25**, 363.

Dyal, J. A., Golub, A. M., and Marrone, R. L. (1967). *Nature (London)* **214**, 720.

Eccles, J. C. (1965). *In* "Anatomy of Memory" (D. P. Kimble, ed.), p. 12. Science and Behavior Books, Palo Alto, California.

Elul, R. (1966). *Nature (London)* **210**, 1127.

Faiszt, J., and Ádám, G. (1968). *Nature (London)* **220**, 367.

Fjerdingstad, E. J. (1969). *J. Biol. Psychol.* **11**, 20.

Fjerdingstad, E. J., ed. (1971). "Chemical Transfer of Learned Information." North-Holland Publ. Amsterdam.

Fjerdingstad, E. J., Nissen, T., and Røigaard-Petersen, H. H. (1965). *Scand. J. Psychol.* **6**, 1.

Fjerdingstad, E. J., Nissen, T., and Röigaard-Petersen, H. H. (1966). *In* "Molecular Basis of Some Aspects of Mental Activity" (O. Walaas, ed.), Vol. 1, p. 165. Academic Press, New York.

Flexner, L. B., and Flexner, J. B. (1966). *Proc. Nat. Acad. Sci. U. S.* **55**, 369.

Flexner, L. B., and Flexner, J. B. (1968). *Science* **159**, 330.

Flexner, L. B., Flexner, J. B., Roberts, R. B., and de la Haba, G. (1964). *Proc. Nat. Acad. Sci. U. S.* **52**, 1165.

Flexner, L. B., Flexner, J. B., and Roberts, R. B. (1967). *Science* **155**, 1377.

Frank, B., Stein, D. G., and Rosen, J. (1970). *Science* **169**, 399.

Gambetti, P., Gonatas, N. K., and Flexner, L. B. (1968). *Science* **161**, 900.

Gay, R., and Raphelson, A. (1967). *Psychon. Sci.* **8**, 369.

Gibby, R. G., Crough, D. G., and Thios, S. J. (1968). *Psychon. Sci.* **12**, 295.

Giurgea, C., Daliers, J., and Mouravieff, F. (1969). *Abstr. Int. Congr. Pharmacol., 4th,* 1969, p. 291.

Glassman, E. (1969). *Annu. Rev. Biochem.* **38**, 605.

Golub, A. M., Epstein, L., and McConnell, J. V. (1969). *J. Biol. Psychol.* **11**, 44.

Golub, A. M., Masiarz, F. R., Villars, T., and McConnell, J. V. (1970). *Science* **168**, 392.

Gordon, M. W., Deanin, G. G., Leonhardt, H. L., and Gwynn, R. H. (1966). *Amer. J. Psychiat.* **122**, 1174.

Grenell, R. G. (1969). Presentation at the meeting of the American Association for the Advancement of Science, Boston, 1969.

Griffith, J. S., and Mahler, H. R. (1969). *Nature (London)* **223**, 580.

Gross, C. R., and Carey, F. M. (1965). *Science* **150**, 1749.

Hebb, D. O. (1949). "The Organization of Behavior." Wiley, New York.

Hechter, O., and Halkerston, I. D. K. (1964). *Perspect. Biol. Med.* **7**, 183.

Hutt, L. D., and Elliott, L. (1970). *Psychon. Sci.* **18**, 57.

Hydén, H. (1959). In "Biochemistry of the Central Nervous System," *Fourth Int. Congr. Biochem., Vienna*, p. 64. Pergamon, Oxford.

Hydén, H. (1967). *Progr. Nucl. Acid Res. Mol. Biol.* **6**, 187.

Hydén, H. (1969). In "The Future of the Brain Sciences" (S. Bogoch, ed.), p. 264. Plenum Press, New York.

Hydén, H., and Lange, P. W. (1968). *Science* **159**, 1370.

Jacobson, M. (1969). *Science* **163**, 543.

James, W. (1890). "Principles of Psychology." Holt, New York.

Janković, B. D., Rakić, L., Veskov, R., and Horfat, J. (1968). *Nature (London)* **218**, 270.

John, E. R. (1967). "Mechanisms of Memory." Academic Press, New York.

Johnston, P. V., and Roots, B. I. (1965). *Nature (London)* **205**, 778.

Kandel, E. R., and Spencer, W. A. (1968). *Psysiol. Rev.* **48**, 65.

Katchalsky, A., and Oplatka, A. (1966). *Neurosci. Res. Program, Bull.* **4**, Suppl., 71.

Katz, J. J., and Halstead, W. C. (1950). *Comp. Psychol. Monogr.* **20**, 1.

Kelly, D. E. (1967). *Anesthesiology* **28**, 6.

Kimble, R. J., and Kimble, D. P. (1966). *Worm Runner's Dig.* **8**, 32.

Korr, I. M., Wilkinson, P. N., and Chornock, F. W. (1967). *Science* **155**, 342.

Krylov, O. A., Kalyuzhnaya, P. I., and Tongur, V. S. (1969). *Zh. Vyssh. Nerv. Deyatel. I. P. Pavlov* **19**, 286.

Lajtha, A., ed. (1970). "Protein Metabolism of the Nervous System." Plenum Press, New York.

Landauer, T. K. (1964). *Psychol. Rev.* **71**, 167.

Lashley, K. S. (1950). In "Physiological Mechanisms in Animal Behavior," *Soc. Exp. Biol. Symp. No 4*, p. 478. Cambridge Univ. Press. London and New York.

Loewenstein, W. R. (1966). *Ann. N. Y. Acad. Sci.* **137**, 441.

Loewi, O. (1921). *Pfluegers Arch. Gesamte Physiol. Menschen Tiere* **189**, 239.

Luttges, M., Johnson, T., Buck, C., Holland, J., and McGaugh, J. (1966). *Science* **151**, 834.

McConnell, J. V. (1962). *J. Neuropsychiat.* **3**, Suppl. 1, 42.

McConnell, J. V. (1965). *Anim. Behav.* **13**, 61.

McConnell, J. V., and Shelby, J. M. (1970). In "Molecular Mechanisms in Memory and Learning" (G. Ungar, ed.), p. 71. Plenum Press, New York.

McConnell, J. V., Shigehisa, T., and Salive, H. (1968). *J. Biol. Psychol.* **10**, 32.

McGaugh, J. L. (1966). *Science* **153**, 135.

McGauch, J. L., and Petrinovitch, L. (1965). *Int. Rev. Neurobiol.* **8**, 139.

Machlus, B., and Gaito, J. (1969). *Nature (London)* **222**, 573.

Miledi, R., and Slater, C. R. (1966). *J. Physiol. (London)* **184**, 473.

Monné, L. (1948). *Advanc. Enzymol.* **8**, 1.

Moore, G. P., Perkel, D. H., and Segundo, J. P. (1966). *Annu. Rev. Physiol.* **28**, 493.

Morrell, F. (1961). *Physiol. Rev.* **41**, 443.

Moscona, M. H., and Moscona, A. A. (1963). *Science* **142**, 1070.

Overton, R. K. (1959). *Psychol. Rep.* **5**, 721.

Penn, R. D., and Loewenstein, W. R. (1966). *Science* **151**, 88.

Perkel, D. H., and Bullock, T. H. (1968). *Neurosci. Res. Program, Bull.* **6**, 221.

Rahmann, H. (1965). *Z. Zellforsch. Mikrosk. Anat.* **67**, 561.

Ramón y Cajal, S. (1911). "Histologie du système nerveux de l'homme et des vertébrés" (Transl. by L. Azoulay). Vol. II. Maloine, Paris.

Rappoport, D. A., and Daginawala, H. F. (1968). *J. Neurochem.* **15**, 991.

Reinis, S. (1965). *Activ. Nerv. Super.* **7**, 167.

Rensch, B., and Rahmann, H. (1966). *Pfluegers Arch. Ges. Physiol.* **290**, 158.

Ribot, T. A. (1881). "Les maladies de la mémoire." Baillière et Fils, Paris.

Roberts, E. (1965). *In* "The Anatomy of Memory" (D. P. Kimble, ed.), p. 292. Science and Behavior Books, Palo Alto, California.

Roberts, R. B., and Flexner, L. B. (1966). *Amer. Sc.* **54**, 174.

Robinson, C. E. (1966). *In* "Molecular Basis of Some Aspects of Mental Activity" (O. Walaas, ed.), Vol. 1, p. 29. Academic Press, New York.

Røigaard-Petersen, H. H., Nissen, T., and Fjerdingstad, E. J. (1968). *Scand. J. Psychol.* **9**, 1.

Rose, S. P. R. (1967). *Nature (London)* **215**, 253.

Rosenblatt, F. (1967). *In* "Computer and Information Sciences" (J. T. Tou, ed.), Vol. II, p. 33. Academic Press, New York.

Rosenblatt, F. (1969). *Proc. Nat. Acad. Sci. U. S.* **64**, 661.

Rosenblatt, F. (1970). *In* "Molecular Mechanisms in Memory and Learning" (G. Ungar, ed.), p. 103. Plenum Press, New York.

Rosenblatt, F., and Miller, R. G. (1966). *Proc. Nat. Acad. Sci. U. S.* **56**, 1423 and 1683.

Rosenblatt, F., Farrow, J. T., and Herblin, W. F. (1966a). *Nature (London)* **209**, 46.

Rosenblatt, F., Farrow, J. T., and Rhine, S. (1966b). *Proc. Nat. Acad. Sci. U. S.* **55**, 548 and 787.

Rosenthal, E., and Sparber, S. B. (1968). *Pharmacologist* **10**, 168.

Sachs, E. (1961). *Fed. Proc., Fed. Amer. Soc. Exp. Biol.* **20**, 339.

Schmitt, F. O. (1962). "Macromolecular Specificity and Biological Memory." MIT Press, Cambridge, Massachusetts.

Schmitt, F. O., and Samson, F. E., Jr. (1969). *Neurosci. Res. Program, Bull.* **7**, 27.

Semon, R. (1904). "The Mneme." Allen and Unwin, London.

Shashoua, V. E. (1968). *Nature (London)* **217**, 238.

Sherrington, C. S. (1906). "The Integrative Action of the Nervous System." Cambridge Univ. Press, London and New York.

Smith, C. E. (1962). *Science* **138**, 889.

Sperry, R. W. (1958). *In* "Biological and Biochemical Bases of Behavior" (H. H. Harlow and C. N. Wolsey, eds.), p. 401. Univ. of Wisconsin Press, Madison.

Sperry, R. W. (1963). *Proc. Nat. Acad. Sci. U. S.* **50**, 703.

Stanford, A. L., Jr., and Lorey, R. A. (1968). *Nature (London)* **219**, 1250.

Szilard, L. (1964). *Proc. Nat. Acad. Sci. U. S.* **51**, 1092.

Telwar, G. P., Chopra, S. P., Geel, B. K., and D'Monte, B. (1966). *J. Neurochem.* **13**, 109.

Ungar, G. (1967a). *Proc. Int. Congr. Coll. Int. Neuropsychopharmacol., 5th*, 1966. p. 169.

Ungar, G. (1967b). *J. Biol. Psychol.* **9**, 12.

Ungar, G. (1968). *Perspect. Biol. Med.* **11**, 217.

Ungar, G. (1970a). *In* "Protein Metabolism of the Nervous System" (A. Lajtha, ed.), p. 571. Plenum Press, New York.

Ungar, G. (1970b). *In* "Molecular Mechanisms in Memory and Learning" (G. Ungar, ed.), p. 149. Plenum Press, New York.

Ungar, G. (1970c). *Int. Rev. Neurobiol.* **13**, 223.

Ungar, G. (1971). *In* "Methods in Pharmacology" (A. Schwartz, ed.) p. 479. Appleton, New York.

Ungar, G., and Chapouthier, G. (1971). *Année Psychol.* **71**, 153.

Ungar, G., and Fjerdingstad, E. J. (1971). *In* "Symposium on Biology of Memory," Hung. Acad. Sci., Budapest, p. 137.

Ungar, G., and Irwin, L. N. (1967). *Nature (London)* **214**, 453.

Ungar, G., and Irwin, L. N. (1968). *In* "Neurosciences Research" (S. Ehrenpreis and O. C. Solnitzky, eds.), Vol. 1, p. 73. Academic Press, New York.

Ungar, G., and Oceguera-Navarro, C. (1965). *Nature (London)* **207**, 301.

Ungar, G., Galvan, L., and Clark, R. H. (1968). *Nature (London)* **217**, 1259.

Ungar, G., Desiderio, D. M., and Parr, W. (1971a). *Nature (London)* (in press).

Ungar, G., Galvan, L., and Chapouthier, G. (1971b). In preparation.

Uttal, W. R. (1969). *Perspect. Biol. Med.* **12**, 344.

von Foerster, H. (1948). "Das Gedächtnis; Eine quantenmechanische Untersuchung." Deuticke, Vienna.

Waxman, S. G., and Pappas, G. D. (1969). *Brain Res.* **14**, 240.

Weiss, P. (1965). *Neurosci. Res. Program, Bull.* **3**, 1.

Wolthuis, O. L. (1969). *Arch. Int. Pharmacodyn. Ther.* **182**, 439.

Wolthuis, O. L., Anthoni, J. F., and Stevens, W. F. (1969). *Acta Physiol. Pharmacol. Neer.* **15**, 93.

Zippel, H. P., and Domagk, G. F. (1969). *Experientia* **25**, 938.

7

γ-Aminobutyric Acid in the Nervous System

MASANORI OTSUKA

I.	Introduction	250
II.	Early History	250
III.	Crustacean Neuromuscular Junction	251
	A. Distribution of GABA in Crustacean Nervous System	251
	B. Action of GABA on Postsynaptic Membrane	257
	C. Release of GABA from Inhibitory Nerves	260
	D. Metabolism of GABA in Crustacean Nervous Tissue	264
	E. Storage and Uptake of GABA	265
IV.	Other Invertebrate Inhibitory Synapses	266
V.	Inhibitory Action of GABA in Nonmammalian Vertebrates	268
VI.	Inhibitory Synapses in Deiters Nucleus	268
	A. Action of GABA on Postsynaptic Membrane	268
	B. Distribution of GABA and Glutamate Decarboxylase	269
	C. Release of GABA	272
VII.	Other Inhibitory Synapses in Mammalian CNS	272
	A. Cerebral Cortex	272
	B. Inhibitory Synapses Blocked by Picrotoxin	273
	C. GABA in Retina	274
VIII.	Metabolism of GABA in Mammalian CNS	274
	A. Enzymes in GABA Pathway	274
	B. Subcellular Distribution of GABA and Related Enzymes	275
	C. Uptake of GABA	276
IX.	Other Amino Acids Related to GABA	277
	A. L-Glutamate	277
	B. Glycine	279
X.	General Comments and Conclusion	280
	A. GABA, L-Glutamate, and Glycine as Neurotransmitters	280
	B. Methodology of Transmitter Identification in CNS	281
	C. Conclusion	282
	References	283

I. Introduction

In peripheral nervous system there are at present three kinds of substances approved with confidence as neurotransmitters, i.e., acetylcholine, catecholamines (norepinephrine and epinephrine), and γ-aminobutyric acid (GABA). GABA has been established most recently as an inhibitory transmitter at crustacean neuromuscular junction. In central nervous system (CNS), particularly of mammals, the identification of neurotransmitters is much more difficult than in peripheral nervous system mainly because of the structural complexity of central nervous tissue. Recently, howver, there has been rather a compelling evidence for acetylcholine as an excitatory transmitter at the central synapses on Renshaw cells of feline spinal cord (Eccles *et al.*, 1954; Kuno and Rudomin, 1966) and also for GABA as an inhibitory transmitter in certain central synapses of mammals (see below). One may now hope, therefore, that most of the important neurotransmitters in mammalian CNS may possibly be revealed in the near future.

The purpose of the present article is to review the evidence for GABA being an inhibitory transmitter in peripheral as well as in central synapses and also to describe the functioning of GABA in neural tissues. A brief discussion will be presented in Section IX concerning the possible role as neurotransmitter of other amino acids related to GABA, particularly of L-glutamate and glycine, in relation to general methodology in transmitter identification.

II. Early History

The unique presence of GABA in mammalian brain was first reported by Roberts and Frankel (1950), Awapara *et al.* (1950), and Udenfriend (1950). The role of GABA in the CNS had been considered mainly from the point of view of intermediary metabolism (Bessman *et al.*, 1953; Roberts and Bregoff, 1953) until 1956, when two groups of workers suggested that GABA may be concerned with the regulation of physiological activity of the brain. Hayashi and Nagai (1956) reported that GABA as well as γ-amino-β-hydroxybutyric acid applied to motor cortex prevents electrically or chemically induced convulsion in dogs. Bazemore *et al.* (1956, 1957) attempted the isolation and chemical identification of Factor I, an agent extractable from mammalian brain which had been shown to inhibit impulse generation in the stretch receptor of crayfish

(Florey, 1954; Elliott and Florey, 1956). They were led to the conclusion that the principal substance showing Factor I activity in the brain extract is GABA, and further suggested that GABA is possibly an inhibitory transmitter in the brain. This suggestion naturally stimulated many physiological experiments to test the action of GABA on postsynaptic membrane at various inhibitory synapses, particularly since it had already been known that both cholinergic and adrenergic mechanisms do not play any important role in crustacean synapses (Katz, 1936; Ellis *et al.*, 1942; Grundfest *et al.*, 1959) as well as in a large number of central synapses of mammals (Perry, 1956; Eccles, 1957; Curtis *et al.*, 1961a). As a result, in crustacean inhibitory synapses GABA was shown to duplicate the actions of natural inhibitory transmitter (Kuffler and Edwards, 1958; Boistel and Fatt, 1958; Kuffler, 1958, 1960; Furshpan and Potter, 1959; Grundfest *et al.*, 1959; Edwards and Kuffler, 1959; Hagiwara *et al.*, 1960; Dudel and Kuffler, 1961). In mammalian CNS, on the other hand, the possibility that GABA functions as an inhibitory transmitter seemed at first less promising (Curtis *et al.*, 1959; Curtis, 1963). Further development will be presented in the following sections.

III. Crustacean Neuromuscular Junction

A. DISTRIBUTION OF GABA IN CRUSTACEAN NERVOUS SYSTEM

1. *Substance I*

Florey (1954, 1960) has shown that crustacean nervous tissues contain an active agent inhibiting the crayfish stretch receptor and heart. This agent was named as Substance I to distinguish it from the mammalian Factor I (Florey, 1960). Substance I was found to be present in inhibitory nerve fibers but lacking in sensory and motor fibers of crabs (Florey and Biederman, 1960). Following the isolation and identification of Factor I from mammalian brain (Bazemore *et al.*, 1956, 1957), Florey and co-workers attempted the chemical identification of Substance I. They were led to the conclusion that Substance I activity in the extracts of crustacean nervous tissues could not be due to GABA for the following reasons: (a) chromatographic analysis demonstrated only traces of GABA present in peripheral and central nervous system of crustacean species, and (b) in order to explain the great activity of their extract it would have been necessary to assume an improbably high concentration of GABA in their inhibitory neurons (Florey, 1960; Florey and Biederman, 1960; Florey and Chapman, 1961). The first reason is incompatible with the later observations (see below). Concerning the second reason, it turned out that GABA is indeed present in surprisingly high concentration in isolated inhibitory axons (Kravitz *et al.*, 1963b).

2. *Distribution of GABA between Excitatory and Inhibitory Axons*

In 1957 Kuffler and his collaborators undertook a project to identify the inhibitory transmitter substance at the crustacean neuromuscular junction (see Eliot *et al.*, 1957). Their principle in survey of the neurotransmitter was simple and plain: The inhibitory transmitter should be present in the inhibitory neurons and it should exert an inhibitory effect when it is applied to the neuromuscular junction. Water extracts of central and peripheral nervous system of lobsters and crabs were fractionated using ion exchange columns, electrophoresis, and paper chromatography. Each fraction was assayed for blocking activity at crayfish neuromuscular junction. As a result of such survey, 10 inhibitory substances were isolated, of which eight were chemically identified. GABA, taurine, and betaine contributed most of the blocking activity of the extract. GABA is physiologically the most active and it contributed 20–65% of the total activity in the extracts. The specific physiological activities of other nine blocking substances are more than 10 times weaker than GABA (Dudel *et al.*, 1963; Kravitz *et al.*, 1963a,b; Potter, 1968).

In the lobster it is possible to isolate single excitatory and inhibitory axons of large sizes. These isolated axons were analyzed for their content of 10 inhibitory substances mentioned above. GABA is the only compound which shows a markedly unequal distribution between excitatory and inhibitory axons. The other nine are more or less evenly distributed between both types of axons (Kravitz *et al.*, 1963b). GABA concentration obtained with an enzymic method is about 0.1 M in three types of inhibitory axons if GABA is freely dissolved in axoplasm, and less than 0.001 M in seven types of excitatory axons. Substrates of GABA metabolism, glutamate and α-ketoglutarate are equally distributed between excitatory and inhibitory axons (Table I) (Kravitz and Potter, 1965; Kravitz *et al.*, 1965). These results strongly suggested GABA's being the inhibitory transmitter at crustacean neuromuscular junction.

The above experiments of Kuffler and his collaborators show an example of success obtained by an elegant combination of microchemical and microphysiological techniques. It is noted that their studies were fa-

TABLE I

ENZYMES AND SUBSTRATES OF GABA METABOLISM IN EXCITATORY AND INHIBITORY
AXONS OF THE LOBSTER [a]

(A) Enzymes (pmoles/cm/hour)	Excitatory	Inhibitory
Glutamate decarboxylase	0	90
GABA-glutamate transaminase	23	32
(B) Substrates (mmoles/liter of axoplasm)		
Glutamate	90	70
α-Ketoglutarate	0.3	0.3
GABA	0.6	100

[a] After Kravitz et al. (1965) and Hall et al. (1970).

cilitated by following three advantages. (a) The large size of efferent axons of the lobster, with a diameter of about 50 μ, eases the dissection and chemical analysis. (b) GABA concentration in the inhibitory axons is very high, i.e., 0.1 M, which may be compared, for example, with the acetylcholine concentration, 0.08 mM, in ventral root of the cat (Evans and Saunders, 1967). (c) Enzymic GABA analysis permits the measurement of as little as 5×10^{-12} moles of the material (Jakoby and Scott, 1959; Hirsch and Robins, 1962). This sensitivity may be compared with the lowest amount of acetylcholine, 3×10^{-12} moles, which can be assayed by the use of cat blood pressure (Kuno and Rudomin, 1966).

3. Abdominal Ganglion of the Lobster

Studies of GABA distribution were then extended to neuronal cell bodies (Otsuka et al., 1967). In the abdominal ganglion of the lobster it is possible to identify 21 pairs of efferent cell bodies with their physiological functions determined. These cell bodies are large and apparently free of synapses. Figure 1A shows the locations of certain physiologically identified cell bodies, inhibitory neurons marked with white, excitatory with black. The muscles innervated by these marked neurons are known. Identified cell bodies were then isolated under the binocular microscope (Fig. 2) and analyzed for their GABA contents. In Fig. 1B, cells with more than 2×10^{-11} moles of GABA are presented in white, those without detectable GABA in black. Comparison of Figs. 1A and B establishes the

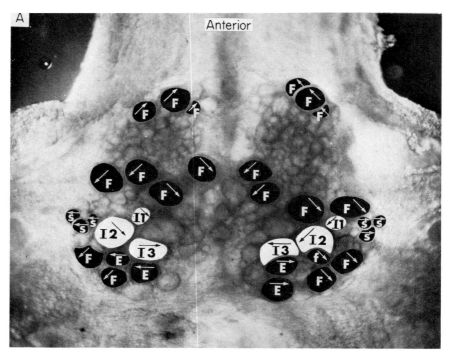

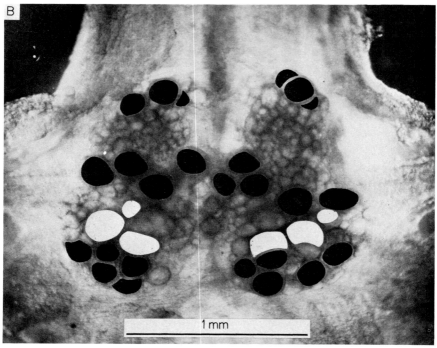

correlation between inhibitory function and a high GABA content, and excitatory function and a low GABA content. An interesting fact is that the three inhibitory cell bodies, named I1, I2, and I3, are always clustered together. These neurons innervate muscles of different or opposing functions. A possible explanation is that these three inhibitory neurons have a common embryological origin. Perhaps in the developing ganglia, certain cells acquire a GABA accumulating mechanism first (chemical differentiation) and then they give rise to the cells which acquire distinct neural connections (anatomical differentiation).

GABA concentration in inhibitory cell bodies is 13–15 mM if GABA is referred to the total volume of the cell body. This value represents the lower limit since GABA is not likely to be equally distributed in all the constituents of the cell body. The rise in the concentration of GABA from cell body to axon of inhibitory neurons is therefore seven fold or less. This may be compared with the distribution of norepinephrine within adrenergic neurons revealed by histochemical means. According to Dahlström (1967), there may be a 10–300-fold increase of norepinephrine concentration in passing from cell body to nerve terminal. In adrenergic neuron it has been suggested that the transmitter is synthesized in the cell body and then transferred to the periphery by axoplasmic flow (Dahlström, 1965). Whether this is also the case in crustacean inhibitory neurons is not known. We know, however, that the inhibitory axon of the lobster is endowed with GABA synthesizing machinery (Kravitz *et al.*, 1965; see Section III,D), and that 10 weeks after an inhibitory axon of the lobster is disconnected from its cell body, the stimulation of the severed axon still produces a good inhibitory junctional potential (IJP) (Otsuka, 1966; cf., Hoy *et al.*, 1967).

GABA concentration in excitatory cell bodies is 1 mM or less. Glutamate is about equally distributed in both inhibitory and excitatory cell bodies (Otsuka *et al.*, 1967).

Fig. 1. Physiological and chemical maps of the third abdominal ganglion of a lobster. In A, physiologically identified inhibitory cell bodies have been marked with white and excitatory cell bodies with black. B is a chemical map of the same ganglion as A; cells containing more than 2×10^{-11} moles of GABA were marked white; others containing no detectable GABA were marked black. F, excitatory cells innervating flexor muscles; f, excitors innervating the superficial flexor muscles; E, excitors of the extensor musculature; s, excitatory cells of the swimmeret muscles. I1, I2, and I3, inhibitory cell bodies. Arrows indicate whether axons are crossed or uncrossed; a diagonal arrow indicates that axon leaves through the third root either anterior or posterior to the ganglion. From Otsuka *et al.* (1967).

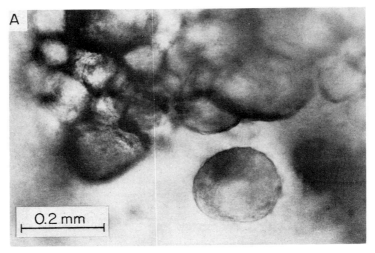

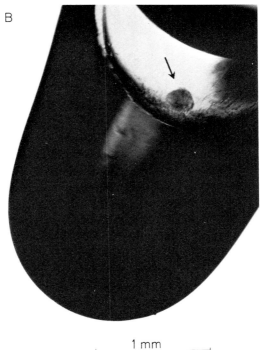

Fig. 2. Single cell body isolated from the abdominal ganglion of the lobster. (A) The cell body at the lower right was separated from its neighbors by free-hand dissection. Its axon was severed, and the cell lies free on the ganglion. From Otsuka *et al.* (1967). (B) The cell body (arrow) has been transferred to a 0.2-ml conical tube with a small amount of saline for further chemical analysis.

B. ACTION OF GABA ON POSTSYNAPTIC MEMBRANE

1. *Postsynaptic Muscle Membrane*

In crustacean muscle both GABA and neural inhibitory transmitter increase the conductance of muscle membrane (Fatt and Katz, 1953; Boistel and Fatt, 1958). Using iontophoretic application from a micropipette, Takeuchi and Takeuchi (1965) showed that the action of GABA is confined to the inhibitory neuromuscular junction. As shown in Fig. 3, GABA produces a relatively large and rapid depolarization only when it is applied to well-circumscribed regions. The focus of GABA sensitive spots coincides with the inhibitory neuromuscular junctions located by recording the extracellular IJP's.

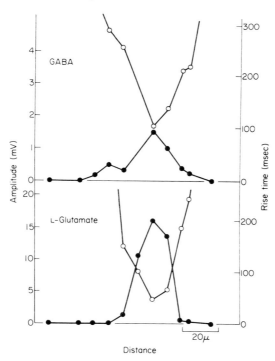

Fig. 3. Distribution of GABA sensitivity and glutamate sensitivity along a fiber of crayfish opener muscle. Membrane potential of the muscle fiber was recorded with an intracellular electrode. ●, amplitude of GABA potential and L-glutamate-induced potential change (glutamate potential) obtained by injecting constant doses of the drugs from a double-barrelled micropipette at different points on the muscle surface. ○, time to the peak of GABA and glutamate potentials. Abscissa, distance along the muscle surface. From Takeuchi and Takeuchi (1965).

The conductance increase of postjunctional muscle membrane of Crustacea produced by both GABA application and inhibitory nerve stimulation is mainly due to the increase in Cl ion permeability (Boistel and Fatt, 1958; Reuben *et al.*, 1962; Takeuchi and Takeuchi, 1967; Motokizawa *et al.*, 1969). The Takeuchis (1967) have shown that under the action of GABA the postsynaptic muscle membrane becomes selectively permeable to anions of relatively small sizes. The contribution of K ions to the GABA-induced conductance increase is less than 0.4%.

One of the crucial criteria for GABA being the inhibitory transmitter is the comparison of the reversal potentials of IJP and GABA-induced potential change (GABA potential). In the experiment of the Takeuchis shown in Fig. 4, IJP's and GABA potential were recorded intracellularly

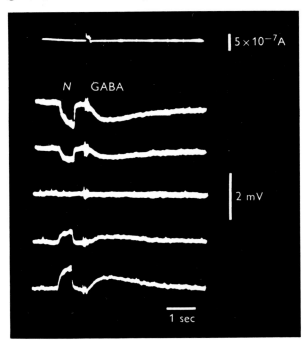

Fig. 4. Reversal potentials of IJP's and GABA potential. Intracellular recordings from a fiber of crayfish opener muscle. Potential changes marked with "N" are IJP's produced by stimulating the inhibitory nerve at 30/second. Potential changes marked with "GABA" were produced by iontophoretic injection of GABA on the sensitive area of the same muscle fiber. The uppermost trace: monitored injection current. Bottom trace was obtained at the resting potential (-70 mV), and the level of the membrane potential was displaced in 2-mV steps in depolarizing direction. The reversal potential in this case was about -66 mV. From Takeuchi and Takeuchi (1965).

from the same muscle fiber, whose membrane potential was varied by injecting current. Both IJP's and GABA potential reversed their sign at the same potential level (Kuffler, 1960; Takeuchi and Takeuchi, 1965).

Electrophoretic injection of GABA into the interior of crayfish muscle fiber produces no appreciable potential change, a fact indicating that the GABA-sensitive receptor is located on the outer surface of the muscle membrane. A steady iontophoretic application of GABA does not produce any marked desensitization of GABA receptor (Takeuchi and Takeuchi, 1965). From the relation between the concentration of GABA applied and the conductance change produced, Takeuchi and Takeuchi (1967) suggested that two molecules of GABA combine with a receptor and produce the conductance increase.

2. Presynaptic Terminals of Excitatory Axon

At the crayfish neuromuscular junction, an inhibitory nerve impulse induces two discrete mechanisms: (a) postsynaptic inhibition, which acts directly on the muscle fiber, raising its Cl permeability and stabilizing the membrane potential near its resting level, and (b) presynaptic inhibition, which acts on the excitatory nerve terminals and decreases the amount of excitatory transmitter released by a nerve impulse (Dudel and Kuffler, 1961). Dudel and Kuffler (1961) supposed that the inhibitory axon exerts the presynaptic inhibition by means of a chemical transmitter. Since a single inhibitory neuron exerts both pre- and postsynaptic inhibitions, it is likely that the same transmitter compound is involved in both mechanisms (Dale, 1935). GABA again duplicates the neural presynaptic inhibition (Dudel and Kuffler, 1961; Dudel, 1963, 1965a,b; Takeuchi and Takeuchi 1966a,b). Both GABA and neural inhibitory transmitter act on the excitatory axon terminals and reduce the release of excitatory transmitter by increasing the Cl conductance of excitatory nerve terminals and thus reducing the size of presynaptic excitatory spike. These presynaptic inhibitory effects of GABA as well as of neural inhibitory transmitter are abolished in Cl-free solution (Takeuchi and Takeuchi, 1966b).

3. Pharmacology of Inhibitory Neuromuscular Junction of Crustacea

Picrotoxin, a CNS stimulant, blocks both presynaptic and postsynaptic inhibitory actions of GABA as well as of neural inhibitory transmitter at crustacean neuromuscular junctions (Robbins and Van der Kloot, 1958; Robbins, 1959; Grundfest et al., 1959; Van der Kloot, 1960; Takeuchi and Takeuchi, 1969). The analysis of dose–response curves showed that picrotoxin depresses the conductance increase produced by GABA in a noncompetitive manner and that the antagonistic action of picrotoxin to GABA was more effective in low Cl^- solution. Based on these observations Takeuchi and Takeuchi (1969) suggested that the attachment of one molecule of picrotoxin to a specific site depresses the Cl conductance increase, possibly by interfering with the ionic gating process at the junctional membrane (cf. Grundfest, 1961). It is interesting to note that picrotoxin does not completely abolish the IJP's or GABA action, but about 10% of the response remains even with high concentration of picrotoxin (Takeuchi and Takeuchi, 1969).

A number of amino and guanido acids related to GABA have inhibitory effects on the crayfish neuromuscular junction (Robbins, 1959; Dudel *et al.*, 1963; Dudel, 1965a,b). β-Guanidino-propionic acid has a presynaptic inhibitory effect similar to GABA but has no direct effect on the conductance of muscle membrane. This guanido acid antagonizes the postsynaptic inhibitory action of GABA, probably by competing with GABA for the receptor (Kuffler, 1960; Dudel, 1965a). Pentobarbital and thiopental diminish the size of IJP and the effect of GABA on the conductance of muscle membrane at crayfish neuromuscular junction (Iravani, 1965a,b).

No drugs are at present known which, like eserine in cholinergic system, potentiate IJP's at crustacean synapses by inhibiting the inactivation process of inhibitory transmitter. Although cesium ions were reported to increase the amplitude of IJP at lobster neuromuscular junction, this effect is probably due to the increase in the amount of released transmitter (Reuben and Grundfest, 1960b).

C. Release of GABA from Inhibitory Nerves

In the preceding paragraphs (Section III,A and B) evidence was presented for GABA's being the inhibitory transmitter at crustacean neuromuscular junction: (a) GABA is present specifically in high concentration in inhibitory neurons, and (b) GABA duplicates the action of neural inhibitory transmitter in increasing Cl permeability of postsynaptic membrane, driving the membrane potential toward the similar reversal potential and being antagonized by picrotoxin. A crucial experiment, i.e., the demonstration that GABA is actually released from inhibitory nerve terminals in response to nerve stimulation, however, has been made only recently (Otsuka *et al.*, 1966; Iversen *et al.*, 1966; Kravitz *et al.*, 1968). Various nerve–muscle preparations of the lobster were dissected out and perfused with a chilled, oxygenated seawater, the ouflow being collected in 25- or 30-minute fractions. Inhibitory and excitatory axons innervating the muscles were stimulated separately at frequencies of 5–20/second. Excitatory junctional potentials (EJP's) and IJP's were monitored intracellularly with a glass microelectrode. GABA was isolated from perfusates by adsorption and selective elution from ion exchange resins and measured by the specific enzymic assay of Jakoby and Scott (1959). Figure 5

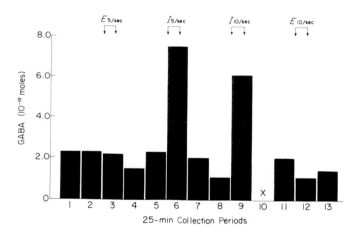

Fig. 5.   The release of GABA in response to inhibitory nerve stimulation in the opener muscle from the crusher claw of the lobster. The nerve–muscle preparation was washed continuously with chilled saline. Ordinate represents the GABA content assayed in 25-minute collection sample. Between arrows, excitatory (marked with E) and inhibitory (marked with I) nerves were stimulated with frequencies indicated in the figure. In this experiment the value obtained for inhibitory nerve stimulation at 5/second was higher than generally observed. The assay failed on one sample, indicated by X in the figure. From Otsuka *et al.* (1966).

shows the results of an experiment performed on the opener muscle of the crusher claw. This muscle is innervated by a single inhibitory and a single excitatory axons. The amount of GABA in the perfusate increased markedly during inhibitory nerve stimulation but not during excitatory nerve stimulation. In this particular experiment, less GABA was collected during inhibitory nerve stimulation at a frequency of 10/second than at 5/second, probably due to the gradual deterioration of the preparation. Although the amounts of GABA collected during inhibitory nerve stimulation were variable, statistical analysis of the results given in Table II shows that the average amount of GABA released in excess of the spon-

TABLE II

GABA Release in Lobster Nerve–Muscle Preparations [a]

Preparation	Duration of collection period (minutes)	Average GABA content of collection periods (10^{-10} moles)				
		Rest	I stimulation		Post I stimulation (rest)	E stimulation 5–10/second
			5/second	10/second		
Opener of crusher claw	25	1.7 ± 0.12 (46)	3.2 ± 0.37 [b] (8)	4.9 ± 0.61 [b] (5)	2.1 ± 0.28 (10)	1.7 ± 0.26 (10)
Opener of cutter claw	25	1.2 ± 0.24 (15)	—	2.2 ± 0.30 [b] (10)	1.7 ± 0.26 (10)	0.80 ± 0.09 (6)
Superficial flexor muscle	30	2.0 ± 0.24 (19)	5.0 ± 0.66 [b] (13)	—	3.4 ± 0.64 [c] (6)	—

[a] Inhibitory (I) or excitatory (E) nerve stimulation was administered for the first 15 minutes (opener muscles) or the entire 30 minutes (superficial flexor muscles). Values are means ± S.E.M.; number of samples indicated in parentheses. After Otsuka *et al.* (1966) and Iversen *et al.* (1966).

[b] $P < 0.01$ when compared with control rest periods.

[c] $P < 0.05$ when compared with control rest periods.

taneous efflux (i.e., net release) was about twice higher during stimulation at 10/second than at 5/second. In the experiments with superficial flexor muscle, the average net release of GABA was 4.4×10^{-10} moles in 30 minutes of inhibitory nerve stimulation at 5/second (Table II). This is only about 4% of the total GABA present in the preparation (cf. Iversen and Kravitz, 1968).

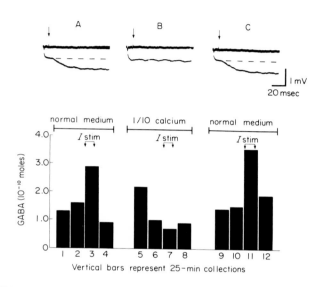

Fig. 6. Effects of low-Ca medium on IJP's and GABA release in the opener muscle from crusher claw of the lobster. The oscilloscope records in the upper part of the figure show extracellularly recorded action potentials of the nerve (upper trace, arrows) and the first part of IJP's simultaneously recorded intracellularly from a muscle fiber (lower trace). In normal medium (A) stimulation of the inhibitory nerve at 7.5/second evoked IJP's in the muscle and was accompanied by a release of GABA (lower part of figure). After exposure of the preparation to a medium containing 1/10 of the normal Ca (B), inhibitory nerve stimulation no longer produced IJP's or GABA release, although action potentials were still recorded from the nerve (upper trace of B). This effect was reversed on return to normal medium (C). From Otsuka, et al. (1966).

Calcium ions are considered to be indispensable for the electrically evoked transmitter release (Harvey and MacIntosh, 1940; Boullin, 1967; Katz, 1969). The experiment shown in Fig. 6 demonstrates the effects of a low-Ca medium on the liberation of GABA. In normal medium, both before and after exposure of the preparation to a Ca-deficient solution, IJP's were recorded and GABA release was demonstrated. In the medium containing 1/10 of the normal Ca, inhibitory nerve stimulation produced no IJP's and no release of GABA, although action potentials could still be recorded from the inhibitory axon.

It may be noted that the principles of the above experiments for demonstrating GABA release is essentially the same as those of Loewi's experiment performed almost 50 years ago for demonstrating acetylcholine release (1921). Yet, a few differences may be indicated. In the experiment on the lobster nerve–muscle preparations, single inhibitory axons were stimulated instead of nerve bundles, and this naturally simplifies the interpretation of the results. Furthermore, GABA was measured by chemical, i.e., enzymic assay instead of bioassay. The concentration of GABA in the perfusates in these experiments was usually less than 10^{-8} M, which is about 1000 times less than the lowest detectable concentration by bioassay (Kuffler and Edwards, 1958; Ash and Tucker, 1967).

The net amount of GABA release per stimulus ranged from $1-5 \times 10^{-14}$ moles. These values are minimum estimates of the amount of GABA released because GABA is removed from the extracellular space by a specific uptake system (Iversen and Kravitz, 1968). There is no information concerning the numbers of inhibitory synapses in the nerve–muscle preparations used in these perfusion experiments. If there were 1000 inhibitory synapses in the superficial flexor muscle, the amount of GABA released per impulse at each synapse would be 5×10^{-17} moles. Takeuchi and Takeuchi (1965) estimated that the minimum amount of GABA required to produce a potential change of the same size as IJP's when applied electrophoretically to GABA sensitive area of crayfish muscle was 4×10^{-15} moles. The difference between these values may not be unreasonable in view of the divergent experimental circumstances as well as the considerable uncertainties involved in these estimates.

D. Metabolism of GABA in Crustacean Nervous Tissue

The metabolism of GABA in lobster nervous tissues has been extensively studied by Kravitz and his collaborators. The pathway of GABA metabolism is shown in Fig. 7. As in mammalian CNS (Baxter and Roberts, 1960), GABA is synthesized from glutamate by glutamate decarboxylase and metabolized to succinate by GABA-glutamate transaminase and succinate semialdehyde dehydrogenase (Kravitz, 1962; Kravitz *et al.*, 1965; Hall and Kravitz, 1967a,b; Molinoff and Kravitz, 1968). The properties of these three enzymes purified from the lobster CNS were studied. There is no evidence for these enzymes being bound to synaptic

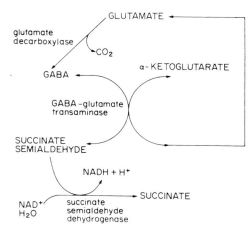

Fig. 7. Pathway of synthesis and degradation of GABA. After Molinoff and Kravitz (1968).

vesicles in the lobster nervous system. All three enzymes can be readily obtained in a soluble form.

Kravitz *et al.* (1965) compared the levels of glutamate decarboxylase, GABA-glutamate transaminase, and their substrates in isolated excitatory and inhibitory axons. The only marked difference found, other than GABA, was in the decarboxylase activity which was more than 100 times higher in inhibitory axons than in excitatory axons (Table I) (Hall *et al.*, 1970). The difference in GABA concentration between excitatory and inhibitory neurons, therefore, appears to be due to the difference in the capacity to synthesize GABA. Interestingly, the activity of glutamate decarboxylase is reduced by about 70% in the presence of 0.1 M GABA, and thus GABA synthesis is balanced approximately by destruction in the homogenate of inhibitory axon. Kravitz *et al.* (1965) suggested that the high glutamate decarboxylase activity and the GABA inhibition together provide a means of stabilizing the high GABA level in the inhibitory axon.

E. Storage and Uptake of GABA

At vertebrate neuromuscular junction as well as at many other chemically transmitting synapses there is an accumulating evidence that a transmitter substance is released from presynaptic terminals in a quantal manner and that synaptic vesicles loaded with transmitter compound are the units of transmitter release (see Katz, 1969; Jones and Kwanbunbumpen, 1970). It is probable that the same is true for GABA release process from the inhibitory axon terminals at crustacean neuromuscular junction. Spontaneous miniature IJP's have been observed at lobster and crayfish neuromuscular junction (Reuben and Grundfest, 1960a; Takeuchi and Takeuchi, 1966b). Electronmicroscopic observations revealed nerve terminals with synaptic vesicles at crayfish neuromuscular junction (Uchizono, 1967, 1968; Atwood and Jones, 1967). However, attempts to isolate a vesicle fraction containing GABA from lobster nervous system has so far been unsuccessful (Kravitz *et al.*, 1965; Kravitz, 1967).

No analogue of acetylcholinesterase of cholinergic synapse, an enzyme which destroys the released GABA in synaptic cleft, is known. GABA-glutamate transaminase is the only enzyme to degrade GABA. This enzyme, however, is probably not responsible for the removal of GABA at crustacean inhibitory synapse, since the enzyme requires α-ketoglutarate for the metabolism of GABA, and it is therefore unlikely that the enzyme is located at the outside surface of the pre- or postsynaptic membrane (Hall and Kravitz, 1967a). Furthermore, inhibitors of the GABA-glutamate transaminase, such as amino-oxyacetic acid or hydroxylamine, do not potentiate IJP's at crustacean neuromuscular junction (Potter, 1963).

Iversen and Kravitz (1968), on the other hand, found a specific GABA uptake process in lobster nerve–muscle preparation. This process is dependent on temperature as well as on sodium ions in the medium. It was suggested that GABA uptake could serve to terminate the transmitter action of GABA by rapidly removing it from synaptic clefts. Morin and Atwood (1969) reported that there is a correlation between GABA uptake and degree of inhibitory innervation in different crustacean neuromuscular preparations. Recently, the principal site of GABA uptake has been found to be the connective tissue and Schwann cells which surround nerve and muscle (Orkand and Kravitz, 1971). At adrenergic synapses, in contrast, there is evidence that catecholamine uptake occurs in sympathetic nerve terminals (see Iversen, 1967).

IV. Other Invertebrate Inhibitory Synapses

The inhibitory action of GABA was particularly well studied on crustacean stretch receptor (Bazemore *et al.*, 1957; Kuffler and Edwards, 1958; Kuffler, 1958, 1960; Edwards and Kuffler, 1959; Hagiwara *et al.*, 1960). Here again, GABA mimics the action of neural transmitter released from the inhibitory axon (or axons) synapsing with the stretch receptor: both GABA and neural inhibitory transmitter inhibit the impulse generation by increasing the membrane conductance of stretch receptor and stabilizing the membrane potential close to the resting potential (Kuffler and Eyzaguirre, 1955; Kuffler, 1958; Kuffler and Edwards, 1958); the reversal potentials of both agents are similar (Kuffler, 1958; Hagiwara et al., 1960); picrotoxin and bicuculline (see Section VII,B) block the actions of GABA and neural inhibitory transmitter (Elliott and Florey, 1956; McGeer et al., 1961; Iwasaki and Florey, 1969; McLennan, 1970). It has been suggested that the increase in K ion permeability is involved in synaptic inhibition of stretch receptor since the reversal potential of IJP altered depending on the K concentration in external medium (Kuffler and Edwards, 1958; Edwards and Hagiwara, 1959). The experiments of Hagiwara et al. (1960), however, showed that the increase in Cl permeability is also important in inhibition of stretch receptor.

Recently, Iwasaki and Florey (1969) convincingly showed the presence of miniature IJP's in crayfish stretch receptor. This finding again strongly supports the quantal release mechanism of the transmitter from inhibitory nerve terminals.

An interesting fact observed by Kuffler and Edwards (1958) is that the blocking action of GABA on impulse generation of stretch receptor declines or disappears while GABA solution still surrounds the cell. This cannot be attributed to the desensitization of GABA receptors since the blocking action reappears on stirring the solution. Apparently, GABA is inactivated by the tissue. Whether the inactivation of GABA is brought about by the GABA uptake, which has been found in stretch receptor (Sisken and Roberts, 1964), is not known.

The action of GABA was compared with that of neural inhibitory transmitter at various other inhibitory synapses of invertebrates: in crayfish heart (Enger and Burgen, 1957; Florey, 1957), in Squilla heart ganglion (Watanabe et al., 1968), in crayfish nerve cord (Furshpan and Potter, 1959), and at insect and earthworm neuromuscular junction (Usherwood and Grundfest, 1965; Hidaka et al., 1969). In general, the action of GABA is common with that of neural inhibitory transmitter in increasing the conductance of cell membrane and/or in being blocked by picrotoxin. Preliminary experiment of Florey (1957) has shown that an inhibitory factor (Substance I) is released into the perfusate of crayfish heart during the electrical stimulation of inhibitory axon supplying the heart ganglion.

V. Inhibitory Action of GABA in Nonmammalian Vertebrates

The action of electrophoretically administered GABA on Mauthner cells of goldfish resembles that of neural inhibitory transmitter, both driving the membrane potential to a similar equilibrium potential and increasing the permeability of cell membrane to various anions of relatively small sizes (Asada, 1963; Diamond, 1968; Roper and Diamond, 1969). Administration of strychnine, however, discriminates the actions of both agents, i.e., it abolishes the neural inhibition but does not affect the action of GABA. This finding suggests following two possibilies: (a) that GABA is not the transmitter of postsynaptic inhibition of Mauthner cells, and/or (b) that strychnine blocks the inhibitory synapses presynaptically (Roper and Diamond, 1969).

Ventral root reflex of the isolated frog or toad spinal cord is depressed by relatively high concentrations of GABA (Curtis *et al.*, 1961b; Fukuya, 1961).

VI. Inhibitory Synapses in Deiters Nucleus

It is well known that certain physiological and pharmacological aspects of synaptic processes in crustacean nervous system are very similar to those in mammalian CNS (Kuffler, 1958, 1960; Eccles, 1964). In view of the strong evidence for GABA as an inhibitory transmitter at crustacean neuromuscular junction, therefore, it is probable that GABA also functions as an inhibitory transmitter at mammalian central synapses. Particularly good evidence has been obtained at two places: inhibitory synapses in Deiters nucleus and in cerebral cortex.

A. Action of GABA on Postsynaptic Membrane

Purkinje neurons of cerebellar vermis of the cat send their axons to the lateral vestibular nucleus of Deiters (Walberg and Jansen, 1961) and form inhibitory synapses with Deiters neurons (Ito and Yoshida, 1966). Obata *et al.* (1967) first examined the action of electrophoretically administered GABA on Deiters neurons of the cat and found that the action of GABA resembles the synaptic inhibition produced by cerebellar cortical stimulation in producing a hyperpolarization and a conductance increase of the membrane of Deiters cells. Inhibitory equilibrium potential of GABA action was found to be similar to that of inhibitory postsynaptic potentials (IPSP's). Inhibitory action of GABA as well as IPSP is not blocked by strychnine (Obata et al., 1967; Bruggencate and Engberg, 1969a,b,c; Obata et al., 1970b). A systemic administration of relatively large dose of picrotoxin, on the other hand, was found to reduce or abolish the neurally induced inhibition of Deiters cells, and similarly, electrophoretic application of picrotoxin blocked the action of GABA (Bruggencate and Engberg, 1969a; Obata et al., 1970b). The action of two GABA analogues, β-alanine and glycine, were examined on Deiters neurons. These amino acids, when administered electrophoretically, exert inhibitory effects similar to, though weaker than, GABA effects. The equilibrium potential of glycine-induced hyperpolarization is similar to that of IPSP's. The inhibitory action of glycine, however, differs from GABA action and neural inhibition since the glycine action is blocked by strychnine but not by picrotoxin (Bruggencate and Engberg, 1969a,b,c; Obata et al., 1970b).

B. Distribution of GABA and Glutamate Decarboxylase

There is a considerable evidence that cerebellar Purkinje neurons are inhibitory (Ito and Yoshida, 1966; Eccles et al., 1967; Ito et al., 1970c). If the chemical transmitter of Purkinje neurons is GABA, as suggested by Obata et al. (1967), one would expect that Purkinje cell bodies in cerebellar cortex may contain GABA in a high concentration. Kuriyama et al. (1966) measured GABA and the enzymes of its metabolism in various layers of rabbit cerebellum and found that the GABA content and glutamate decarboxylase activity are higher in the layer containing Purkinje cell bodies than in other molecular or granular layers, or white matter. Obata (1969) dissected out Purkinje cell bodies from cerebellum of the cat and rat and measured their GABA contents. GABA concentration assessed for these isolated Purkinje cell bodies is 5–8 mM compared with that of spinal motoneurons being about 1 mM (Obata, 1969; Obata et al., 1970a; Otsuka et al., 1971; cf. Table III). High GABA values obtained in these experiments for Purkinje cell layer or for isolated Purkinje cell bodies may be attributed to Purkinje cell bodies themselves containing high concentrations of GABA or to presynaptic terminals of basket cells which are known to form inhibitory synapses on Purkinje cells, or to both (Kuriyama et al., 1966; cf. Eccles et al., 1967).

Recent experiments in our laboratory strongly suggest that GABA is specifically concentrated in Purkinje axon terminals synapsing with Deiters cells (Obata et al., 1970a; Otsuka et al., 1971). GABA analyses were

TABLE III

GABA Analysis on Single Nerve Cell Bodies Isolated from Cat CNS [a]

Type of nerve cells	GABA content (10^{-14} moles)	Volume (10^{-12} liters)	GABA concentration (mM)	
Spinal motoneurons	2.8 ± 0.7	31.5 ± 3.2	0.9 ± 0.2	(10)
Oculomotor neurons	7.8 ± 1.9	16.8 ± 2.5	5.0 ± 0.8	(8)
Ventral Deiters cells	13.0 ± 1.7	50.0 ± 7.5	2.7 ± 0.2	(9)
Dorsal Deiters cells	36.2 ± 6.7	55.8 ± 6.7	6.3 ± 0.8	(10)
Cerebellar nuclei cells	5.0 ± 1.0	8.5 ± 1.5	6.0 ± 1.1	(8)
Purkinje cells	3.1 ± 0.6	4.7 ± 0.4	6.6 ± 1.0	(8)
Betz cells	2.3 ± 0.3	9.2 ± 0.7	2.5 ± 0.3	(8)

[a] Each value represents the mean $\pm$ S.E.M. The figures in parentheses indicate the number of determinations. After Miyata *et al.* (1970) and Otsuka *et al.* (1971).

made on large nerve cells dissected out from dorsal and ventral parts of Deiters nucleus of the cat. By the use of enzymatic cycling method of Lowry *et al.* (1961) in combination with the enzymatic GABA assay of Jakoby and Scott (1959), it is now possible to determine GABA in an amount of as little as 2×10^{-14} moles (Otsuka *et al.*, 1971). Using this micromethod, GABA contents of individual isolated Deiters cells were determined. As shown in Table III and Fig. 8, average GABA concentration in dorsal Deiters cells was 6.3 mM, seven times higher than that of spinal motoneurons. Average GABA level in ventral Deiters cell, on the other hand, was 2.7 mM. Since the isolated nerve cell preparations assayed in these experiments contained very probably presynaptic terminals adhered to the cell bodies, high GABA values obtained for dorsal Deiters cells may be due to GABA being present at high concentrations in nerve terminals. It is known that Purkinje neurons of cerebellar vermis send their axons to the dorsal part of Deiters nucleus but they do not send their fibers to the ventral part of the nucleus (Walberg and Jansen, 1961). On the basis of this information, an attempt was made to eliminate these Purkinje axon terminals from the dorsal Deiters cells by denervation. Results of these experiments are summarized in Fig. 8. GABA concentrations in the isolated dorsal Deiters cells were greatly reduced after the removal of cerebellar vermis while those of the ventral Deiters cells were unaffected by the denervation. The results presented in Fig. 8 may satisfactorily be explained by assuming that GABA is concentrated within Purkinje axon terminals originating from cerebellar vermis and

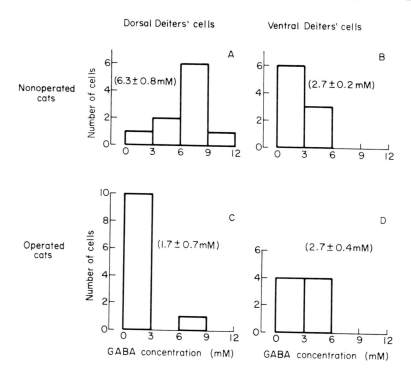

Fig. 8. Histograms of GABA concentrations in single isolated Deiters cell bodies from normal and operated (cerebellar vermis removed) cats. (A) Dorsal Deiters cells and (B) ventral Deiters cells from normal cats. (C) Dorsal and (D) ventral Deiters cells from operated cats. In each histogram, numbers in parentheses represent a mean value of GABA concentration and S.E.M. From Otsuka *et al.* (1971).

synapsing with dorsal Deiters cells. Since the volume occupied by the inhibitory terminals is probably a minor portion of the total volume of an isolated cell preparation (cf. Uchizono, 1968), GABA concentration in the nerve terminals may be considerably higher than 6.3 mM assessed for the GABA level of dorsal Deiters cells in the normal cat.

Similarly determined GABA concentrations in isolated cerebellar nuclei cells of the cat showed high values (Table III) (Obata *et al.*, 1970a; Otsuka *et al.*, 1971). Since it is known that Purkinje neurons form inhibitory synapses with cerebellar nuclei cells (Ito *et al.*, 1970c), GABA may again be concentrated in Purkinje axon terminals attached to the nerve cell bodies of cerebellar nuclei.

In crustacean nervous system, the activity of GABA synthesizing enzyme, glutamate decarboxylase, is more than 100 times higher in inhibitory axons than in excitatory axons (Kravitz *et al.*, 1965; Hall *et al.*, 1970). In mammalian CNS, too, there exists a certain parallelism between the distribution patterns of GABA and glutamate decarboxylase activity (Albers and Brady, 1959; Roberts and Eidelberg, 1960; see, however, Section VIII,A). In this connection Fonnum *et al.*, (1970) measured the activity of glutamate decarboxylase in the dorsal and ventral parts of Deiters nucleus of the cat and found that the activity of the enzyme is 2.5 times higher per dry weight in the dorsal than in the ventral part and, further, that the enzyme activity in the dorsal part is greatly reduced while that in the ventral part unaffected by the removal of cerebellar vermis. These observations of Fonnum *et al.* are quite in parallel with our above-mentioned results of GABA analyses on Deiters cells.

C. Release of GABA

In the cat, Deiters nuclei as well as intracerebellar nuclei are located adjacent to the fourth ventricle. Therefore, if GABA is released from Purkinje axon terminals forming inhibitory synapses in these nuclei, one would expect that the released GABA may diffuse out into the fourth ventricle. This was examined by Obata and Takeda (1969) who perfused the fourth ventricle of the cat and analyzed the GABA contents of the perfusates. During cerebellar cortical stimulation at 200/second GABA output increased to about three times of the resting output.

Thus, experimental evidence presented in Section VI altogether strongly supports GABA as an inhibitory neurotransmitter of Purkinje neurons synapsing with dorsal Deiters cells.

VII. Other Inhibitory Synapses in Mammalian CNS

A. Cerebral Cortex

Evidence in favor of GABA being an inhibitory transmitter in cerebral cortical inhibition is essentially the same as in Deiters nucleus described in Section VI and will therefore be described only briefly. The action of iontophoretically administered GABA on cortical, pericruciate neurons of the cat resembles IPSP's evoked by cortical surface stimulation in producing a hyperpolarization and a conductance increase of cell membrane, in increasing the membrane permeability to Cl ions and in driving the membrane potential to a similar equilibrium potential (Krnjević and Schwartz, 1967; Dreifuss *et al.*, 1969). Average GABA concentration in isolated Betz cell bodies of the cat is 2.5 mM, being higher than in spinal motoneurons, a fact suggesting that GABA may be concentrated in certain inhibitory presynaptic terminals attached to the Betz cell bodies (Table III) (Otsuka et al., 1971). Furthermore, the output of endogenous GABA from the posterior lateral gyrus of the cat increased markedly during cortical inhibition produced by electrical stimulation of the cortical surface or the lateral geniculate nucleus, and the increase in GABA efflux during stimulation was dependent on the presence of Ca ions in the perfusing medium (Mitchell and Srinivasan 1969; Iversen et al., 1970; cf. Jasper et al., 1965).

B. INHIBITORY SYNAPSES BLOCKED BY PICROTOXIN

At many invertebrate inhibitory synapses, picrotoxin specifically blocks the action of GABA and neural inhibition, and this provides one of the criteria for transmitter identification at these synapses (see Sections III, B and IV). In mammalian CNS, too, picrotoxin depresses or abolishes the synaptic inhibition at several places: postsynaptic inhibition in Deiters and other vestibular neurons (see Section VI,A; Ito et al., 1970b), oculomotor neurons (Ito et al., 1970a), and in spinal motoneurons (Kellerth and Szumski, 1966; Kellerth, 1968), presynaptic inhibition in spinal cord (Eccles et al., 1963; cf. Schmidt, 1963) and in brain stem nuclei (Shende and King, 1967; Banna and Jabbur, 1968). Iontophoretically administered picrotoxin also blocks the inhibitory action of GABA on mammalian central neurons (Bruggencate and Engberg, 1969a; Galindo, 1969; Obata and Highstein, 1970; Obata et al., 1970b). Whether GABA functions as neurotransmitter at these picrotoxin-sensitive inhibitory synapses of mammalian CNS is a quite interesting problem, because, if so, picrotoxin would serve as an useful and experimentally easy criterion for identifying the nature of synaptic transmission. A fact consistent with this thought is that considerably high concentrations of GABA were found in isolated oculomotor neurons of the cat, suggesting that GABA may be concentrated in presynaptic terminals adhered to the cell bodies (Table III) (Miyata et al., 1970).

Curtis and Ryall (1966) reported that in feline spinal cord the electrical excitability of primary afferent terminals was lowered by GABA and that this finding did not support the transmitter role of GABA in presynaptic inhibition because the primary afferent terminals are depolarized and, consequently, their excitability is increased in presynaptic inhibition (Eccles, 1964). However, other investigators reported that the electrical excitability of primary afferent terminals in the spinal cord as well as in cuneate nucleus was increased under the action of GABA (Eccles *et al.*, 1963; Schmidt, 1963; Davidson and Southwick, 1970).

Quite recently, bicuculline, another CNS stimulant, was introduced as a specific antagonist of GABA by Curtis *et al.* (1970a). This drug antagonizes the depressant action of GABA on mammalian central neurons as well as on crustacean stretch receptor and also reduces the neurally evoked inhibition of Deiters and pericruciate cortical neurons. Spinal pre- and postsynaptic inhibitions are not affected by bicuculline (Curtis *et al.*, 1970a,b,c; McLennan, 1970). Further evidence is, however, required before one could conclude whether or not bicuculline may serve as a pharmacological criterion for GABA-mediated synaptic inhibition (Godfraind *et al.*, 1970).

C. GABA in Retina

Considerable interest attaches to the role of GABA in retina. Kuriyama *et al.* (1968b) analyzed the cellular layers of rabbit retina and found that GABA as well as glutamate decarboxylase activity occurs mainly in the ganglion cell layer. GABA exerts inhibitory effects on the retinal ganglion cells of the frog and cat (Kishida and Naka, 1968; Straschill and Perwein, 1969). Rat retina possesses an efficient uptake mechanism of GABA (Goodchild and Neal, 1970).

VIII. Metabolism of GABA in Mammalian CNS

A. Enzymes in GABA Pathway

The pathway of the synthesis and degradation of GABA in mammalian brain has been extensively studied (for review, see Roberts, 1956, 1968; Elliott and Jasper, 1959; Kravitz, 1967; Roberts and Kuriyama, 1968). The GABA pathway in mammalian CNS is essentially the same as that in crustacean nervous system shown in Fig. 7. Three relevant enzymes, glutamate decarboxylase, GABA-glutamate transaminase, and succinate semialdehyde dehydrogenase of mammalian brain, have been purified, and studies on their properties have been carried out (Albers and Koval, 1961; Waksman and Roberts, 1965: Susz *et al.*, 1966).

It has been suggested that the GABA pathway serves as an important shunt to the Krebs cycle in mammalian brain (Roberts, 1956; McKhann *et al.*, 1960; Balázs *et al.*, 1970). In this connection, it must be noted that

GABA concentration in certain parts of nervous system is quite low, e.g., less than 0.1 mM in spinal ganglia or spinal roots (Graham *et al.*, 1967; Otsuka *et al.*, 1971) compared with 9.7 mM in substantia nigra (Fahn and Côté, 1968). Therefore, if GABA pathway plays a significant role for producing energy, its importance would be variable depending on the type of nerve cells.

Glutamate decarboxylase is found chiefly in the gray matter in mammalian CNS (Roberts, 1956; Lowe *et al.*, 1958; Albers and Brady, 1959). It was shown that the concentration of GABA in brain could be correlated with the activity of glutamate decarboxylase. Therefore, as in the case of crustacean nervous system, it is probable that the steady-state levels of GABA in mammalian CNS normally are governed by the glutamate decarboxylase activity (Roberts and Eidelberg, 1960). However, in the cat spinal cord and roots, the distribution pattern of glutamate decarboxylase is not quite in parallel with that of GABA. A considerable activity of this enzyme was found in ventral roots of spinal cord, indicating the presence of glutamate decarboxylase unrelated to GABA as neurotransmitter (Graham and Aprison, 1969; cf. Haber *et al.*, 1970). Glutamate decarboxylase is inhibited by certain hydrazides. Systemic administration of semicarbazide, for example, causes a decrease in glutamate decarboxylase activity and a consequent lowering of GABA level in the brain (Killam and Bain, 1957; Baxter and Roberts, 1960).

GABA-glutamate transaminase is found mainly in the gray matter of CNS, but it occurs also in other nonneural tissues (Bessman *et al.*, 1953; Roberts and Bregoff, 1953; Salvador and Albers, 1959). It has been suggested that GABA-glutamate transaminase may play an important role in blood–brain barrier which restricts the passage of GABA from blood to brain (van Gelder, 1967). This hypothesis, however, is incompatible with the recent observation that GABA still cannot penetrate the blood–brain barrier after the transaminase is inhibited by amino-oxyacetic acid (Fisher *et al.*, 1966; Hespe *et al.*, 1969). A specific histochemical method for GABA-glutamate transaminase has been developed (van Gelder, 1965a). Since the activity of this enzyme is high in cholinergic neurons, the transaminase is apparently not specific for the neurons which release GABA (van Gelder, 1965b) (cf., Table I).

B. Subcellular Distribution of GABA and Related Enzymes

Extensive studies have been made on the subcellular distribution of GABA and related enzymes in brain homogenates. The results of these studies indicate that glutamate decarboxylase is predominantly localized in synaptosomes (Weinstein *et al.*, 1963; Salganicoff and de Robertis, 1965; Balázs *et al.*, 1966; Fonnum, 1968). Neal and Iversen (1969) recently showed that as much as 80% of glutamate decarboxylase in cortical homogenates could be recovered in particles which were tentatively identified as synaptosomes. These results, therefore, suggest that GABA synthesis occurs mainly in nerve endings.

Variable recoveries of particle-bound GABA, on the other hand, have been reported (Elliott and van Gelder, 1960; Weinstein *et al.*, 1963; Mangan and Whittaker, 1966). In the experiments of Neal and Iversen (1969), for example, 40–60% of the total GABA in cortical homogenates could be recovered in synaptosomal fractions. Neal and Iversen suggest that the lower recoveries may be due to the leakage of GABA from particles during homogenization and centrifugation. Question arises whether GABA and glutamate decarboxylase are bound to synaptic vesicles. Although a specific association of GABA and glutamate decarboxylase with a synaptic vesicle fraction obtained by hypotonic rupture of synaptosomes has been reported (Kuriyama *et al.*, 1968a; Whittaker, 1968), it is difficult to get an exact estimate for the proportions contained in synaptic vesicles because the loss and redistribution of GABA and the enzyme may occur during the fractionation procedures (Salganicoff and de Robertis, 1965; Mangan and Whittaker, 1966; Neal and Iversen, 1969).

The enzymes in GABA-metabolizing pathway, GABA-glutamate transaminase and succinate semialdehyde dehydrogenase, appear to have a mitochondrial localization (Salganicoff and de Robertis, 1965; Waksman *et al.*, 1968).

C. Uptake of GABA

If GABA is an inhibitory transmitter in mammalian CNS, one may expect the existence of some mechanism for rapid removal of GABA from the synaptic site of action. It is thought improbable that GABA-glutamate transaminase is responsible for this mechanism (see discussion in Section III,E; Krnjević and Schwartz, 1968), although hydroxylamine, an inhibitor of the transaminase, occasionally potentiated the synaptic inhibition in Deiters neurons (Obata *et al.*, 1967). A specific GABA uptake process has been demonstrated in mammalian brain slices (Elliott and van Gelder, 1958; Tsukada *et al.*, 1963; Nakamura and Nagayama, 1966; Iversen and Neal, 1968). This is a sodium- and temperature-dependent process, and it occurs only in central nervous tissue but not in liver or kidney. A good correlation was found to exist for the various regions of the brain between the endogenous GABA levels and the activity of GABA uptake (Hökfelt *et al.*, 1970). Varon *et al.* (1965) have shown that synaptosomal particles isolated from the mouse brain accumulate GABA in the presence of Na ions in the medium. A hypothesis has been proposed that the presynaptic terminals take up the released GABA at mammalian inhibitory synapses (Sisken and Roberts, 1964; Kravitz, 1967; Iversen and Neal, 1968), but this remains to be established (see Section III,E). Certain mercurials inhibit the uptake of GABA as well as of other amino acids in rat brain slices. Electrophoretic application of these mercurials potentiates the depressant action of GABA on spinal neurons but does not modify the synaptic inhibition of Renshaw cells (Curtis *et al.*, 1970d).

IX. Other Amino Acids Related to GABA

A. L-Glutamate

1. *Invertebrate Neuromuscular Junction*

a. Action of L-Glutamate. There is a considerable, though not conclusive, evidence that L-glutamate is an excitatory transmitter at neuromuscular junction of arthropods (for review, see Kravitz, 1967; Kravitz *et al.*, 1970). It has been observed that L-glutamate induces a contraction and depolarization of crustacean muscle in relatively low concentrations (Robbins, 1958, 1959; Elliott and van Gelder, 1958; van Harreveld and Mendelson, 1959). Takeuchi and Takeuchi (1964), using the method of iontophoretic application, showed that glutamate sensitive spots on the opener muscle of the crayfish are restricted to the junctional areas located by extracellularly recording EJP's (Fig. 3). As to the pharmacological criterion, almost no drugs, except L-glutamate itself, are known to affect the glutamate action. Continuous electrophoretic administration of small doses of L-glutamate to a sensitive spot on the opener muscle potentiates the effects of a test dose of glutamate as well as the neurally evoked EJP's. A steady application of larger doses of glutamate, on the other hand, produces desensitization of the receptors and inhibits both the effects of a test dose of glutamate and the EJP's (Takeuchi and Takeuchi, 1964). Based on these observations, Takeuchis concluded that the receptors which respond to L-glutamate are identical with normal neuroreceptors. Because of the technical difficulties it was not possible to compare exactly the reversal potentials of glutamate action and of EJP's in crustacean muscles (cf. Takeuchi and Takeuchi, 1964; Ozeki *et al.*, 1966).

Brief iontophoretic application of L-glutamate on insect muscle fibers also results in a transient depolarization (Usherwood and Machili, 1968; Usherwood *et al.*, 1968; Beránek and Miller, 1968). Glutamate sensitive areas are similarly restricted to the excitatory synaptic sites. It was shown that the glutamate sensitivity of insect muscle fibers remains after denervation, excluding the possibility that glutamate might act presynaptically on excitatory axon terminals inducing the release of excitatory transmitter therefrom. Furthermore, after denervation the glutamate receptors can be found over the entire surface of muscle fibers of the locust (Usherwood, 1969). Beránek and Miller (1968) reported that the reversal potentials for both L-glutamate action and miniature EJP's in locust muscles lies between -10 and -25 mV.

L-Glutamate has apparently the optimum configuration for excitatory action on invertebrate muscles. For example, D-glutamate has no excitatory action, and L-aspartate has a quite weak action on arthropod muscles (van Harreveld, 1969; Robbins, 1959; Takeuchi and Takeuchi, 1964; Usherwood and Machili, 1968; Kravitz *et al.*, 1970).

b. Distribution, Release, and Uptake of Glutamate. In contrast to GABA, which shows a marked asymmetric distribution, glutamate is found in roughly equal concentrations in excitatory and inhibitory neurons of the lobster (Kravitz *et al.*, 1963b, 1965; Otsuka *et al.*, 1967). This is, however, not necessarily the reason for rejecting glutamate as the excitatory transmitter (see Kravitz *et al.*, 1970).

Glutamate release with excitatory nerve stimulation has been reported in many invertebrate nerve–muscle preparations (Kerkut *et al.*, 1965; Usherwood *et al.*, 1968; Kravitz *et al.*, 1970). In lobster nerve–muscle preparation, the amount of glutamate released in excess of the background efflux during excitatory nerve stimulation was of the same order of magnitude as the GABA release with inhibitory nerve stimulation (Kravitz *et al.*, 1970).

There is a sodium-dependent glutamate uptake in lobster nerve–muscle preparation (Iversen and Kravitz, 1968).

2. *Vertebrate Central Synapses*

Evidence for glutamate as an excitatory transmitter in vertebrate central synapses is weaker than in invertebrate neuromuscular junction. Although L-glutamate exerts an excitatory action on vertebrate central neurons (Curtis and Watkins, 1960; Krnjević and Phillis, 1963), this action is shared by many other related compounds (van Harreveld, 1959). For example, in amphibian spinal cord, the excitatory action of N-methyl-D-aspartate is 70 times, and that of kainic acid is 300 times stronger than L-glutamate (Curtis et al., 1961b; Konishi et al., 1970). It has been reported that in the spinal motoneuron the equilibrium potential for the depolarizing action of L-glutamate was at a different level from that of excitatory postsynaptic potential (Curtis, 1965). However, the method employed in this study is inadequate for a strict comparison of the reversal potentials (Curtis et al., 1968a).

Distribution pattern of L-glutamate in vertebrate spinal cord and roots has been extensively studied (Graham et al., 1967; Rizzoli, 1968; Duggan and Johnston, 1970). If glutamate is the excitatory transmitter released at the terminals of primary afferent fibers in the spinal cord (Graham et al., 1967), one would expect that glutamate is more concentrated in dorsal than in ventral roots. Although this is in fact the case in many species, the concentration ratio between dorsal and ventral roots is less than 2, and the distribution pattern of L-glutamate within the spinal cord is rather homogeneous (Graham et al., 1967).

B. GLYCINE

Aprison and Werman (1965) first suggested that glycine might be a postsynaptic inhibitory transmitter in the feline spinal cord. Electrophoretically applied glycine produces a hyperpolarization accompanied by an increase in membrane conductance of the spinal motoneurons of the cat (Werman et al., 1968; Curtis et al., 1968a; cf. Curtis and Watkins, 1960). GABA and β-alanine have a similar but weaker hyperpolarizing action on the motoneurons. The reversal potential for these hyperpolarizations is close to that of IPSP's. Alterations in intracellular concentrations of K^+, Cl^-, and other various anions affect the IPSP's and the actions of the neutral amino acids in the same fashion, suggesting that similar alterations in ion permeabilities of spinal motoneurons are involved in IPSP's and the amino acid actions.

Similar inhibitory effects of glycine have also been observed on spinal interneurons (Bruggencate and Engberg, 1968; Werman et al., 1968; Curtis et al., 1968b), on Deiters neurons (Bruggencate and Engberg, 1969a,b; Obata et al., 1970b), and on other brain stem neurons (Galindo et al., 1967; Hösli et al., 1969).

A remarkable evidence in favor of glycine being an inhibitory transmitter of postynaptic inhibition of spinal motoneurons is that both neurally evoked inhibition and the inhibitory actions of glycine and β-alanine, but not that of GABA, are blocked reversibly by strychnine (Curtis *et al.*, 1968a,b). Recently, a doubt was raised on the validity of this evidence (Roper and Diamond, 1969). In the goldfish, strychnine administered systemically in amounts adequate to suppress completely the physiological inhibition of the Mauthner cells had little or no effect on the inhibitory action of electrophoretically administered glycine on these neurons (cf. Roper and Diamond, 1970; Curtis and Johnston, 1970). In the cat spinal cord, however, intravenous administrations of strychnine depressed the recurrent IPSP's and the glycine action to a similar extent (Larson, 1969).

Another evidence for glycine being an inhibitory transmitter is its uneven distribution in the nervous system of different species (Graham *et al.*, 1967; Davidoff *et al.*, 1967; Aprison *et al.*, 1969; Duggan and Johnston, 1970). In cat, for example, ventral gray matter contains the highest mean glycine concentration, i.e., 7.1 μmoles/gm wet weight compared with spinal roots containing 0.6 μmoles/gm. Furthermore, the loss of interneurons in the ventral and dorsal gray matter produced by aortic occlusion is accompanied by a parallel decrease in glycine concentration (Davidoff *et al.*, 1967), suggesting a high concentration of glycine in inhibitory spinal interneurons. It is, however, to be noted that in dorsal root ganglia containing presumably only excitatory neurons (Eccles, 1964), glycine level is relatively high, 1.9 μmoles/gm (Duggan and Johnston, 1970).

Recently, Hopkin and Neal (1970) demonstrated an increase in ^{14}C-glycine output from rat spinal cord slices during electrical stimulation. Temperature- and sodium-dependent uptake mechanism for glycine was found in the spinal cord (Neal and Pickles, 1969). These findings are consistent with a neurotransmitter role of glycine.

Little is known about glycine action in invertebrate nervous system. Although crustacean nervous tissues contain glycine, it has a negligibly weak action on crayfish neuromuscular junction or stretch receptor (Edwards and Kuffler, 1959; Potter, 1968).

X. General Comments and Conclusion

A. GABA, l-Glutamate, and Glycine as Neurotransmitters

There is now little doubt that GABA is the inhibitory transmitter compound at crustacean neuromuscular junction. GABA seems to meet all the criteria for identification of transmitter: (a) It is specifically concentrated in the inhibitory neurons, (b) it reproduces the postsynaptic membrane processes evoked by the natural inhibitory transmitter, and (c) it is released from the inhibitory axon terminals in response to nerve stimulation. There is also a very good evidence for GABA as an inhibitory transmitter in mammalian CNS. The evidence in mammalian CNS may appear less clear-cut than that in crustacean neuromuscular junction. But it is a usual practice in neurophysiology that a fact established with a firm evidence in simple preparations of lower animals is accepted with less complete evidence in experimentally difficult, higher centers.

The case for L-glutamate as an excitatory transmitter at arthropods neuromuscular junction is also considerably strong. That L-glutamate appears to be ubiquitous in the nervous system is not contra-indicating, but not indicating either, the transmitter role of L-glutamate. In the spinal cord the evidence for L-glutamate as an excitatory transmitter is yet weak and that for glycine as an inhibitory transmitter is considerable. The distributions of these amino acids within the spinal cord are rather homogeneous (Graham et al., 1967), and therefore, it would be very difficult to show these amino acids being released from some particular excitatory or inhibitory neurons.

B. METHODOLOGY OF TRANSMITTER IDENTIFICATION IN CNS

Since the criteria of transmitter identification in CNS have already been critically reviewed (e.g., Eccles, 1964; Werman, 1966; Aprison and Werman, 1968; Hebb, 1970), only a few additional remarks will be discussed.

So far as three known neurotransmitters, acetylcholine, norepinephrine, and GABA, are concerned, the existing data are consistent with the hypothesis that a transmitter compound is present in much higher concentration in the neurons which release the compound than in neurons which do not release this transmitter (e.g., Loewi and Hellauer, 1938; von Euler, 1956; Kravitz et al., 1963b; Kravitz and Potter, 1965; Otsuka et al., 1967, 1971). If this is also true for other transmitters, this will be a useful guide for the survey of new transmitters. On the other hand, if L-glutamate is a neurotransmitter, then the hypothesis can no more be generalized. It is possible that nervous system utilizes an ordinary metabolite as neurotransmitter by developing a specific release mechanism and postsynaptic receptors.

In case a transmitter suspect is ubiquitous in the nervous tissues, then as discussed for glutamate and glycine in the preceding paragraph, the interpretation of the release experiments becomes difficult because in mammalian CNS it is difficult to functionally isolate, stimulate, and perfuse a particular inhibitory or excitatory pathway.

Pharmacological analyses permited to discriminate two types of inhibitory actions on central neurons: (a) glycine-type action, which is antagonized by strychnine but little affected by picrotoxin, and (b) GABA-type action, which is antagonized by picrotoxin but relatively resistant to strychnine (Bruggencate and Engberg, 1969a; Obata *et al.*, 1970b). The specificity of pharmacological actions, however, is rarely absolute. Thus, it was reported that in certain cases the inhibitory action of glycine is antagonized by picrotoxin and that the GABA action is reduced by strychnine (Kawai and Yamamoto, 1967; Davidoff and Aprison, 1969; Davidoff *et al.*, 1969). Such cross antagonism is not quite unexpected in view of the closely related structures of these amino acids.

In order that a drug may be used as a pharmacological criterion for transmitter identification, it is essential that the site of action of the drug is known. On the other hand, it is difficult to determine whether a certain drug affects the synaptic transmission presynaptically or postsynaptically unless the transmitter is known.

A conclusion of such considerations described above is that there is no perfect criterion for transmitter identification in CNS.

C. Conclusion

Average GABA content of whole brain of the mouse is about 4 μmoles/ gm wet tissue (Weinstein *et al.*, 1963). If GABA is mostly concentrated in neurons which release GABA, then assuming the upper limit of intraneuronal GABA concentration being 40 mM, we are led to the conclusion that more than 1/10 of the total volume of CNS would be occupied by the neurons whose transmitter is GABA. Such consideration suggests that GABA may be more important than acetylcholine or norepinephrine as neurotransmitters in mammalian CNS. On the basis of such assumption, we could expect the development of at least two important fields in relation to GABA.

First, it would be highly desirable that methods are developed for visualizing GABA or related enzymes in tissue sections, such as the fluorescence histochemical technique for catecholamines. No such histochemical method for GABA or glutamate decarboxylase is at present available. However, the enzymic assay of GABA is now sensitive enough to permit the analysis of single neurons of mammalian CNS (Otsuka *et al.*, 1971). So far the available evidence is consistent with the hypothesis that GABA serves only as an inhibitory transmitter. Therefore, the studies of GABA distribution in nervous system might be a particularly valuable way to map certain inhibitory pathways.

Second, only a few drugs are known to affect the GABA-mediated synaptic transmission. Development of numerous such drugs is hoped to open up new vistas in the studies of CNS.

ACKNOWLEDGMENTS

The author is grateful to Professors A. Takeuchi and M. Kotani and Drs. T. Hironaka and Y. Miyata for many valuable comments on this manuscript. He also wishes to thank Miss Y. Tanaka, Miss T. Kajiwara, and Mr. N. Ishii for unfailing assistance in the preparation of this manuscript. The investigations made by the author and his colleagues in the Department of Pharmacology, Faculty of Medicine, Tokyo Medical and Dental University were supported by grants from U.S. Public Health Service NB–07440 and from the Ministry of Education of Japan.

REFERENCES

Albers, R. W., and Brady, R. O. (1959). *J. Biol. Chem.* **234**, 926.

Albers, R. W., and Koval, G. J. (1961). *Biochim. Biophys. Acta* **52**, 29.

Aprison, M. H., and Werman, R. (1965). *Life Sci.* **4**, 2075.

Aprison, M. H., and Werman, R. (1968). *In* "Neurosciences Research" (S. Ehrenpreis and O. C. Solnitzky, eds.), Vol. 1, p. 143. Academic Press, Oxford.

Aprison, M. H., Shank, R. P., and Davidoff, R. A. (1969). *Comp. Biochem. Physiol.* **28**, 1345.

Asada, Y. (1963). *Jap. J. Physiol.* **13**, 583.

Ash, A. S. F., and Tucker, J. F. (1967). *J. Pharm. Pharmacol.* **19**, 240.

Atwood, H. L., and Jones, A. (1967). *Experientia* **23**, 1036.

Awapara, J., Landua, A. J., Fuerst, R., and Seale, B. (1950). *J. Biol. Chem.* **187**, 35.

Balázs, R., Dahl, D., and Harwood, J. R. (1966). *J. Neurochem.* **13**, 897.

Balázs, R., Machiyama, Y., Hammond, B. J., Julian, T., and Richter, D. (1970). *Biochem. J.* **116**, 445.

Banna, N. R., and Jabbur, S. J. (1968). *Nature (London)* **217**, 83.

Baxter, C. F., and Roberts, E. (1960). *In* "The Neurochemistry of Nucleotides and Amino Acids" (R. O. Brady and D. B. Tower, eds.), p. **127**. Wiley, New York.

Bazemore, A., Elliott, K. A. C., and Florey, E. (1956). *Nature (London)* **178**, 1052.

Bazemore, A., Elliott, K. A. C., and Florey, E. (1957). *J. Neurochem.* **1**, 334.

Beránek, R., and Miller, P. L. (1968). *J. Physiol. (London)* **196**, 71P.

Bessman, S. P., Rossen, J., and Layne, E. C. (1953). *J. Biol. Chem.* **201**, 385.

Boistel, J., and Fatt, P. (1958). *J. Physiol. (London)* **144**, 176.

Boullin, D. J. (1967). *J. Physiol. (London)* **189**, 85.

Bruggencate, G. T., and Engberg, I. (1968). *Brain Res.* **11**, 446.

Bruggencate, G. T., and Engberg, I. (1969a). *Pflügers Arch. Gesamte Physiol. Menschen Tiere* **312**, R121.

Bruggencate, G. T., and Engberg, I. (1969b). *Brain Res.* **14**, 533.

Bruggencate, G. T., and Engberg, I. (1969c). *Brain Res.* **14**, 536.

Curtis, D. R. (1963). *Pharmacol. Rev.* **15**, 333.

Curtis, D. R. (1965). *In* "Studies in Physiology" (D. R. Curtis and A. K. McIntyre, eds.), p. 34. Springer-Verlag, Berlin, Göttingen, and Heidelberg.

Curtis, D. R., and Johnston, G. A. R. (1970). *Nature* (*London*) **225**, 1258.

Curtis, D. R., and Ryall, R. W. (1966). *Exp. Brain Res.* **1**, 195.

Curtis, D. R., and Watkins, J. C. (1960). *J. Neurochem.* **6**, 117.

Curtis, D. R., Phillis, J. W., and Watkins, J. C. (1959). *J. Physiol.* (*London*) **146**, 185.

Curtis, D. R., Phillis, J. W., and Watkins, J. C. (1961a). *J. Physiol.* (*London*) **158**, 296.

Curtis, D. R., Phillis, J. W., and Watkins, J. C. (1961b). *Brit. J. Pharmacol.* **16**, 262.

Curtis, D. R., Hösli, L., Johnston, G. A. R., and Johnston, I. H. (1968a). *Exp. Brain Res.* **5**, 235.

Curtis, D. R., Hösli, L., and Johnston, G. A. R. (1968b). *Exp. Brain Res.* **6**, 1.

Curtis, D. R., Duggan, A. W., Felix, D., and Johnston, G. A. R. (1970a). *Nature* (*London*) **226**, 1222.

Curtis, D. R., Duggan, A. W., Felix, D., and Johnston, G. A. R. (1970b). *Nature* (*London*) **228**, 676.

Curtis, D. R., Duggan, A. W., and Felix, D. (1970c). *Brain Res.* **23**, 117.

Curtis, D. R., Duggan, A. W., and Johnston, G. A. R. (1970d). *Exp. Brain Res.* **10**, 447.

Dahlström, A. (1965). *J. Anat.* **99**, 677.

Dahlström, A. (1967). *Naunyn-Schmiedebergs Arch. Pharmakol. Exp. Pathol.* **257**, 93.

Dale, H. H. (1935). *Proc. Roy. Soc. Med.* **28**, 319.

Davidoff, R. A., and Aprison, M. H. (1969). *Life Sci.* **8**, 107.

Davidoff, R. A., Graham, L. T., Shank, R. P., Werman, R., and Aprison, M. H. (1967). *J. Neurochem.* **14**, 1025.

Davidoff, R. A., Aprison, M. H., and Werman, R. (1969). *Int. J. Neuropharmacol.* **8**, 191.

Davidson, N., and Southwick, C. A. P. (1970). *J. Physiol.* (*London*) **210**, 172P.

Diamond, J. (1968). *J. Physiol.* (*London*) **194**, 669.

Dreifuss, J. J., Kelley, J. S., and Krnjević, K. (1969). *Exp. Brain Res.* **9**, 137.

Dudel, J. (1963). *Pflügers Arch. Gesamte Physiol. Menschen Tiere* **277**, 537.

Dudel, J. (1965a). *Pflügers Arch. Gesamte Physiol. Menschen Tiere* **283**, 104.

Dudel, J. (1965b). *Pflügers Arch. Gesamte Physiol. Menschen Tiere* **284**, 81.

Dudel, J., and Kuffler, S. W. (1961). *J. Physiol.* (*London*) **155**, 543.

Dudel, J., Gryder, R., Kaji, A., Kuffler, S. W., and Potter, D. D. (1963). *J. Neurophysiol.* **26**, 721.

Duggan, A. W., and Johnston, G. A. R. (1970). *J. Neurochem.* **17**, 1205.

Eccles, J. C. (1957). "The Physiology of Nerve Cells." Johns Hopkins Press, Baltimore, Maryland.

Eccles, J. C. (1964). "The Physiology of Synapses." Springer-Verlag, Berlin, Göttingen, and Heidelberg.

Eccles, J. C., Fatt, P., and Kotetsu, K. (1954). *J. Physiol.* (*London*) **126**, 524.

Eccles, J. C., Schmidt, R., and Willis, W. D. (1963). *J. Physiol.* (*London*) **168**, 500.

Eccles, J. C., Ito, M., and Szentágothai, J. (1967). "The Cerebellum as a Neuronal Machine." Springer-Verlag, Berlin, Göttingen, and Heidelberg.

Edwards, C., and Hagiwara, S. (1959). *J. Gen. Physiol.* **43**, 315.

Edwards, C., and Kuffler, S. W. (1959). *J. Neurochem.* **4**, 19.

Eliot, C. R., Kaji, A., Seeman, P., Ubell, E., Kuffler, S. W., and Burgen, A. S. V. (1957). *Biol. Bull.* **113**, 344.

Elliott, K. A. C., and Florey, E. (1956). *J. Neurochem.* **1**, 181.

Elliott, K. A. C., and Jasper, H. H. (1959). *Physiol. Rev.* **39**, 383.

Elliott, K. A. C., and van Gelder, N. M. (1958). *J. Neurochem.* **3**, 28.

Elliott, K. A. C., and van Gelder, N. M. (1960). *J. Physiol. (London)* **153**, 423.

Ellis, C. H., Thienes, C. H., and Wiersma, C. A. G. (1942). *Biol. Bull.* **83**, 334.

Enger, P. E. S., and Burgen, A. S. V. (1957). *Biol. Bull.* **113**, 345.

Evans, C. A. N., and Saunders, N. R. (1967). *J. Physiol. (London)* **192**, 79.

Fahn, S., and Côté, L. J. (1968). *J. Neurochem.* **15**, 209.

Fatt, P., and Katz, B. (1953). *J. Physiol. (London)* **121**, 374.

Fisher, M. A., Hagen, D. Q., and Colvin, R. B. (1966), *Science* **153**, 1668.

Florey, E. (1954). *Arch. Int. Physiol.* **62**, 33.

Florey, E. (1957). *Naturwissenschaften* **44**, 424.

Florey, E. (1960). *In* "Inhibition in the Nervous System and Gamma-Aminobutyric Acid" (E. Roberts *et al.*, eds.), p. 72. Pergamon, Oxford.

Florey, E., and Biederman, M. A. (1960). *J. Gen. Physiol.* **43**, 509.

Florey, E., and Chapman, D. D. (1961). *Comp. Biochem. Physiol.* **3**, 92.

Fonnum, F. (1968). *Biochem. J.* **106**, 401.

Fonnum, F., Storm-Mathisen, J., and Walberg, F. (1970). *Brain Res.* **20**, 259.

Fukuya, M. (1961). *Jap. J. Physiol.* **11**, 126.

Furshpan, E. J., and Potter, D. D. (1959). *J. Physiol. (London)* **145**, 326.

Galindo, A. (1969). *Brain Res.* **14**, 763.

Galindo, A., Krnjević, K., and Schwartz, S. (1967). *J. Physiol. (London)* **192**, 359.

Godfraind, J. M., Krnjević, K., and Pumain, R. (1970). *Nature (London)* **228**, 675.

Goodchild, M., and Neal, M. J. (1970). *J. Physiol. (London)* **210**, 182P.

Graham, L. T., and Aprison, M. H. (1969). *J. Neurochem.* **16**, 559.

Graham, L. T., Shank, R. P., Werman, R., and Aprison, M. H. (1967). *J. Neurochem.* **14**, 465.

Grundfest, H. (1961). *In* "Biophysics of Physiological and Pharmacological Actions" (A. M. Shanes, ed.), p. 329. Publ. No. 69, Amer. Ass. Advance. Sci., Washington, D.C.

Grundfest, H., Reuben, J. P., and Rickles, W. H., (1959). *J. Gen. Physiol.* **42**, 1301.

Haber, B., Kuriyama, K., and Roberts, E. (1970). *Science* **168**, 598.

Hagiwara, S., Kusano, K., and Saito, S. (1960). *J. Neurophysiol.* **23**, 505.

Hall, Z. W., and Kravitz, E. A. (1967a). *J. Neurochem.* **14**, 45.

Hall, Z. W., and Kravitz, E. A. (1967b). *J. Neurochem.* **14**, 55.

Hall, Z. W., Bounds, M. D., and Kravitz, E. A. (1970). *J. Cell Biol.* **46**, 290.

Harvey, A. M., and MacIntosh, F. C. (1940). *J. Physiol. (London)* **97**, 408.

Hayashi, T., and Nagai, K. (1956). *Abstr. Commun., XX*th *Int. Physiol. Congr.*, p. 410.

Hebb, C. (1970). *Annu. Rev. Physiol.* **32**, 165.

Hespe, W., Roberts, E., and Prins, H. (1969). *Brain Res.* **14**, 663.

Hidaka, T., Ito, Y., Kuriyama, H. and Tashiro, N. (1969). *J. Exp. Biol.* **50**, 417.

Hirsch, H. E., and Robins, E. (1962). *J. Neurochem.* **9**, 63.

Hökfelt, T., Jonsson, G., and Ljungdahl, Å. (1970). *Life Sci.* **9**, 203.

Hopkin, J. M., and Neal, M. J. (1970). *Brit. J. Pharmacol.* **40**, 136P.

Hösli, L., Tebēcis, A. K., and Filias, N. (1969). *Brain Res.* **16**, 293.

Hoy, R. R., Bittner, G. D., and Kennedy, D. (1967). *Science* **156**, 251.

Iravani, J. (1965a). *Naunyn-Schmiedebergs Arch. Exp. Phathol. Pharmakol.* **251**, 265.

Iravani, J. (1965b). *Naunyn-Schmiedebergs Arch. Exp. Phathol. Pharmakol.* **251**, 375.

Ito, M., and Yoshida, M. (1966). *Exp. Brain Res.* **2**, 330.

Ito, M., Highstein, S. M., and Tsuchiya, T. (1970a). *Brain Res.* **17**, 520.

Ito, M., Highstein, S. M., and Fukuda, J. (1970b). *Brain Res.* **17**, 524.

Ito, M., Yoshida, M., Obata, K., Kawai, N. and Udo, M. (1970c). *Exp. Brain Res.* **10**, 64.

Iversen, L. L. (1967). "The Uptake and Storage of Noradrenaline in Sympathetic Nerves." Cambridge Univ. Press, London and New York.

Iversen, L. L., and Kravitz, E. A. (1968). *J. Neurochem.* **15**, 609.

Iversen, L. L., and Neal, M. J. (1968). *J. Neurochem.* **15**, 1141.

Iversen, L. L., Kravitz, E. A., and Otsuka, M. (1966). *J. Physiol. (London)* **188**, 21P.

Iversen, L. L., Mitchell, J. F., Neal, M. J., and Srinivasan, V. (1970). *Brit. J. Pharmacol.* **38**, 452P.

Iwasaki, S., and Florey, E. (1969). *J. Gen. Physiol.* **53**, 666.

Jakoby, W. B., and Scott, E. M. (1959). *J. Biol. Chem.* **234**, 937.

Jasper, H. H., Kahn, R. T., and Elliott, K. A. C. (1965). *Science* **147**, 1448.

Jones, S. F., and Kwanbunbumpen, S. (1970). *J. Physiol. (London)* **207**, 31.

Katz, B. (1936). *J. Physiol. (London)* **87**, 199.

Katz, B. (1969). "The Release of Neural Transmitter Substances." Liverpool Univ. Press, Liverpool.

Kawai, N., and Yamamoto, C. (1967). *Experientia* **23**, 822.

Kellerth, J.-O. (1968). *In* "Structure and Function of Inhibitory Neuronal Mechanisms" (C. von Euler, S. Skoglund, and U. Söderberg, eds.), p. 197. Pergamon, Oxford.

Kellerth, J.-O., and Szumski, A. J. (1966). *Acta Physiol. Scand.* **66**, 146.

Kerkut, G. A., Leake, L. D., Shapira, A., Cowan, S., and Walker, R. J. (1965). *Comp. Biochem. Physiol.* **15**, 485.

Killam, K. F., and Bain, J. A. (1957). *J. Pharmacol. Exp. Ther.* **119**, 255.

Kishida, K., and Naka, K.-I. (1968). *J. Neurochem.* **15**, 833.

Konishi, S., Shinozaki, H., and Otsuka, M. (1970). Unpublished observation.

Kravitz, E. A. (1962). *J. Neurochem.* **9**, 363.

Kravitz, E. A. (1967). *In* "The Neurosciences" (G. C. Quarton, T. Melnechuk, and F. O. Schmitt, eds.), p. 433. Rockefeller Univ. Press, New York.

Kravitz, E. A., and Potter, D. D. (1965). *J. Neurochem.* **12**, 323.

Kravitz, E. A., Kuffler, S. W., Potter, D. D., and van Gelder, N. M. (1963a). *J. Neurophysiol.* **26**, 729.

Kravitz, E. A., Kuffler, S. W., and Potter, D. D. (1963b). *J. Neurophysiol.* **26**, 739.

Kravitz, E. A., Molinoff, P. B., and Hall, Z. W. (1965). *Proc. Nat. Acad. Sci. U. S.* **54**, 778.

Kravitz, E. A., Iversen, L. L., Otsuka, M., and Hall, Z. W. (1968). *In* "Structure and Function of Inhibitory Neuronal Mechanisms" (C. von Euler, S. Skoglund, and U. Söderberg, eds.), p. 371. Pergamon, Oxford.

Kravitz, E. A., Slater, C. R., Takahashi, K., Bownds, M. D., and Grossfeld, R. M. (1970). *In* "Excitatory Synaptic Mechanisms" (P. Andersen and J. K. S. Jansen, eds.), p. 85. Scandinavian University Books, Oslo.

Krnjević, K., and Phillis, J. W. (1963). *J. Physiol. (London)* **165**, 274.
Krnjević, K., and Schwartz, S. (1967). *Exp. Brain Res.* **3**, 320.
Krnjević, K., and Schwartz, S. (1968). *In* "Structure and Function of Inhibitory Neuronal Mechanisms" (C. von Euler, S. Skoglund, and U. Söderberg, eds.), p. 419. Pergamon, Oxford.
Kuffler, S. W. (1958). *Exp. Cell Res., Suppl.* **5**, 493.
Kuffler, S. W. (1960). *Harvey Lect.* **54**, 176.
Kuffler, S. W., and Edwards, C. (1958). *J. Neurophysiol.* **21**, 589.
Kuffler, S. W., and Eyzaguirre, C. (1955). *J. Gen. Physiol.* **39**, 155.
Kuno, M., and Rudomin, P. (1966). *J. Physiol. (London)* **187**, 177.
Kuriyama, K., Haber, B., Sisken, B., and Roberts, E. (1966). *Proc. Nat. Acad. Sci. U. S.* **55**, 846.
Kuriyama, K., Roberts, E., and Kakefuda, T. (1968a). *Brain Res.* **8**, 132.
Kuriyama, K., Sisken, B., Haber, B., and Roberts, E. (1968b). *Brain Res.* **9**, 165.
Larson, M. D. (1969). *Brain Res.* **15**, 185.
Loewi, O. (1921). *Pflügers Arch. Gesamte Physiol. Menschen Tiere* **189**, 239.
Loewi, O., and Hellauer, H. (1938). *Pflügers Arch. Gesamte Physiol. Menschen Tiere* **240**, 769.
Lowe, I. P., Robins, E., and Eyerman, G. S. (1958). *J. Neurochem.* **3**, 8.
Lowry, O. H., Passonneau, J. V., Schulz, D. W., and Rock, M. K. (1961). J. *Biol. Chem.* **236**, 2746.
McGeer, E. G., McGeer, P. L., and McLennan, H. (1961). *J. Neurochem.* **8**, 36.
McKhann, G. M., Albers, R. W., Sokoloff, L., Mickelsen, O., and Tower, D. B. (1960). *In* "Inhibition in the Nervous System and Gamma-Aminobutyric Acid" (E. Roberts *et al.*, eds.), p. 169. Pergamon, Oxford.
McLennan, H. (1970). *Nature (London)* **228**, 674.
Mangan, J. L., and Whittaker, V. P. (1966). *Biochem. J.* **98**, 128.
Mitchell, J. F., and Srinivasan, V. (1969). *Nature (London)* **224**, 663.
Miyata, Y., Obata, K., Tanaka, Y., and Otsuka, M. (1970). *J. Physiol. Soc. Jap.* **32**, 377.
Molinoff, P. B., and Kravitz, E. A. (1968). *J. Neurochem.* **15**, 391.
Morin, W. A., and Atwood, H. L. (1969). *Comp. Biochem. Physiol.* **30**, 577.
Motokizawa, F., Reuben, J. P., and Grundfest, H. (1969). *J. Gen. Physiol.* **54**, 437.
Nakamura, R., and Nagayama, M. (1966). *J. Neurochem.* **13**, 305.
Neal, M. J., and Iversen, L. L. (1969). *J. Neurochem.* **16**, 1245.
Neal, M. J., and Pickles, H. G. (1969). *Nature (London)* **222**, 679.
Obata, K. (1969). *Experientia* **25**, 1283.
Obata, K., and Highstein, S. M. (1970). *Brain Res.* **18**, 538.
Obata, K., and Takeda, K. (1969). *J. Neurochem.* **16**, 1043.
Obata, K., Ito, M., Ochi, R., and Sato, N. (1967). *Exp. Brain Res.* **4**, 43.
Obata, K., Otsuka, M., and Tanaka, Y. (1970a). *J. Neurochem.* **17**, 697.
Obata, K., Takeda, K., and Shinozaki, H. (1970b). *Exp. Brain Res.* **11**, 327.
Orkand, P. M., and Kravitz, E. A. (1971). *J. Cell Biol.* **49**, 75.
Otsuka, M. (1966). Unpublished observation.
Otsuka, M., Iversen, L. L., Hall, Z. W., and Kravitz, E. A. (1966). *Proc. Nat. Acad. Sci. U. S.* **56**, 1110.
Otsuka, M., Kravitz, E. A., and Potter, D. D. (1967). *J. Neurophysiol.* **30**, 725.
Otsuka, M., Obata, K., Miyata, Y., and Tanaka, Y. (1971). *J. Neurochem.* **18**, 287.

Ozeki, M., Freeman, A. F., and Grundfest, H. (1966). *J. Gen. Physiol.* **49**, 1335.

Perry, W. L. M. (1956). *Annu. Rev. Physiol.* **18**, 279.

Potter, D. D. (1963). Unpublished data. Cited in Hall and Kravitz (1967a).

Potter, D. D. (1968). *In* "Structure and Function of Inhibitory Neuronal Mechanisms" (C. von Euler, S. Skoglund, and U. Söderberg, eds.), p. 359. Pergamon, Oxford.

Reuben, J. P., and Grundfest, H. (1960a). *Biol. Bull.* **119**, 335.

Reuben, J. P., and Grundfest, H. (1960b). *Biol. Bull.* **119**, 336.

Reuben, J. P., Girardier, L., and Grundfest, H. (1962). *Biol. Bull.* **123**, 509.

Rizzoli, A. A. (1968). *Comp. Biochem. Physiol.* **26**, 1131.

Robbins, J. (1958). *Anat. Rec.* **132**, 492.

Robbins, J. (1959). *J. Physiol. (London)* **148**, 39.

Robbins, J., and Van der Kloot, W. G. (1958). *J. Physiol. (London)* **143**, 541.

Roberts, E. (1956). *Progr. Neurobiol.* **1**, 11.

Roberts, E. (1968). *In* "Structure and Function of Inhibitory Neuronal Mechanisms" (C. von Euler, S. Skoglund, and U. Söderberg, eds.), p. 401. Pergamon, Oxford.

Roberts, E., and Bregoff, H. M. (1953). *J. Biol. Chem.* **201**, 393.

Roberts, E., and Eidelberg, E. (1960). *Int. Rev. Neurobiol.* **2**, 279.

Roberts, E., and Frankel, S. (1950). *J. Biol. Chem.* **187**, 55.

Roberts, E., and Kuriyama, K. (1968). *Brain Res.* **8**, 1.

Roper, S., and Diamond, J. (1969). *Nature (London)* **223**, 1168.

Roper, S., and Diamond, J. (1970). *Nature (London)* **225**, 1259.

Salganicoff, L., and de Robertis, E. (1965). *J. Neurochem.* **12**, 287.

Salvador, R. A., and Albers, R. W. (1959). *J. Biol. Chem.* **234**, 922.

Schmidt, R. F. (1963). *Pflügers Arch. Gesamte Physiol. Menschen Tiere* **277**, 325.

Shende, M. C., and King, P. B. (1967). *J. Neurophysiol.* **30**, 947.

Sisken, B., and Roberts, E. (1964). *Biochem. Pharmacol.* **13**, 95.

Straschill, M., and Perwein, J. (1969). *Pflügers Arch. Gesamte Physiol. Menschen Tiere* **312**, 45.

Susz, J. P., Haber, B., and Roberts, E. (1966). *Biochemistry* **5**, 2870.

Takeuchi, A., and Takeuchi, N. (1964). *J. Physiol. (London)* **170**, 296.

Takeuchi, A., and Takeuchi, N. (1965). *J. Physiol. (London)* **177**, 225.

Takeuchi, A., and Takeuchi, N. (1966a). *J. Physiol. (London)* **183**, 418.

Takeuchi, A., and Takeuchi, N. (1966b). *J. Physiol. (London)* **183**, 433.

Takeuchi, A., and Takeuchi, N. (1967). *J. Physiol. (London)* **191**, 575.

Takeuchi, A., and Takeuchi, N. (1969). *J. Physiol. (London)* **205**, 377.

Tsukada, Y., Nagata, Y., and Hirano, S. (1963). *J. Neurochem.* **10**, 241.

Uchizono, K. (1967). *Nature (London)* **214**, 833.

Uchizono, K. (1968). *In* "Structure and Function of Inhibitory Neuronal Mechanisms" (C. von Euler, S. Skoglund, and U. Söderberg, eds.), p. 33. Pergamon, Oxford.

Udenfriend, S. (1950). *J. Biol. Chem.* **187**, 65.

Usherwood, P. N. R. (1969). *Nature (London)* **223**, 411.

Usherwood, P. N. R., and Grundfest, H. (1965). *J. Neurophysiol.* **28**, 497.

Usherwood, P. N. R., and Machili, P. (1968). *J. Exp. Biol.* **49**, 341.

Usherwood, P. N. R., Machili, P., and Leaf, G. (1968). *Nature (London)* **219**, 1169.

Van der Kloot, W. G. (1960). *In* "Inhibition in the Nervous System and Gamma-Aminobutyric Acid" (E. Roberts *et al.*, eds.), p. 409. Pergamon, Oxford.

van Gelder, N. M. (1965a). *J. Neurochem.* **12**, 231.

van Gelder, N. M. (1965b). *J. Neurochem.* **12**, 239.

van Gelder, N. M. (1967). *Progr. Brain Res.* **29**, 259.

van Harreveld, A. (1959). *J. Neurochem.* **3**, 300.

van Harreveld, A., and Mendelson, M. (1959). *J. Cell. Comp. Physiol.* **54**, 85.

Varon, S., Weinstein, H., Kakefuda, T., and Roberts, E. (1965). *Biochem. Pharmacol.* **14**, 1213.

von Euler, U. S. (1956). "Noradrenaline." Thomas, Springfield, Illinois.

Waksman, A., and Roberts, E. (1965). *Biochemistry* **4**, 2132.

Waksman, A., Rubinstein, M. K., Kuriyama, K., and Roberts, E. (1968). *J. Neurochem.* **15**, 351.

Walberg, F., and Jansen, J. (1961). *Exp. Neurol.* **3**, 32.

Watanabe, A., Obara, S., and Akiyama, T. (1968). *J. Gen. Physiol.* **52**, 908.

Weinstein, H., Roberts, E., and Kakefuda, T. (1963). *Biochem. Pharmacol.* **12**, 503.

Werman, R. (1966). *Comp. Biochem. Physiol.* **18**, 745.

Werman, R., Davidoff, R. A., and Aprison, M. H. (1968). *J. Neurophysiol.* **31**, 81.

Whittaker, V. P. (1968). *In* "Structure and Function of Inhibitory Neuronal Mechanisms" (C. von Euler, S. Skoglund, and U. Söderberg, eds.), p. 487. Pergamon, Oxford.

8

The Electrical Activity of the Normal Brain

MARY A. B. BRAZIER[1]

I. Introduction—The Phenomenon as Observed 292
II. The EEG of Normal Man 293
   A. Adults 293
   B. Children 296
   C. Reaction of the EEG in the Normal Adult to Metabolic Disturbances 297
   D. EEG in Normal Sleep 297
III. Neuronal Mechanisms Underlying the EEG 300
IV. The Effect of Peripheral Stimulation on the Electrical Activity of the Brain 306
   A. Responses Evoked by Somato-Sensory Stimulation 307
   B. Potentials Evoked in the Thalamus and Cortex of Man by Peripheral Stimulation 308
   C. Visually Evoked Responses 309
   D. Responses Evoked by Acoustic Stimuli 312
   E. Habituation of the Brain's Response to Sensory Stimulation . . . 313
   F. Potential Changes Evoked by Expectancy: The Contingent Negative Variation 314
V. Neuronal Mechanisms Underlying the Evoked Potential 316
VI. Summary 317
   References 317

[1] The work of this investigator is supported by (Career Award) # 5–K6–NB–18608 from the National Institutes of Health and Grant NS 09774 from USPHS.

I. Introduction — The Phenomenon as Observed

The study of the electrical activity of the brain, which early gained the name of electroencephalography, has developed in three major stages: In the first, dating from the initial discovery in 1875 (Caton, 1875), all the work was on lower animals; then from 1929, the year when the first work on man was published (Berger, 1929), emphasis was laid on the development of electroencephalography as a clinical test, i.e., recordings being made from the scalp and assessed by visual inspection. After World War II, when scientists all over the world returned to their laboratories, the third era opened, the era in which neurophysiologists recognized that in the electrical activity of the brain lay a clue to its physiology and its function. The neurophysiologists brought with them the urge to quantify and to use the aid that the new technology has provided in the form of analyzers and computers, but they also brought other outstanding developments in technique, such as the successful recording from within individual cells and the achievement of safe recording, not only from the scalp, but from the brain itself through indwelling electrodes. This has opened new aspects of the brain's electrical activity in its relation to behavior, both normal and abnormal. Running like a thread through all these periods was the curiosity of the basic neurophysiologist to know what the intimate neuronal mechanisms were that resulted in this phenomenon of wavetrains.

When two electrodes are attached to the skull of animals, including man, a potential difference between them is found which, when suitably amplified, is seen to fluctuate, indicating changing current flow. As the discoverer of the EEG (Caton) described it in 1875, "Feeble currents of varying direction pass through the multiplier when the electrodes are placed on two points of the external surface, or one electrode on the grey matter, and one on the surface of the skull."

This was not the only phenomenon that this early investigator observed; he noted that there was a standing difference of potential between the external surface of the gray matter and "the surface of a section through it" (Caton, 1875) and that this difference which was "in constant fluctuation" (Caton, 1877) gave a major deflection when a sensory stimulus was applied to the animal (Caton, 1887).

Thus, four major characteristics of the brain's electrical activity have been known for nearly 100 years: the oscillatory EEG, the transcortical potential gradient with the transient changes in it evocable by activation of sensory pathways, and the concomitant change in background oscillations that such sensory stimulation elicits (Beck, 1891). A fifth was uncovered by Grey Walter in 1964 (W. G. Walter *et al.*, 1964), i.e., the contingent negative variation (CNV) described below.

In the years that have followed these early discoveries (Brazier, 1961), the number of empirical observations that have been made on this phenomenon would fill the shelves of a library, hence, in a review of this length only the essence of some can be distilled.

II. The EEG of Normal Man

A. ADULTS

In man the fluctuating potential difference of the most prominent waves recorded between leads on the unshaved scalp is commonly between 50 to 100 millionths of a volt, or about a tenth the magnitude of electrocardiographic potentials. These waves are most prominent at the back of the head over the visual association areas of the brain; waves recorded there were designated "alpha waves" by Berger (1930) (Fig. 1). The alpha waves disappear momentarily when the eyes are opened or when a sudden sensory stimulus is applied. This desynchronization is known as alpha blocking and one can hardly improve on the description given by its discoverer (Beck) in 1891: "During stimulation of the eye with light, rhythmic oscillations that have been previously described disappeared. However this phenomenon was not the consequence of light stimulation specifically, for it appeared with every kind of stimulation of other afferent nerves".

Since a similar phenomenon was found in man (Berger, 1930), many studies have been undertaken to explain the underlying physiological mechanisms. Careful investigation revealed that mere sensory stimulation was not the principal cause of blocking for, on continued stimulation, the alpha waves returned. It was then suggested by many workers that attention to the stimulus was a necessary condition, but even that now needs further refinement. Recent work has brought evidence that, for alpha blocking, the quality of novelty in the stimulus is all important—a finding which relates to Information Theory (Shannon, 1948) and to the orienting response of the Pavlovian school (Sokolov, 1960). According to Information Theory, information is equated with statistical unexpectedness, i.e., novelty of some component in the total ensemble of sensory stimuli that ceaselessly bombard our nervous system (Brazier, 1967a), and ac-

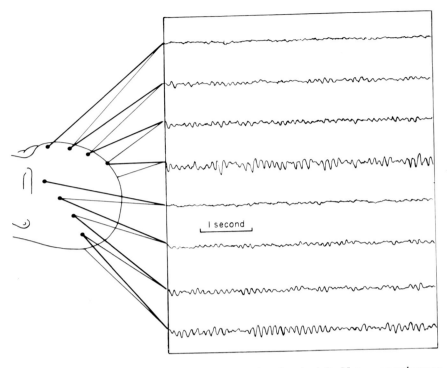

Fig. 1. Typical electroencephalogram of a fully relaxed adult. Note preponderance of alpha rhythm in the posterior part of the head. (From Brazier, 1968a.)

cording to Pavlovian theory, the most potent evocator of the orienting reflex is a novel stimulus.

Alpha is, by common consent, defined as activity in the frequency range from 8 to 13 Hz, faster frequencies being named beta rhythms. To be more exact, the waveform recorded by the electroencephalograph is a complex composed of waves of many frequencies with shifting phase relationships and varying amplitudes.

In the normal brain when the subject is awake and relaxed, but not alerted, the type of rhythm differs in recordings from the various areas of the scalp. The beta type of rhythm is more commonly found in the frontal part of the brain while the strongest centers of alpha activity are usually located in the parieto-occipital regions from which their field may spread over the whole scalp (Fig. 2). However, almost all variations are met with, and the above statement applies only to the great majority of normal records. The early hypothesis that the alpha rhythm is generated solely in the occipital poles is no longer so rigidly maintained, the incidence of alpha foci having been demonstrated in other parts of the brain although they are rare in the frontal regions.

The search for the generator, or generators of this prominent rhythm in man has had to be pursued in the main through gross models, with exploration of the more intimate neuronal mechanisms being made in lower animals (as described below) (Pollen, 1969).

To a newcomer to the field the search for a model of the generators, based only on recordings from the scalp, may seem a hopeless task and the number of generators required almost infinite. Nevertheless, an extremely parsimonious model consisting of two generators oscillating with a phase difference between them has been proposed by Rémond (1969), which could account for many of the characteristics of the alpha rhythm, including the shift in phase of the rhythms as they spread over the scalp, giving the appearance of "traveling waves" (Petsche and Sterc, 1968; Petsche and Rappelsberger, 1970). This is a model for the phenomenon

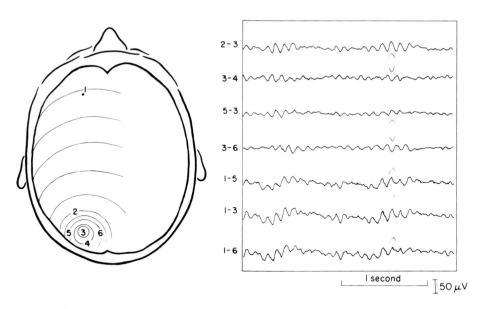

Fig. 2.   Plot to illustrate the field of an alpha rhythm centering at electrode 3. Negativity of a peak of the wave causes a downward deflection when electrode 3 is on grid 1 of the input to the electroencephalograph (as in linkages 3–4 and 3–6) and an upward deflection when it is on grid 2 (as in linkages 2–3, 5–3, 1–3). All electrodes in the occiput are negative to a distant electrode (1) on the far front of the head (Brazier, unpublished data).

as seen on the scalp of man and is based on physical spread of electrical potential and does not claim to cover neuronal transmission of electrical effects in the depth of the brain.

B. CHILDREN

Many studies of the ontogeny of the brain's rhythms have established that, although the EEG is present at birth and *in utero* (Lindsley, 1939), the frequencies of the occipital regions are lower than in the adult (Fig. 3). These rhythms increase in rate, at first rapidly and then more slowly, until at about 13 years of age the range of frequencies resembles that of the adult (Corbin and Bickford, 1955; Ellingson, 1964). Thus, in young children's records the band of frequencies between 4 and 7 Hz (named theta) is a normal rhythm. An outstanding feature of the records of normal children is their great variability from day to day, in contrast to the comparative stability of the adult's record.

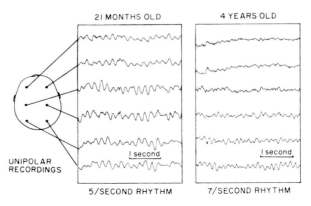

Fig. 3. The electroencephalogram in childhood. Two samples, taken at different ages, to illustrate the change in frequency with increasing age. The chart also illustrates the point that in infancy the dominant rhythm is not restricted to the occiput, as it tends to be later in childhood and in the adult (From Brazier, 1968a).

The lack of stability of the immature brain makes it more susceptible to seizures (Dreyfus-Brisac and Monod, 1964; Purpura, 1969b), and the EEG patterns have a different relationship to the clinical signs from those found in adults. It is not surprising that no direct correlation has been found between the electroencephalogram and skeletal maturity, and it is of interest that there is no correlation with the intelligence quotient in normal children.

C. Reaction of the EEG in the Normal Adult to Metabolic Disturbances

Variations in the content of the blood circulating in the brain are reflected in the EEG, the two principal components, i.e., oxygen and blood sugar, being the most influential. Hypoxia and hypoglycemia both result in slowing of the rhythms and eventual depression of the voltage. Overbreathing with resultant hypocapnia causes cerebral vasoconstriction and hypoxia. It follows that the EEG is also an index of cerebral blood flow and of metabolic disturbances such as are present in hyper- and hypothyroidism or are caused by drugs (Brazier, 1964a).

D. The EEG in Normal Sleep

The EEG is very sensitive to lapses in alertness, even moderate drowsiness causing a slight slowing of the alpha rhythm with a change in amplitude and the gradual appearance of theta activity (i.e., 6 or 7 waves/second). Interestingly enough, Berger (1938), who studied so many of the characteristics of the EEG, never pursued the effects of sleep beyond this stage.

As the subject passes from drowsiness to light sleep, the alpha rhythm drops out and the general range of frequencies lies between 2 and 7/second. It is at this light level of sleep that a response in the form of a sharp wave can be evoked at the vertex by a stimulus too weak to awaken the subject.

If the subject is undisturbed and allowed to reach a deeper level, theta and even slower waves (delta) take over the record but are interrupted from time to time by prominent "spindles," i.e., bursts of waves in the 12–16/second frequency band. These are found not only at the scalp but in deep structures of the human brain (Brazier, 1968b). This striking wave pattern appears only in this midlevel of sleep to which it has given the name "spindling stage." But it may not be wise to estimate depth of sleep by waveforms found in scalp recordings; spindles occurring in deep structures of the human brain in sleep are not necessarily accompanied by the same wave pattern on the scalp (Fig. 4). It is in this phase of sleep that a stimulus, and notably an acoustic one, evokes a wave at the vertex followed by a spindle (Fig. 5). The discoverers of this phenomenon (Davis et al., 1939) named it the K complex. As a matter of fact, later work showed that the same response could be elicited at certain levels of anesthesia (Brazier, 1955) and that it is not an EEG phenomenon specifically tied to normal sleep nor, indeed, to an acoustic stimulus for it can be evoked, for example, by a pin prick.

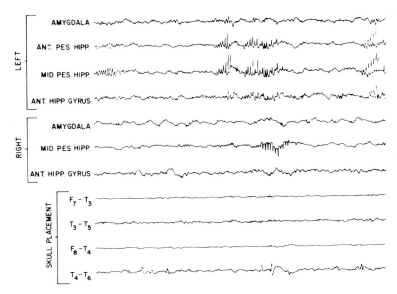

Fig. 4. Sleep spindles occurring in limbic structures of man simultaneously with low-voltage fast activity in skull leads. Abbreviations: ant, anterior; pes hipp, pes hippocampus; hipp. gyrus, hippocampal gyrus. F7 and F8, frontal leads, left and right respectively. T_3 and T_4, anterior temporal leads (International Placements). (Brazier, unpublished data.)

At a stage of sleep in which this responsiveness is lost, very slow waves of high voltage dominate the record. On the scalp these are found to have potential gradients centering around the vertex or, at times, forward of this (Brazier, 1949). Although these conspicuous waves drew most attention from electroencephalographers, it had early been remarked in both lower animals (Derbyshire *et al.*, 1936) and in man (Brazier, 1949, 1966b) that they did not persist throughout a night of normal sleep but gave way from time to time to a beta type of activity. Little interest was shown in these fluctuations of the EEG throughout a night of sleep until the added observation was made by Aserinsky and Kleitman in 1953 that the low amplitude beta phases were accompanied, in the sleeper, by rapid eye movements. Since then great numbers of hypotheses have been launched as to the cognitive function accompanying these EEG phases, an early popular one being that dreaming accompanies the low voltage phase (now named, for the muscle movements, REM). Attractive as this proposal was to psychologists, psychiatrists, and the press, no such clear-cut relation of dreaming to REM sleep has survived critical work (Clemente,

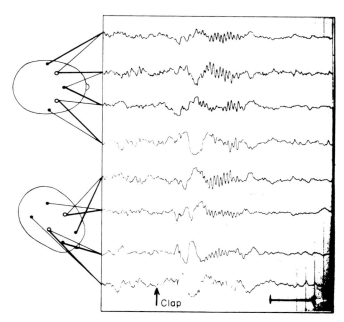

Fig. 5. The effect of an acoustic stimulus on the electroencephalogram of man during sleep. Response shows a slow wave followed by a "spindling" train of faster waves, the center of the disturbance being at the vertex and spreading widely over the scalp. Horizontal line indicates 1 second. (From Brazier, 1955.)

1967), for dream recall may be obtained on waking from any variety of EEG waveforms (Foulkes, 1962). As a consequence, the neuronal activity correlated with dreaming remains unknown. Unfortunately, as Dement (1967), one of the outstanding workers in this field, has observed, some of the early postulates, since disproved, have been incorporated in textbooks. There is no evidence that the rapid eye movements occur as a scanning response to dream imagery, or that REM deprivation plays a causal role in the development of neuroses.

Fortunately, for research on sleep, rather similar EEG changes occur in the lower animals, and this has led to a search in many laboratories for the brain mechanisms involved. Many of the outstanding results have come from Moruzzi who, with his collaborators (Batini *et al.*, 1959; Moruzzi, 1963) has shown the level of sleep that is accompanied by rapid eye movements to depend on the integrity of the pontile reticular system, for it is prevented from developing if the pons is transected or if local lesions are made in the medial pontile tegmentum.

The brain mechanisms underlying the REM level of sleep appear, therefore, to contrast with those operating at other levels which can be related to inhibitory influences in the nonspecific thalamo-cortical system (Jouvet, 1967).

III. Neuronal Mechanisms Underlying the EEG

The very early suggestion that EEG waves were envelopes of action potentials gave way as soon as extracellular and intracellular recordings from cortical cells became possible. The elucidation of post-synaptic potentials furnished the widely accepted view that in their characteristics lies the mechanism for the surface waves of the EEG, a suggestion made long ago by Bremer (1958).

The exact neuronal mechanisms at the membrane level have still to be defined in a model that suits all the available data, but there is fairly general agreement that neocortical potentials are generated by post-synaptic activity and paced from the thalamus.

This hypothesis developed from the long-held view, derived from the work of Morison and Dempsey (Dempsey and Morison, 1942); in the 1940's, and of many workers since, that the medial and intralaminar nuclei of the thalamus are the critical subcortical centers for synchronization of neocortical activity. That view was based on the demonstration that slowly repeated stimulation of medial (nonspecific) nuclei in the intralaminar regions of the thalamus, at low rates not far different from that of the animal's own cortical potentials, can bring their rhythms into step and pace them to the exact repetition rate of the stimulus pulse. The phenomenon was named "the recruiting response."

Dempsey and Morison's classic discovery of the recruiting response, reported in a long series of papers at the time, had immense importance for neurophysiologists seeking the neuronal mechanisms underlying the synchronized activity of the EEG at the surface, for here was an artificial way of creating such synchrony which they could pace by stimulation in the nonspecific nuclei of the thalamus, provided they kept the stimulation rate within the range of normal EEG waves. In the early 1940's successful recording from inside individual neurons had not yet developed, and it is 20 years later that we find explanations at the unit level, principally in the work of Purpura (1959), Purpura and Shofer (1964), Purpura *et al.*, (1964), Creutzfeldt (1969), and Creutzfeldt *et al.* (1966a,b).

When intracellular recordings were made from nerve cells in the nonspecific thalamus simultaneously with recruiting responses at the cortex, a clear sequence of alternating excitatory and inhibitory postsynaptic potentials was found.[2] The long-lasting IPSP that followed each excitatory stimulus was the pacemaker for the recruiting response of summated EPSP's; this response could not be evoked by faster stimulation rates when the inhibitory phase was curtailed.

When similar intracellular recordings were made from neocortical neurons during recruiting responses, this alternation of EPSP and IPSP was also present, but not so stereotyped in its temporal patterns (Purpura and Shofer, 1964; Purpura et al., 1964), owing, the authors suggested, to the greater complexity of synaptic organizations at the cortical level.

The data are illustrated in Fig. 6, taken from the work of Purpura and Shofer (1963). The classic, synchronized recruiting response at the cortex is seen in the upper trace (A). The incidence of each stimulus that was delivered to the medial thalamus is indicated by the small blips on each trace. The first of these barely evokes a change at the cortex, but at this slow rate of stimulation (7/second), the response develops. In the thalamic site recorded in B, the first stimulus inhibits an on-going discharge and a large down-going IPSP is seen, indicating hyperpolarization of the cell. On repetition the sequence EPSP–IPSP then develops. At other thalamic sites variations of this EPSP–IPSP alternation are seen. The duration of the IPSP's varies from about 80 to 150 msec, and it is this period range that determines the stimulus rate that can evoke the synchronized response at the cortex, i.e., 6 to 12/second.

A second feature of the EEG (often called alpha-blocking) has received considerable attention during the last 20 years. In 1949 Moruzzi and Magoun demonstrated that the desynchronization of the EEG caused by sensory stimulation (as described by Beck in 1891) could also be evoked by high-frequency stimulation of the midbrain reticular formation and that the pathway to the cortex lay through mesial nonspecific nuclei in

---

[2] An excitatory post-synaptic potential (EPSP) is a nonpropagated local response of the membrane of the receiving nerve cell. It is an electrotonic potential that falls off exponentially with increasing distance from the junctional point. The EPSP reflects a graded depolarization of the cell membrane that can sum on repetition as it has no refractoriness. An inhibitory post-synaptic potential (IPSP), in contrast, reflects an increase of the negative potential difference across the membrane of the cell—a hyperpolarization of the postjunctional membrane temporarily preventing the neuron from firing. An outstanding feature of IPSP's is their long duration. For further explanation, see Brazier (1968a, 1969).

the thalamus. This they called "the ascending reticular system." Intra-cellular recording (Maekawa and Purpura, 1967) has revealed that the effect of high-frequency stimulation is to prevent the development of the inhibitory post-synaptic potential, thus removing the pacemaking influence that its long-lasting hyperpolarization exercises in the unstim-ulated EEG or in the recruiting response. The result is a blockade of the recruiting response and an increase in excitatory synaptic activity which is reflected, behaviorally, in alerting of the animal.

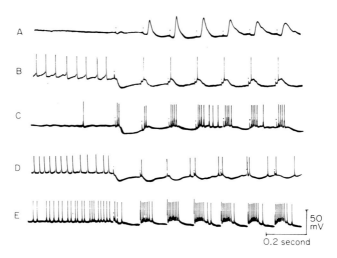

Fig. 6. Patterns of intracellularly recorded activities of thalamic neurons during cortical recruiting responses evoked by 7/second medial thalamic stimulation. (A) Characteristics of surface-negative recruiting responses (motor cortex) elicited through-out the experiment from which the intracellular records (B–E) were obtained. (B) Neuron in ventral anterior region of thalamus exhibiting prolonged IPSP following first stimulus, then EPSP–IPSP sequences with successive stimuli. (C) Relatively qui-escent ventrolateral neuron develops double discharge with first stimulus; note alterna-tion in IPSP amplitude. (D) Neuron with discharge characteristics similar to that shown in B. (E) Neuron in intralaminar region exhibiting an initial prolonged IPSP that in-terrupts spontaneous discharges. The second and all successive stimuli evoked prolonged EPSP's with high-frequency repetitive discharges that are terminated by IPSP's. (From Purpura and Shofer, 1963.)

The data are illustrated in Fig. 7 (also taken from Purpura and Shofer, 1963). In the uppermost trace (A) a low rate of medial thalamic stimula-tion produces the typical EPSP–IPSP sequence and on cessation evokes marked hyperexcitability. High-frequency stimulation begins at the first arrow and after an initial brief hyperpolarization, evokes prolonged summation of EPSP's and high-frequency discharge. A second phase of high-frequency stimulation produces an even greater degree of depolarization by facilitation of EPSP's. Only some time after stimulation ceases does the cell recover enough to resume its pacemaking alternation of EPSP and IPSP.

The accumulated evidence supports the hypothesis that EEG waves are attributable to the summation of EPSP–IPSP sequences from a relatively large population of elements (Purpura, 1969a). This hypothesis does not

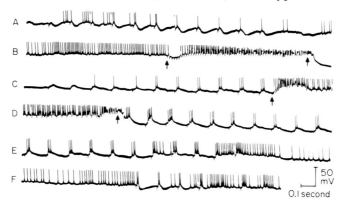

Fig. 7.   Effects of repeated high-frequency medial thalamic stimulation on a ventro-medial thalamic neuron exhibiting a typical EPSP–IPSP sequence during low-frequency stimulation. A–E: continuous record. A: 7/second medial thalamic stimulation; note prominent IPSP's. Following cessation of this stimulation the unit exhibits a phase of hyperexcitability (B); at first arrow in B, a prolonged IPSP is initiated by the first stimulus of the high-frequency (60/second) repetitive train. Successive stimuli after the IPSP evoke summating EPSP's associated with high-frequency spike attenuation. D: Second period of 7/second medial thalamic stimulation, after repolarization, initiates only prolonged, slowly augmenting EPSP's. Changes in stimulus frequency between arrows in C and D induce high-frequency repetitive discharges superimposed on depolarization whose magnitude is related to stimulus frequency. F: Several seconds later; note reappearance of IPSP's during low-frequency medial thalamic stimulation. (From Purpura and Shofer, 1963.)

require the presence of recurrent collaterals or of inhibitory interneurons in the thalamo-cortical pathways, although intrathalamic interaction is indubitable.

One recently proposed hypothesis (Andersen and Andersson, 1968; Andersen, 1966), however, is in disagreement. Based largely on the finding of spindling activity in specific thalamic relay nuclei (as well as in the classically recognized nonspecific nuclei), Andersen and Andersson (1968) attribute the major synchronizing influence to a recurrent inhibitory system in the thalamus and postulate the presence of recurrent axon collaterals acting through inhibitory interneurons to result in an "intra-thalamic synchronizing mechanism." The experimental data supporting this view come, however, from studies of barbiturate spindles in cats, and the analogy of these to the alpha activity in man is an assumption as yet unproven. Moreover, barbiturate is a great synchronizer.

For the alpha rhythm of man, the major postulate of a close relationship between wavetrains in nonspecific thalamus and cortex receives support from simultaneous recordings made with indwelling electrodes, as illustrated in Fig. 8.

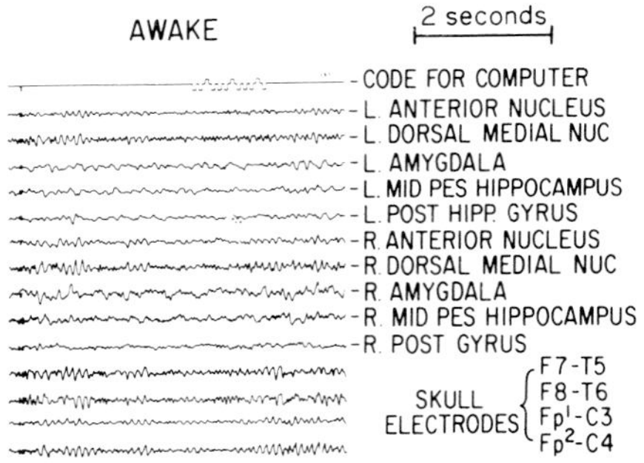

Fig. 8. Simultaneously recorded EEG's from thalamic, limbic, and cortical sites in man. Note the similarity of activity in cortex as recorded by skull electrodes and thalamus (left and right anterior nuclei; left and right dorsal medial nuclei). The activity remains independent in the limbic structures (amygdala, pes hippocampus, and hippocampal gyrus of both hemispheres). (From Brazier, 1968a.)

Direct recording from deep centers in man has revealed that the spindles of normal sleep and those produced by barbiturates are very widely distributed within the brain, the distribution being markedly different from that of the alpha rhythms of the subject when awake. Suggestive as these findings in the human brain may be, it must be remarked that no search through the various nuclei of the thalamus is possible in man, and one can make only the broad conclusion that, when viewed at large, the synchronizing mechanisms for the spindle phenomenon and the alpha system within the brain of man are dissimilar.

In cats, the search for histological evidence of recurrent collaterals of neurons in the relay system to the cortex is more successful than that for an interneuron with inhibitory properties. Some electrophysiological support for the latter activity is provided by the authors of this hypothesis (Andersen and Andersson, 1968) and by some others (Marco and Brown, 1966) but considered unconfirmed as yet by other investigators. There is some agreement, however, on the proposal that an inhibitory neuron plays some part (Creutzfeldt, 1971, 1969). Creutzfeldt's model is illustrated in Fig. 9, which depicts activity in inhibitory neurons (colored black) as playing on relay nuclei in the thalamus, in which (as seen on the right) hyperpolarization is recorded intracellularly. This alternation of

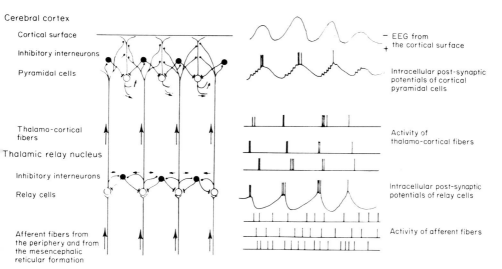

Fig. 9. Proposed model for the mechanism underlying wavetrains in the EEG. Random inflow from the periphery discharges relay cells in the thalamus whose main axons project to the cortex but whose collaterals activate inhibitory interneurons causing a relatively long hyperpolarization after each discharge (as shown by the intracellular recordings on the right). The grouping of the excitatory discharges, paced by the inhibitory pauses, leads to smooth surface waves. The inhibitory neurons at the cortical level are apparently not involved in this pacemaking influence. (From Creutzfeldt, 1971, by permission.)

EPSP and IPSP results in the pacing seen in the activity of thalamo-cortical fibers. The model also envisages inhibitory neurons at the cortical level playing onto the soma of pyramidal cells whose dendrites are receiving excitation from nonspecific afferents.

Alpha occurs in man only in the waking state. Spindling occurs only in sleep or under the influence of certain anesthetics of which barbiturates are the outstanding example.

IV. The Effect of Peripheral Stimulation on the Electrical Activity of the Brain

When the sensory receptors for any of the body's afferent systems are stimulated, changes take place in the electrical activity of the brain, not only in the cerebral cortex but throughout all systems (Cooper *et al.*, 1965), including the lower brainstem, the thalamus, and the memory circuits of the limbic system (Brazier, 1964b).

In ordinary life, the random bombardment from our sensory receptors is so mixed and continuous that specific isolated responses assignable to any individual event cannot be detected in the EEG. The mass effect is a marked change in the on-going rhythmic activity which, in man, is a desynchronization of the familiar alpha rhythm, paralleling the effect found in animals in the last century by the discoverers (Caton, 1877; Beck, 1891) of the electroencephalogram, a phenomenon they called "the functional current."

A specific response in man to a single stimulus can only be detected provided the stimuli are artificially intense, and even then, a very careful search over the scalp may be needed before the optimal placement of the electrodes is found for detecting it in any given individual.

In an attempt to overcome this difficulty, neurophysiologists (Brazier and Casby, 1952; Brazier and Barlow, 1956) introduced the techniques of the radar engineers and the use of computers. In this procedure a specified stimulus is given repeatedly; the resultant responses of the brain that are time-locked to this stimulus are summed and stored in some memory system (usually on magnetic tape or in a computer's storage). Because the interval between stimulus and response remains approximately constant, at least for the first few stimuli, the voltages of the waveforms occurring at this interval from the stimulus will, on summing, give a representative average, whereas the background EEG activity, not time-locked to the stimulus, will, on averaging, still show a random distribution.

This is the engineers' method for increasing the signal-to-noise ratio, the "signal" in this case being the time-locked evoked potential, and the "noise," the random activity in the EEG. This technique is successful even when the individual responses to sensory stimuli are of lower amplitude than the background EEG and are completely masked in a single recording.

With this wholly artificial way of inducing the brain to respond, a series of potential changes can be elicited by stimulation of the individual sensory receptors: visual, auditory, somato-sensory, or olfactory. The pattern of evoked potential change differs for each of the sensory systems and is recorded optimally from different areas on the human scalp. The visually evoked response is the most readily found for, although the primary visual receiving area in the striate cortex is tucked away in the calcarine fissure, the area of responsivity (area 19) is extensive on the cortical convexity and readily tapped by scalp electrodes. The acoustically evoked response is more closely hidden from scalp electrodes, the receiving area being, in man, deep in Heschl's gyrus.

Although the initial deflection for the response of each sensory system is found on the scalp over the cortical receiving area for that sense, a late component of the waveform, and often its most prominent one, is found at the vertex, whatever the initiating sense modality may be. The latency to this wave, though variable, is approximately 150 msec from the stimulus.

A. RESPONSES EVOKED BY SOMATO-SENSORY STIMULATION

In 1913 Pravdich–Neminsky demonstrated that a sharp deflection occurred in the EEG recorded from the cortex of the dog following an electrical stimulus to the sciatic nerve. This was the first demonstration of an

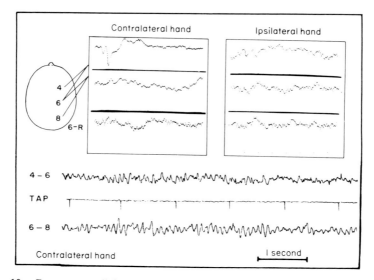

Fig. 10. Responses to light tapping of the volar surface of the hand, recorded at the scalp in normal man and averaged by computer. Note large evoked response in contralateral sensori-motor area and small response ipsilaterally, with a suggestion of a late wave over the association area. Length of sweeps: 200 msec; 90 responses averaged. Below is a section of the EEG from which the computation was taken (Brazier, 1967b).

evoked response to a peripheral stimulus. The search at the scalp of man for a similar response to a single stimulus failed, and it was only when Dawson (1947) adapted Galambos' technique (Galambos and Davis, 1943) of superimposing successive sweeps of the cathode-ray beam that the time-locked responses emerged from the background EEG. Dawson demonstrated this in man by electrical stimulation of the ulnar nerve. Since then, computers have come to our aid providing us with the average curve derived from many responses. No longer is it necessary to use the extremely unphysiological stimulus of an electric shock to a nerve which, with its massively synchronized volley, may force synapses that might not, in more normal conditions, be traversed. By computer averaging, the response to a gentle tapping of the hand can be recorded by electrodes on the scalp overlying the sensori-motor cortex of man (Fig. 10).

B. Potentials Evoked in the Thalamus and Cortex of Man by Peripheral Stimulation

In any study of cortical responses to peripheral stimulation, it is of interest to know the events in the thalamic relay. This is one area in which

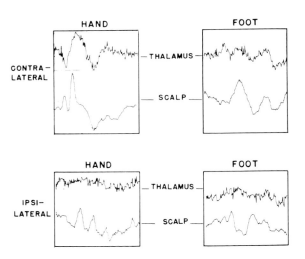

Fig. 11. Simultaneous recordings of responses (averaged) in the ventral posterior lateral nucleus of the thalamus and in scalp electrodes over the sensori-motor area in man. The stimulus in every case was a light tap, in the charts on the left to the hand, in those on the right to the foot. Note specificity of response of this thalamic site and wider response at the scalp with lengthened latency for response to tapping of the foot. Length of sweeps: 125 msec. (From Brazier, 1966a.)

we have no data from normal man and, therefore, have to draw on the rather rare occasions on which such studies have been made on patients.

Such opportunities as we have had to seek these responses simultaneously in thalamus and scalp have made clear how highly localized are responding neurons in the human thalamus.

In Fig. 11 are the results recorded from one site in the ventral posterior thalamic nucleus chosen for its response to tapping of the contralateral hand. In the two charts on the left one sees at the scalp the clearly defined primary response to contralateral tapping and the related thalamic response. As in Fig. 10, the scalp is seen to give some response to ipsilateral stimulation, but the thalamus does not. On the right, one sees that the same scalp linkage shows responses, with longer latencies, to both contralateral and ipsilateral tapping of the foot although this position in the thalamic nucleus is silent.

The responses illustrated were evoked by light tapping of the hand or foot. Others have used percutaneous electrical stimulation, for example, Pagni (1967), who has timed the latencies from various stimulation points (face, median nerve, nerves of the foot). He also was unable to evoke a response in the thalamus from ipsilateral stimulation other than very late components.

C. Visually Evoked Responses

The response to a brief but very intense flash of light can sometimes be detected by eye in the EEG of man recorded from the occipital scalp and can even be seen in the EEG of the neonate (Ellingson, 1960). With the greatly increased definition that computer averaging can give, it becomes clear that the component of the response seen in the raw trace is not the primary response of shortest latency but a later wave of higher amplitude.

It has, of course, been known for some years (Adrian, 1943; V. J. Walter and Walter, 1949) that at certain optimal flash rates the phenomenon of "driving" can be evoked (Fig. 12), a procedure that proves to be an irritant in some types of epilepsy in which, as a consequence, the EEG is activated into a seizure pattern.

When a number of individual responses are averaged by a computer in order to deemphasize the on-going EEG potentials that may mask the evoked response in man, many details emerge. The earliest potential change has a latency usually between 25 and 35 msec, from the flash (Cobb and Dawson, 1960; Brazier, 1958); this is then followed by many

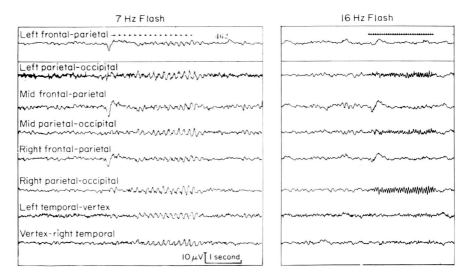

Fig. 12. An example of EEG responses in a normal subject to flickering light of two different frequencies. F, frontal; P, parietal; O, occipital lead. The large slow wave seen in the leads from the front of the head (left F–P, mid F–P, right F–P) are eyeblink potentials at the onset of the flicker. (From Brazier, 1968a.)

other components, that of highest amplitude usually peaking at about 100 to 150 msec from the flash. This is the only one usually detectable in the ink-written EEG trace. In many subjects the subsequent potential changes become oscillatory in waveform and resemble a stimulus-locked after-discharge (Cigánek, 1965; Barlow, 1960; Brazier, 1960). Current researchers are investigating whether this is a locking into the stimulus of the subject's own alpha or whether a different neuronal mechanism has been activated. Figure 13 illustrates a typical averaged response to flash as recorded from a central-to-occipital linkage on one hemisphere of a normal man.

All the pioneer work on this response was done with brief intense flashes of light, an event we experience almost only when facing the photographer's flashbulb. Modern research has therefore turned to the use of stimulation by a pattern, usually with black and white contours or edges, or some pattern like a checkerboard (Spehlman, 1965). Care has to be exerted to have equivalent luminence when comparing patterns, for the response is sensitive to intensity (Vaughan and Hull, 1965), but when this is controlled, it has been possible to elicit apparently significant differences in waveform (John *et al.*, 1967). Observers have also been able

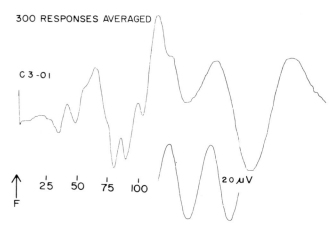

Fig. 13. Average waveform of 300 responses to flash recorded from a central-to-occipital linkage in a normal man. The various components of the waveform have different fields on the surface of the scalp and therefore give their maximum amplitude at different sites on the head. Relative negativity at the occiput is recorded downwards. The abscissa in milliseconds. (From Brazier, 1968a.)

to detect differences in the waveform of the response when contours were presented out of focus for the individual and when sharpened (Harter and White, 1968). The response of a myopic individual changes when he wears corrective lenses.

The primary route for these visually evoked impulses is via the lateral geniculate nucleus. However, since one's visual experiences are not ephemeral but leave memory traces, one might expect that they also enter the limbic system where increasing evidence indicates that the memory circuits lie. The opportunity having been presented to record directly from indwelling electrodes in limbic structures in man, the occasion to test this hypothesis has been provided. Results show clear responses in the human hippocampus, maximally present posteriorly (Brazier, 1964b, 1970). The latencies differ from those recorded at the occipital scalp, as also do the waveforms.

Another category of evoked responses in the visual system is the so-called "lamda wave" first described by Evans (1952) and Gastaut (1951). These consist of bursts of sharp waves occurring in the occipital area following each saccadic eye movement, for example, when the subject is reading. They appear in the pause after that eye movement during which fixation of gaze is being made on the next line of script.

D. Responses Evoked by Acoustic Stimuli

The response in man to acoustic stimuli has been studied less extensively than the other sense modalities. The primary response (only recordable from the exposed cartex) occurs with a shorter latency from the stimulus than is found in the visual system where a delay for chemical reactions in the retina lengthens the latency. As with the other senses, attention and distraction have some effect on the waveform (Wilkinson and Morlock, 1967), specifically, of the late vertex response. An empirical observation has been reported, with no clue yet as to the possible underlying neuronal mechanisms, of a change in waveform of the late component of the auditory response to a toneburst depending on whether the subject is requested to pay attention to its pitch or to its loudness (Gardiner and Walter, 1969).

The acoustically evoked primary response is impossible to detect in recordings from scalp electrodes. The only component that can usually be defined, even in averages of many, is the late vertex wave (Borsanyi and Blanchard, 1964) common to the response to stimulation of all sensory modalities; the vertex-negative peak of the diphasic response occurs usually about 150 msec after a click. In nearly all subjects a brief deflec-

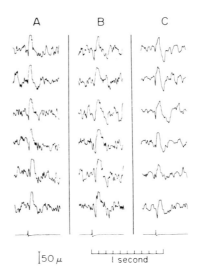

Fig. 14. Successive responses to single clicks recorded from three human subjects. The electrodes were placed directly in the brain. In subjects A and B the electrodes were on the insular cortex, in C they were deep to the superior temporal gyrus. (From Chatrian *et al.*, 1960.)

tion of very short latency appears in the record, but this has been shown to be a myogenic reaction to the sound (Bickford *et al.*, 1964).

In patients examined during brain operations, responses to clicks recorded directly from the cortical surface close to the Sylvian fissure were found to vary in latency from 8 to 16 msec (Chatrian *et al.*, 1960), but these small current flows do not reach through the skull to scalp linkages (Fig. 14).

E. Habituation of the Brain's Response to Sensory Stimulation

The technique of computer averaging, introduced into electroencephalography in 1952 (Brazier and Casby, 1952), has been widely adopted for searching for responses of small amplitude masked by background EEG waves of much higher amplitude. There is, however, an assumption underlying the method that often goes unrecognized. The assumption is that the potentials one is averaging are normally distributed, i.e., that they have a Gaussian distribution.

Unfortunately, experiment has shown that this is not necessarily so. When a stereotyped unchanging stimulus is presented at constant intervals, the response gradually wanes (Bogacz *et al.*, 1960, 1962; Brazier, 1963; Ber-

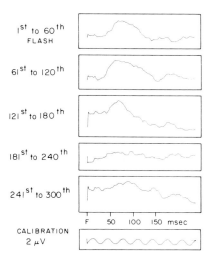

Fig. 15. Decrease in hippocampal (posterior pes hippocampus) response to flash in man during a monotonous unbroken series of 300 stimuli, averaged in samples of 60 each (From Brazier, 1967b.)

gamasco *et al.*, 1964), not only at the cortex (where it is the late nonspecific components that change most) but in structures deep in the brain that are involved with sensory experience, though not directly with its initial signal (Brazier, 1967a.) This is one more example of the importance of "novelty" for the information-carrying properties of the brain. An example is shown in Fig. 15 of the serial decrease in response to monotonously repeated flash from electrodes in the hippocampus in man (Brazier, 1967b).

If one pauses for a moment here to consider what may be the intimate neuronal mechanisms concerned with these grossly recorded evoked responses, one recognizes that they are compound excitatory post-synaptic potentials and, as such, may be examined in the light of simple neuronal circuits where some direct evidence can be obtained as to the behavior of EPSP's on monotonous repetitive stimulation.

This has recently been very clearly demonstrated by Bruner and Tauc (1966) in the comparatively simple nervous system of *Aplysia*. These investigators found diminution of the compound EPSP of the giant ganglion cell of this animal to repetitious monotonous stimulation, either mechanical or electrical. The magnitude of the original response could immediately be restored, as it can in man, by a change in stimulus frequency or introduction of some additional but novel stimulus (such as scratching the skin).

It is clear, then, that a property of nervous systems, whether simple or complex, is to give a changing response to unchanging stimuli, and this fact must be recognized by all who use an averaging technique to extract these signals.

F. POTENTIAL CHANGES EVOKED BY EXPECTANCY: THE CONTINGENT NEGATIVE VARIATION

Until 1964 all the known specific changes in potential at the cortex were evoked by physiological or electrical stimuli. The long-held hope that some more subtle function could be reflected in the EEG was at last achieved by Grey Walter, whose original contributions to the whole field of the brain's electrical activity exceed those of any other investigator.

By liberating himself from the restraint the majority of EEGers put on their results through the use of R–C coupled amplifiers that cut out all slow potential shifts and by the wise use of computer averaging, Grey Walter was able to demonstrate what he later named the "contingent negative variation" or CNV (W. G. Walter *et al.*, 1964).

Using direct-coupled amplifiers, he was able to demonstrate a brief diphasic wave followed by a prolonged increase in surface negativity at the vertex of the human head when the subject had been conditioned or warned to expect a second stimulus. An interesting feature of this non-specific response is that if the subject is required to make a motor movement in response to the expected second stimulus, or some purely mental decision concerning it, the negativity that has been building up during the period of expectancy collapses and is, in fact, followed by a brief surface positivity. No negative shift occurs between the two stimuli if no warning to expect the second one is given. Figure 16 illustrates the original finding. At first the CNV was thought to be related to a motor response to the second stimulus, but later, W. G. Walter (1965) was able to show that a purely semantic stimulus is effective in eliciting a CNV and no overt motor response is necessary. The CNV is therefore not the exact analog of the negative shift or "readiness potential" that Kornhüber and Deeke (1965) were the first to show preceded a motor movement that evoked a "motor potential" at the cortex. W. G. Walter (1967) has named this the "intention wave" and has designed an experimental paradigm

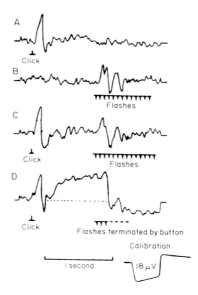

Fig. 16.   Contingent negative variation. (A) response to clicks; (B) to flicker; (C) clicks followed by flicker; (D) clicks followed by flicker terminated by the subject pressing a button as instructed. Increasing negativity shown in an upward direction. (From W. G. Walter *et al.*, 1964.)

that differentiates it from the CNV of expectancy. Clearly, physiological correlates had been found for some phenomena previously described only in the psychological realm of discourse, namely, "expectancy" and "intention."

V. Neuronal Mechanisms Underlying the Evoked Potential

Several attempts to devise a model of the neuronal activity responsible for the sequence of components of the cortical response have been made. One of considerable interest is that of Creutzfeldt *et al.* (1966) and Creutz-

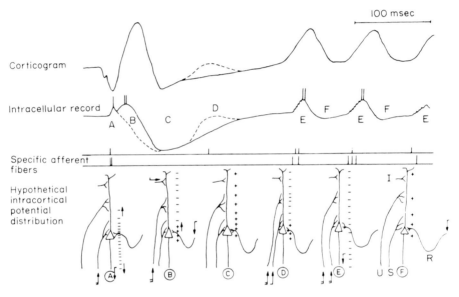

Fig. 17. Proposed model of activity in cortical neurons responsible for peripherally evoked responses at the cortex. Top trace: Response at cortex recorded with gross electrodes (positivity downwards). 2nd trace: Intracellular from a pyramidal cell (EPSP's upward, IPSP's downward). 3rd and 4th traces: Activity in two afferent fibers. Bottom section depicts the hypothesis: In A, the specific afferent volley (S) produces EPSP's, i.e., depolarizes soma and deeper parts of the neuron; surface is therefore relatively positive to this deep negativity. (B) Negativity spreads upwards to surface, enhanced by arrival of impulses in nonspecific afferent (U) and by inhibitory recurrent collateral (R). Surface now negative to depth. (C) The inhibitory action spreads over the whole neuron, and surface again becomes positive. (D, E, and F) negative–positive swings caused by alternating dominance of depolarization from nonspecific afferents (U) synapsing on apical dendrites and hyperpolarization from hypothetical inhibitory recurrent collateral (R). (From Creutzfeldt and Kuhnt, 1967.)

feldt and Kuhnt (1967), who view the initial deflection as EPSP's at the soma, evoked by impulses in the specific afferents and making the surface relatively positive to deep depolarization, which, however, spreads electrotonically up the dendrites, their negativity being reinforced by incoming activity over nonspecific afferents. In this way, the surface becomes relatively negative to the depth where an inhibitory recurrent collateral is viewed as hyperpolarizing the soma. An alternation of the dominance of excitatory and inhibitory influences is held responsible for the sequence of potential changes that follow at the surface (Fig. 17). The hypothesis is ingenious but awaits anatomical and electrophysiological evidence of a recurrent inhibitory collateral operating in the neocortex.

VI. Summary

A condensed review has been given of some of the most outstanding characteristics of the electrical activity of the brain in its normal states and some of the currently contributory models of the neuronal mechanisms underlying the current flows that are recordable outside the skull.

REFERENCES

Adrian, E. D. (1943). *Lancet* **2**, 33.
Andersen, P. (1966). *In* "The Thalamus" (D. P. Purpura and M. D. Yahr, eds.), pp. 143–151. Columbia Univ. Press, New York.
Andersen, P., and Andersson, S. A. (1968). "Physiological Basis of the Alpha Rhythm." Appleton, New York.
Aserinsky, E., and Kleitman, N. (1953). *Science* **118**, 273.
Barlow, J. S. (1960). *Electroencephalogr. Clin. Neurophysiol.* **12**, 317.
Batini, C., Moruzzi, G., Palestini, M., Rossi, G. F., and Zanchetti, A. (1959). *Arch. Ital. Biol.* **97**, 1.
Beck, A. (1891). *Rozpr. Wydz. Mat.-Przyr. Polsk. Akad. Um. Ser. 2*, **1**, 186.
Bergamasco, B., Bergamini, L., and Mobelli, A. M. (1964). *Riv. Patol. Nerv. Ment.* **85**, 565.
Berger, H. (1929). *Arch. Psychiat. Nervenkr.* **87**, 527.
Berger, H. (1930). *J. Psychol. Neurol.* **40**, 160.
Berger, H. (1938). *Arch. Psychiat. Nervenkr.* **108**, 407.
Bickford, R. G., Jacobson, J. L., and Cody, T. R. (1964). *In* "Sensory Evoked Response in Man" (R. Katzman, ed.), pp. 204-218. N. Y. Acad. Sci., New York.
Bogacz, J., Vanzulli, A., Handler, P., and Garcia-Austt, E. (1960). *Acta Neurol. Latino-amer.* **6**, 353.
Bogacz, J., Vanzulli, A., and Garcia-Austt, E. (1962). *Acta Neurol. Latino-amer.* **8**, 244.
Borsanyi, S. J., and Blanchard, C. L. (1964). *Arch. Otolaryngol.* **80**, 149.

Brazier, M. A. B. (1949). *Electroencephalogr. Clin. Neurophysiol.* **1**, 195.

Brazier, M. A. B. (1955). *In* "Neuropharmacology" (H. A. Abramson, ed.), pp. 107-144. Josiah Macy, Jr. Found., New York.

Brazier, M. A. B. (1958). *In* "Reticular Formation of the Brain" (H. H. Jasper *et al.*, eds.), pp. 151-168. Little, Brown, Boston, Massachusetts.

Brazier, M. A. B. (1960). *In* "Moscow Colloquium on Electroencephalography of Higher Nervous Activity" (H. H. Jasper and G. D. Smirnov, eds.), pp. 347–358. *Electroencephalogr. Clin. Neurophysiol. Suppl.* 13.

Brazier, M. A. B. (1961). "A History of the Electrical Activity of the Brain. The First Half-Century." Pitman, London.

Brazier, M. A. B. (1963). *In* "Brain Mechanisms" (G. Moruzzi, A. Fessard, and H. H. Jasper, eds.), pp. 349-366. Elsevier, Amsterdam.

Brazier, M. A. B. (1964a). *Clin. Pharmacol. Ther.* **5**, 102.

Brazier, M. A. B. (1964b). *Ann. N. Y. Acad. Sci.* **112**, 33.

Brazier, M. A. B. (1966a). *In* "Kortiko-Viszerale Physiologie, Pathologie und Therapie" (R. Baumann and K. Fichtel, eds.), pp. 363-372. Akademie Verlag, Berlin.

Brazier, M. A. B. (1966b). *In* "Anesthesiology of the Nervous System" (J. B. Dillon and C. M. Ballinger, eds.), pp. 106-128. Univ. of Utah Press, Salt Lake City, Utah.

Brazier, M. A. B. (1967a). *In* "Mechanisms of Orienting Reaction in Man" (L. Cigánek, V. Zikmund, and E. Kellerova, eds.), pp. 339-346. Slovak Acad. Sc., Bratislava.

Brazier, M. A. B. (1967b). *In* "The Evoked Potentials" (W. A. Cobb and C. Morocutti, ed.), pp. 1–8. *Electroencephalogr. Clin. Neurophysiol. Suppl.* 26.

Brazier, M. A. B. (1968a). "The Electrical Activity of the Nervous System," 3rd rev. ed. Williams & Wilkins, Baltimore, Maryland. Pitman, London.

Brazier, M. A. B. (1968b). *Electroencephalogr. Clin. Neurophysiol.* **25**, 309.

Brazier, M. A. B. (1969). *In* "The Structure and Function of Nervous Tissue" (G. H. Bourne, ed.), Vol. 2, pp. 409–421. Academic Press, New York.

Brazier, M. A. B. (1970). *Exp. Neurol.* **26**, 354.

Brazier, M. A. B., and Barlow, J. S. (1956). *Electroencephalogr. Clin. Neurophysiol.* **8**, 325.

Brazier, M. A. B., and Casby, J. U. (1952). *Electroencephalogr. Clin. Neurophysiol.* **4**, 201.

Bremer, F. (1958). *Physiol. Rev.* **38**, 357.

Bruner, J., and Tauc, L. (1966). *Nature (London)* **210**, 37.

Caton, R. (1875). *Brit. Med. J.* **2**, 278.

Caton, R. (1877). *Brit. Med. J.* **1**, Suppl. 62.

Caton, R. (1887). *9th Int. Med. Congr.*, Vol. 3, p. 246.

Chatrian, G. E., Petersen, M. C., and Lazarte, J. A. (1960). *Electroencephalogr. Clin. Neurophysiol.* **12**, 479.

Cigánek, L. (1965). *Electroencephalogr. Clin. Neurophysiol.* **18**, 625.

Clemente, C., ed. (1967). "Physiological Correlates of Dreaming." *Exp. Neurol. Suppl.* 4.

Cobb, W. A., and Dawson, G. D. (1960). *J. Physiol. (London)* **152**, 108.

Cooper, R., Winter, A. L., Crow, H. J., and Walter, W. G. (1965). *Electroencephalogr. Clin. Neurophysiol.* **18**, 217.

Corbin, H. P. F., and Bickford, R. G. (1955). *Electroencephalogr. Clin. Neurophysiol.* **7**, 15.

Creutzfeldt, O. D. (1969). *In* "Basic Mechanisms of the Epilepsies" (H. H. Jasper, A. Ward, and A. Pope, eds.), pp. 397-410. Little, Brown, Boston, Massachusetts.

Creutzfeldt, O. D. (1971). *In* "Aktuelle Probleme der Neuropsychologie" (M. Haider, ed.). Huber, Stuttgart.

Creutzfeldt, O. D., and Kuhnt, U. (1967). *In* "The Evoked Potentials" (W. Cobb and Morocutti, eds.), pp. 29–41. *Electroencephalogr. Clin. Neurophysiol. Suppl.* 26.

Creutzfeldt, O. D., Watanabe, S., and Lux, H. D. (1966a). *Electroencephalogr. Clin. Neurophysiol.* **20**, 19.

Creutzfeldt, O. D., Lux, H. D., and Watanabe, S. (1966b). *In* "The Thalamus" (D. P. Purpura and M. D. Yahr, eds.), pp. 209-230. Columbia Univ. Press, New York.

Davis, H., Davis, P. A., Loomis, A. L., Harvey, E. N., and Hobart, G. (1939). *J. Neurophysiol.* **2**, 500.

Dawson, G. D. (1947). *J. Neurol., Neurosurg. Psychiat.* **10**, 134.

Dement, W. (1967). *In* "Physiological Correlates of Dreaming" (C. Clemente, ed.), pp. 38–55. *Exp. Neurol. Suppl.* 4.

Dempsey, E. W., and Morison, R. S. (1942). *Amer. J. Physiol.* **135**, 293.

Derbyshire, A. J., Rempel, B., Forbes, A., and Lambert, E. F. (1936). *Amer. J. Physiol.* **116**, 577.

Dreyfus-Brisac, C., and Monod, N. (1964). *In* "Neurological and Electroencephalographic Correlative Studies in Infancy" (P. Kellaway and I. Petersen, eds.), pp. 250-257. Grune & Stratton, New York.

Ellingson, R. J. (1960). *Electroencephalogr. Clin. Neurophysiol.* **12**, 663.

Ellingson, R. J. (1964). *Progr. Brain. Res.* **9**, 26.

Evans, C. C. (1952). *Electroencephalogr. Clin. Neurophysiol.* **1**, 111.

Foulkes, D. (1962). *J. Abnorm. Soc. Psychol.* **65**, 14.

Galambos, R., and Davis, H. (1943). *J. Neurophysiol.* **6**, 39.

Gardiner, M. F., and Walter, D. O. (1969). *In* "Averaged Evoked Potentials" (E. Donchin and D. B. Lindsley, eds.), pp. 335-342. NASA.

Gastaut, Y. (1951). *Rev. Neurol.* **84**, 640.

Harter, M. R., and White, C. T. (1968). *Vision Res.* **8**, 701.

John, E. R., Herrington, R. M., and Sutton, S. (1967). *Science* **155**, 1439.

Jouvet, M. (1967). *Physiol. Rev.* **47**, 117.

Kornhüber, H. H., and Deeke, L. (1965). *Pflüger's Arch. Gesamte Physiol. Menschen Tiere* **284**, 1.

Lindsley, D. B. (1939). J. *Genet. Psychol.* **55**, 197.

Maekawa, K., and Purpura, D. P. (1967). *J. Neurophysiol.* **30**, 360.

Marco, L. A., and Brown, T. S. (1966). *Nature (London)* **210**, 1388.

Morison, R. S., and Dempsey, E. W. (1942). *Amer. J. Physiol.* **135**, 281.

Moruzzi, G. (1963). *Harvey Lect.* **58**, 233.

Moruzzi, G., and Magoun, H. W. (1949). *Electroencephalogr. Clin. Neurophysiol.* **1**, 455.

Pagni, C. S. (1967). *In* "The Evoked Potentials" (W. Cobb and C. Morocutti, eds.), p. 147–155. *Electroencephalogr. Clin. Neurophysiol. Suppl.* 26.

Petsche, H., and Rappelsberger, P. (1970). *Electroencephalogr. Clin. Neurophysiol.* **28**, 592.

Petsche, H., and Sterc, J. (1968). *Electroencephalogr. Clin. Neurophysiol.* **25**, 11.

Pollen, D. A. (1969). *In* "Basic Mechanisms of the Epilepsies" (H. H. Jasper, A. Ward, and A. Pope, eds.), pp. 411-420. Little, Brown, Boston, Massachusetts.

Pravdich-Neminsky, V. V. (1913). *Zentralbl. Physiol.* **27**, 951.

Purpura, D. P. (1959). *Int. Rev. Neurobiol.* **1**, 47.

Purpura, D. P. (1969a). *In* "The Interneuron" (M. A. B. Brazier, ed.), pp. 467-496. Univ. of. Calif. Press, Los Angeles, California.

Purpura, D. P. (1969b). *In* "Basic Mechanisms of the Epilepsies" (H. H. Jasper, A. Ward, and A. Pope, eds.), pp. 481-505. Little, Brown, Boston, Massachusetts.

Purpura, D. P., and Shofer, R. J. (1963). *J. Neurophysiol* **26**, 495.

Purpura, D. P., and Shofer, R. J. (1964). *J. Neurophysiol.* **27**, 117.

Purpura, D. P., Shofer, R. J., and Musgrave, F. S. (1964). *J. Neurophysiol.* **27**, 133.

Rémond, A. (1969). *In* "Advances in EEG Analysis" (D. O. Walter and M. A. B. Brazier eds.), pp. 29–49. *Electroencephalogr. Clin. Neurophysiol. Suppl.* 27.

Shannon, C. W. (1948). *Bell Syst. Tech. J.* **27**, 379 and 623.

Sokolov, E. N. (1960). *In* "Central Nervous System and Behavior" (M. A. B. Brazier, ed.), Vol. 3, pp. 187-276. Joisah Macy, Jr. Found., New York.

Spehlman, R. (1965). *Electroencephalogr. Clin. Neurophysiol.* **19**, 560.

Vaughan, H. G., and Hull, R. C. (1965). *Nature (London)* **206**, 720.

Walter, W. G. (1965). *J. Psychosom. Res.* **9**, 51.

Walter, W. G. (1967). *In* "The Evoked Potentials" (W. Cobb and C. Morocutti, eds.), pp. 123–130. *Electroencephalogr. Clin. Neurophysiol. Suppl.* 26.

Walter, W. G., Cooper, R., Aldridge, V. J., McCallum, W. C., and Winter, A. L. (1964). *Nature (London)* **203**, 380.

Walter, W. J., and Walter, W. G. (1949). *Electroencephalogr. Clin. Neurophysiol.* **1**, 57.

Wilkinson, R. T., and Morlock, H. C. (1967). *Electroencephalogr. Clin. Neurophysiol.* **23**, 50.

9

The Blood–Brain Barrier

HUGH DAVSON

I. Introduction 323
    A. Morphology 323
    B. Historical Aspects 326

II. Drainage of the Cerebrospinal Fluid—Arachnoid Villi 330
    A. Valvular Action 331
    B. Equivalent Lymphatic System 332

III. The Secretion of the Cerebrospinal Fluid—Choroid Plexuses . . . 332

IV. Chemistry of the Cerebrospinal Fluid 336
    A. Protein 337
    B. Noncolloidal Constituents 337

V. Rate of Secretion of Cerebrospinal Fluid 341
    A. Subarachnoid Drainage 341
    B. Drainage from Aqueduct 341
    C. Clearance of Injected Substances 342

VI. Passage of Infused Material from Blood to Cerebrospinal Fluid 344
    A. Kinetics 345
    B. Slowly Equilibrating Substances 347
    C. Ions 347
    D. Complexities 347

VII. Penetration into Brain 350
    A. Lipid Solubility 350
    B. Reflexion Coefficients 350
    C. Antipyrine and Salicylic Acid 352
    D. Complete Mathematical Analysis 353
    E. Simpler Treatments 353

VIII. Permeability of the Choroid Plexus 356
    Reflexion Coefficients 357

IX. Slowly Equilibrating Substances 358

X. Extracellular Space of Brain 358
   A. Sink Action 360
   B. Ventricular Perfusion 360
   C. Infusion–Perfusion 361
   D. Silicone Perfusion 361

XI. Brain–Cerebrospinal Fluid Exchanges 362
   A. Transependymal Exchanges 362
   B. Fluid Exchanges 364
   C. Transpial Exchanges 364
   D. The Dura 365

XII. Active Transport Outwards 366
   A. Halogen Anions and Thiocyanate 366
   B. Sulfate 367
   C. Transport out of Brain 367
   D. Organic Bases 368

XIII. Morphology of the Blood–Brain Barrier 369
   A. Brain Capillaries 369
   B. Choroid Plexus 373
   C. Ependyma and Pia-Glia 373

XIV. Significance of the Blood–Brain Barrier 376
   A. CSF–Brain Exchanges 377
   B. Active Transport 378
   C. Regional Variations in Concentration 378
   D. Freshly Secreted Fluid 382
   E. Resting Potentials 383

XV. Mechanism of Homeostasis 384
   Carrier Mechanism 384

XVI. The Cerebrospinal Fluid and Brain Potentials 387
   A. Brain Surface Potentials 388
   B. Choroid Plexus 388
   C. Brain and Plexus 389
   D. Relation to Cerebral Blood Flow 389

XVII. Acid–Base Parameters 391
   A. Paradoxical Changes in pH 392
   B. Permeability to Bicarbonate 392
   C. Respiratory Alkalosis and Acidosis 392
   D. Brain pH, etc. 395

XVIII. Some Special Features of the Blood–Brain Barrier System . . . 398
   A. Facilitated Transfer of Sugars 398
   B. Amino Acids 402
   C. Proteins 407

XIX. Modifications of the Barriers 410
   A. Proteins 410
   B. Crystalloids 411
   C. Direct Exchanges between Blood and Brain 414
   D. Rate of Secretion of Cerebrospinal Fluid 415

XX. Ontogeny of the Blood–Brain Barrier 420
    A. Drainage Route 420
    B. Blood–Brain Uptake 421
    C. Chemical Composition of Cerebrospinal Fluid 424
    D. Secretory Processes 428
    E. Morphology 428
XXI. Special Regions of the Brain 429
    A. Fenestrated Capillaries 430
    B. Ependymal Specialization 431
XXII. Peripheral Nerve 431
    A. Perineurium 432
    B. Blood–Nerve Barrier 433
    Appendix *by K. W. Welch* 435
    References 437

I. Introduction

The concept of the blood–brain barrier derives from the classical studies of Ehrlich (1887), Lewandowsky (1900), and Goldmann (1909, 1913) on vital staining; in essence, they found that many dye stuffs, when injected into the blood, would stain most tissues of the body but not the brain and spinal cord. In some way, then, the central nervous tissue was being protected from the presence of foreign materials in the blood. The concept has passed through several vicissitudes, during which it has been fundamentally modified, e.g., by von Monakow and by Stern, and has been actually denied an existence as a physical entity (e.g., by Edström, 1958), but the present writer can confidently affirm the general validity of the concept, if by blood–brain barrier is meant a physical restraint on the passage of material from the vascular system of the central nervous tissue into the extracellular space surrounding it.

A. Morphology

We shall see, immediately, that the exchanges between blood and central nervous parenchyma are more complex than those between blood and other tissues, such as skeletal muscle, by virtue of the presence of the cerebrospinal fluid, which bathes the tissue both internally and externally. It is therefore important that the essential anatomical features of this relationship be emphasized now, while later morphological details, bearing on specific points, will be dealt with as the occasion arises.

Schematically, the situation may be represented by Fig. 1, in which the brain tissue is shown as being effectively surrounded by cerebrospinal fluid. This is formed by the *choroid plexuses*, which are vascular evaginations into the ventricles and covered by the ependymal lining of these cavities. It is essentially this ependymal lining—called in this context the *choroidal epithelium*—that is responsible for the active transport processes that culminate in the production of a fluid that passes continuously into the ventricles. From the ventricles, the fluid passes into the subarachnoid space, i.e., the space between the pial lining of the surface of the brain and chord and the arachnoid membrane lining the dura.

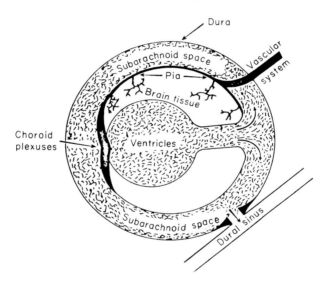

Fig. 1. Illustrating the relationships between CSF on the one hand and the blood and nervous tissue on the other. (Davson, 1963.)

1. *Trans-Choroidal Exchanges*

Thus, one means of exchange of material between blood and brain and cord is through the choroid plexuses. A given substance in the blood may be expected to pass into the secreted cerebrospinal fluid and to be carried in the general bulk flow through the ventricles and over the external surface of the brain and cord. During its passage, it will be able to pass across the ependyma into the adjacent central nervous parenchyma. In studying the passage of material from blood to brain and cord, we must investigate the permeability characteristics of the choroidal blood vessels, their epithelial limiting layer separating the plexuses from the ventricular cavities, and also, the permeability characteristics of the ependymal lining of the remainder of the ventricles

2. Direct Capillary Exchanges

A more obvious area of exchange between blood and central nervous parenchyma is the capillary circulation of this tissue, which is largely derived from the arteries passing in the pia-arachnoid and plunging deep into the tissue (Fig. 2).

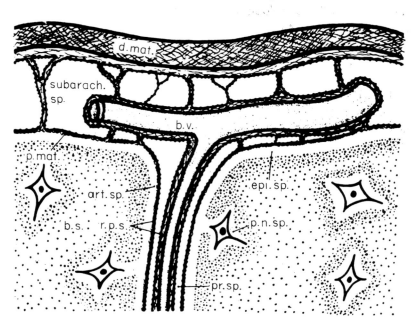

Fig. 2. Illustrating relation of meninges to blood vessel penetrating nervous tissue. b.v., blood vessel; p. mat., pia mater; art. sp., artefact space; b.s., brain substance; epi. sp., epispinal space of His; p.n.sp., perineuronal space; pr. sp., perivascular space; r.p.s., reticular perivascular sheath. (Millen and Woollam, 1962.)

3. Trans-Meningeal Exchanges

Finally, two additional loci of exchange must be envisaged although their importance is not completely clear. First, the pial tissue itself is in obviously close relationship with the cerebrospinal fluid on the one hand and the brain and cord tissue on the other so that exchanges between blood in the pia and these adjacent compartments may be important and, at any rate, cannot be ignored as a possibility. Secondly, the dura is supplied by blood vessels, and after intravenous injection of dye stuffs, it is found that this tissue is not protected by the blood–brain barrier; hence, if the brain and cord are to be protected from the presence of foreign substances in the blood, there must be some restraint on their diffusion imposed by the membranes separating the tissue of the dura from the cerebrospinal fluid since, as we have seen, access to the cerebrospinal fluid might well allow access to the central nervous parenchyma across the pial lining. The membranes separating the dura from the cerebrospinal fluid are a mesothelial lining belonging to the dura and the arachnoid membrane fitting closely to this mesothelium.

B. Historical Aspects

Ehrlich (1887) in his studies of vital staining noted that, when the animal was injected with a variety of dyes, practically all tissues were stained while the brain, but not the dura, was spared. Later, Lewandowsky (1900) showed that the Prussian blue reagents[1] failed to pass into the brain and cord, and he formulated clearly the concept of a blood–brain barrier (*Bluthirnschranke*), i.e., the existence of a restraint on the passage of material from blood to central nervous parenchyma. Goldmann's experiments were based on the acid dyestuff, trypan blue; this, when injected into the blood, failed to stain the brain and also failed to appear in measurable concentration in the cerebrospinal fluid. It stained the other tissues of the body, such as muscle, and it also stained the dura and the connective tissue of the choroid plexus, and these additional observations emphasize the significance of the choroidal epithelium and the arachnoid membrane as participating in the barrier opposed to the penetration of this dyestuff from blood into the central nervous parenchyma. Goldmann (1913) extended the concept of the blood–brain barrier when he injected trypan blue into the cerebrospinal fluid and now found that the brain and cord were stained. Thus, the barrier had been circumvented, and it seemed that the ependymal linings to the ventricles and, possibly also, the pial linings to the surface of the brain and cord were ineffective barriers to the passage of trypan blue from the cerebrospinal fluid into the tissue.

---

[1] The reagents are potassium ferrocyanide and ferric ammonium citrate; on acidification they give a blue precipitate of insoluble ferric ferrocyanide.

1. *The Goldmann–Stern Hypothesis*

Goldmann concluded from his 1913 experiment, according to which trypan blue injected into the cerebrospinal fluid passed into the brain tissue, but not when injected into the blood, that the normal mode of exchange between blood and brain was by way of the choroid plexuses and the cerebrospinal fluid. Passage directly across the capillaries of the central nervous parenchyma was insignificant because of the virtual absoluteness of the blood–brain barrier here. The choroid plexuses could be regarded as analogous with the placenta, modulating or completely inhibiting the exchanges between blood and the cerebrospinal fluid. This concept, which was described as the "way through the fluid" (*Weg über den Liquor*) was developed by von Monakow (1920) and, more explicitly, by Lina Stern and her collaborators. Thus, Stern and Gautier (1921) carried out the first really systematic study of the penetration of a variety of substances from the blood into the cerebrospinal fluid. A given substance was injected into the blood; in order that the substance should not be too rapidly excreted, the kidneys were removed. After a time, the cerebrospinal fluid was withdrawn, and a qualitative test was applied to the fluid to determine whether the substance had penetrated. Among the substances that could penetrate the blood–cerebrospinal fluid barrier were bromide, thiocyanate, strychnine, morphine, atropine, and bile salts, while iodide, ferrocyanide, salicylate, curare, adrenaline, bile pigments, eosin, and fluorescein were said to be invariably absent from the cerebrospinal fluid. In a second paper (1922) Stern and Gautier studied the effects of a variety of substances on the central nervous system after intravenous injection and were able to establish a correlation between penetration into the cerebrospinal fluid and influence on the nervous system. For example, intravenous bromide had a depressant effect on rabbits and could be found, after intravenous injection, in both cerebrospinal fluid and nervous tissue. Again, thiocyanate increased the excitability of cats and could be similarly found in both fluid and nervous tissue. Iodide and ferrocyanide, on the other hand, had no nervous influence after intravenous injection and were found to be absent from the cerebrospinal fluid and nervous tissue. These authors then injected these substances into the subarachnoid space and found that, in general, they all passed into the brain tissue and produced characteristic neurological effects.

Stern and Gautier arrived at the plausible conclusion, previously adumbrated by Goldmann and von Monakow, that passage from blood

to brain tissue took place by way of the cerebrospinal fluid as an intermediary, and the cerebrospinal fluid was regarded as the sole nutrient medium for the central nervous tissue. The blood–brain barrier, or *barrière
hémato-encéphalique* of Stern and Gautier was therefore regarded as a
complex, consisting of an absolute prohibition of penetration from blood
into the central nervous parenchyma by way of the capillary circulation,
together with a restraint which could vary from absolute prohibition,
as with ferrocyanide, to moderately rapid penetration as with bromide,
exerted by the choroid plexuses. The theory is now of only historical
interest, but the experimental work was of value in emphasizing the cooperation between choroid plexuses and parenchymal capillaries that must
be necessary if passage from blood into the parenchyma is to be controlled.
Thus, it would be useless to restrain the passage of iodide from blood
into the brain by way of the blood capillaries if there were a free passage
across the choroidal epithelium since the experiments of Stern and Gautier had shown that iodide, once in the cerebrospinal fluid, passed readily
into the brain tissue.

2. *Modern Concept*

To anticipate a great deal of recent work, we may outline the modern
concept of the blood–brain barrier as in Fig. 3; according to this, the total
exchanges between blood and brain—and it is these that should be
embraced by the term blood–brain barrier[2]—are determined by the following.

1. (a) Exchanges across the blood in the brain capillaries and the extracellular space. (b) Exchanges between extracellular fluid of the nervous
tissue and the surrounding cells of the brain parenchyma, neurons, and
glial cells.

2. (a) Exchanges between blood in the choroidal capillaries and the
cerebrospinal fluid, mediated across the choroidal epithelium and involving a bulk flow of fluid as well as diffusional exchanges. (b) Exchanges

---

[2] It is so usual to limit the meaning of the blood–brain barrier to the exchanges across
the blood vessels of the brain parenchyma and the extracellular space that I shall, in
general, restrict its meaning here accordingly. However, so far as the title of this article
is concerned, it is obvious that it must embrace the limitations imposed on exchanges
between blood on the one hand and cerebrospinal fluid and brain and cord tissue on the
other, i.e., the whole gamut of relationships between blood, extracellular fluid, intracellular fluid, and cerebrospinal fluid.

between cerebrospinal fluid and the brain tissue across the ependyma of the ventricles. (c) Exchanges between cerebrospinal fluid and the brain tissue across the pia and its adjacent layer of glial cells, i.e., the pia-glia.

3. (a) Exchanges between blood in the dural capillaries and the dural tissue. (b) Exchanges between dural tissue and the subjacent cerebrospinal fluid. (c) Exchanges between cerebrospinal fluid and subjacent nervous tissue across pia and glia.

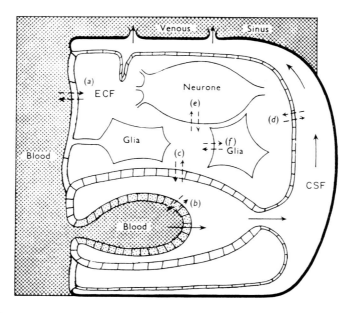

Fig. 3. Diagram of fluid compartments of the blood–brain–CSF system. Continuous arrows represent proven directions of fluid flow. Interrupted arrows indicate where diffusion of water and solutes may occur between the different compartments, namely, (a) across the blood–brain barrier, between brain capillaries and extracellular fluid; (b) across the epithelia of the choroid plexuses; (c) across the ependyma; (d) across the pia-glial membranes; (e) and (f) across the cell membranes of neurons and glial cells. Thick line represents the arachnoid-dural enclosure of the system. (Davson and Bradbury, 1965a.)

The relative importance of these loci of exchange will vary according to the substance considered. We may now proceed to discuss special features of the processes involved before attempting an integrated picture of the mechanisms concerned in the exchanges of certain specific molecules and ions.

II. Drainage of the Cerebrospinal Fluid—Arachnoid Villi

The cerebrospinal fluid is formed continuously, and it is therefore important to know the mechanism by which it is removed from the ventricles and subarachnoid spaces. Weed (1914) showed that it was the *arachnoid villi*, i.e., evaginations of the arachnoid tissue into the dural sinuses of the cortical surface of the brain, that were most probably the site of removal (Fig. 4). Weed considered that the endothelial lining of the dural sinus remained intact as a cap over the herniating arachnoid tissue so that passage of cerebrospinal fluid would have to occur through this endothelium, and Weed postulated that an important force driving fluid into the blood was the difference of colloid osmotic pressure between

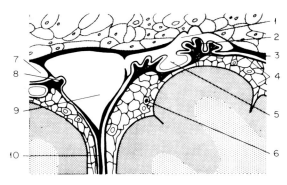

Fig. 4.   Section through superior sagittal sinus showing lacunae laterales. (Davson, 1967, after Hafferl, 1953.) 1. Lacuna lateralis. 2. Arachnoid granulation. 3. Dura mater. 4. Arachnoid and subarachnoid. 5. Opening of cerebral vein. 6. Cerebral artery. 7. Lacuna lateralis. 8. Arachnoid granulation. 9. Superior sagittal sinus. 10. Falx cerebri.

the plasma and the virtually protein-free cerebrospinal fluid operating across this endothelial cap which was supposed to act as a membrane impermeable to plasma proteins. It was argued, however (Davson, 1956), that, if there were a serious restraint on the exit of plasma proteins, which appear in the freshly secreted fluid in a measurable concentration (p. 337), these would accumulate in the fluid and eventually bring drainage to a halt. It was considered that the only feasible mechanism of drainage would be through pores large enough not to exert measurable restraint on the plasma proteins; thus, Courtice and Simmonds (1951) injected tagged proteins into the cerebrospinal fluid and analyzed the animal's blood and lymph. Their results showed, without doubt, that the plasma proteins do escape directly from the subarachnoid space into the blood and not by phagocytosis, the mechanism that must be invoked if the lining membrane of the villus is, indeed, impermeable to proteins.

A. Valvular Action

The concept of a relatively unrestricted flow of large molecules out of the villi is confirmed by the studies of Welch and Friedman (1960) and Welch and Pollay (1961), who showed, histologically, that the villi could be considered as aggregates of tubes opening directly into the lacunae laterales of the dural sinus provided that the pressure in the subarachnoid space was high enough. When the pressure was too low, the system collapsed so that the system acted as a valvular mechanism ensuring that flow would be from subarachnoid space to blood, thereby preventing back-flow of blood into the cerebrospinal fluid should the pressure in the blood vessel become greater than that in the subarachnoid space (Fig. 5). This concept was supported by experiments on isolated pieces of dura containing villi, which showed that such a valvular mechanism did, indeed, operate, while there was little or no obstruction to the passage of particles as large as 7.5 μ in diameter.

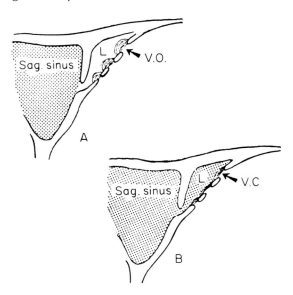

Fig. 5. Diagrammatic illustration of the situation and function of the arachnoid villi. When the meningeal pressure is sufficiently greater than that in the sinus the villus meshwork is open as in (A). When the meningeal pressure is below that in the sinus, reflux of blood is prevented by collapse of the villus (B). (Welch and Friedman, 1960.)

B. Equivalent Lymphatic System

In general, studies in which proteins and other large molecular-weight substances have been injected into the cerebrospinal fluid confirm the view that there is little or no restraint on the movement of fluids, and of all its constituents, out of the subarachnoid space, the physical force determining this being the difference in hydrostatic pressures of cerebrospinal fluid (CSF) and dural sinus, which is normally positive and favoring outward flow. Because of this feature, we may regard the CSF as the equivalent of a lymphatic system, carrying away from the cranial and spinal systems substances that would not be able to leave at significant rates by the alternative route through the blood capillaries of the brain and cord parenchyma.[3a] Kinetically, this creates an interesting situation, namely, one in which the penetration of a given substance into the brain and cerebrospinal fluid may be restricted but its egress will be unrestricted.[3b]

III. The Secretion of the Cerebrospinal Fluid—Choroid Plexuses

The choroid plexuses were early implicated in the formation of the cerebrospinal fluid, although the evidence adduced in support of the concept was highly suspect. Today, most reliance is placed on the circum-

---

[3] (a) The possibility that absorption of cerebrospinal fluid may occur across the ependyma into the vascular system of the brain has been discussed by Sahar *et al.* (1969a). They injected kaolin into the cisterna magna of cats, thereby blocking communication between ventricles and subarachnoid space. Under these conditions absorption of perfused fluid still occurred although a higher pressure was required to induce this. It is not clear from their paper, however, to what extent absorption consisted of retention in the expanding ventricles (Sahar *et al.*, 1969a, p. 643). In another study (Sahar *et al.*, 1969b), the uptake of protein from ventricles into brain was measured as a function of distance from the surface when the protein was perfused through the ventricles; they considered that passage into the brain was an index to flow of CSF, but this could have been due to diffusion, and it is interesting that the concentration profile is very similar to one predicted by Welch (1969) on the basis of diffusion through intercellular channels.

(b) Shabo and Maxwell (1968a,b), on the basis of electron microscopy of the arachnoid villi, have argued that the membrane separating cerebrospinal fluid from blood is intact, and they have claimed that absorption of protein is by phagocytosis. In this event the colloid osmotic pressure of the cerebrospinal fluid would be an important factor determining rate of drainage, yet Davson *et al.* (1971) have shown that, even when the cerebrospinal fluid is replaced by the animal's own plasma or by equivalent solutions of dextrans, the altered resistance to outflow can be accounted for entirely on the basis of the altered viscosity.

stance that the fluid is produced within the ventricles rather than in the subarachnoid space since occlusion of the aqueduct of Sylvius leads to high pressure with dilatation of the ventricles (hydrocephalus). However, the unequivocal proof that the fluid is *exclusively* formed within the ventricles and *only* by the choroid plexuses has not been forthcoming so that dogmatic statements in this respect must be avoided.

In four discrete regions the pia becomes modified into highly vascularized bodies which project into the ventricles and constitute the choroid plexuses. Essentially, in these regions, namely, the roofs of the third and fourth ventricles and the walls of the lateral ventricles, the wall consists of only two membranes, the ependyma and the pia; and it is the outpouching of the pia, together with its highly developed vascularization, that forms the choroid plexus, which is thus lined by ependyma or, as it is called here, the choroidal epithelium. On cross section, then, the plexus appears as a fold of epithelium with a core of highly vascularized connective tissue (Fig. 6). This association of a vascular connective tissue core with an epithelial lining is the expected arrangement for an organ producing fluid; we may presume that a filtrate of plasma is formed in the connective tissue and that the epithelial lining actively transports salt to produce the difference of osmotic pressure that will cause a flow of fluid from connective tissue core to ventricles. The ultrastructure of the epithelium supports this view of its function. (Maxwell and Pease, 1956; Wislocki and Ladman, 1958; Tennyson and Pappas, 1961; Carpenter, 1966; Brightman and Reese, 1969). The light microscopist described the cells as having a "brush-border," and the nature of this border is revealed in the electron microscope as a series of microvilli, i.e., extensions of the apical cytoplasm covered by plasma membrane (Fig. 7).

Another feature is the manner in which the membranes of the cells show the so-called basal infoldings, i.e., the invagination of the plasma membrane to separate the cytoplasm into compartments. Similar invaginations occur in epithelia well recognized for their transport of fluid secretions, e.g., the proximal convoluted tubule that continuously absorbs some 90% of the glomerular filtrate, the ciliary epithelium producing the ocular fluid, the epithelium of the salt gland, and so on.

The blood capillaries, too, share a feature of those associated with secretory activity, namely, the presence of the so-called fenestrae, attenuations of the cytoplasm of the endothelial cell to the point that the plasma membranes covering the internal and external aspects of the cell are closely apposed and partially obliterated so that only a layer some 60 Å thick separates the contents of the capillary from the extracellular

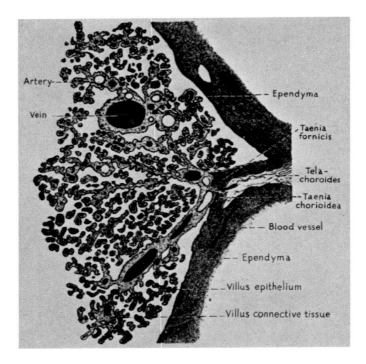

Fig. 6.   Choroid plexus. (Clara, 1953.)

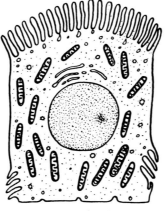

Adult choroid plexus

Fig. 7.   Illustrating basal infoldings of the plasma membrane. (Tennyson and Pappas, 1961.)

space (Rhodin, 1962). These Type II capillaries (Majno, 1965) are found in endocrine glands, the renal glomerulus, the ciliary body, salivary glands, intestinal villus, and so on, regions where a generally high permeability might be required.

As with other secretory epithelia, the walls of adjacent cells contain "junctional complexes" of Farquhar and Palade (1963), including the

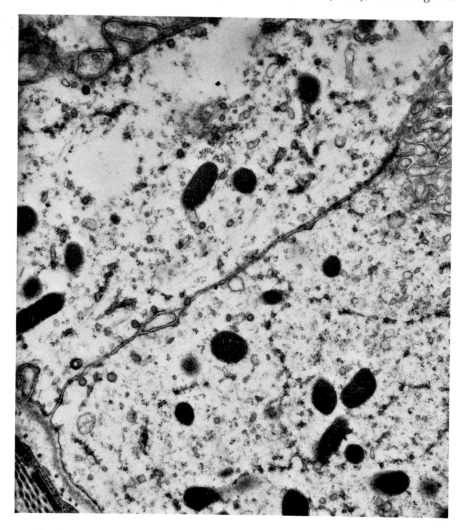

Fig. 8. Section through two choroidal epithelial cells showing intercellular cleft. Normal rabbit. ×30,000. (Burgess and Segal, 1970.)

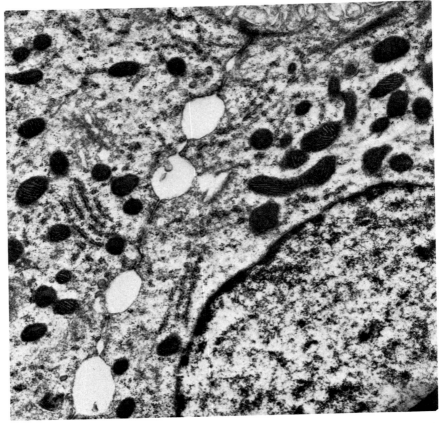

Fig. 9. Section through two choroidal epithelial cells showing intercellular cleft with engorgements resulting from treatment with Diamox. × 30,000. (Burgess and Segal, 1970.)

tight junction or zonula occludens at the apical ends. It is interesting that the intercellular clefts in the normally secreting choroid plexus are narrow; when secretion is inhibited, the spaces become enlarged to give vesicle-like expansions [Figs. 8 and 9 (from Burgess and Segal, 1970)].

IV. Chemistry of the Cerebrospinal Fluid

The chemistry of the cerebrospinal fluid is of obvious interest in the context of the blood–brain barrier since the composition must be related to that of the extracellular fluid of the brain and cord, with which it comes into close diffusional relationships in the ventricles and subarachnoid spaces. In fact, it may well be argued that the cerebrospinal and extracellular fluids are very closely similar in composition (Wallace and Brodie, 1939, 1940; Davson, 1958; Bradbury and Davson, 1965; Fencl *et al.*, 1966; M. W. Cohen *et al.*, 1968).

A. PROTEIN

The average protein concentrations in the fluids of the rabbit are 6500 mg/100 gm for plasma and 31 mg/100 gm for CSF.

Comparable figures are found in other species including man. Electrophoretic analysis of the proteins shows them to be apparently identical with those in the plasma although their proportions in the two fluids are not the same. Thus Spina-Franca (1960) gives the following values for the ratios of the percentages in CSF and serum: albumin, 1.0; α-globulin, 0.9; β-globulin, 1.6; γ-globulin, 0.6.

When ventricular, cisternal, and lumbar fluids of man are compared, the total protein concentrations increase in this order (Hunter and Smith, 1960; Hill *et al.* 1958, 1959). In general, it appeared from the Hill *et al.* study that the higher concentration in the lumbar fluid was due to the appearance of more albumin and, to a less extent, α_1- and γ-globulins. It seems likely, therefore, that the fluid as primarily secreted has proteins in characteristic proportions that are not necessarily those in the plasma; on its passage through the ventricles and subarachnoid spaces additional proteins diffuse from the tissue into the fluid, the amounts of the different types depending, perhaps, on the ease with which these escape from the blood into the tissue, or from the blood in the pia into the subarachnoid space, and also on the breakdown of cells in the tissue.[4]

B. NONCOLLOIDAL CONSTITUENTS

Table I illustrates the concentrations of the main constituents of the rabbit's plasma and cerebrospinal fluid. The ratios, i.e., concentration in CSF/concentration in plasma (R_{CSF}), have been compared with cor-

---

[4] A small percentage of the total protein of CSF migrates more rapidly than albumin and has been called *pre-albumin* by Esser and Heinzler (1952); it was thought not to be in plasma but is present, constituting some 0.5% of the total proteins (Schultze *et al.*, 1956). From light-scattering data its molecular weight is 61,000 and its carbohydrate content and amino acid composition are different from those of serum albumin. The concentration is greatest in the ventricles, less in the cisterna magna, and least in the lumbar region (Steger, 1953).

TABLE I

Concentrations of Various Solutes (mEq/kg H_2O) in CSF and Plasma of the Rabbit, and Distribution Ratios[a]

Substance		Plasma	CSF	R_{CSF}	R_{Dial}
Na		148	149	1.005	0.945
K		4.3	2.9	0.675	0.96
Mg^b		2.02	1.74	0.92	0.80
Ca^b		5.60	2.47	0.45	0.65
Cl		106	130	1.23	1.04
HCO_3		25	22	0.92	1.04
^{82}Br		1	0.71	0.71	0.96
^{131}I	High	13	2.6	0.20	0.85
	Low	0.25	0.0025	0.01	0.85
$^{14}CNS^c$	High	8.25	4.50	0.545	0.73
	Low	1.77	0.071	0.04	0.60
Glucose		8.3	5.35	0.64	0.97
Urea		8.35	6.5	0.78	1.00
Osmolality		298.5	305.2	1.02	0.995
pH		7.46	7.27	—	—

[a] R_{CSF} = concentration in CSF/concentration in plasma, and R_{Dial} = concentration in dialysate/concentration in plasma (Davson, 1967).

[b] From Bradbury (1971).

[c] From Pollay (1966).

responding ratios for a dialysate of plasma (R_{Dial}). In general, the fluid differs from a plasma dialysate, the main deviations being the low concentrations of HCO_3^-, K^+, $SO_4^=$, urea, glucose, and amino acids, and the relatively high concentrations of Cl^-, Na^+, and Mg^{++}. When different species are compared, the same general features are revealed although the discrepancies from a plasma dialysate often vary; thus, in man the value of R_{CSF} for Mg^{++} is 1.39 (Hunter and Smith, 1960) compared with only 0.92 in the rabbit. In the monkey Bito (1969) found a ratio of 1.66, indicating a very large deviation from R_{Dial} which, because of binding to plasma proteins, is only about 0.80. In the rat, Chutgow (1968) found a R_{CSF} ratio of 1.05. The results, then, show that the fluid is not a simple filtrate from plasma, as originally argued by Merritt and Fremont-Smith (1937) so that it is to be described as a secretion.

1. Electrochemical Potential

As to which ions are actively transported and which move passively along gradients of electrochemical potential can only be assessed by measuring the potential across the choroid plexuses. In general, there is a small positivity of the cerebrospinal fluid in relation to the blood (Loeschke, 1956a,b) but this can by no means account for the distributions of, say, K^+ and Cl^-, especially when the effects of fluctuations in plasma concentrations of these ions are studied since these have little or no effect on the concentrations in the cerebrospinal fluid and, thus, produce large alterations in the value of R_{CSF} without affecting the potential significantly. It is this immunity of the cerebrospinal fluid from alterations in plasma concentration of certain of its constituents that is of greatest interest when studying the chemistry of the fluid, revealing, as it does, accurate homeostatic mechanisms that maintain the composition of the cerebrospinal fluid and, therefore presumably, of the extracellular fluid of brain and cord, within strict limits.

2. Homeostasis in Cerebrospinal Fluid Composition

Bekaert and Demeester (1951a,b, 1952) raised the plasma-K^+ by injection of isotonic KCl, or by inducing a hyperthermia with dinitrophenol, and they found a negligible rise in concentration in the cerebrospinal fluid. Again, Cooper *et al.* (1955) infused KCl into dogs, and although the plasma-K^+ rose from 3.9 to 10.7 mEq/liter, the concentration in the cerebrospinal fluid rose only from 3.07 to 3.36 mEq/liter, a rise that was statistically insignificant.[5] Lowering the plasma K^+, by injection of insulin or glucose (Bekaert and Demeester, 1951a) or by treatment with DOCA, likewise had a very small or negligible effect on fluid K^+. Bradbury and Kleeman (1967) made animals chronically hypo- or hyperkalaemic and followed the concentrations in cerebrospinal fluid, brain, and skeletal muscle. Some results are shown in Table II, and it will be seen that in hypokalaemia the concentration of K^+ in the cerebrospinal fluid is actually greater than in plasma since the hypokalaemia has not been reflected in a pronounced fall in cerebrospinal fluid concentration. Whereas the concentration in skeletal muscle rises and falls in hyper- and hypokalaemia respectively, the concentration in brain remains remarkably

---

[5] Kemeny *et al.* (1965) have shown that the dog's CSF is not completely immune to raised plasma levels of K^+, the concentration in CSF (Y) depending on the plasma concentration (X) in accordance with the regression equation $Y = 4.02 - 0.27(X - 7.54)$.

TABLE II

CONCENTRATIONS OF K$^+$ IN PLASMA AND CSF (mEq/LITER) AND IN MUSCLE AND BRAIN (mEq/kg) OF RABBITS DIETED FOR 3 WEEKS [a]

	Plasma	CSF	Muscle	Brain
Control	4.15	2.83	111	95.4
Low K$^+$	1.58	2.72	72.2	94.5
High K$^+$	7.09	3.02	110	94.9

[a] Bradbury and Kleeman (1967).

constant. Studies on Mg^{++}, Ca^{++}, and pH illustrate the same phenomenon in so far as acute and chronic changes in the plasma levels of these ions are reflected in only small changes in concentration in the cerebrospinal fluid. Thus, Fig. 10 from Oppelt *et al.* (1963) shows the response of the dog's cerebrospinal fluid to an actual rise in the plasma concentration of Mg^{++}. Studies with isotopic ^{28}Mg showed that the failure to respond to the altered plasma level was not just due to a low permeability of the

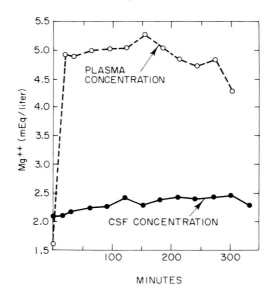

Fig. 10. CSF and plasma magnesium concentrations during intravenous infusion of MgCl$_2$ and MgSO$_4$. (Oppelt *et al.* 1963.)

blood–CSF barrier to the ion; in fact, the computed transfer constant was 0.0005 minute^{-1} compared with 0.0073 minute^{-1} for ^{24}Na found by Wang (1948) in the dog.[6]

V. Rate of Secretion of Cerebrospinal Fluid

The rate of production of CSF is an important parameter in the discussion of the blood–brain barrier. Thus, if the brain is to receive material from the CSF, the laws of diffusion indicate that the higher the concentration gradient between the CSF and the tissue, the more rapid the net flux of material to the tissue; the more sluggish the flow, the smaller will be the average concentration gradient during a given period. Similarly, if the CSF is receiving material from the brain, the more rapid the flow, the lower the average concentration in the CSF and the larger the concentration gradient.

A. Subarachnoid Drainage

The earliest attempts at measuring the rate of formation of the fluid consisted in simply allowing it to drain. Thus, Riser (1929) recorded that, if a cannula is inserted into the cisterna magna of a dog, in the first half-hour 10–20 ml flow out, apparently 75% of the total. After the second half-hour the rate of leakage settles down to an average rate of loss of about 30 ml/24 hours, i.e., 0.021 ml/minute, a value agreeing with that of Frazier and Peet (1914), namely, 0.023 ml/minute. Again, Greenberg *et al.* (1943) in their study of penetration of isotopes into the dog's CSF, found an average rate of drip of 0.2 ml/hour/kg. For a 10-kg dog this would be 2 ml/hour or approximately 0.03 ml/minute. The main objection to this drip technique is that the cerebrospinal fluid pressure has to be kept at a negative value in order to maintain a regular drip, and this may cause some exudation from other structures than the choroid plexuses.

B. Drainage from Aqueduct

An improvement in technique was made by Flexner and Winters (1932), who placed a cannula in the aqueduct of Sylvius of the cat. To

---

[6] The situation with regard to pH is complex, as we shall see, owing to the ready diffusibility of CO_2 across the blood–brain and blood–CSF barriers (p. 391).

prevent leakage around the cannula the latter was surrounded by a bal-
loon that could be inflated after insertion. The cannula made connection
with a graduated tube, which was connected to a reservoir of saline that
permitted the maintenance of a constant pressure of 110 mm H_2O in
the ventricles. The formation of the fluid in the ventricles was reflected
by the movement of a bubble in the graduated tubing. On average, the
fluid was formed at the rate of 12.1 ml/day; this ignores the fluid formed
by the fourth ventricle, and if allowance is made for its contribution,
(it is 25% smaller than the others) a figure of 15 ml/day or 0.015 ml/min-
ute is reached. Flexner (1933) computed that the total volume of the
cat's cerebrospinal fluid was about 4.4 ml; consequently, a rate of formation of 0.015 ml/minute corresponds to a renewal rate of 0.34%/minute.

C. Clearance of Injected Substances

Injection of a substance into the cerebrospinal fluid and measurement
of its rate of disappearance from the fluid could give a measure of the
rate of drainage of the fluid and, thus, a measure of its rate of production.
This would only be true if the injected substance were unable to diffuse
across the ependymal and other linings of the cavities containing the cerebrospinal fluid. Proteins, inulin, and high-molecular weight dextrans
have been used in this context, the losses across the ependyma and pia-
glia being considered to be negligible compared with the escape by the
normal drainage mechanism through the arachnoid villi. Davson *et al.*
(1962) found that the fall in concentration of inulin, in 1 hour after injection into the cisterna magna, was some 17% and this corresponded to a
rate of renewal of the fluid, i.e., of the production of an inulin-free fluid
diluting the existing fluid, of 0.3%/minute. Similarly, in the dog, Rothman *et al.* (1961) computed a renewal rate of 0.2%/minute from the rate
of removal of inulin or dextran, while in man Sweet *et al.* (1950) found
a half-life for disappearance of injected protein corresponding to a drainage rate of some 0.4%/minute.

1. *Ventriculo-Cisternal Perfusion*

An improvement of this technique, based on the clearance of a foreign
molecule too large to pass directly into the brain tissue in significant
amounts, is given by continuous perfusion of the ventricles by means of
cannulae inserted into the lateral ventricles and in the cisterna magna.
The technique of perfusion was developed by Royer (1950) and Leusen

(1950) in their studies of exchanges between cerebrospinal fluid and brain. Pappenheimer *et al.* (1962) applied it to the goat, measuring the inflow and outflow concentrations of inulin during perfusion at a constant and known rate. With the passage of time the concentration in the outflowing fluid rises to reach a steady-state level after about 60 minutes (Fig. 11). The rate of secretion, K_f, is given by

$$K_f = K_x[(C_{In} - C_{Out})/C_{Out}]$$

where C_{In} and C_{Out} are the inflowing and outflowing concentrations of inulin or other marker molecule, e.g., dextran, and K_x is the rate of perfusion.

The results of measurements, on several species, employing this technique, are summarized in Table III. The absolute rate of production of fluid increases with the size of the brain from 2.2 μl/minute for the rat to 370 μl/minute in man. Expressed as a percentage of the total volume of cerebrospinal fluid, the rates are not greatly different, varying from 0.6%/minute in the rabbit to 0.37%/minute in man. Thus, the efficacies of the

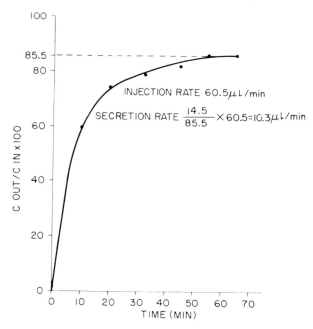

Fig. 11. Showing the change in concentration of dextran in the outflowing fluid (C_{Out}) during ventriculo-cisternal perfusion in the rabbit expressed as % of the inflowing concentration (C_{In}). (Davson, 1967.)

TABLE III

RATES OF SECRETION OF CSF IN VARIOUS SPECIES

Species	μl/minute	%/minute	μl/minute/mg c.p.
Rat	2.2	—	—
Rabbit	10.1	0.63	0.43
Cat	20	0.45	0.5
	22	0.50	0.55
	22	0.50	0.55
Dog	50	0.40	0.625
	66	—	0.77
	47	—	—
Goat	164	0.65	0.36
Man[a]	520	0.37	0.29

[a] Rubin *et al.* (1966) used ventriculo-cisternal perfusion to measure secretion rate in humans; they found 370 μl/minute. In children, Cutler *et al.* (1968b) found a rate of 350 μl/minute.

CSF of different species in promoting exchanges with the brain parenchyma are not likely to be greatly different if only the percentage rate of renewal is taken into account. A better index would be rate of renewal per unit weight of brain, in which case the rates for rat, rabbit, and man would be in the order 2.5, 1.0, and 0.5 μl/gm/minute.

VI. Passage of Infused Material from Blood to Cerebrospinal Fluid

Having outlined the main features governing the production and drainage of the CSF, we may proceed to consider the passage of material from blood into this fluid; a study of the kinetics of this process will bring into prominence the importance of exchanges between the CSF and the brain. In Fig. 12 are shown the results of maintaining a steady concentration of several substances in the blood and measuring the concentration in the cerebrospinal fluid as a function of time after establishing this steady blood concentration. The animal was intact and unanesthetized until the moment came to remove its cerebrospinal fluid, and since removal of fluid disturbs the system, only one measurement was made on any given animal. Thus to obtain a given point on a curve some six animals had to be studied and the mean values for plasma and cerebrospinal fluid concentrations were taken. It will be seen from Fig. 12 that the rate of equilibration increases with increasing lipid solubility, indicating the presence of a barrier with physical features similar to those of the plasma membrane separating the cytoplasm from the outside medium of a cell.

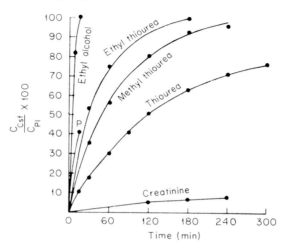

Fig. 12.   Penetration of different substances of increasing lipid solubility into rabbit's CSF. P, propyl thiourea. (Davson, 1967.)

A. KINETICS

The curves are remarkably regular when we consider the complexity of the system since the material in the blood may pass into the fluid directly in the secreted fluid and indirectly from the blood vessels of the brain parenchyma and across the ependymal lining of the ventricles and the pia-glial lining of the subarachnoid spaces. In Fig. 13, the points for penetration of methyl thiourea have been plotted semilogarithmically, giving a good straight line indicating that the process can be described by a simple two-compartment equation of the form:

$$dC/dt = k_{In}\ C_{Plasma} - k_{Out}\ C_{CSF} \tag{1}$$

which on integration, with C_{Plasma} constant, gives:

$$\ln[1 - (C_{In}/rC_{Out})] = - k_{Out}\ t \tag{2}$$

$$\text{or } 1 - (C_{In}/rC_{Out}) = e^{-k_{Out}\,t} \tag{2'}$$

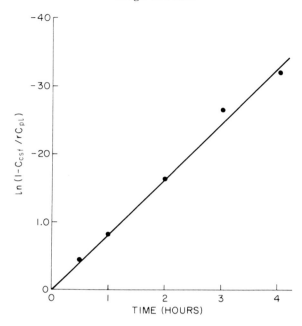

Fig. 13. Penetration of methyl thiourea into rabbit's CSF. The logarithmic function has been plotted against time. (Davson, 1967.)

where r is the steady-state ratio C_{In}/C_{Out} at infinite time. This will be unity when k_{In} equals k_{Out}, and in fact, the experimental results of Fig. 12 indicate that the steady-state levels are indeed equal to unity for alcohol and the thioureas.

The simple kinetic behavior in a complex situation would be explained in several ways. It could be argued that the Stern-Gautier hypothesis was correct so that the only means of influx from blood to cerebrospinal fluid was through the choroid plexuses. We may make the simple assumption that the freshly secreted fluid contains the substance in a concentration r times the concentration in the plasma, where r may be equal to unity, when the substance is highly lipid soluble, and so penetrates rapidly across the epithelial cells, or less than unity, when lipid solubility is low. In this case the amount entering in unit time will be $K_f r C_{Plasma}$ and the amount leaving, if exchanges with brain are indeed forbidden, will be simply $K_f C_{CSF}$. Thus,

$$dS/dt = K_f r C_{Plasma} - K_f C_{CSF} \tag{3}$$

$$dC/dt = (K_f/V)\, r C_{Plasma} - (K_f/V) C_{CSF} \tag{4}$$

i.e.,

$$dC/dt = k_{In}C_{Pl} - k_{Out}\,C_{CSF}$$

with k_{In} being equal to the product of r and the inflow constant for production of cerebrospinal fluid. We shall see, however, that influx in the newly secreted fluid is not necessarily the only pathway, so that additional pathways from the brain parenchyma will make k_{In} greater than $r \times K_f$.

B. SLOWLY EQUILIBRATING SUBSTANCES

With creatinine, the concentration in the cerebrospinal fluid approaches a steady state with a value of only some 10% of that in the plasma; with other substances such as sucrose, p-aminohippurate, inulin, and serum albumin, the steady-state levels are probably even lower. Figures 14 and 15 show the equilibration of CSF with sucrose and γ-globulin after intravenous injection.

C. IONS

In Fig. 16 the penetration of certain ions into the cerebrospinal fluid is shown; with sodium the behavior is very similar to that of thiourea, the process following a two-compartment equation with the steady-state ratio, $r = C_{CSF}/C_{Plasma}$ approximately unity as indicated by the straight line relationship between $\ln(1 - C_{CSF}/rC_{Plasma})$ and time. With ${}^{82}Br$ and ${}^{42}K^+$ steady-state ratios of considerably less than unity are approached and this corresponds with the steady-state values found with nonradioactive ions (Table I). The kinetics of equilibration of these two ions do not follow a simple two-compartment equation; thus, the initial rate for Br^- is actually faster than that for ${}^{24}Na$, yet Br approaches a steady-state of about 0.7 while ${}^{24}Na$ approaches a value of unity; inspection of Eq. (2) shows that no such situation could arise on a simple two-compartment basis.

D. COMPLEXITIES

It would be fruitless to discuss further the kinetics of penetration into the CSF without considering the penetration into the nervous tissue; thus, as indicated earlier, we may expect that when a substance is injected into the blood it will pass not only into the CSF through the choroid plexuses but also directly into the brain. At any given moment the concentration of

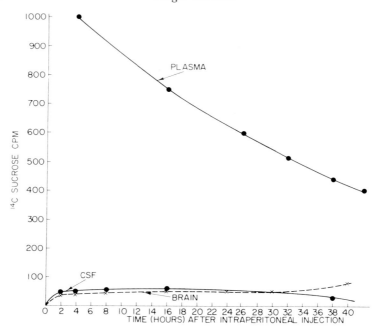

Fig. 14.   Penetration of ^{14}C-sucrose into CSF and brain after intraperitoneal injection into nephrectomized rats. Note that the CSF concentration passes through a maximum indicating that the steady-state distribution ratio is considerably less than unity. The tendency for the brain concentration to rise after some 30 hours may be due to intracellular penetration, either as sucrose or as a ^{24}C-metabolite. (After Reed and Woodbury, 1963.)

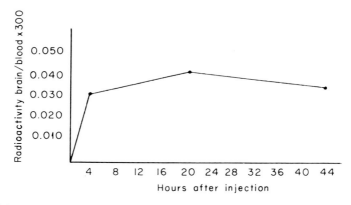

Fig. 15.   Relation of radioactivity of brain/serum from 23 cats at different time intervals after intravenous injection of ^{131}I γ-globulin. The greatest relative activity was found at 20–24 hours and was never more than 1 to 1.5%. (Hochwald and Wallenstein, 1967a.)

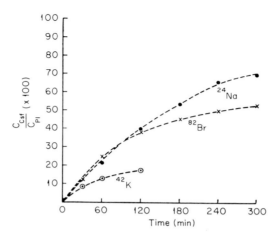

Fig. 16. Penetration of some ions into CSF. (After Davson, 1955a.)

the substance in the cerebrospinal fluid may be above that in the extra-cellular fluid of the brain, in which case there will be net losses into the brain during the approach to the steady state. Alternatively the concentration may be greater in the extracellular fluid of brain, in which case the cerebrospinal fluid will gain substance from two sources, namely, the choroid plexuses and the brain across the ependyma and pia. Finally, during the approach to the steady state one state of affairs may prevail during the early phase of penetration to be reversed during the later phase. Clearly, these exchanges will complicate the kinetic analysis although under some conditions the simple two-compartment equation will be followed. The behavior of ^{42}K could be accounted for qualitatively on the assumption that it passed directly into the cerebrospinal fluid in the newly secreted fluid at a concentration $r \times C_{Plasma}$, where r is the steady-state ratio R_{CSF} of approximately 0.7; the isotope would also pass directly into the brain extracellular space from the brain capillaries, but because of the large reservoir of inactive K^+ in the nervous tissue, the isotope would exchange rapidly with the intracellular contents so that the concentration in the extracellular fluid could be well below that in the CSF, and this would favor losses from cerebrospinal fluid to brain and would account for the rapid slowing off in equilibration of the cerebrospinal fluid. As time proceeded the reverse situation could arise so that in the later phases of equilibration the CSF would be gaining from the brain and the steady-state level of 0.7 would be slowly achieved (Bradbury and Kleeman, 1967).

VII. Penetration into Brain

Figure 17 shows the curves of penetration of ^{24}Na, thiourea, and ethyl thiourea into brain and cerebrospinal fluid. With ^{24}Na the curves for both brain and cerebrospinal fluid tend to overlap, indicating that both compartments equilibrate with blood plasma at about the same rate, and it could well be that exchanges between cerebrospinal fluid and extracellular fluid of brain are very small during the whole process of equilibration. If this were so, the simple two-compartment equation of p. 345 would apply since the only source of influx could now well be that in the secreted fluid. With thiourea and ethyl thiourea the rates of equilibration with brain are considerably more rapid than with cerebrospinal fluid, and under these conditions it is certain that the cerebrospinal fluid will be gaining material from the brain. With ethyl alcohol an exact kinetic comparison between brain and cerebrospinal fluid is not easy since passage into the brain is so rapid that complete equilibration is achieved within the few minutes necessary to establish the steady level in the blood.

A. Lipid Solubility

As with penetration into the CSF, the lipid solubility of the substance plays a dominant role in determining speed of equilibration; thus, the lipid solubilities of thiourea, ethyl thiourea, and ethyl alcohol measured by their ether–water partition coefficients are in this order. Again, Mayer *et al.*, studies (1959) gave relative rates in the order acetamide > barbital > *N*-acetyl-4-aminopyrine > salicylic acid, and their heptane–water partition coefficients were in the order 0.01, 0.005, 0.004, and 0.001, respectively. Finally, Crone (1965), employing the technique of analysis of arterial and cerebral venous blood, i.e., the "indicator dilution technique," obtained the values for permeability constants of the brain capillaries shown in Table IV. Here, the assumption is made that uptake into the cerebrospinal fluid was negligible by comparison with that into the brain during the period of measurement.

B. Reflexion Coefficients

By estimating the amount of water withdrawn from the brain and CSF when the blood was made hypertonic with different solutes, Fenstermacher and Johnson (1966) obtained a series of reflexion coefficients, on the assumption that the reflexion coefficient of raffinose was unity, as follows, formamide, 0.31; urea, 0.44; glucose, 0.89; sucrose, 0.98; raffinose, 1.00.

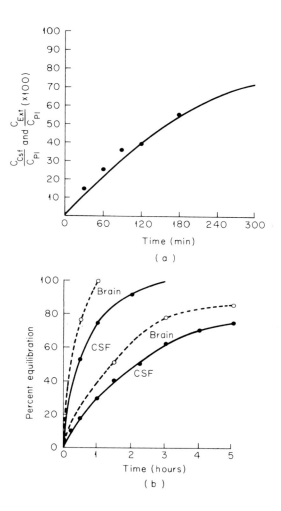

Fig. 17 (a) Penetration of ^{24}Na into CSF (smooth curve) brain and extracellular H_2O (points). Ordinates: $\dfrac{\text{concentration in CSF } (C_{CSF}) \text{ or brain extracellular } H_2O \ (C_{Ext})}{\text{concentration in plasma } (C_{Pl})} \times 100.$

Abscissae: time in minutes. (Davson, 1955a.) (b) Penetration of ethyl thiourea (upper curve) and thiourea, (lower curves) into brain (dotted curves) and CSF (full curves) of the rabbit. Note that concentration in brain is always higher than in CSF. (Davson *et al.*, 1963.)

TABLE IV

PERMEABILITY CONSTANTS (IN cm/SECOND) DEDUCED FROM ANALYSIS OF INFLOWING AND
OUTFLOWING BLOOD OF BRAIN [a]

Substance	Permeability constant cm/second $\times$ 10[5]
Fructose	0.16
Glycerol	0.21
Thiourea	0.29
Propylene glycol	0.38
Urea	0.44
Antipyrine	3.3
Ethanol	>10

[a] Crone (1965).

C. ANTIPYRINE AND SALICYLIC ACID

A number of other studies on the passage from blood to both brain
and cerebrospinal fluid concur in showing that when penetration is relatively rapid the brain equilibrates more rapidly than the cerebrospinal
fluid, while the reverse occurs with slowly penetrating substances. Thus,
Figs. 18 and 19 show the equilibration of the rapidly penetrating antipyrine and the slowly penetrating salicylic acid (Mayer *et al.*, 1959).

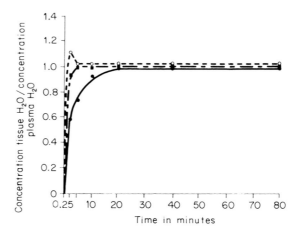

Fig. 18.   Penetration of antipyrine into liver ($\bigcirc$), brain ($\blacksquare$) and CSF ($\bullet$) from blood.
(Mayer *et al.*, 1959.)

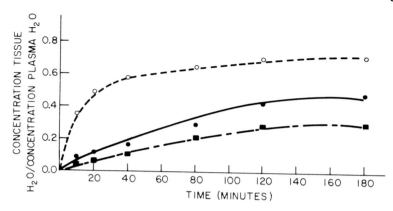

Fig. 19. Penetration of salicylic acid into liver (○), brain (■) and CSF (●) from blood. (Mayer *et al.*, 1959.)

D. COMPLETE MATHEMATICAL ANALYSIS

Hence, in setting up equations to describe the passage of material into the CSF we must envisage the CSF acting as a drain or sink for the brain or, alternatively, acting as an additional source to that provided by the transcapillary influx directly into the tissue. A complete mathematical analysis of the processes of equilibration of brain and cerebrospinal fluid with any given substance is complex and has been achieved by Welch (1969). This treatment is given in the Appendix, and here it is sufficient to note that it is based on influx in the primary secretion, as described above: influx into the brain extracellular space from the capillaries, exchanges between the extracellular space and the intracellular fluid of the tissue, and finally, diffusion through the brain extracellular fluid in accordance with the Fick diffusion equation, without any significant barrier to diffusion between cerebrospinal fluid and the tissue. Figure 20 shows the experimental points for penetration of ^{24}Na into the rabbit's brain and CSF and the calculated curve based on Welch's equations using computer analysis for choice of appropriate parameters.

E. SIMPLER TREATMENTS

Under certain conditions the treatment may be much simpler. Thus, we have seen how the equilibration of a rapidly penetrating substance like ethylthiourea seems to follow a simple two-compartment curve, and and this is doubtless due to the circumstance that at any given moment

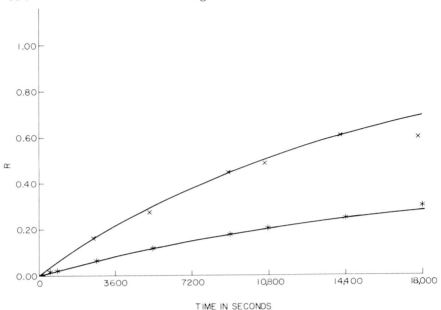

TIME IN SECONDS

Fig. 20. Penetration of ^{24}Na into CSF and brain. Counts per unit volume of CSF/ counts per unit volume of plasma water (+) and counts per unit volume of brain water/ counts per unit volume of plasma water (*) are shown at several times after the establishment of a steady plasma level. The lines are solutions of Eq. (4), etc. (Appendix) and its integrals for $D = 1.64 \times 10^{-5}$ cm^2 second^{-1}, $C = \pi/2$, $V = 2.5$ cm^3, $y = 6.67 \times 10^{-5}$ second^{-1}, $K = 17.6 \times 10^{-5}$ second^{-1}, $l = 0.2$ cm, $K_i = 7.5 \times 10^{-3}$ second^{-1}, $K_o = 4.29 \times 10^{-3}$ second^{-1}. The calculated permeability coefficient for the cerebral capillaries is 8.4×10^{-8} cm second^{-1}. (Courtesy K. Welch.)

the concentration in the extracellular fluid of the brain is not greatly different from that in the plasma. Under these conditions the influx will be given by

$$K_f C_{\text{Plasma}} + K_d C_{\text{Plasma}}$$

where K_d is the transfer constant for exchanges across the ependyma and pia. The outflux will be given by

$$K_f C_{\text{CSF}} + K_d C_{\text{CSF}}$$

Thus,

$$dS/dt = (K_f + K_d)(C_{\text{Plasma}} - C_{\text{CSF}})$$

which is identical with Eq. (1) with k_{In} equal to k_{Out} equal to $K_f + K_d$.

1. *Sodium in Perfused System*

A rather more complex situation was tackled by Davson and Pollay (1963b) to cover the equilibration of ^{24}Na between plasma and the artificially perfused ventricles. Here, the concentration of ^{24}Na is below that in the brain extracellular fluid and only gradually approaches this. The penetration into perfusion fluid follows the more complex double exponential equation

$$\frac{C_{\text{Out}}}{C_{\text{Plasma}}} = R + \frac{k_d}{k_d - k_1} e^{-k_b t} - \left(\frac{k_1 - k_x}{k_1} + \frac{k_d}{k - k_1} \right) e^{-k_1 t}$$

where $k_1 = k_x + k_d + k_f$, k_d and k_b are coefficients defining the rates of exchange between brain and CSF (k_d) and between blood and brain (k_b), and k_x is the rate of perfusion. The initial rapid rise corresponds to the influx in the newly secreted fluid while the slower rise corresponds to penetration from blood into brain; in fact, its slope is a reasonable measure of the rate of equilibration of the brain with the blood, i.e., of the blood–brain barrier (Fig. 21).

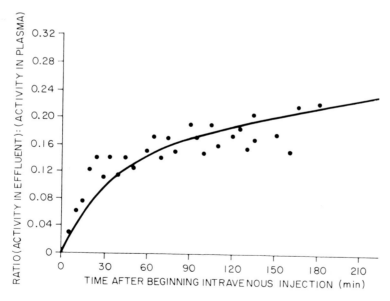

Fig. 21. Penetration of ^{24}Na from blood into fluid perfusing the ventricular system of the rabbit. Points are experimental while curve is theoretical. (After Davson and Pollay, 1963b.)

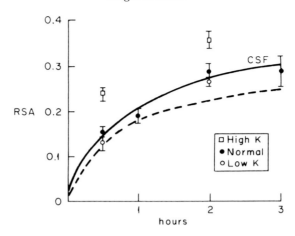

Fig. 22. Penetration of ^{42}K into cisternal CSF of the rabbit expressed as relative specific activity (RSF) against time. The theoretically obtained interrupted line was computed in accordance with the equation: $(RSA) = 1 - 0.8Ie^{-0.022t} - 0.19e^{-1.96t}$. Limits are standard errors. (Bradbury and Kleeman, 1967.)

2. *Potassium in Intact Animal*

Figure 22 shows the result of a similar treatment for the equilibration with ^{42}K in the intact animal by Bradbury and Kleeman (1967). In this case k_x, the rate of perfusion, has been put equal to zero. However, this equation is only an approximation since it takes no account of the exchanges between intracellular and extracellular compartments, so Welch's treatment, although requiring computer solutions, is preferable.

VIII. Permeability of the Choroid Plexus

Welch and Sadler (1966) measured the uptake of isotopically labeled substances in the blood drawn from the cannulated vein of an exposed lateral ventricle; the labeled substances were included in the pool of fluid bathing the plexus. From the estimated blood flow and the measured concentration in the blood, the uptake was computed; and from the measured area of the exposed epithelial cells, permeability constants were calculated. The values are shown in Table V. It is interesting that there is a measurable permeability to inulin, suggesting the presence of porous leaks in the epithelium.

TABLE V

PERMEABILITY CONSTANTS FOR PENETRATION INTO THE CHOROID PLEXUSES[a]

Substance	k' (cm/second $\times$ 10^6)
Urea	11.6 $\pm$ 2.2
Creatinine	6.9 $\pm$ 1.4
Mannitol	6.7 $\pm$ 1.3
Sucrose	5.0 $\pm$ 1.0
Inulin	2.7 $\pm$ 1.3

[a] Welch (1965) and Welch and Saddler (1966).

REFLEXION COEFFICIENTS

E. M. Wright and Prather (1970) studied the penetration of the isolated frog choroid plexus, separating two Ringer's solutions, by a large number of solutes by measuring the reflexion coefficients, which were themselves related indirectly to the streaming potentials developed when the Ringer's solution on one side was made hypertonic by adding the substance to be examined. Thus, on adding an impermant solute, such as sucrose or raffinose, the osmotic flow caused the development of a streaming potential which was linearly proportional to the degree of hyperosmolality. If another substance, which penetrated the plexus, was studied, the streaming potential for a given concentration was less than that developed with sucrose, and the ratio of the two gave the reflexion coefficient, which thus varied from unity when the substance did not penetrate, to zero when penetration was very rapid. In this way the authors confirmed the importance of lipid solubility in determining rate of transport. For example, the reflexion coefficients for urea, thiourea, methyl thiourea, and ethyl thiourea were 0.56, 0.50, 0.26, and 0.11, respectively, and this is the inverse order of the values of k_{In} or k_{Out} deduced from studies of penetration into the rabbit's CSF (Davson, 1955a; Kleeman et al., 1962). In general, the behavior of the isolated choroid plexus is similar to that of other tissues limited by an epithelial membrane, e.g., the gall bladder (E. M. Wright and Diamond, 1969).

IX. Slowly Equilibrating Substances

Certain substances, when a steady level is maintained in the plasma, reach only very small concentrations in the CSF and brain even after very long periods; these substances, like sucrose, p-aminohippurate, inulin, etc., are lipid insoluble and relatively large molecular weight substances. As such they may be expected to remain extracellular so that, so far as brain is concerned, the uptake in the steady state may appear low only because of the small value of the extracellular space. Thus, if this constituted only 2% of the total weight of the brain, then the steady-state level, expressed as concentration/gm brain/concentration/gm plasma would be only 0.02 at equilibrium. This would not account for the low steady-state ratio for the CSF, however. A low ratio could be reached, nevertheless, if penetration into the secretion were very slow, in which case the influx would be given by $k_f r C_{\text{Plasma}}$, where r might be as low as 0.01. If there were no exchanges with the nervous tissue the final steady-state ratio would be 0.01 in this case. In fact, exchanges do occur so that with sucrose and inulin, for example, the steady-state level of about 0.02 is compounded of a low value of r together with some influx from the brain. The cerebrospinal fluid is acting as a sink for the brain and preventing the concentration in its extracellular fluid from rising to the value in the plasma.

To examine the situation more precisely we must measure the volume of the extracellular fluid of the brain. Only when this is known can we say, from the chemical analysis of the brain, what the concentration in this fluid is likely to be. Here we run into difficulties not encountered with other tissues of the body since the marker whose distribution between tissue and plasma is used as a measure of extracellular space is, in this case, very slowly penetrating.

X. Extracellular Space of Brain

It will be recalled that this is measured by maintaining a fixed concentration in the plasma of an "extracellular tag," e.g., $^{35}SO_4^{=}$, ^{14}C-sucrose, ^{14}C-inulin, and estimating the concentration in the tissue at equilibrium, when the space is given by

$$\frac{\text{mEq/100 gm tissue}}{\text{mEq/100 gm plasma dialysate}} \times 100$$

The important points to ascertain are (a) that the system has achieved equilibrium or a steady state and (b) that the tag has remained extracellular. In skeletal muscle an equilibrium[7] is achieved fairly rapidly, but even here there is considerable uncertainty as to the true extracellular space because different tags can lead to different spaces. This is indicated by Fig. 23, where it is seen that the inulin space is considerably less than the sucrose space. In the central nervous system the situation is more complex since, even when a steady state between plasma and tissue levels has been achieved (and because of the blood–brain barrier this takes much longer), the sink action of the cerebrospinal fluid may maintain the con-

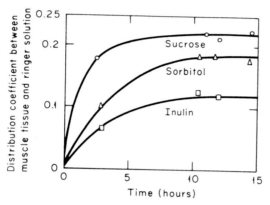

Fig. 23. Time course of uptake of sucrose, sorbitol, and inulin by frog voluntary muscle indicating decreasing volumes of distribution in this order. (Ling and Kromash, 1967.)

centration of the tag in the extracellular fluid well below that in the plasma or its dialysate and so give an erroneously low figure for the extracellular space. This was demonstrated by Davson and Spaziani (1959), who showed that the sucrose-space of brain, determined after maintaining a steady level in the plasma for 2 hours was only some 2%, while after incubation of the isolated tissue in a sucrose medium it was 15%. By contrast, the sucrose space for muscle of some 18% was achieved after only some 15 minutes of maintaining a steady level in plasma. Thus, under *in vivo* conditions, the extracellular tag fails to achieve the same con-

[7] A true equilibrium between plasma and extracellular fluid is not always achieved because flow of lymph may carry away the fluid before complete equilibration. This point has been examined by Johnson (1966), who found that the inulin and sucrose spaces were in the ratio of 0.88 when measured *in vivo*, and he considered that the discrepancy was due to this cause.

centrations in extracellular fluid and plasma. Later studies on rats from Woodbury's laboratory fully confirmed the failure to reach a space of more than some 2% for sucrose and inulin, while the study of Barlow *et al.* (1961) with $^{35}SO_4$ likewise gave a figure of only 2–4%.

A. Sink Action

It was argued by Davson (1963) that the cause for these low estimates resided in the sink action of the cerebrospinal fluid. Thus, although diffusion from blood into the tissue may be slow, given enough time the concentration should reach that in the plasma or its dialysate to give a volume of distribution of some 10% if the value obtained with excised tissue is correct. There is no doubt from studies on penetration of sucrose, inulin, sulphate, etc., into the cerebrospinal fluid that, after several hours, the concentration in this fluid will be very much less than in plasma. Thus, after 6 hours Barlow *et al.* found the sulphate concentration only 9% of that in plasma while the true steady-state level, measured with inactive sulphate, was found by Van Harreveld *et al.* (1966) to be only 17% in the rabbit and 24% in cats. Similarly, Reed and Woodbury (1963) found that after 24 hours the concentration of inulin in cerebrospinal fluid was only 1–2% of that in plasma. Thus, the concentration gradients would favor losses from brain extracellular fluid to cerebrospinal fluid; the situation is illustrated by Fig. 24 [from Davson and Bradbury (1965b)].

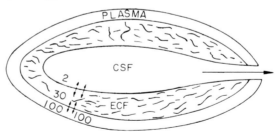

Fig. 24. Illustrating the manner in which the CSF may impose a low concentration on an extracellular tag. (Davson and Bradbury, 1965b.)

B. Ventricular Perfusion

Clearly, a better way to measure the extracellular space would be to present the tag by a nonvascular route. This was done by Davson and Spaziani (1959) when they examined excised tissue, but it is preferable, because of inadequate oxygenation of mammalian tissue, to use an *in vivo* technique. Goldmann and Stern and Gautier had shown that substances presented by way of the cerebrospinal fluid would pass relatively rapidly into the tissue, although excluded when presented through the blood; and a number of recent studies in which a steady level of the tag has been maintained in the cerebrospinal fluid have led to much higher estimates of extracellular space. Thus, Davson *et al.* (1961) found a space for spinal cord of 12%; Rall *et al.* (1962), using inulin perfused at a constant concentration through the ventricles of the dog computed a space of 12%.

C. Infusion–Perfusion

It was pointed out by Bito *et al.* (1966), however, that even this method of presentation would not necessarily give a true picture of the correct equilibrium distribution since the blood vessels of the brain would be acting as a sink for the tissue. Only because the substances considered diffuse slowly across the blood–brain barrier is it possible to obtain these high values. Nevertheless, some losses will presumably occur, and the best way is to perfuse the ventricles with an artificial CSF containing a known concentration of, say, sucrose, and infuse the animal intravenously with sucrose to give the same concentration in its plasma. Under these conditions there should be no sinks and a true equilibrium should be obtained. Bito *et al.* showed that the iodide space rose from about 14%, with ventriculo-cisternal perfusion alone, to some 18%, with combined ventriculo-cisternal perfusion and intravenous infusion. In a similar way Woodward *et al.* (1967) and Oldendorf and Davson (1967) found values of 13.5–14.5% and 10% for the sucrose spaces in rat and rabbit respectively, while Cutler *et al.* (1968a) found a sulphate space of 12% in the cat.

D. Silicone Perfusion

Finally, by perfusing the ventriculo-cisternal system of the rabbit with silicone fluid, Davson and Segal (1969) showed that the sucrose space, obtained with intravenous infusion of ^{14}C-sucrose for 1.5 hours, increased from a mean of 1.5% for the control animal to 6.4% for the silicone-perfused animal. By contrast, the ^{24}Na space of brain was unaffected, as we should expect since in the normal intact animal the rates of equilibration of CSF and brain are so nearly equal that large sinks in either direction are not likely to arise.

XI. Brain–Cerebrospinal Fluid Exchanges

A. TRANSEPENDYMAL EXCHANGES

The concept of a sink-action of cerebrospinal fluid on brain, or of brain on the cerebrospinal fluid implies the possibility of free exchanges across the ependyma and piaglia. Qualitative evidence for a high permeability of these linings is provided by the classical studies of Goldmann and Stern and Gautier already alluded to, while more quantitative analyses are those of Bakay (1960) and of Rall *et al.* (1962). Bakay measured transport of ^{24}Na from blood to brain and from CSF to brain and computed, on the basis of the relative areas of ependyma and the capillaries of brain, that permeability across the ependyma was some 30 times as high as across the brain capillaries. Rall *et al.* (1962) maintained a steady level of inulin in the dog's ventricles by perfusion, and they analyzed the brain at successive depths after a given time, as illustrated by Fig. 25. They computed that the fall in concentration along the brain could be accounted for by simple diffusion without any significant restraint across the ependyma. More recently, Pollay and Kaplan (1970) have perfused the aqueduct of Sylvius with an artificial CSF containing ^{14}C-urea and ^{14}C-creatinine and measured the uptake into the adjacent brain as a function of distance from the ependymal surface. The variation of concentration with distance at a

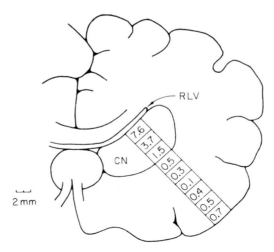

Fig. 25. Showing inulin concentration as per cent of perfusate is tissue blocks from caudate nucleus outward. CN, caudate nucleus; RLV, right lateral ventricle. (Rall *et al.*, 1962.)

given time followed a profile that could be calculated on the basis of the standard Fick diffusion equation for a thin sheet, thus, once again showing that there is no significant barrier at the ependymal interface since in this event there would have been an abrupt fall in concentration on passing from CSF to the first millimeter or so of tissue. Pollay and Kaplan computed a diffusion coefficient that was very much smaller (10–38%) than that in free solution. Since Davson and Spaziani (1959) had found little difference in diffusion coefficients computed from diffusion through brain slices and those given for free diffusion in water, it seems unlikely that the more complex diffusion path could account for the differences found by Pollay and Kaplan, and they are almost certainly due to the removal of the solutes across the blood–brain barrier. This would act as a "distributed sink," cause a reduction in the magnitudes of the concentrations along the whole profile, and give an erroneously low value for the diffusion coefficient.

1. Sodium Flux

That the fluxes across the ependyma can be very high is indicated by a study of Davson and Pollay (1963b) on the passage of ^{24}Na from brain into the perfused ventricles. The animal had received an injection some 48 hours earlier so that its brain was completely equilibrated with the isotope. On perfusing with an artificial cerebrospinal fluid, the emerging fluid was originally very active since it was the animal's own CSF. As dilution with the inactive fluid continued, a steady state was reached, with the activity in the effluent some 30% of that in the animal's plasma. The ^{24}Na in the effluent was derived from the brain and the choroid plexuses; the amount entering in a minute from the latter source was probably equivalent to the amount of CSF secreted during that time, and the remainder was derived from the brain. The computed flux from the brain was 1.65 $\mu mole/cm^2/minute$. This compares with a flux of 1.3 $\mu mole/cm^2/minute$ for the muscle capillary, a membrane with a very high permeability. Thus, the ependyma must be classed as a highly permeable and nonselective interface between CSF and brain.[8]

---

[8] Perfusion of the ventricles with an artificial CSF and measurement of the change in concentration of the perfusate as it leaves at the cisterna magna gives a measure of the loss of material and, so, might be used as a measure of transependymal permeability. A variety of such studies have been reported (Heisey *et al.*, 1962; Davson and Pollay, 1963a; Bradbury and Davson, 1964; Bering and Sato, 1963), and from them estimates of the flux across the ependyma and choroid plexus may certainly be made. The limiting

B. Fluid Exchanges

Bering and Sato (1963) concluded from their experiments on dogs, made hydrocephalic by kaolin injections, that over half of the total production of fluid came from the subarachnoid spaces rather than the ventricles. Pollay and Curl (1967) perfused the aqueduct of Sylvius with an artificial CSF and found that there was some dilution of the perfusate, presumably by a fluid formed in the adjacent nervous tissue, since the choroid plexuses had been bypassed. The production was considered to represent perhaps as much as a third of the total; Diamox inhibited the flow by some 29–53%. This finding suggests that there is a continuous production of extracellular fluid within the brain and that it finds its way into the cavities of the cerebrospinal system. A movement in the reverse direction was claimed by Sahar *et al.* (1969b) in cats with an experimental obstructive hydrocephalus; their evidence was based on an observed passage of labeled protein out of the ventricles into the adjacent tissue. However, the movement of protein does not necessarily betoken flow of fluid, and it is interesting that the concentration profile in the brain is similar to that predicted by Welch (1969) on the basis of passive diffusion without flow.

C. Transpial Exchanges

The absence of a well-defined capillary bed in the pia suggests that direct exchanges between blood and the subarachnoid CSF are unlikely to be significant. There is some evidence that the large vessels permit some exchange, however, since Schaltenbrand and Putnam (1927) observed fluorescein escaping from these vessels into the surrounding fluid after an intravenous injection of the fluorescent dye. Van Harreveld and Ahmed (1968) have shown that intravenously injected ^{131}I appears in the fluid perfused over the surface of the brain, and they attribute this to escape from the pial vessels, but until diffusion from the underlying brain tissue can be excluded as the source of the ^{131}I,[9] we must hesitate to accept this

factor in escape, however, is probably the rate of escape *from* the nervous tissue and into the choroid plexuses, i.e., the relative rates are a reasonable measure of the combined blood–CSF and blood–brain barriers rather than of the ependymal barrier. Thus, the losses of sugars may be reduced by competition, indicating facilitated transfer (Bradbury and Davson, 1964).

[9] Van Harreveld *et al.* (1966) observed that the concentration of sulphate in the CSF obtained after protracted withdrawal, was higher than that in the normal fluid, and they concluded that they were withdrawing fluid that was derived from the cortical subarachnoid space with a higher concentration of sulphate. A similar phenomenon was observed

interpretation. With a gas like H_2, escape from the pial vessels has been demonstrated by Stosseck and Acker (1969), a point that must be born in mind when estimating blood flow from wash-out curves.

D. THE DURA

The barrier between blood and the central nervous system seems not to include the substance of the dura since the classical studies with trypan blue showed that this was stained after intravenous injection. Measurements with ^{22}Na have likewise shown a rapid uptake (Davson and Segal, 1971) so that we may expect the barrier between dural blood vessels and subarachnoid fluid to be the mesothelium of the dura, or the arachnoid membrane, or both. Rodriguez-Peralta (1957) observed that the mesothelium did not take up fluorescent acridine dyes from the blood but it did from the CSF and he argued that this layer of cells had a one-way permeability to the dye. As pointed out earlier (Davson, 1967) the interpretation of these experiments with acridine dyes is by no means unequivocal, and a one-way permeability to the dye is unlikely.

The existence of a barrier between CSF and dura is illustrated by the early observation of Spatz (1934) that the dura is not stained by trypan blue after introduction into the cerebrospinal fluid. As to what cellular layer constitutes the barrier between subarachnoid fluid and the substance of the dura, there is no direct evidence. The electron microscopy of the arachnoid, as described by Nelson et al. (1961), suggests that the arachnoid, adjacent to the dura, is not an uninterrupted layer of cells. There is said to be no regularity in the structure so that at given points CSF "cisterns" penetrate deeply into the layer of cells and reach the surface, i.e., the fluid can apparently come into direct contact with the dural mesothelium. If this description is correct, it seems that it is the dural mesothelium that constitutes the barrier to diffusion.[10]

with intravenously injected ^{131}I (Van Harreveld and Ahmed, 1968), but the more likely explanation is that the choroid plexuses were producing an abnormal fluid under these conditions of acute and prolonged reduction of intracranial pressure, in a similar way to the formation of the plasmoid aqueous humour of the eye.

[10] The ultrastructural relations between arachnoid and dura are worthy of further investigation. Waggener and Beggs (1967) have contributed some useful facts; they state that the contact between dura and arachnoid is distinctive, without junctions between the cells of the two tissues, a 200-Å gap between the layers being maintained. They quarrel with the classical description of the inner surface layer of the dura as "mesothelial"; the cells are squamous but their cytological characteristics are those of fibroblasts. The

XII. Active Transport Outwards

A. HALOGEN ANIONS AND THIOCYANATE

Examination of Fig. 16 shows that penetration of bromide into CSF is initially more rapid than that of ^{24}Na, but later, there is a slowing down, and at the steady state in the rabbit the ratio: concentration in CSF/concentration in plasma is 0.71; in man it is much lower, i.e., 0.37 (Hunter *et al.*, 1954). An analysis of the kinetic aspects of this transport suggested that Br^- was being converted to some new product in the brain and in this form it diffused away into the blood; in this way the brain was acting as a permanent sink for the anion (Davson, 1956). A similar explanation was invoked for the even more anomalous behavior of I^- and CNS^-, described by Wallace and Brodie (1940). This view seemed to be supported by the finding that ^{131}I and CNS^- disappeared very rapidly from the CSF after injection into the cisterna magna (Davson, 1955b). That active processes were involved was strikingly demonstrated by Pappenheimer *et al.* (1961) when they showed that *p*-aminohippurate and Diodrast were absorbed from the perfused ventricles against a gradient of concentration between the artificial CSF and blood; furthermore, the absorption of the one could be competitively inhibited by the presence of the other. This absorption was attributed to an active process across the choroid plexus of the IVth ventricle. Subsequent studies showed that I^- and CNS^- were absorbed by the same mechanism, but in the rabbit the process was not confined to the choroid plexus of the IVth ventricle (Pollay and Davson, 1963). *In vitro* studies with the isolated plexus carried out by Becker (1961) and Welch (1962) showed that these two ions could be accumulated in the tissue to concentrations well above those in the medium. In addition to I^- and CNS^-, it was shown by Bito *et al.* (1966) that Br^- was also actively transported and there is no reason to doubt that this is the cause for the low steady-state distribution of this ion, as well as of the much lower distributions for I^- and CNS^-.

authors regard the outermost layer of the arachnoid as a continuous cellular sheet which might well constitute the barrier between dura and subarachnoid space. Reese (1971) agrees with this view and emphasizes the gradual transition in structure of the dura as one progresses deeper toward the arachnoid, the fibroblast-like cells becoming more and more tightly arranged. The outermost layer of the arachnoid is, according to him, a complete sheet of cells whose intercellular clefts are closed by tight junctions. It is important to appreciate that the transition from dura to arachnoid is not abrupt so that many injections or perfusions that are thought to be subdural might well have been intradural.

B. SULFATE

We have seen that the steady-state distribution of $SO_4^=$ between CSF and plasma gives a value of R_{CSF} of 0.17 in the rabbit and 0.24 in the cat; this could be due to a low permeability of the choroid plexus epithelium to this large anion, in which case there is no need to invoke active transport. However, Cutler et al. (1968c) have shown that the outflux of the ^{35}S-labeled ion, during ventriculo-cisternal perfusion, was reduced by increasing the concentration of the inactive sulfate, or of thiosulfate, while it was unaffected by increasing the plasma level of [35]SO_4. Experiments on isolated plexuses showed tissue/medium ratios of about 3, suggesting accumulation against a concentration gradient (Robinson et al., 1968a), a characteristic that developed in the fetal rabbit and cat (Robinson et al., 1968b).

C. TRANSPORT OUT OF BRAIN

On the basis of the active transport of I^-, CNS^-, and Br^- by the choroid plexuses, we may probably explain the low steady-state ratios; furthermore, it was argued by Reed et al. (1965), Bito et al. (1966), and Pollay (1966) that the low ^{131}I and CNS^- spaces of brain were due to the sink

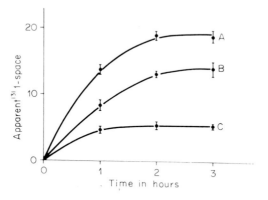

Fig. 26. Apparent ^{131}I space of brain during ventriculo-cisternal perfusion with artificial CSF under three different conditions. (A) During combined ventriculo-cisternal perfusion and intravenous infusion with ^{131}I-containing fluids. (B) During ventriculo-cisternal perfusion with a fluid containing [131]I. (C) During intravenous infusion of ^{131}I when the ventriculo-cisternal fluid contained no [131]I. In all cases active transport of ^{131}I was inhibited by perchlorate. Ordinate: apparent ^{131}I space of brain expressed as (activity per gram tissue/activity per gram reference fluid) × 100. Abscissa: time in hours from beginning of perfusion (curves A and B) or infusion (curve C.) (Bito et al., 1966a.)

action created by the low levels of these ions in the CSF. Thus, after several hours of intravenous infusion, the iodide space of brain is only 4%. If the ^{131}I is presented by way of the CSF, the space increases to some 12%, and if it is presented by both routes simultaneously, it rises to some 18% (Fig. 26). Again, if active transport is inhibited by increasing the concentration of inactive I$^-$ or CNS$^-$ in the blood, then the ^{131}I or CNS$^-$ space increases (Reed *et al.*, 1965; Pollay, 1966; Bito *et al.*, 1966). Studies on the ligatured spinal cord, however, failed to give the high ^{131}I spaces that would be expected when the sink action is effectively removed (Bito *et al.*, 1966), and experiments in which the spinal subarachnoid space was perfused with an artificial cerebrospinal fluid, containing ^{131}I, indicated the active removal of the isotope (Lorenzo and Cutler, 1969). Since the fluid was not exposed to a choroid plexus, the active process must have been carried out either by the dura or by the capillaries of the cord parenchyma.[11] Evidence supporting an active transport by brain capillaries is conflicting. Bito *et al.* failed to achieve a significant increase in ^{131}I space of brain when the ventricles were perfused with ^{131}I-containing fluid and the active transport processes were poisoned by perchlorate. Yet, if the brain capillaries were indeed actively transporting the isotope back into the blood, such an increase would have been expected. However, Ahmed and Van Harreveld (1969), using the combined ventricular and blood presentation of the isotope to the brain developed by Bito *et al.*, were able to obtain considerably larger ^{131}I spaces in the perchlorate-poisoned animal than in the animal not so treated. Thus, in the perchlorate-treated animals the mean ^{131}I space was 16.8%, whereas in the unpoisoned animals it was only 10.2%. Clearly, the perchlorate is preventing the active removal of the isotope from the brain, so that the sink action of the CSF is not the sole cause of the low ^{131}I space of brain.

D. Organic Bases

Schanker *et al.* (1962) have shown that some quaternary ammonium compounds, e.g., N'-methylnicotinamide, hexamethonium, etc., are

---

[11] L. A. Coben and Smith (1969) also concluded that the cord contained an actively absorbing site for ^{131}I; they perfused the isolated subarachnoid space and showed that inactive iodide reduced the extraction of the isotope. Alternatively, on intravenous injection, the uptake of ^{131}I into spinal CSF was low in spite of separating the cord from the cranial system; thus, the low concentration in the CSF was not due to action by the choroid plexuses.

rapidly eliminated from the CSF, exhibiting the phenomenon of competitive inhibition. Serotonin and norepinephrine also seem to be actively transported by the choroid plexuses (Tochino and Schanker, 1965). The *in vitro* accumulation of these bases is inhibited by serum and CSF, and it would seem that the factor responsible is choline (Tochino and Schanker, 1966). Of some interest is the finding of Ashcroft *et al.* (1968) that 5-hydroxyindol-3-ylacetic acid and 3-methoxy-4-hydroxyphenylacetic acid are both actively transported by the choroid plexus of the fourth ventricle of the dog, since these compounds are the acid metabolites of 5-hydroxytryptamine and of dopamine respectively, both of which are probably central transmitters. Probenecid inhibited the active transport. In this connection it should be noted that 5-hydroxytryptamine passes rapidly from blood to brain in the rat, and the usual failure to observe this is its rapid conversion to 5-hydroxyindoleacetic acid (Bulat and Supek, 1968).

In general, these active mechanisms may be considered as developments that permit the rapid removal of certain substances from the CSF and thus increase its sink action. This emphasizes the function of the CSF as a substitute for the lymphatic pathway found in other tissues.[12]

XIII. Morphology of the Blood–Brain Barrier

The passage of solutes from the capillaries of the central nervous system is far more restricted and selective than that from the capillaries of, say, skeletal muscle; and the question arises as to what morphological feature this selectivity may be attributed to, and it is natural, in this respect, that we should seek it in some difference between cerebral and muscle capillaries.

A. BRAIN CAPILLARIES

In general, the capillaries of the two tissues are remarkably similar and fall into the same class on the basis of Bennet's *et al.* (1958) or Majno's (1965) classifications. Thus, they are both nonfenestrated and have intact and well-defined basement membranes.

---

[12] Csáky and Rigor (1968) have shown that isolated choroid plexus can concentrate glucose and galactose, a process that is inhibited by lack of Na^+ and various inhibitors. Perfusion of the ventricles by recirculating an artificial CSF showed an uphill transport into the blood. The system is saturated by such low concentrations of glucose, however, that it seems unlikely that it serves any useful role in sugar transport.

1. *Glial End-Feet*

Early anatomists and physiologists were struck by the numerous end-feet of astrocytes that made contact with the endothelial cells, through close apposition of their respective basement membranes, to make what appeared to be a closely investing covering for the capillary (Fig. 27), and it was considered that it was this layer that gave the blood–brain barrier its special features. In fact, it was argued by De Robertis (1965)

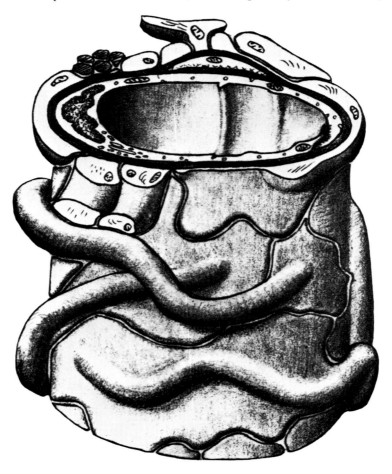

Fig. 27. Three-dimensional schematic drawing of cerebral capillary. On front side only the astrocyte processes are indicated. Above, in cross section, the two layers covering the endothelial cells are indicated, namely the astrocyte processes (light) and the processes of other cells (shaded). (Wolff, 1963.)

that the only pathway from capillary to neuron was through the cytoplasm of the astrocytes. This view was supported by the experiment of Clemente and Holst (1954) when they showed that massive doses of x-rays were followed by breakdown of the blood–brain barrier, in the sense that trypan blue penetrated the brain after intravenous injection; associated with this there was degeneration of the astrocytic end-feet. Further support was given by Gray's statement (1961) that the membranes of adjacent end-feet made the close type of contact called zonulae occludentes, a contact that would certainly make the astroglial covering of the capillary similar in its permeability properties to an epithelium.

2. Horseradish Peroxidase

However, Reese and Karnovsky's (1967) study, using horseradish peroxidase as a marker for penetration through capillaries, has shown that the capillary endothelium is likely to act as a barrier to diffusion independently of the astrocytic covering. Horseradish peroxidase is a protein of relatively low molecular weight (40,000) corresponding to a diameter of 50–60 Å. This may be identified in a tissue by its reaction products with H_2O_2 and 3-3'-diaminobenzidene, the product reacting with OsO_4 to give dense electron staining. The molecule is sufficiently small to escape from the muscle capillary, and hence, after an intravenous injection, its pathway outwards should be identifiable in the electron microscope. Karnovsky (1967) found, in cardiac capillaries, that the marker was concentrated in the intercellular clefts, indicating that this was its main, if not exclusive, pathway out of the capillary. This was interesting since earlier electron-microscopical studies of capillaries had shown that the clefts were apparently sealed by tight junctions or zonulae occludentes (Muir and Peters, 1962; Luft, 1965; Bruns and Palade, 1968), a form of seal that would definitely have inhibited the passage of horseradish peroxidase and of the smaller inulin molecule.

3. Intercellular Clefts

Karnovsky reexamined the intercellular clefts and observed that when the tissue was stained with uranyl acetate, the commonest observation was a region of close approximation of the two cell membranes, but very rarely was there actual fusion, a space of up to 40 Å between the outer leaflets being observed. In some regions there was, indeed, fusion, as in Fig. 28, but if the same region was sectioned at a different level, this disappeared, indicating that the junction was not a complete belt or zonula but only a button or macula.

Thus, the high permeability of the muscle capillary is due to the presence of open pathways between cells of about 30 Å diameter. These are partially interrupted by maculae occludentes but in such a way as only to make the pathway more devious. When Reese and Karnovsky (1967) examined brain capillaries, they found no escape of horseradish peroxidase into the tissue; however, the marker did not accumulate between the base-

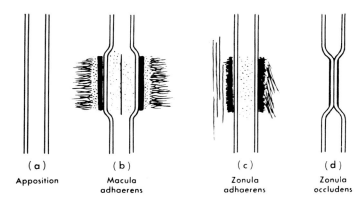

(a)	(b)	(c)	(d)
Apposition	Macula	Zonula	Zonula
	adhaerens	adhaerens	occludens

Fig. 28.   Illustrating fusion of adjacent cell membranes to form a tight junction. (Brightman and Palay, 1963.)

ment membrane and the glial end-feet as would be expected were the latter the functional barrier. The marker was retained in the lumen of the capillary, its passage through the cell clefts being blocked now by zonulae occludentes which, in these capillaries, were variable in number and type, sometimes one would run the whole length of the cleft.

4. *Tight Junction*

It would seem, then, that the morphological basis for the blood–brain barrier, i.e., the low capillary permeability of cerebral capillaries, is the tight junction that seals completely the intercellular clefts. Solutes leaving the capillary must therefore cross this junction or, failing this, must pass through the endothelial cells. This requirement would account for the importance of lipid solubility in the kinetics of the barrier as revealed by Figs. 12 and 18.

B. CHOROID PLEXUS

The capillaries of the choroid plexuses do not show any barrier action, in the sense that trypan blue passes into the connective tissue of the plexus and is only held up by the choroidal epithelium whose intercellular clefts are sealed by tight junctions. Brightman (1967) has shown that horseradish peroxidase passes out of the choroid plexus capillaries through the intercellular clefts.

C. EPENDYMA[13] AND PIA-GLIA

Physiological studies in which substances are injected into the ventricular and subarachnoid fluids have shown that both ependyma and pia-glia are far less selective than the blood–brain barrier, so we might expect that the ependymal and pia-glial cells would not be joined laterally by tight junctions, i.e., the route for passage would be between these cells rather than through them. In the electron microscope Brightman and Palay (1963) and Tennyson and Pappas (1962) described tight junctions between adjacent ependymal cells, but the experimental studies of Brightman (1965a) with ferritin particles, of molecular diameter some 100 Å, showed that these could pass out of the ventricles, when they were seen in the intercellular clefts of the ependyma. Similarly, the particles, when injected into the subarachnoid space, passed between the pia-glial lining cells into the subjacent brain parenchyma (Brightman, 1965b). It would seem, then, that the tight junctions are not effective barriers, and could well be similar to the tight junctions described in the capillaries of muscle, i.e., not true tight junctions but gap junctions characterized by very close apposition of adjacent membranes but not complete fusion to that there remained a central electron-lucent gap some 20–30 Å wide sufficient to permit the passage of very large molecules, such as inulin.

3. *Gap-Junctions*

Brightman and Reese (1969) have reexamined the junctions of the central nervous system, and have shown that those between ependymal cells, previously described as "tight" or zonulae occludentes, are, in fact, of the gap-junction type, so that, when the tissue is treated with uranyl

---

[13] The detailed light microscopy of the ependyma has been described by Fleischhauer (1957, 1961). Millen and Woollam (1961) have described the light microscopy of the pia mater.

acetate before dehydration, the junctions appear seven-layered with a
median slit of constant width continuous with the remaining interspace
(Figs. 29 and 30). On the external surface of the brain there is a layer of
specialized astrocytes and the pia, i.e., the *pia-glia*. As described by Brightman and Reese, the most superficial layers of the brain consisted of a
network of interdigitating sheet-like processes limited by a basement
membrane. Lying next to this basement membrane was the layer of pial
mesothelial cells. Adjacent mesothelial cells were separated by gap-junctions, as were also the underlying astrocytic processes. Thus, the intercellular relationships of the limiting glial sheath of the brain are similar

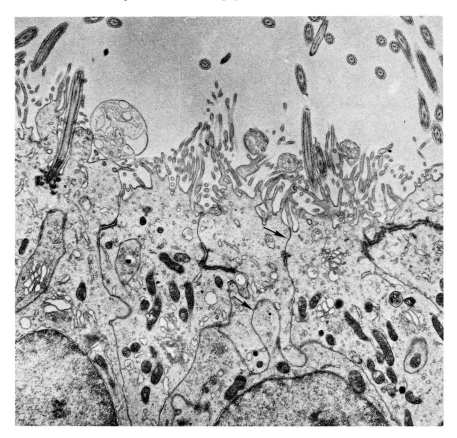

Fig. 29. The internal surface of the brain is formed by the folds of ependymal plasmalemma projecting into the cerebral ventricle (top). The four contiguous ependymal
cells are joined, at their apices and below, by junctions heretofore interpreted as "tight"
(arrows). OsO$_4$. Mouse. ×16,000. (Brightman and Reese, 1969.)

to those of the astrocytic processes surrounding the capillaries. In both cases the underlying intercellular clefts of the parenchyma are in communication with the overlying basement membrane, either directly through open, relatively wide clefts or by way of narrow slits in gap-junctions. Horseradish peroxidase, injected into the ventricles, passed through the intercellular clefts into the parenchyma of the brain; similarly, when per-

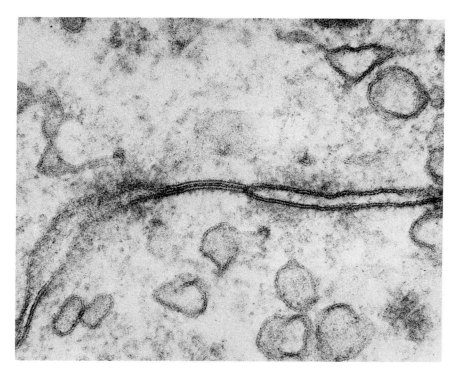

Fig. 30. In tissue treated with uranyl acetate before dehydration such "tight" junctions appear as seven-layered gap junctions bisected by a median slit of constant width (left) that is continuous with the remaining interspace (right). OsO_4. Mouse. $\times 310,000$. (Brightman and Reese, 1969.)

fused through the subarachnoid space it passed into the interstitial spaces of the brain parenchyma by way of the intercellular clefts and gap-junctions of the superficial astrocytic layer. The possible relationships between blood, brain, and CSF are illustrated schematically by Fig. 31. This indicates the relatively free communication between ventricular and subarachnoid fluids by way of intercellular clefts.

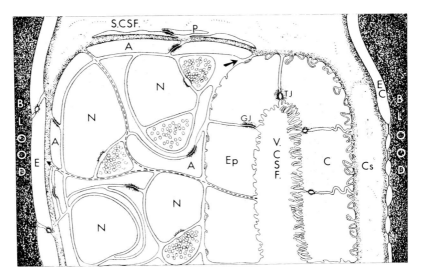

Fig. 31.　Schema of blood, and CSF relationships in the mouse. A, astrocyte process; C, choroid plexus epithelium; Cs, choroid plexus stroma; E, endothelium of parenchymal vessel; EC, endothelium of choroid plexus vessel; Ep, ependyma; GJ, jap junction; N, neuron; P, pia; S.CSF., cerebrospinal fluid of subarachnoid space; TJ, tight junction; V.CSF., cerebrospinal fluid of ventricles.

The dashed line follows two typical open pathways connecting ventricular CSF with the basement membrane of parenchymal blood vessels and with the basement membrane of the surface of the brain. Peroxidase is seen within these pathways. Where peroxidase cannot cross cellular layers such as the parenchymal vascular endothelium (E) and the epithelium of the choroid plexus (C), the component cells are joined by tight junctions. The thick arrow (top) indicates a "functional leak" whereby substances crossing the fenestrated endothelium of the choroid plexus can pass along the choroidal stroma to enter the parenchyma of the brain at the root of the choroid plexus. A "leak" in the opposite direction could also occur, as indicated by the arrow point. (Brightman and Reese, 1969.)

XIV. Significance of the Blood–Brain Barrier

The general picture that has emerged is one of a highly selective passage of solutes from blood into the secreted CSF, and into the extracellular fluid of brain and spinal cord. This selectivity ensures that certain substances exchange with plasma only very slowly indeed, while others, either by virtue of their lipid solubility or through their affinity for certain carriers in the membrane, exchange more rapidly. Associated with these two exchanges with blood there is a relatively unrestricted and unselective exchange between extracellular fluid and CSF. This latter exchange implies that, for restraint on the passage from blood to brain to be effective, there must be a corresponding restraint on passage from blood to CSF. Thus, raising the concentration of K+ in the blood plasma causes little or no change in the concentration in the brain; if passage into the CSF were rapid, the rise in concentration in the cerebrospinal fluid would lead to diffusion from here into the brain and so make the selectivity of the blood–brain barrier profitless.

A. CSF–Brain Exchanges

This exchange between the two compartments can be easily demonstrated by perfusing the ventricles with artificial CSF with different concentrations of K+ in them. The results of such an experiment are shown in Fig. 32, where the concentration of K+ in the effluent is plotted against time from the beginning of the perfusion. With high concentrations of K+, the steady-state level in the effluent is lower than in the inflowing

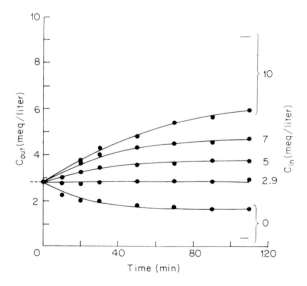

Fig. 32. The concentration of K+ in the outflowing perfusion fluid, C_{Out}, at various times after the start of perfusion of fluids, of different K+ content, from lateral ventricle to cisterna magna of the rabbit. The interrupted line on the ordinate represents the normal concentration of K+ in rabbit CSF. The numbers at the right-hand side of the figure indicate the values of C_{In}, the concentration of K+ in the inflowing fluid. The short horizontal marks bracketed to the curves marked 10 and 0 are the values of C_{Out} that would have been observed, with these values of C_{In}, had there been no losses of K+ to the tissue. (Bradbury and Davson, 1965.)

fluid owing to a steady loss of K^+ to the tissue. By contrast, with no K^+ in the fluid, the steady-state level in the effluent contains some 1.8 mEq/liter, indicating a loss of K^+ from brain to the perfusing fluid. Only when the concentration in the perfusing fluid was 2.9 mEq/liter was there no change in concentration during flow through the ventricles; this concentration is considerably less than in blood plasma but is equal to that in the normal rabbit's CSF.

B. Active Transport

It must be emphasized that a mere restraint on the passage of solute from blood into brain will not usually be sufficient to establish significant deviations from the equilibrium distribution of solutes between plasma and CSF or extracellular fluid of the tissue. Thus, the concentration of K^+ in CSF is normally below that in a dialysate of plasma, and active processes must be operating to maintain this concentration at lower electrochemical potential than in plasma. The nature of the active processes will be discussed briefly later, and for the moment we may accept their necessity. If the choroid plexuses secreted a fluid with low concentration of K^+, while the capillaries of the brain and cord merely produced an extracellular fluid by filtration from plasma as in other parts of the body, then the newly secreted CSF, passing through the ventricles and subarachnoid spaces, would, because of the possibility of relatively unrestricted diffusion between CSF and brain and cord, gain K^+ from the extracellular fluid of these tissues. Thus, the concentrations in the steady state would be in the order plasma > extracellular fluid > CSF. Furthermore, the concentration of K^+ in the freshly secreted fluid of the ventricles would be less than that in the cisterna magna and cortical and spinal subarachnoid spaces. It is of some interest, therefore, to determine the changes in concentration of certain solutes as the CSF passes on its journey from the ventricles to its final place of absorption from the cortical subarachnoid space.

C. Regional Variations in Concentration

In a relatively early study Davson (1958) showed that the concentrations of Cl^- and glucose, both solutes with markedly different concentrations in the CSF from those in plasma (Table I), did not vary measurably as small samples were withdrawn in rapid succession from the cisterna magna. It was argued that the first sample would represent fluid that had just left the ventricles and, probably also, some ventricular fluid, while later samples would come from more remote subarachnoid regions. Davson (1958) suggested on this basis and on that of a survey of the classical literature on this point that the CSF and extracellular fluid of brain were similar in composition, in which case active transport processes were probably operating to determine the concentrations of these and other solutes in both, i.e., that the extracellular fluid of brain could not be viewed as a mere filtrate or dialysate of plasma but rather as a secreted fluid.[14]

1. *Fluid from Different Regions*

A more satisfactory approach is to withdraw, as nearly simultaneously as possible, fluid directly from a lateral ventricle, the cisterna magna, and the cortical and spinal subarachnoid spaces. For this a larger animal than the rabbit is necessary and Bito and Davson (1966) chose the dog, analyzing the fluids for Na^+, K^+, Cl^-, Ca^{++}, HCO_3^-, urea, and glucose. In general, the results indicated a remarkable uniformity in composition so far as Na^+, Cl^-, Ca^{++}, HCO_3^-, and glucose were concerned, thus confirming the earlier work of Davson (1958). The behavior of K^+ was of special interest. As Table VI shows, the concentration in the dog's lateral ventricle was 2.93 ± 0.08 mEq/liter; that in the cisterna magna was not significantly different, namely, 2.98 ± 0.06, but the concentration in the cortical subarachnoid fluid was *lower*, namely, 2.65 ± 0.10 ($P < 0.001$). Thus, the fluid, on passing over the surface of the brain, had become less like a dialysate of plasma than the freshly secreted fluid of the ventricles. Clearly, the concentration in the extracellular fluid of the cerebral cortex was contributing to lower the concentration of K^+ in the CSF. By no stretch of the imagination, then, can the extracellular fluid be considered as a passive filtrate of plasma; rather, it is secreted at a lower concentration of K^+ than that in the CSF. Studies on Mg^{++} illustrate essentially the same phenomenon (Bito, 1969; Bito and Myers, 1970); thus, the plasma concentration in monkeys was 1.18 ± 0.07 and the cisternal concentration was 1.86 ± 0.05 mEq/kg H_2O, indicating the secretion of a fluid containing a considerably higher concentration than in plasma or its dialysate. This is a fairly general feature of the Mg

---

[14] There are instances, such as with urea, where passive processes may account for deviation from equilibrium. Nevertheless the active transport of such ions as Na^+ and Cl^- has to be invoked to provide the flow of CSF that will produce the discrepancies from equilibrium.

TABLE VI

MEAN CONCENTRATION OF K^+ (mEq/kg H_2O) IN PLASMA AND CSF OF DOGS [a]

	Plasma$_1$ [b]	Plasma$_2$	Plasma$_3$	Cist. mag.	cort. subarach	Ventr.	Lumbar
Dogs	4.56 ± 0.12 (16)	4.57 ± 0.14 (16)	3.97 ± 0.12 (12)	2.98 ± 0.06 (15)	2.65 ± 0.10 (8)	2.93 ± 0.08 (15)	3.22 ± 0.08 (8)
Cort Subarach/Cist. Mag.						0.86 ± 0.02	$P < 0.001$
Ventr./Cist. Mag.						0.98 ± 0.01	$P > 0.1$
Lumbar/Cist. Mag.						1.06 ± 0.01	$P < 0.001$

[a] Numbers in parentheses indicate numbers of animals from which a given fluid was taken (Bito and Davson, 1966).

[b] Plasma$_1$ is from blood withdrawn before anaesthesia; Plasma$_2$ from blood withdrawn immediately after anaesthesia, and Plasma$_3$ from blood withdrawn after all CSF had been taken. P is the probability that the observed ratio would occur by chance.

distribution in mammals, although in the rabbit the deviation from a dialysate is not so large (Davson, 1955a, 1967). The cortical subarachnoid fluid had an even higher concentration, namely, 2.00 mEq/kg H_2O so that once again the concentration in the "older" fluid is more discrepant from equilibrium than that in the "younger."

a. Urea. The concentration of urea in the CSF is less than in plasma (Table I); this could be due to active transport, as with K^+, but the bulk of experimental evidence suggests that this solute is handled passively, the low concentration being due to a low permeability of the choroidal epithelial cells to urea so that during the process of secretion of the fluid some molecular sieving takes place. If the brain capillaries handle urea similarly, we may expect the concentration in the extracellular fluid to be approximately equal to that in a dialysate of plasma, and this seems to be true (Kleeman, *et al.*, 1962). Hence, the concentration in the cortical subarachnoid fluid should be higher than that in the ventricles or cisterna magna. In fact, Bradbury and Stubbs (1963) found a concentration of 20 mg/100 ml in human ventricular fluid and 26 mg/100 ml in cisternal fluid, while Bito and Davson (1966), in their study of the dog and cat, found the figures shown in Table VII. The rise on passing from

TABLE VII

MEAN CONCENTRATION OF UREA (mg/100 ml H_2O) IN PLASMA AND CSF OF SIX DOGS AND SIX CATS[a]

Species	Plasma	Cist. mag.	Cort. subarach.
Dogs	25.4 ± 2.4	21.3 ± 2.3	24.4 ± 2.3
Cats	69.4 ± 10.5	39.9 ± 3.9	50.3 ± 4.2

Distribution Ratios

Dogs	Cort. subarach./cist. mag.	1.15 ± 0.03	$P < 0.01$
	Cist. mag./plasma	0.84 ± 0.03	$P < 0.01$
	Cort. subarach./plasma	0.96 ± 0.02	$P > 0.1$
Cats	Cort. subarach./cist. mag.	1.27 ± 0.01	$P < 0.001$

[a] Plasma of dogs was from blood drawn immediately after anaesthesia, that of cats withdrawn before anaesthesia (Bito and Davson, 1966).

cisterna magna to cortical subarachnoid fluid in the cat is very striking; the change in the dog is not so large, but this is because the concentration in cisternal fluid is not so discrepant from that in plasma.

D. Freshly Secreted Fluid

It is of great interest to determine the chemical composition of the CSF as soon as it is formed; thus, ventricular fluid, although a "younger" fluid than that in the cortical subarachnoid space, has nevertheless been exposed to the brain for some time (the "half-life" of the lateral ventricular fluid may be 30 minutes) (Tubiana *et al.*, 1951). Ames pioneered studies of this sort by exposing the cat's lateral choroid plexus, covering it with oil and collecting the drops of fluid as they formed. The results of some analyses are shown in Table VIII from Ames *et al.*

TABLE VIII

Concentrations of Ions (mEq/kg H_2O) in Plasma, Plasma Ultrafiltrate. Choroid Plexus Fluid, and Cisterna Magna Fluid of the Cat [a]

	Cl	Na	K	Ca	Mg
Plasma	132	163	4.4[b]	2.62	1.35
Plasma ultrafiltrate	136	151	3.3	1.83	0.95
Choroid plexus fluid	138	158	3.28	1.67	1.47
Cisterna magna fluid	144	158	2.69	1.50	1.33

[a] Ames *et al.* (1964).
[b] Value for K^+ in plasma considered too high because of white cells, etc., being present.

(1964). The fluid collected from the surface in this way is sufficiently different from a plasma ultrafiltrate to indicate that active transport processes have been at work in forming it so that any suggestion that the CSF is formed as a simple filtrate of plasma, which is later modified by exchanges with the central nervous tissue, cannot be sustained. On comparing the freshly secreted fluid with that from the cisterna magna, it will be seen that the concentration of chloride has risen to the value characteristic of bulk CSF, while that of Mg^{++} has fallen a little but is still some 35% higher than in a plasma ultrafiltrate.

1. *Potassium*

The results obtained with K^+ are probably misleading; thus, it will be seen that the concentration in the newly secreted fluid is 3.28 mEq/liter, which is very close to the 3.3 mEq/liter found in the plasma ultrafiltrate. This would suggest that the fluid, as freshly secreted, was in equilibrium with plasma and only later acquired the lower value found in the cisternal fluid, namely, 2.69 mEq/liter. While the drop from 3.28 to 2.69 mEq/liter may be correct, the finding that the fluid, as secreted, has the same concentration as in a plasma filtrate is probably an artefact, due to the sustained anesthesia which results in a very low plasma concentration of K^+ (Bradbury and Davson, 1965). Since the concentration of K^+ in the CSF is hardly affected by that in the plasma, it is understandable that, under these particular conditions, the freshly formed fluid has the same concentration as that in a plasma filtrate, but there is no reason to believe that, if the plasma level had been higher, the concentration in the freshly formed fluid would have been correspondingly higher. The rise in concentration found on passing from freshly formed fluid to cisternal fluid is presumably a reflection of exchanges with the extracellular fluid of brain which has a lower concentration. Thus, only by the time the CSF has been in the cortical subarachnoid space can the concentration be said to represent fairly that in the extracellular fluid.

2. *Glucose*

The concentration of glucose in the cerebrospinal fluid is about 60% of that in the plasma. This was originally attributed to consumption by the adjacent tissue, but the failure to find large differences in concentration when ventricular and subarachnoid fluids were compared (Bito and Davson, 1966) suggested that this was not an important factor and that the fluid, as secreted, probably had a low concentration of glucose. This was confirmed by direct analyses of the fluid secreted from the exposed choroid plexus (Sadler and Welch, 1967).

E. RESTING POTENTIALS

The evidence thus suggests that the extracellular fluid of brain is similar in composition to that of the CSF, but not identical with it since certain exchanges take place during its passage through the system. This brings into focus the physiological significance of the blood–brain barrier, which may now be regarded as not just the reflexion of a restraint on passage of solutes from blood to nervous tissue but as a control mechanism that leads to the maintenance of levels of various ions and nonelectrolytes in the extracellular fluid that are different from those in the extracellular fluids of other tissues, in particular, low glucose, low K^+, and high Mg^{++}. The two ions K^+ and Mg^{++} have significant effects on excitability of neurons, and it may well be that these particular concentrations hold excitability at a lower level than if the neurons were surrounded by a plasma filtrate. More important, of course, is the homeostatic mechanism that holds these levels constant in the face of considerable variations in plasma concentration.

Measurements of the resting potentials of central neurons should be be able to confirm the view that the environment of the neuron, or glial cell, is more similar to that of the CSF than to plasma or its filtrate. Nicholls and Kuffler (1964) showed that the glial cells of the leech gave resting potentials of the order of 75 mV, which varied with external concentration of K^+ in accordance with the Nernst equation so that the suggestion that they contained a high concentration of Na^+ rather than K^+ and thus acted as an external medium for the neurons was disposed of. M. W. Cohen *et al.* (1968) proceeded to show that the glial cells of the mudpuppy (*Necturus*) likewise had K-dependent resting potentials, and they showed that, when the level of K^+ in the blood was raised by a factor of about 5, the rise in level in the CSF was much smaller; and the resting potential behaved as though its environmental K^+ had risen in accordance with the rise in the CSF rather than that in the plasma. The value of this homeostatic mechanism in protecting the brain from the effects of large variations in plasma K^+ concentration is shown by the simple expedient of injecting KCl into the CSF a procedure that leads to epileptiform discharges in conscious cats (Zuckermann and Glaser, 1968).

XV. Mechanism of Homeostasis

Carrier Mechanism

The secretion of a fluid with the concentrations of some solutes virtually independent of those in the plasma could be achieved, theoretically, by the involvement of a system of carriers that, by virtue of their specific affinities for given solutes, not only permitted their entry into the secretion but limited their rate by virtue of the restricted numbers of sites available for transport. Thus, at a sufficiently high concentration the carriers would be saturated, and if transport were confined to this carrier mechanism, a limit to the amount of the given solute that could be transported in unit time would be reached. Such a mechanism would exhibit a *transport maximum* but not a uniform rate of transport over a wide range of concentration; over a certain range the amount carried by the carriers would increase with increasing concentration of solute in the plasma, to reach a plateau at saturation.

1. *Potassium*

Where K^+ is concerned, we have seen that the dependence on plasma concentration is very small, whether the plasma concentration is raised chronically or lowered, so that an additional mechanism is probably operative. Thus, examination of the dependence of the concentration of K^+ in the freshly secreted fluid from the choroid plexuses gave Fig. 33 (Ames *et al.*, 1965a), showing a definite tendency for the concentration to fall at low plasma levels. Again, when Bradbury and Kleeman (1967) studied the influx of ^{42}K into the CSF as a function of the concentration of inactive K^+ in the plasma, they found that this was depressed by high concentrations of K^+, as would be expected of saturating a carrier mechanism, but not to the extent that would give the homeostasis required.[15] If the outflux from the CSF were governed by a similar, but inverse, mechanism, an adequate homeostatic mechanism could be achieved.

a. Outflux of ^{42}K. Measurements of outflux of ^{42}K are carried out by perfusing the ventricles with an artificial CSF containing the isotope; the efflux measured under these conditions, however, is largely determined by losses to adjacent cells so that efflux across the choroid plexuses and the capillaries of the brain, in which we are interested, is obscured. Thus, Bradbury and Davson (1965), Katzman *et al.* (1965), and Cserr (1965) could find little evidence of suppression of efflux of ^{42}K by increasing the concentration of inactive K^+ in the perfusion medium. However, Bradbury and Štulcová (1970) estimated the net losses to the blood by measuring the amount of ^{42}K that had remained in the brain during a period of perfusion; the amounts entering and leaving in the perfusion fluid

---

[15] Leiderman and Katzman (1953) showed that the influx of ^{42}K into rat brain was reduced at high plasma concentrations of K^+; Domer (1961) in a semiquantitative study found that the amount of ^{42}K entering the perfused cat's ventricles from the blood could be reduced by increasing the amount of inactive K^+ in the intravenous injection. Bradbury and Davson (1965) found that the influx of ^{42}K from plasma into the perfused rabbit ventricles was reduced to 60–80% by raising the plasma K^+ by about 100%.

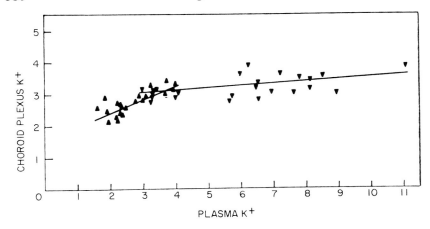

Fig. 33. Variation of concentration of K+ in freshly secreted cerebrospinal fluid with plasma concentration. Ordinate and abscissa: mEq/kg H_2O. (Ames *et al.*, 1965a.)

were known, so by subtraction, the amount leaving by choroid plexuses and the blood vessels of the brain could be obtained. Using this measure of outflux, they found that the efflux of ^{42}K was, in fact, accelerated by raising the concentration of inactive K+. In Fig. 34 the estimated outflux of K+, determined by the estimated losses of ^{42}K, has been plotted as a function of the concentration of K+ in the medium. If a simple noncarrier process were involved, the relation between outflux of K+ and the concentration of K+ would be linear. In fact, there is an S-shaped relationship, with a sharp increase in efflux, on raising the concentration from 3 to 6 mEq/liter. Such an acceleration suggests a carrier mechanism with two sites on it such that it is more efficient as a carrier when both sites are occupied than when only one is. A similar system has been described in the erythrocyte by Sachs and Welt (1967).

b. Combined Action. We may presume that the level of K+ in the CSF and also, presumably in the extracellular fluid of the brain, is held virtually independent of the level in the plasma by the combined actions of the two control mechanisms: (a) that operating from blood to CSF (and brain), consisting of a carrier whose efficiency, measured in terms of the fraction of the plasma concentration carried in unit time, decreases with increasing plasma concentration and (b) a control mechanism that shows an increased carrier efficiency with increasing concentrations of K+. It remains to be proved that similar mechanisms are operative in controlling the concentrations of other solutes, such as Ca++, Mg++, Cl−, $HCO_3^−$, and H+.

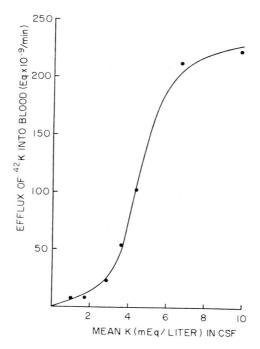

Fig. 34. The relation of the efflux of ^{42}K from CSF across the barrier to the mean concentration of potassium in CSF. (Bradbury and Štulcová, 1970.)

XVI. The Cerebrospinal Fluid and Brain Potentials

A potential between the surface of the brain and a remote indifferent electrode has been known to exist for a long time and has been called by the neurophysiologist the DC potential; characteristic shifts of this have been associated with neuronal activity. Loeschke (1956a) described a potential between a glass pipette electrode inserted into the cisterna magna and another electrode on the surface of the body; only when the electrode had penetrated the arachnoid membrane did the potential develop. It was called a transmeningeal potential and was considered to be the consequence of the restraint to ionic movements across the arachnoid membrane. The polarity was such that the CSF was positive by some 12 mV. Loeschke (1956b) showed that the potential became more positive if the P_{CO_2} of the blood was increased. In the cat, Mottschall and Loeschke (1963) found a smaller positive potential of 5.3 mV, but on raising the P_{CO_2} the shift was towards *negative* values.

A. Brain Surface Potentials

Tschirgi and Taylor (1958) placed one electrode on the surface of the brain and another in the jugular blood; the brain electrode was usually 1–5 mV *negative* in respect to blood, but in its sensitivity to P_{CO_2} of the blood and to metabolic acidosis it was very similar to the cisternal potential of Loeschke. Tschirgi and Taylor considered that the potential was across the blood–brain barrier and that this barrier was behaving as a hydrogen electrode; and the more recent studies of Held *et al.* (1964) and Severinghaus (1965) have confirmed the dependence on the H^+ concentration of the blood, although behavior is not that of an ideal H^+ electrode (Fig. 35). Increasing the concentration of K^+ in the CSF also modified the potential, making it more negative, and it was claimed that the potential was only responsive to alterations in CSF K^+ and blood H^+ ion concentration so that alterations of blood K^+ or CSF H^+ ion concentration were without effect. This asymmetry, if confirmed, would be surprising, and it is interesting that Cameron and Kleeman (1970) have shown that the potential does vary with plasma K^+.

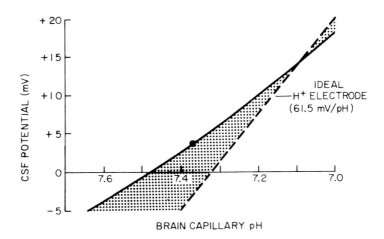

Fig. 35. CSF potential versus brain capillary pH. (Severinghaus, 1965.)

B. Choroid Plexus

The origin of the potential is presumably across the choroid plexuses; at any rate, Welch and Sadler (1965) inserted a glass pipette electrode into individual epithelial cells of the exposed rabbit's choroid plexus and measured the potential between this and another electrode which was either in the pool of artificial CSF or was in the connective tissue of the choroid plexus. On the average the potential between inside of the cell and the ventricular fluid was 64 mV, the inside of the cell being negative, as with a neuron or other epithelial cells. The difference between the inside of the cell and the stroma of the plexus was less, namely, 50 mV, so that the potential across the epithelium must have been some 14 mV, the ventricular side being positive. This is in remarkably good agreement with that measured directly by Loeschke (1956a).

C. Brain and Plexus

In a system like the cerebrospinal one where the extracellular fluid of the nervous tissue is in close diffusional relation with the CSF it is unlikely that a potential could be sustained across the choroid plexus without a corresponding mechanism to maintain a potential across the blood–brain barrier, or vice versa. Thus, we must seek the cause in the ionic relationships between blood, on the one hand, and the cerebrospinal and extracellular fluids on the other; moreover, we must not ignore the shunt across the arachnoid villi which, as we have seen, offer no resistance to the passage of ions. Whatever the origin of the potential, a great deal must be lost because of this short-circuiting.

D. Relation to Cerebral Blood Flow

Woody et al. (1970) and Besson et al. (1970) were impressed by the circumstance that, in the cat and monkey, the brain dc potential, measured with an electrode in the cisterna magna or on the surface of the brain, or by an electrode within the tissue or ventricle, responded to inhalation of 6–30% CO_2 by a negative shift, whereas in the rabbit and dog the shift is positive (Fig. 36). They were struck, too, by the close correlation between the cerebral changes in blood flow caused by various maneuvers, including altered P_{CO_2}, and the shift in potential. Thus, increased P_{CO_2} increased blood flow in all four species, but the potential shifts were in the reverse direction. The onset of the shift in potential coincided very exactly with the onset of a change in cerebral blood flow. On the other hand, this negative shift in the cat and monkey was usually preceded by a small positive shift and this was associated in time with a measurable decrease in pH of the surface of the brain. It would seem, then, that in the cat and monkey the positive response to high P_{CO_2} is swamped by the

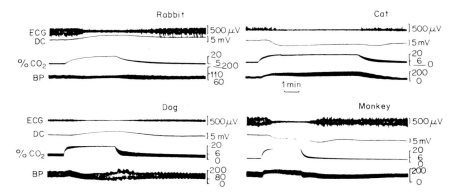

Fig. 36. Comparison of brain dc potential shift following 20% CO_2 administration in rabbit (Nembutal), dog (Nembutal), cat (chloralose), and monkey (Nembutal). Electrocorticogram (ECG) and brain steady potential (DC) recorded from suprasylvian cortex of cat, middorsal cortex of rabbit and dog, and precentral cortex of monkey. Simultaneous recording of expiratory CO_2 level, measured continuously at trachea, is also shown, as is blood pressure. Same recording techniques used in all preparations; reference on posterior lateral skull. Note positive dc shift in rabbit and dog and negative shift in cat and monkey. Positive is up. ECG shows reduction of cortical activity during administration of CO_2. (Woody et al., 1970.)

succeeding negative shift which is associated with an increase in cerebral blood flow. When the cerebral blood flow in the cat and monkey was altered, by the aid of drugs, the potential shifts were in accordance with the altered blood flow; thus, epinephrine, which increases the flow, caused a negative shift and acetylcholine caused a positive shift in potential. In the dog and rabbit the effects were variable but usually opposite to those in the cat and monkey so that the relation between blood flow and potential is different in the dog and rabbit and not so well defined. In general, drugs that might be expected to modify neuronal activity, such as strychnine, had little or no effect on the response to altered P_{CO_2}; moreover, it was suggested that some of the effects of the dc potential, which had hitherto been ascribed to neuronal activity, might have been due to altered blood flow. Thus, stimulation of the reticular formation with its associated "arousal" is accompanied by negative dc shift and also by an increase in cerebral blood flow.

Mechanism

The association between the two phenomena, potential shift and cerebral blood flow, is interesting but it is not necessarily causal; if it is, it can be that the dilatation of the small vessels alters the permeability of the brain capillaries permitting an ion, such as H^+ or K^+, to influence the potential across the capillary more or less effectively; certainly hypercapnia modifies the blood–brain barrier (Cameron et al., 1970). Alternatively, the concentration of an ion in the extracellular fluid may be dependent on rate of blood flow; thus, the effects of anoxia or heart failure are striking and rapid in onset and could, perhaps, be best explained on the basis of an accumulation of a metabolic product at the blood–extracellular fluid interface. In this connexion the work of Siesjö and his collaborators (Section XVII) on the changes in lactate and pyruvate in brain and CSF following alterations in blood flow, fluid pressure, and so on, are of special interest.

XVII. Acid–Base Parameters

The pH of CSF is more acid than that of arterial plasma; As Table IX shows, this is due to both a higher P_{CO_2} and lower concentration of bicarbonate, the P_{CO_2} being equal to that of venous blood (Bradley and Semple, 1962; Posner et al., 1965). It is reasonable to assume that the pH of the cerebrospinal fluid, and of the extracellular space of brain, is

TABLE IX

Acid–Base Parameters of Human Arterial Plasma and CSF[a]

pH		P_{CO_2} (mm Hg)		HCO_3^- (mEq/liter)	
Blood	CSF	Blood	CSF	Blood	CSF
7.414	7.311	38.3	47.9	23.4	22.9

[a] Posner et al. (1965).

controlled by active transport mechanisms, and studies on the effects of alterations in bicarbonate concentration in the blood confirm this, in the sense that these alterations are not followed by corresponding alterations in the fluid. This leads to some paradoxical effects on the pH of the fluid.

A. Paradoxical Changes in pH

Thus, Cestan *et al.* (1925) injected HCl into the blood, thereby reducing the bicarbonate concentration; the blood became more acid but the CSF became more alkaline, and this was because of the failure of the concentration of bicarbonate in the CSF to fall correspondingly. In order that the plasma pH might remain within limits compatible with life, the tension of carbon dioxide in the blood was reduced, by hyperventilation, and since the blood–CSF barrier is rapidly permeable to carbon dioxide (Coxon and Swanson, 1965), this means that the tension in the CSF was correspondingly reduced. Thus, the CSF had a low tension of carbon dioxide with an approximately normal bicarbonate concentration, giving an alkaline response, while the blood had lowered tension and lowered bicarbonate concentration and, thus a slightly acid response, if any.

B. Permeability to Bicarbonate

More recent studies have confirmed the low permeability of both the blood–CSF and blood–brain barriers to bicarbonate (Siesjö, 1965), while the studies of Gesell and Hertzman (1926) showed the converse effects of raising the plasma bicarbonate concentration, in which the CSF became more acid. When Robin *et al.* (1958) maintained the arterial P_{CO_2} constant during administration of $NaHCO_3$, the paradoxical pH shift did not occur.

C. Respiratory Alkalosis and Acidosis

The response to alterations in blood pH brought about by either hyper- or hypoventilation are less paradoxical, the direction of the pH change in the CSF usually being the same as that of the blood, but there is evidence for homeostasis whereby the changes in pH of the fluid are restricted to narrower limits. Thus, when hyperventilation was maintained in the dog for several hours, compensatory mechanisms seemed to come into play restricting the degree of alkalinity of the cerebrospinal fluid [Fig. 37 (from Leusen, 1965)] due to the maintenance of a relatively higher P_{CO_2} which followed from the greater lactic acid production by the brain under these conditions (Van Vaerenbergh *et al.*, 1965).

A number of studies of chronic acidosis or alkalosis have brought into prominence the intervention of homeostatic mechanisms that tend to maintain the pH of the CSF constant. Thus the lines in Fig. 38 [from Mitchell *et al.* (1965)] show the values of the concentration of bicarbonate in the CSF that would be necessary to maintain a constant pH in the face of altering arterial P_{CO_2}. Three values of pH are chosen, namely, 7.298, 7.354, and 7.326. The plotted points are derived from measurements on human subjects; the closeness with which they fall on the lines indicates that homeostasis is brought about by variations in the concentration of bicarbonate. The normal value of R_{CSF} for man is about 0.85, and this will vary if the cerebrospinal fluid and arterial pH are changed relatively since, other things being equal, the concentration of HCO_3^- in the fluids

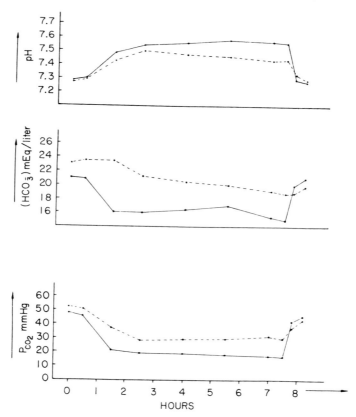

Fig. 37. Acid–base balance in the dog between arterial blood and CSF during prolonged experimental respiratory alkalosis produced by hyperventilation. Hyperventilation started after collection of the first two CSF and blood samples and stopped at $7\frac{1}{2}$ hours. Last two samples were taken during spontaneous respiration. – – – – CSF; ——— blood (plasma). (Leusen, 1965.)

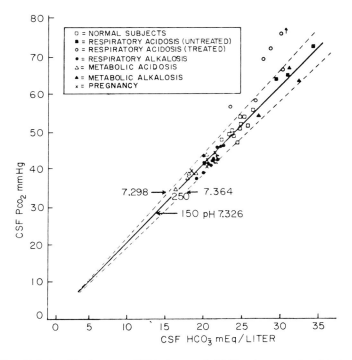

Fig. 38. Relationship between CSF P_{CO_2} and HCO_3^- in normal subjects and patients with abnormal acid–base balance. Central iso-pH line represents normal mean CSF pH (7.326); outer lines indicate 2 SD from the mean. (Mitchell *et al.*, 1965.)

will vary with $[H^+]$ and P_{CO_2}, in accordance with the Law of Mass Action as follows:

$$K'_{1\text{Plasma}} = \frac{[H^+]_{\text{Plasma}} \times [HCO_3^-]_{\text{Plasma}}}{S_{\text{Plasma}} \times (P_{CO_2})_{\text{Plasma}}}$$

$$K'_{1\text{CSF}} = \frac{[H^+]_{\text{CSF}} \times [HCO_3^-]_{\text{CSF}}}{S_{\text{CSF}} \times (P_{CO_2})_{\text{CSF}}}$$

S_{Plasma} and S_{CSF} being the solubility coefficients of CO_2 in plasma and cerebrospinal fluid respectively.

The predicted relationship is given by the curve of Fig. 39, while the actual results are given by the plotted points and crosses. Thus, there seems to be a tendency for the ratio, R_{CSF}, to be held at a value consistent with passive adaptation to altered pH, but the actual ratio is always one that demands active transport since the passive distribution, correspond-

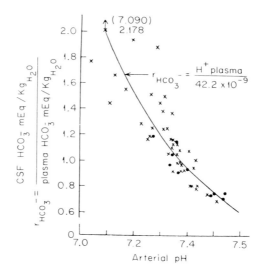

Fig. 39. Relationship between R_{CSF} for HCO_3^- and arterial pH in subjects with metabolic acidosis and alkalosis. Solid line represents predicted relationship. ●, data of Mitchell et al. ×, other data. (Mitchell et al., 1965.)

ing to the observed difference of potential between CSF and blood of 3 mV in human lumbar fluid (Severinghaus, 1964), would demand a ratio of about 1.10. As to whether these adaptive alterations in bicarbonate concentration in the CSF are to be be attributed to active processes or not has been discussed by Loeschke and Sugioka (1969), who have measured the alterations in pH at the surface of the choroid plexus of the IVth ventricle during acute and chronic alterations in the composition of the blood. As we might expect, alterations leading to a change in blood P_{CO_2} result in an immediate change in pH, owing to the rapid penetration of CO_2 across the choroidal epithelium. As in the study of bulk fluid, the changes in local CSF pH are held down to very small amounts, because of passive restraints on, or of active processes in, the transport of bicarbonate.

D. BRAIN pH, ETC.

The main thesis of this chapter is the close relationship between CSF and extracellular fluid of brain, and we must expect the acid–base parameters of the CSF to be strongly influenced by those in the brain parenchyma; in fact, we may expect a dominant influence by the latter since the metabolic activities of the cells must contribute an enormous potential for influencing H^+ ion concentration. The physiological importance of this relationship is nowhere better exhibited than in the influence of blood and CSF pH on the respiratory rate and cerebral circulation. A detailed description of these aspects is, unfortunately, beyond the scope of this chapter, and the reader is referred to fairly recent symposia (Luyendijk, 1968; Brooks *et al.*, 1965) and reviews (Pappenheimer, 1965-1966; Davson, 1967). According to the studies of Pappenheimer and his colleagues, the respiratory responses of the conscious animal to alterations in pH of the CSF are precisely those that would be expected were the extracellular fluid of brain, bathing the respiratory center, in a dynamic steady state with the plasma on the one hand and the CSF on the other. In view of the more rapid exchanges between CSF and extracellular fluid, it follows that it is the pH of the CSF that exerts a dominant influence on the respiratory rate.

1. *Active Transport of H^+*

As to the factors controlling the brain pH, the situation is obviously highly complex. If the brain cells are similar to those of muscle and peripheral nerve, we may expect an active transport of H^+ ions out of the cells—or one of OH^- ions inwards—to maintain the lower pH inside the cell than that required of a passive distribution normally observed (Caldwell, 1968). Evidence for the intervention of some such cellular buffering process was provided by Pontén (1966), who found that the buffering capacity of brain in response to altered P_{CO_2} of the blood was much higher than could be accounted for by the known concentration of bicarbonate in the system and was about equal to that of arterial blood, which, as is known, utilizes the hemoglobin-buffer system to amplify the buffering capacity of the HCO_3^- in the blood. Kjälquist *et al.* (1969b) showed that this buffering capacity was influenced by the anesthetic used, the capacity being greater in rats under nitrous oxide than under phenobarbital, thus emphasizing that the process was influenced by metabolic events. Whether this is simply an intervention of active transport, requiring metabolic energy, or whether the modification of metabolism modifies the lactate and pyruvate in the system, influencing the acid–base parameters in this way, is not yet clear.

2. *Lactate and Pyruvate*

The steady production of the relatively strong acids, pyruvic and lactic, will obviously be an important factor in determining the concentration of bicarbonate in the extracellular phase of the brain and, thence, in the CSF. And until alterations in these rates, in response to acidosis and alkalosis, are understood, it will not be easy to define the nature of the active mechanisms controlling the bicarbonate concentration. Recent work from Siesjö's laboratory is making some progress in this direction. Thus, they measured the lactate and pyruvate concentrations in cisternal CSF of cats and related these to the corresponding concentrations in brain tissue, along with the ATP, ADP, and phosphocreatine and creatine concentrations. Figure 40 [from Granholm and Siesjö (1969)] shows the effects of arterial P_{CO_2}, induced by hyper- or hypoventilation, on lactate and pyruvate in CSF and brain. The steep rises in concentration at low arterial CO_2 tensions are striking. By contrast, there were no measurable effects on the other parameters studied, i.e., ATP, ADP, etc., concentra-

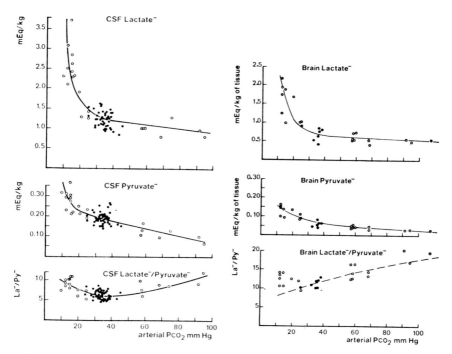

Fig. 40. The influence of changes in the arterial P_{CO_2} on the lactate and pyruvate concentrations and the lactate/pyruvate ratios in cisternal cerebrospinal fluid (left) and cerebral cortical tissue (right) of cats. The broken line (bottom right) is the theoretical change of the lactate/pyruvate ratio, assuming a pH-dependent equilibrium between the lactate/pyruvate and the $NADH/NAD^+$ systems at constant NAD reduction. (Granholm and Siesjö, 1969.)

tions. It was considered by these authors that the alterations in lactate/ pyruvate ratio observed were reflexions of the NADH/NAD system and thus indicated the degree of tissue hypoxia; since these are pH dependent, we may predict that alkalosis will induce an effective anoxia by shifting the NADH/NAD ratio. The observed changes in lactate/pyruvate ratio fitted the predicted ones reasonably well except in the region of steep rise at low CO_2 tensions (Fig. 40, bottom right). As many workers have emphasized, an additional factor that may be dominant in determining the levels of lactate and pyruvate will be the cerebral blood flow. Thus, this depends acutely on arterial P_{CO_2} (see, for example, Posner *et al.*, 1969) so that hyperventilation, by reducing the arterial P_{CO_2}, may lead to an acute reduction in cerebral blood flow producing an anoxic condition. At any rate, Plum and Posner (1967) found an increase in cerebrospinal fluid lactate to result from hyperventilation.

XVIII. Some Special Features of the Blood–Brain Barrier System

Having sketched the main outlines of the relations between blood and the tissues of the brain and spinal cord, we may now examine some special features.

A. FACILITATED TRANSFER OF SUGARS

In several systems, notably the human erythrocyte, and ascites tumor cell, the transport of sugars, although not active in the sense that movement against concentration gradients does not occur, is carrier mediated in the sense that simple permeability kinetics are not ordinarily applicable. Thus, in the simple system, the permeability coefficient is independent of the concentration of solute employed. Nor is it affected by the simultaneous permeation of other solutes. In these other systems, the permeability coefficient does depend on concentration and is influenced by the simultaneous penetration of chemically related substances. The kinetics can be described in terms of movement on a carrier, for which the solute in question has a specific affinity. When different hexoses are compared, it is found that the computed affinities for the carrier are different; again, competition between solutes is observed, so that the penetration of one may be inhibited by the presence of another. When sugars are moved against a concentration gradient, as with absorption from the intestine, a similar specificity is observed, so that carriers have been invoked to describe the kinetics of this process, but in addition, one or more stages must be linked with a chemical reaction that permits the movement uphill of the actively transported solute. The concentration of glucose in normal CSF is lower than in plasma (Table I), and this is also true of the freshly secret fluid (Section XIV,D,2); the low concentration could be due to active processes driving the molecule out of the choroid plexus cells back into the blood, or it could be due to restricted diffusion into these cells by virtue of a low permeability coefficient. Thus, the choroid plexus would be acting as a "molecular sieve," in a manner similar to the way in which it restricts the passage of protein, inulin, and other slowly permeating molecules into the fluid. In general, the studies of Geiger *et al.* (1954), Bradbury and Davson (1964), Fishman (1964), Crone (1965), Le Fevre and Peters (1966), Eidelberg *et al.* (1967), Bidder (1968), and Atkinson and Webb (1969) concur in showing that transport into both CSF and brain is carrier mediated so that Atkinson and Webb (1969), for example, found that the kinetics of penetration of glucose from blood into CSF were described by a Michaelis–Menten type of equation, with the transfer constant, k_{In}, replaced by $V_{max}/(K_m + C_{Plasma})$, V_{max} being the maximum rate of penetration and K_m the dissociation constant for the sugar carrier complex, its reciprocal being a measure of the affinity for the carrier.

1. Penetration in Freshly Secreted Fluid

Of particular interest is a study of Welch *et al.* (1969) in which penetration into the freshly secreted fluid was measured. Under these conditions the concentration of sugar in the fluid is a direct measure of the influx from the blood, uncomplicated by exchanges between the brain parenchyma. With a simple noncarrier mediated type of permeability we may expect the influx to vary linearly with the plasma level, and in fact, this occurred up to a plasma level of 14 mM (235 mg/100 ml); at higher plasma levels there was self-inhibition, suggesting saturation of the carrier mechanism, but at still higher levels the reverse occurred, as though the increase in plasma concentration favored penetration to a greater extent than expected of the increased concentration alone. Under appropriate conditions it could be shown that the different sugars enhanced each other's transport. This cooperation between solutes has been attributed to the presence of two carrier sites in the membrane, the presence of one solute increasing the affinity of the other, either for the same solute or for another; and in this way we may explain both cooperative and inhibitory actions.

2. *Isolated Frog Plexus*

Recently, Prather and Wright (1970) have employed their streaming potential technique to obtain reflexion coefficients for some 41 different sugars and related compounds. The rate of transport v_r, is given by $1/k(1 - \sigma)$ RTC, where k is a parameter that cannot be exactly determined but may well be the same for the different solutes. If this is true, the variation in the rate of transport with concentration of sugar in the medium may be determined, the deviation from linearity indicating carrier mediated transport. The results confirmed the more direct measurements in showing stereospecificity in rate of transport; thus, σ for D-arabinose was 0.98, indicating near impermeability, while for L-arabinose it was 0.52, indicating a permeability comparable with that of urea. The rates of penetration were the same independently of the direction of transport, indicating a passive form of transport; as Fig. 41 shows, the sugars compete with each other, the slope of the Lineweaver–Burk plot for D-xylose alone being less than for D-xylose plus D-glucose. Again, difluorodinitrobenzene inhibited transport of sugars; a similar compound, fluorodinitrobenzene, had been shown to be an inhibitor of facilitated transport of sugar across the erythrocyte membrane, presumably by blocking access to the carrier (Bowyer and Widdas, 1958).

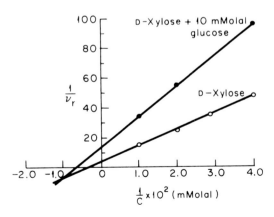

Fig. 41. Inhibition of D-xylose transport by D-glucose. The reciprocal of the relative rate of transport (v_r) as the ordinate is plotted against the reciprocal of concentration for D-xylose both in the presence and absence of 10 mmolal glucose. All results in this graph were obtained in one choroid plexus. (Prather and Wright, 1970.)

3. *Blood–Brain Transfer*

So far as passage from blood into brain tissue is concerned, the evidence for carrier mediation has been discussed by Le Fevre and Peters (1966). Certainly there is competition for penetration, e.g., between D-glucose and D-mannose, but not between D-galactose and D-xylose, the latter sugars showing no evidence for carrier based transport. As Le Fevre and Peters point out, however, it seems likely that they do, indeed, use the same mechanism, but their affinity being so low, the kinetics of penetration become identical with those for noncarrier mediated permeability; the authors base this contention on the high degree of selectivity for sugars shown by the blood–brain barrier, for example, fructose is virtually excluded (Klein *et al.*, 1946), and it is difficult to conceive of a membrane that would differentiate between fructose and glucose on the basis of anything else than some form of chemical affinity. Further evidence favoring facilitated transfer across the blood–brain barrier is provided by Crone's studies employing the indicator-dilution technique (Section VII,A); thus, 3-methylglucose and D-glucose both showed saturation phenomena and mutual inhibition; the penetration of D-mannose, D-galactose, D-arabinose, and D-ribose was slower than that of D-glucose, and it was not possible to distinguish differences in their relative rates; we may assume that the affinities of these sugars were much less than those of D-glucose and 3-methylglucose (Agnew and Crone, 1967). Insulin accelerates the transport of many sugars into skeletal muscle, but it seems to have no effect on transport from blood to brain (Park *et al.*, 1957).[16]

4. *CSF–Brain Relations*

In general, it would seem that passage of sugars into the CSF and brain is a passive process; it is carrier mediated in the sense that the membrane possesses special affinities for the sugars that permit these large water-soluble molecules to pass with some ease through the lipid membranes of the cells constituting the barriers. The permeability of glucose is not so rapid that the freshly secreted CSF has the same concentration as that in plasma. The fact that there are no large alterations in concentration as the fluid passes through the ventricles and subarachnoid space suggests that the extracellular fluid, likewise, has a lower concentration

---

[16] Bronstead (1969) has shown that ouabain reduces the influx and efflux of glucose between blood and the perfused ventricles of the cat, an effect that could not be mimicked by replacement of all the K^+ in the perfusion fluid by Na^+.

than that in plasma. The low concentration here is probably a steady-state condition resulting from utilization by neurons and glia; the importance of the permeability of the blood–brain barrier in this connection is shown by the failure of intravenous fructose to relieve the convulsions due to low glucose, the penetration of fructose being very slow as indicated above.[17]

B. Amino Acids

The concentration of a given amino acid in the blood plasma, at any moment, is the result of the interaction of a number of factors so that it may well alter from hour to hour. The concentration in the CSF will depend on the concentration in the plasma and the kinetics of transport across the barriers of the central nervous system; particularly important may well be the exchanges with the central nervous parenchyma since, *in vitro* at any rate, the brain accumulates many amino acids to concentrations well above those in the medium. In addition, the amino acids will be involved in the constant turnover of protein in the brain so that altogether the situation with respect to any given amino acid is highly complex.

1. *Normal CSF–Plasma Distribution*

The concentrations of individual amino acids in CSF and plasma of dogs, the fluids being drawn at the same time, are shown in Table X. In general, the total concentration is considerably lower than in plasma. This is true of most of the individual acids, with the exceptions of glutamine and glutamic acid, and this is presumably related to the importance of these compounds in the metabolism of the brain. Thus glutamic acid, alanine, γ-aminobutyric acid (GABA) and glutamine—the amide of glutamic acid—are all synthesized within the brain. Altogether, some 80% of the total free amino acids of brain seem to be made up of glutamic and aspartic acids and their derivatives, and this may be connected with the fundamental role of GABA and others of these compounds in transmission within the central nervous system. The concentrations of individual acids in brain and plasma of rats are shown in Table XI; the concentrations of many are fairly close in plasma and brain water. Because of the close association between CSF and brain extracellular fluid, we may ex-

---

[17] The glucose content of brain has been discussed recently by Mark *et al.* (1968); it is very low in the rat (about 0.75 moles/kg), but this species seems to be an exception.

TABLE X

CONCENTRATIONS OF AMINO ACIDS (μmoles/gm H_2O) IN PLASMA AND CSF OF DOGS[a]

Amino acid	Plasma	CSF
Alanine	0.29	0.13
Arginine	0.11	0.04
Aspartic acid	0.02	n.m.
Cystine	0.18	0.02
Glutamic acid	0.13	0.16
Glutamine	n.m.	0.03
Glycine	0.29	0.23
Histidine	0.07	0.09
Isoleucine	0.10	n.m.
Leucine	0.12	0.06
Lysine	0.23	0.18
Methionine	0.03	n.m.
Phenylalanine	0.04	0.07
Serine	0.27	0.05
Threonine	0.13	0.02
Tyrosine	0.05	0.05
Valine	0.04	0.01
Total	2.11	0.80

[a] Bito et al. (1966b).

pect the concentrations in these two fluids to be similar, in which event we may expect some cellular accumulation of the amino acids. Certainly there is a large literature demonstrating the power of isolated slices of brain to accumulate amino acids (for a summary, see Lajtha, 1968; Neame, 1968).

2. Exchanges between Blood and CSF

Quantitative studies on passage of amino acids from blood to CSF are only fairly recent. Wiechert (1963) measured the net uptakes of a variety of amino acids 10 minutes after a single intravenous injection; the blood–CSF barrier, estimated in this way, showed a relative impermeability to GABA, glycine, aspartic acid, and threonine, while penetration of glutamic acid was relatively rapid.

TABLE XI

CONCENTRATIONS OF AMINO ACIDS IN PLASMA AND BRAIN OF RATS [a]

Amino Acid	Plasma (μM/ml)	Brain (μM/gm)
Taurine	0.24	4.9
Aspartic acid	0.02	2.6
Threonine	0.22	0.52
Serine	0.33	0.90
Glutamine	0.66	5.0
Glutamic acid	0.10	9.0
Citrulline	0.13	—
Glycine	0.28	1.1
Alanine	0.37	0.82
Valine	0.19	0.12
Methionine	0.05	0.07
Isoleucine	0.08	0.05
Leucine	0.13	0.10
Tyrosine	0.05	0.06
Phenylalanine	0.08	0.05
Ornithine	0.03	—
Histidine	0.04	0.05
Arginine	0.09	0.08
Hydroxyproline	0.07	—
Proline	0.19	0.13
Lysine	0.28	0.24
GABA	—	2.1

[a] Carver (1965).

3. *Exchanges between Blood and Brain*

As with the CSF, kinetic studies of net uptake show wide variations in rate; thus, Kamin and Handler (1951) were unable to measure any net uptake of glutamic or aspartic acid by the dog's brain after 2–4 hours of intravenous infusion, but there was a limited uptake of ʟ-histidine, ʟ-arginine, and ʟ-methionine. Several other studies suggested that uptake of amino acids by brain from the blood was very slow; for example, Fried-berg and Greenberg (1947) were unable to measure any uptake of glycine, glutamic acid, histidine, lysine, or alanine by brain after intravenous injection. With some amino acids, nevertheless, penetration is very rapid; thus, Chirigos et al. (1960) found penetration of tyrosine as rapid as into muscle, and since tyrosine is not metabolized by brain, the interpretation is not complicated by this factor. The D isomer was taken up much more slowly. Again L-tryptophan was taken up more rapidly than D-tryptophan (Guroff and Udenfriend, 1962). A number of investigators showed, also, that there was competition between amino acids for transport into the brain; thus, Guroff and Udenfriend found competition between phenylalanine and tyrosine, while lysine, alanine, serine, threonine, arginine, glutamic acid, and glutamine had no effect on uptake of tyrosine. It was considered that the reduction in the concentration of endogenous tyrosine in the brain, caused by injection of leucine, was a manifestation of competitive action. Phenylalanine penetrates rapidly into brain. It also, presumably by competition, reduces the level of serotonin in brain so that it may well be that the cerebral manifestations of phenylketonuria are related to the accumulation of phenylalanine in the blood that occurs in this condition, due to its failure to be converted into tyrosine.[18]

a. Isotope Exchanges. Thus, the studies on net uptake of amino acids indicate barriers of varying degrees to the individual amino acids, and the high degree of specificity thus manifest, together with competitive phenomena, indicate carrier mediated transport. When labeled amino acids were injected into the blood, the rate of uptake was generally much higher. Thus, Lajtha (1958) found that inactive lysine penetrated with a transfer constant in the region of 0.002 minutes^{-1} whereas Lajtha et al. (1957) found that ^{14}C-lysine penetrated with a constant of 0.14 minute^{-1}, a rate of exchange some 20 times that of ^{24}Na. The difference is due to the presence of a carrier mechanism that is saturated or near saturated at the levels of plasma lysine used to measure the net uptake with the inactive amino acid. Using the labeled acid, the actual concentration in plasma was no higher than that of endogenous lysine. An additional factor is exchange diffusion, whereby a labeled molecule exchanges with an unlabeled one. This results in transport of the label but no net transport of the amino acid since the carrier has only exchanged a labeled for an unlabeled molecule. Whether the depression in the levels of amino acids in brain that follows the raising of the plasma level of another is due entirely to suppression of influx by competition has been discussed by Roberts

---

[18] The subject of mental changes in the amino acidurias has been reviewed by Nyhan and Tocci (1966).

(1968), and his conclusion is that, in addition to suppression of uptake, for example, that of valine by phenylalanine, there is an enhancement of the utilization of amino acids by the brain.[19]

4. *Efflux of Amino Acids*

An amino acid injected into the subarachnoid space will pass into the blood in the general bulk drainage process; it will also be absorbed by the capillaries of the nervous tissue. Lajtha and Toth (1961, 1963) considered that an active transport outwards might well exist, but the evidence for this was that, when they raised the concentration of a given amino acid in the blood above that in the CSF, the concentration in the latter continued to fall. But, as argued earlier (Davson, 1967), this could represent a loss by flow through the arachnoid villi; this would be independent of the concentration in the blood. Levin *et al.* (1966) perfused the ventricles of cats with different amino acids; the losses were small, e.g., that of glutamic acid, and this presumably reflected the low permeability of the choroid plexuses and the capillaries of the brain. The losses showed mutual competition; for example, the absorption of glutamine fell from 3.8 to 0.6 μmoles/hour on adding GABA to the medium.

5. *Relation to Metabolism*

To summarize a highly complex and still inadequately investigated subject, it appears that the exchanges of amino acids between blood and brain involve carrier mediated processes. Active transport, in the sense of an accumulation against a gradient of electrochemical potential, occurs across the cellular membranes of neurons and glia, if work on isolated tissue can be transposed to *in vivo* conditions; definite proof of active transport across the blood–brain and blood–CSF barriers is lacking, and it may be that the control over influx and efflux is mediated entirely through the passive permeabilities of the limiting barriers. According to Lajtha (1968), the metabolism of the individual acids is closely controlled by the transport mechanisms, the metabolic processes being limited in rate by substrate availability.

[19] The apparent failure of DOPA to pass from blood to brain is not due to an impermeability of the brain capillaries to this metabolic intermediate but to the presence of a decarboxylase in the brain capillary walls that converts it to dopamine, which is then metabolized locally by monoamine oxidase. Thus, inhibition of the DOPA-decarboxylase allows intravenously presented DOPA to accumulate in the brain (Owman and Rosengren, 1967).

C. PROTEINS

As indicated earlier, the protein concentration in CSF is low; when ventricular, cisternal, and lumbar fluids are compared, the concentration rises in this order, suggesting that the freshly secreted fluid has a very low concentration and that protein passes from the cerebral and spinal tissue into the fluid during its life in the system. These additions could represent escape from "defective" capillaries or from breakdown of tissue. Table XII shows the relative proportions of the different components; these were the same for CSF derived from the three sources, but only when the lumbar fluid contained a low concentration of total protein. When the lumbar fluid had a high concentration, but still within the normal limits, the proportions changed, indicating that the relatively high concentration in the lumbar fluid is not just due to absorption of water. The high concentration was due, in general, to the appearance of more albumin and, to a less extent, α_1- and γ-globulins. In general, we may envisage the normal secretion of a primary CSF containing the constituent proteins in characteristic proportions, which are not necessarily those in the original plasma; on its passage through the CSF additional proteins diffuse from the tissue into the fluid, the amounts of the different types depending on the ease with which these escape from the blood and on breakdown of material in the tissue. This view is supported by the finding of considerably larger concentrations of protein in the fluid loculated below a spinal block (Hill *et al.*, 1959; Tveten, 1965). In communicating hydrocephalus, where the blockage to outflow of CSF is probably in the arachnoid villi, Tveten (1965) found that the concentration of protein was high, presumably because, in this condition, the openings out of the arachnoid villi had become sufficiently small to exert a restraint on the outflux of the protein molecules; the CSF was being partially filtered.

1. *Lumbar Fluid*

The higher concentration of protein in the lumbar fluid could be due to a more permeable blood–spinal than a blood–cerebral barrier to protein, but the more sluggish circulation in the spinal space seems much more likely to be the explanation; Hochwald *et al.* (1969) measured the influx of labeled albumin from blood into the artificial CSF, perfusing either the ventricles (ventriculo-cisternal perfusion) or the isolated spinal subarachnoid space. The net uptakes were about the same, but their estimates of the areas of the cat's ventriculo-cisternal and spinal subarach-

TABLE XII

PROTEINS IN VENTRICULAR, CISTERNAL, AND LUMBAR FLUIDS [a]

Site	Total	Prealbumin	Albumin	Globulins				
				α_1	α_2	β	γ	
Ventricle	17.1 ± 9.9	6.3 ± 1.8	46.6 ± 6.5	8.1 ± 1.7	7.9 ± 2.8	19.1 ± 2.0	10.3 ± 3.7	
Cistern	18.3 ± 4.3	4.6 ± 1.6	44.6 ± 7.3	6.7 ± 1.0	9.5 ± 3.7	21.3 ± 4.5	13.4 ± 4.0	
Lumbar	21.0 ± 7.3	5.5 ± 1.1	45.0 ± 6.0	6.8 ± 2.6	9.6 ± 2.3	21.6 ± 4.7	11.1 ± 2.7	
	39.5 ± 4.8	3.9 ± 0.8	46.4 ± 3.6	6.3 ± 2.4	10.5 ± 2.6	18.8 ± 3.7	12.6 ± 3.7	
	59.1 ± 3.8	3.3 ± 1.2	53.6 ± 5.6	5.9 ± 1.6	8.6 ± 1.2	17.6 ± 1.2	10.0 ± 2.5	

[a] Total proteins are given as mg/100 ml, while the fractions are given as percentages of the total (Hill *et al.*, 1958).

noid areas gave 11 and 60 cm² respectively, so that the ventriculo-cisternal barrier was definitely the more permeable. This could have been due to the presence of the choroid plexuses, but even if allowance was made for their area, the ventriculo-cisternal system came out as the more permeable.

2. *Turnover of Labeled Protein*

Other studies with labeled proteins have led to the view that the normal levels of proteins in the CSF are determined by exchanges with the blood during the process of secretion and, subsequently, during flow through the system. Thus, Frick and Scheid-Seydel (1958a,b, 1960) injected labeled albumin and γ-globulin into human subjects and determined the specific activities in serum and fluid at different intervals. It required some three days for a dynamic steady state to be achieved between blood and the fluid, but because of the breakdown of protein in the serum and its replacement by inactive protein, the specific activity in the serum was some 20% less than that in cerebrospinal fluid. With γ-globulin some 100 hours were required. Because of the higher specific activities in cerebrospinal fluid, it was concluded that, at any rate in the normal subject, the proteins were entirely derived from the blood. With a pathological elevation of the γ-globulins, however, the specific activity in the CSF could be only 10% of that in blood, suggesting an origin from a pool not readily accessible to blood. Hochwald and Wallenstein (1967a) found, in cats, that 4 hours after an intravenous injection of γ-globulin, the γ-globulin entering the ventriculo-cisternal perfusion fluid had a specific activity of only 0.8 times that in the plasma, suggesting that during this time the labeled γ-globulin had not equilibrated with that in the brain tissue; after 20–48 hours the specific activities were the same. It is interesting that Diamox, which inhibits the secretory mechanism, reducing the rate of flow by some 60%, caused the ratio of specific activities in fluid and plasma to fall from 0.8 to 0.5 when perfusion was initiated 4 hours after the intravenous injection. This suggests that a considerable fraction of the γ-globulin entering from the blood comes directly in the secretion. Essentially similar results were obtained with labeled albumin (Hochwald and Wallenstein (1967b). In subacute sclerosing leukoencephalitis (SSLE) the γ-globulin of the CSF is elevated; Cutler *et al.* (1967) found that, although in control human subjects the specific activities of fluid and plasma became equal (relative specific activity of fluid = 1) some days after an intravenous dose of labeled γ-globulin, in the SSLE subjects the specific activity in cerebrospinal fluid was only 20–40% of that in plasma, showing that the brain was supplying the γ-globulin, i.e., that it was coming from a pool not readily accessible to the plasma.

XIX. Modifications of the Barriers

The exchange of material between blood on the one hand and CSF and nervous tissue on the other can be modified experimentally or pathologically. The modification may take the form of a decrease in selectivity associated with a general increase in permeability, in which case it is customary to say that there has been a "breakdown" of the barrier; alternatively, and much more rarely, the rate of exchange may be inhibited. This is seen typically in the reduced exchanges consequent on the inhibition of the secretion of the cerebrospinal fluid. Since the normal concentrations of the various solutes in the CSF represent steady states, determined by secretory processes and passive exchanges throughout the system, modification of the permeability of the barriers may well be reflected in changes in the steady-state concentrations; and the more discrepant the concentration of a given solute from that in the plasma, the more obvious will be the effects of altered permeability.

A. PROTEINS

This is manifest with respect to the protein concentration in the CSF; the normal concentrations in ventricle, cisterna magna, and lumbar sac are low, being only a small fraction of the plasma concentration. In meningitis, the protein concentration may rise to many hundreds of milligrams/100 ml, and a variety of studies on the separate proteins and their relative proportions indicate that they are largely derived from plasma. The increased permeability of the barriers is also revealed by the presence of proteins, such as macro-α-globulin, β-lipoprotein, and fibrinogen, that are normally excluded. The elaboration and release of larger quantities of a specific protein by the nervous tissue will also modify the protein composition of the CSF, and this seems to be the cause for the specific rise in γ-globulin concentration in multiple sclerosis. Inhibition of formation of CSF, as with Diamox, might be expected to decrease the concentration of protein in the CSF since the influx in the new secretion is reduced; however, the more sluggish flow through the system allows more time for protein to accumulate from the adjacent tissues so that ultimately one might expect a rise in protein concentration.

B. Crystalloids

An increase in passive permeability of the blood–CSF and blood–brain barriers will militate against the effects of active transport processes so that it is likely that a serious breakdown in the barriers will modify the concentrations of such solutes as Cl^-, K^+ and Mg^{++} and bring them closer to those characteristic of a dialysate of plasma. Nobécourt and Voisin (1903) and, later, Mestrezat (1911) pointed out that the concentration of chloride in the CSF in meningitis was characteristically lower than normal. Later, H. Cohen (1927) found a definite fall in the concentration of magnesium in the meningitic cerebrospinal fluid. Thus, the average values for normal serum and CSF were 2.56 and 3.28 mg/100 ml respectively; in meningitis the average values were 2.7 and 2.5 mg/100 ml. Inorganic phosphorus, on the other hand, showed the reverse behavior, being elevated in meningitis. Cohen formulated a so-called "Law of Meningitis", to the effect that, in this condition, the concentrations of those substances that were in excess over those in the plasma, namely, magnesium and chloride, would fall, while the concentrations of those substances that were in deficiency, namely, inorganic phosphorus, potassium, and protein, would rise. This is what we would expect of a breakdown of the barrier, namely, the movement of the concentration towards equilibrium.

1. *Chloride*

So far as Cl^- was concerned, it appeared from a more exact study that this agreement with theoretical expectation was illusory. For example Linder and Carmichael (1928) showed that, although the concentration of chloride in the CSF was quite definitely below normal in meningitis, so was that of the plasma, the ratio concentration in CSF/concentration in plasma being hardly altered (1.12 in normal subjects and 1.11 to 1.16 in meningitis). A more extensive investigation of S. L. Wright et al. (1930) and of Fremont-Smith et al. (1931) led to the same conclusion, the mean normal ratio obtained by the last-mentioned authors being 1.16 whilst in various meningitic conditions it was 1.13 to 1.18, although in all the conditions the absolute value of the chloride concentration in the CSF was low (372–422 mg/100 ml compared with the normal average of 440 mg/100 ml). This contradiction was shown by Bradbury *et al.* (1963) to be illusory, however, since the value of the normal Cl⁻ ratio depends on the absolute level of this ion in the plasma. Thus, when the plasma concentration was low in normal human subjects, the value of R_{CSF} tended to be higher than the average (Fig. 42), so that the finding of a "normal" value of R_{CSF} in patients with a low plasma Cl⁻ was, in fact, an indication that the concentration of Cl⁻ in the CSF of these patients was pathologically low. Thus, when the concentration of Cl⁻ in the CSF is plotted against concentration of Cl⁻ in plasma, it becomes at once clear from Fig. 42 that the meningitis patients (open circles) have values of CSF Cl⁻ that are below the average, and their values of R_{CSF} are, in fact, low by comparison with normal subjects with corresponding low plasma Cl⁻.

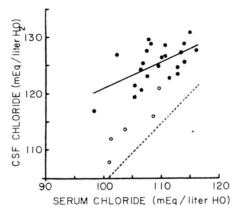

Fig. 42.   Chloride in CSF as a function of serum chloride. Full circles and line normal human subjects; open circles and broken line, patients with T. B. meningitis. (Bradbury *et al.*, 1963.)

2. *Potassium*

If Cohen's Law is to be strictly applied, we may expect a rise in the concentration of potassium in the CSF in meningitis. In a group of humans, Kral *et al.* (1929) found an average ratio of 0.54 for the distribution of potassium, and in two cases of meningitis the ratios were 0.58 and 0.30. On the other hand, Lowenthal (1954) has found what appears to be a definite correlation between the concentration of potassium in the CSF and the concentration of protein; thus, with protein concentrations less than 19 mg/100 ml, the potassium concentration was 2.90 mEq/liter;

with protein concentrations between 60 and 200 mg/100 ml, the potassium concentration was 3.46 mEq/liter, and with protein concentrations between 200 and 500 mg/100 ml, the potassium concentration was some 4.35 mEq/liter. A similar correlation, moreover, had been reported by Ragazzini (1952).

3. Calcium and Magnesium

According to Hunter and Smith (1960), the behavior of these alkali earth cations is in accordance with Cohen's Law. Mg^{++}, it will be recalled, is, in the fluids of most species, in higher concentration than would be expected of a plasma dialysate, while the concentration of Ca^{++} is lower; the normal values and those for tubercular meningitis are shown in Table XIII.

TABLE XIII

CONCENTRATIONS OF Ca^{++} AND Mg^{++} IN LUMBAR, CISTERNAL, AND VENTRICULAR FLUIDS IN NORMAL AND T.B. MENINGITIC HUMAN SUBJECTS [a]

	Calcium (mEq/liter)			Magnesium (mEq/liter)		
	Lumbar	Cisternal	Ventricular	Lumbar	Cisternal	Ventricular
Normal	2.32	2.24	2.28	2.20	2.14	2.24
Meningitic	2.7	2.4	2.25	1.66	2.02	2.08

[a] Hunter and Smith (1960).

4. Bromide

The steady-state level of bromide in the CSF is lower than in a plasma dialysate; thus, in man the value of R_{CSF} is 0.37; as indicated earlier, the evidence suggests that the low concentration in the fluid is determined by active transport outwards across the choroid plexuses and if Ahmed and Van Harreveld's work (1969) on ^{131}I may be extended to bromide, by an active transport across the capillaries of the brain and cord. In meningitis the value of R_{CSF} rises, and the phenomenon is the basis of the "Bromide Test" of Walter (1925).

C. Direct Exchanges between Blood and Brain

Damage to the brain, such as that caused by x-irradiation, stab wounds, thermocoagulation, and so on, results in the taking up of intravenously injected trypan blue or labeled protein, presumably because the damage is primarily to the capillaries of the central nervous system. It must be appreciated that there are two aspects of this breakdown; an increased permeability will increase the rate at which substances pass out of the vascular system, while damage to the cells will increase the size of the compartment into which the solute may pass. Most studies on uptake of dyes have failed to distinguish between the two. In a quantitative study Bakay *et al.* (1959) showed that, after ultrasonic irradiation of the brain, there was a massive increase in the uptake of trypan blue and $^{32}PO_4$ by the irradiated regions. That the increased uptake of $^{32}PO_4$ revealed a genuine increase in the permeability of the blood–brain barrier to inorganic phosphate, rather than an increased turnover of the isotope in metabolism, is indicated by the linear dependence of the uptake on plasma concentration, a situation that was not found in normal animals. Furthermore, as with other types of injury, it was found that, if the $^{32}PO_4$ was given intracisternally, the damaged region did not take up more isotope than the controls, whereas, as indicated above, increased uptake occurred after intravenous administration (Bakay *et al.*, 1959). As these authors point out, the much more vigorous uptake of $^{32}PO_4$ by tumors, described by Selverstone and Moulton (1957), may well be a reflexion of a defective barrier rather than of increased turnover of ^{32}P alone.[20]

1. *Hypercapnia*

Clemedsen *et al.* (1958) found that inhalation of 7–30% CO_2 caused staining of intravenous injected trypan blue in the brains of rats and guinea pigs. The lesions were associated with hemorrhages, and the remark-

---

[20] Increased uptake by a tumor is not confined to $^{32}PO_4$, but is revealed probably by any substance that does not penetrate the barrier easily; thus, the accumulation of ^{203}Hg-labeled chloromerodin (Neohydrin) may be a reflexion only of a breakdown of the blood-brain barrier. This agent is employed in tumor scanning because it emits a useful gamma radiation that may be detected with considerable accuracy; it accumulates in brain tumors. Other substances are ^{131}I-labeled protein (RISA) or polyvinyl pyrrolidone (Pitlyk *et al.*, 1963); a recent innovation is technetium-99m which has the advantage of a short half-life and emits only gamma radiation (Harper *et al.*, 1964). The general subject has been reviewed by Blahd *et al.* (1965).

able feature was their rapid reversibility on discontinuing the inhalation, so if trypan blue was given intravenously just a few minutes after exposure there was no staining (and there were no hemorrhages observable post mortem). Goldberg *et al.* (1963) exposed cats to 25% CO_2 and showed an increased rate of uptake of $^{35}SO_4$ but not of urea; presumably, this was because the breakdown of the barrier would show up most with a slowly penetrating substance like $^{35}SO_4$ rather than with urea which penetrates more rapidly, and is taken up by all the cells of the brain. When the up-take of labeled albumin was studied, Cutler and Barlow (1966) found that there were pronounced regional differences in uptake, the greatest being by the thalamus, colliculi, and medulla, and the smallest by the white matter and cerebral cortex. In a quantitative study, Cameron *et al.* (1970) showed that, in rabbits, the uptake of ^{14}C-sucrose by the rabbit's brain increased when they inhaled 18% CO_2; the effect was manifest as an increase in *rate of uptake* rather than simply an expanded "sucrose-space", since hypercapnia had no effect on the "sucrose-space" measured by perfusing the ventricles with the labeled sucrose. During the mea-surements, which lasted from 45 minutes to 3 hours, the arterial blood pH decreased from a control value of 7.43 to one of 7.14–7.11, i.e., there was a definite respiratory acidosis. To what extent the effect of hypercap-nia is secondary to the dilatation of the cerebral blood vessels that takes place (Wolff and Lennox, 1930) is not known, but the rapid reversibility of the effect suggests that this is an essential element in the phe-nomenon.[21]

D. RATE OF SECRETION OF CEREBROSPINAL FLUID

To the extent that the sink-action of cerebrospinal fluid on the compo-sition of the brain extracellular fluid, or the reverse, is important we may expect modifications of the rate of secretion of CSF to influence the steady-state levels of solutes in the various compartments. In this respect the effects of inhibitors of secretion are of interest, but much more so by virtue of the light the effects of inhibitors may throw on the mechanism of secretion. Since the composition of the extracellular fluid is controlled

[21] Most of the insults to the central nervous system employed for studying a break-down of the blood–brain barrier lead to the condition of cerebral edema, a subject on which a large literature has accumulated. The interested reader may be referred to the monograph of Bakay and Lee (1965) and the symposium edited by Klatzo and Seitel-berger (1967).

by active processes, we may expect inhibitors of secretion of CSF to have some influence on the flow of this extracellular fluid if, as argued by Bering and Sato (1963), Reed and Woodbury (1963), and Pollay and Curl (1967), there is, indeed, a continuous bulk interchange between extracellular fluid and CSF; in addition, an inhibition of the active transport processes might be expected to modify the concentrations of such ions as K^+ in the extracellular fluid.

1. *Acetazoleamide*

The rate of secretion of CSF may be reduced by the carbonic anhydrase inhibitor, acetazoleamide, or Diamox. After intravenous injection there is a reduction of about 60% in the rate, as determined by the rate of drip from the cisterna magna (Tschirgi *et al.*, 1954) or by dilution of inulin in the perfused ventricles (Davson and Pollay, 1963a; Oppelt *et al.*, 1964; Rubin *et al.*, 1966; Cutler *et al.*, 1968b). The inhibition of secretion is accompanied by a reduction in the concentration of chloride in the CSF, so that the value of R_{CSF} fell from 1.17 to 1.13; this is not just due to a more sluggish rate of flow since Davson and Spaziani (1962) found that the concentration in hypothermic rabbits was normal in spite of a considerable reduction in rate of secretion. Associated with the fall in Cl^- there was a rise in HCO_3^- (Davson and Luck, 1957; Kjällquist *et al.*, 1969b). In the freshly secreted fluid, Ames *et al.* (1965b) found no change of concentration; since the high concentration in the CSF seems to be built up later during the fluid's stay in the ventricles, it would seem that Diamox affects this later process, i.e., it may cause a reduction in the concentration in the brain extracellular fluid.

a. Intracellular Acidosis. The inhibition of secretion is in line with the effects of Diamox on other systems, e.g., the bird's salt gland, gastric secretion, formation of the aqueous humour, and so on, but the involvement of carbonic anhydrase in the active transport processes is not always easy to envisage, and it may be, as Maren (1967) has argued, that the effect is obtained by modification of the composition of the cell's internal pH, the abnormality of this reducing the secretory cell's power for active transport of such ions as Na^+ and Cl^-. In support of this is the finding of Kjällquist *et al.* (1970) that Diamox causes a large reduction in the CO_2-buffering capacity of the brain, a reduction that they attribute to an inhibition of the active removal of H^+ from the cells. Thus, the cells of the brain would be suffering from an "intracellular acidosis" that might well affect their powers of carrying out other functions; if the effects extended to the cells of the choroid plexuses, the influence on secretion of CSF might become intelligible.[22]

2. Other Drugs and Hormones

Table XIV shows the effects of a variety of agents, which are known to affect active transport in other systems, on rate of secretion of cerebrospinal fluid in the rabbit; many of these, such as ouabain, spirolactone, amiloride, amphotericin, and vasopressin, caused a significant reduction

TABLE XIV

EFFECTS OF VARIOUS INHIBITORS ON THE RATE OF SECRETION OF CSF[a]

Inhibitor	n	Secretion rate (μl/min)	Inhibition (%)	P
Control	23	12.9 ± 0.7		
Diamox	10	4.6 ± 1.1	64	> 0.001
Ouabain	6	5.8 ± 0.7	55	> 0.001
Diamox + ouabain	7	4.0 ± 0.5	69	> 0.001
Spirolactone	5	3.7 ± 0.8	71	> 0.001
Amiloride	8	6.4 ± 0.9	50	> 0.001
Amphotericin	10	3.8 ± 0.8	70	> 0.001
Vasopressin	8	6.4 ± 0.7	50	> 0.001
Choline chloride	6	9.6 ± 1.1	26	0.05
18% CO_2	5	10.0 ± 1.6	22	0.1
Puromycin	5	11.0 ± 1.0	8	0.3
Actinomycin D	5	12.7 ± 1.4	1	0.9
Cycloheximide	5	10.4 ± 1.4	19	0.2

[a] Limits are S.E. n equals number of animals. P is the probability that the observed difference would have occurred by chance (Davson and Segal, 1971).

in rate of secretion, although it is interesting that Domer (1969a) found that the *anti*-aldosterone, spironolactone, *increased* the rate of secretion in the cat. Of other diuretics studied by Domer in addition to Diamox, aminometradine, mersalyltheophylline, hydrochlorothiazide, chlorothia-

[22] Shaywitz et al. (1969) point out that Diamox does not affect the dynamics of the CSF in very young animals, and this is because their brains (choroid plexuses and glial cells) do not contain carbonic anhydrase.

zide, triamterine, and ethacrynic acid, all caused significant inhibition.[23]
In Table XV the effects of the same drugs on the rate of equilibration of
^{22}Na with the brain are shown, and it is remarkable that the differences are insignificant. This is a surprising finding since one might expect the control processes, postulated to account for the homeostasis in
the composition of both cerebrospinal and extracellular fluids, would be

TABLE XV

EFFECTS OF VARIOUS INHIBITORS ON THE PENETRATION OF ^{22}Na FROM THE BLOOD INTO
THE BRAIN DURING 75 MINUTES OF VENTRICULO-CISTERNAL PERFUSION [a]

Inhibitor	n	Equilibration achieved at 75 min (%)	Difference (%)	P
Control	23	24.10 ± 0.96		
Diamox	5	22.26 ± 1.37	—8.3	0.25
Ouabain	6	21.62 ± 1.85	—10.3	0.15
Diamox + ouabain	7	21.16 ± 0.94	—12.2	0.05
Spirolactone	5	21.24 ± 0.86	—11.9	0.10
Amiloride	7	24.19 ± 1.62	—0.4	0.75
Amphotericin B	9	23.78 ± 0.79	—1.3	0.5
Vasopressin	7	78.47 ± 1.57	+18.1	0.08
Choline	6	20.80 ± 1.41	—13.7	0.05
18% CO_2	5	24.2 ± 1.90	+0.4	
Puromycin	5	24.0 ± 1.1	—0.4	0.2
Actinomycin D	5	21.0 ± 0.9	—12.9	0.1
Cycloheximide	5	23.4 ± 1.8	—0.3	0.5

[a] Limits are S.E. n equals number of animals. P is the probability that the observed
difference would have occurred by chance (Davson and Segal, 1971).

affected by the same agents. So far as the turnover of ^{22}Na in the brain
is concerned, however, these drugs have little or no influence, by contrast
with their inhibition of the secretion of CSF. It may be, then, as argued by
Davson and Segal (1971), that the exchanges of Na$^+$ across the blood–
brain barrier do not involve a flow of fluid, as postulated by Bering and

[23] Domer (1969a) also studied the effects of diuretics on the rate of passage of ^{42}K
into the perfused ventricle; inhibition of secretion was not necessarily associated with a
reduced influx of the isotope. In this connection it may be mentioned that Domer (1969b)
found that intra-arterial histamine increased the influx of ^{42}K from blood to perfusion
fluid, an effect that was blocked by diphenylhydramine.

Sato and Pollay and Curl. Thus, exchanges of Na^+ doubtless involve active transport, and as such are probably inhibited by poisons such as ouabain, but because the net flow of ions from blood to extracellular fluid is negligible, inhibition of the processes controlling the exchange of Na^+ will not necessarily be revealed as a measurable alteration in the rate of equilibration of ^{22}Na between blood and the tissue. Thus, the concentration of Na^+ in the red cell is controlled by active transport, but inhibition of this by ouabain does not bring about a marked inhibition of the exchange of ^{22}Na between the outside and inside of the cell. With the CSF, or the fluid secreted by the salt gland of the bird, on the other hand, the active transport of Na^+ is involved in a net flow of the ion, and water, from blood to the secretions. Inhibition of this may be expected to reduce the influx of ^{22}Na from blood into these secretions, as indeed, it does. Hence, the results on the effects of inhibitors rather favor the presence of a stagnant extracellular fluid in the central nervous parenchyma, and this is consistent with the dynamics of the barriers, as analyzed by Welch (1969), which postulate the absence of significant flow between parenchyma and CSF.

3. Pressure

When outflow from the ventricles is blocked, large pressures associated with expansion of the cavities may develop, and it is of interest to determine whether these pressures eventually reduce the rate of secretion of CSF. In general, the studies of Heisey et al. (1962) and of later workers, e.g., Cutler et al. (1968b), using the perfused ventricles for study of rate of secretion, revealed no reduction in rate when the pressure was experimentally varied from a negative value to 20 cm H_2O. In animals made hydrocephalic experimentally by injection of kaolin into the cisterna magna, a procedure that blocked communication between ventricles and subarachnoid space, Hochwald et al. (1969) found that rate of production of CSF, as measured by dilution of fluid perfused from one lateral ventricle to the other, was reduced from a control value of 15 to one of 2.7 $\mu l/$ minute; in dogs, a value of 33.3 $\mu l/$minute was obtained which compares with Bering and Sato's value of 47 $\mu l/$minute for normal dogs. Histologically Hochwald et al. showed that there was destruction and denudement of the cells lining the choroid plexuses and ventricular wall, so that it seems likely that the effects are not so much a reduction of secretion by virtue of an opposed hydrostatic pressure but by destruction of the secretory organs. When the hydrocephalus was due to vitamin A deficiency in calves, however, Calhoun *et al.* (1967a, b) found no significant change in rate of secretion; this ruled out an excess secretion as a causative factor in the hydrocephalus as well as showing that the high pressures developed in the ventricles (up to 50 cm H_2O) do not *reduce* secretion.

XX. Ontogeny of the Blood–Brain Barrier

The ontogenetic development of the blood–brain barrier is obviously related to the development of the CSF as a characteristic secretion, so that any information on this aspect of the cerebrospinal system will be just as relevant as information on the changes in the kinetics of passage of material from blood into the nervous tissue. Unfortunately, there are only scattered studies bearing on the ontogenetic aspects of the cerebrospinal system, and most of these are only of a qualitative kind.

A. DRAINAGE ROUTE

Thus, Weed's classical study (1917) on pig embryos was devoted to showing that the stage when the choroid plexuses develop, about the 14-mm embryo, corresponds to the stage when Prussian blue reagents are able to escape from the medullary tube into the adjacent mesenchyme, i.e., it seemed that some form of drainage mechanism developed at the point when bulk formation of fluid began, and he suggested that the specialized thinning of the roof of the wall of the IVth ventricle—the area membranacea inferior—was actually ruptured by the developing pressure resulting from secretion of CSF.[24] Similar results were described by H. Cohen and Davies (1937, 1938) in chick embryos although in several

---

[24] Brocklehurst (1969) has examined human embryos with a view to following the development of communication between the internal and external cerebrospinal fluids. This seems to occur between the seventh and eighth weeks, the inferior membranaceous area showing imperfections at this stage and allowing the passage of dextrans, etc., into the subarachnoid spaces after injection into the ventricle. The lateral connections, corresponding to the foramina of Luschka, only appear at 26 weeks. The view that the developing pressure ruptures the roof of the fourth ventricle is not supported by Brocklehurst, and he shows that the suggestion that spina bifida might arise through failure of the development of communication between internal and external fluids is unsound since the condition may occur in embryos as small as 5 and 7 mm, i.e., immediately after the time for normal neuropore closure and before the development of the choroid plexuses (Lemire *et al.*, 1965; Patten, 1953).

other species, including the rabbit, this coincidence between development of the plexuses and of communication between the internal and external fluids was not observed.

B. Blood–Brain Uptake

So far as direct uptake of material from blood is concerned, Behnsen (1926, 1927) observed that trypan blue, injected into young mice, was accumulated extensively in the nervous tissue, and he concluded that the blood–brain barrier was not fully developed in these immature animals. In very young animals the staining of the central nervous system was extensive, and it was only by the seventh to eighth week that the staining picture became indistinguishable from that in the adult animal. Behnsen considered that the defects in the blood–brain barrier manifest in the young mouse were essentially exaggerations of those normally observed in the adult, in the sense that they were expansions of those localized areas, like the area postrema, that normally permit the dyestuff to leave the blood stream. Stern and Peyrot (1927) arrived at an essentially similar conclusion as a result of their studies of the uptake of Prussian blue reagents by the brains of the rabbit, rat, mouse, cat, and dog, the uptake being extensive at birth and decreasing until the eyes opened when the adult picture was obtained. The guinea pig was an exception in showing adult features at birth, presumably because of its more advanced state of development, since a study of fetal animals showed that only when their lids were still sealed and their hair was undeveloped, would penetration from blood to CSF and nervous tissue occur.

1. Kernicterus

Again, Spatz (1934) attributed the frequent association of kernicterus, i.e., jaundice of the brain nuclei, with hemolytic and other forms of jaundice in the newborn to the immaturity of the blood–brain barrier in the human fetus. Thus, in the jaundiced adult the brain, except for the dura, is free from bilirubin whereas in the jaundiced newborn infant the brain as well as other tissues is usually stained.

2. Quantitative Studies

More quantitative studies were carried out by Bakay (1953) on the uptake of $^{32}PO_4$ by the brains of fetal and postnatal rabbits; these showed a steady decrease in the uptake, 24 hours after injection into the blood-stream, on progressing from fetal animals to the seventh postnatal week when the uptake corresponded with the adult value. In a later study, Bakay (1960) found a greater uptake of ^{24}Na by the fetal kitten's brain than the mother's after allowance was made for the much smaller activity in the fetal blood resulting from the blood–placental barrier. Other studies along the same lines are those of Roberts *et al.* (1959) on the flux of ^{14}C-glutamic acid, of Kuttner *et al.* (1961) on the metabolically inert α-aminoisobutyric acid, and of Lajtha (1957) on Cl$^-$ and CNS$^-$, and their results agree in attributing greater uptakes by fetal or young animals than in the adult.

3. *Metabolic Fate*

As Dobbing (1968), has emphasized, however, great care must be taken in the interpretation of this kind of study since the fetal and early postnatal brain is undergoing rapid changes that are reflected in higher metabolism and in alterations in the sizes of the water and solute compartments. Thus, the uptake of ^{32}PO$_4$ by brain, although doubtless its rate is governed by the blood–brain barrier, in total amount reflects incorporation into the organic phosphates. A highly metabolic tissue will incorporate more labeled phosphate, and more rapidly, than a less metabolic one. Thus, it would be more convincing evidence in favor of a developing barrier if the uptake after intraventricular injection remained the same and independent of age.

4. *Extracellular Space*

With ions such as Cl$^-$ and Na$^+$ the uptake will be influenced by the volume of the extracellular space, and since this decreases with age during fetal and early postnatal life, allowance for this must be made. The study of Vernadakis and Woodbury (1965) takes into account these changes in morphology. They confirmed the decrease in chloride space with development described by Vernadakis and Woodbury (1962); they showed that there was a progressive decrease in rate of equilibration of ^{35}Cl and ^{14}C-inulin with brain in the rat. The changes from the 8- to the 32-day-old animals are shown in Fig. 43; analysis of the curves indicated half-lives of 315, 135 and 120 minutes for 32-, 17-, and 8-day-old rats, respectively, so that there has been not only a decrease in inulin space but also in the rate of equilibration of inulin with this space.

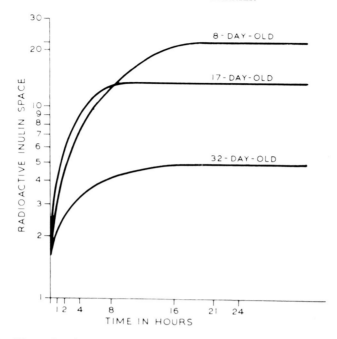

Fig. 43. Illustrating decrease in inulin space with increasing age of rats. Individual curves show increase in volume of distribution in brain with time after a single parenteral injection. (Davson, 1967, after Vernadakis and Woodbury, 1965.)

5. Sink Action of CSF

However, we have seen that the steady-state inulin space, obtained when a constant level of inulin has been maintained in the blood for a long time, is not a measure of the true volume of distribution, because of the sink-action of the CSF. Thus, a smaller sink action due to, say, a slower rate of secretion, could account for the effect of immaturity. Hence, a constant blood–brain barrier, but a variable rate of secretion and a variable extracellular space, as revealed by the choride and sodium spaces might well account for the observations. This scepticism is demanded by the observations of Gröntoft (1954), Grazier and Clemente (1957), and Millen and Hess (1958), all of whom were unable to confirm the staining of the brain by trypan blue in fetal animals.[25] In a more recent

[25] Millen and Hess (1958) found that the barrier to trypan blue in 2-8 day-old rats was just as effective as in adults; Grazier and Clemente made their injections through the wall of the maternal uterus and found no penetration into the central nervous system even in animals 12 days after conception. Gröntoft's studies were on dead human fetuses using Broman's technique (1950) of intra-arterial perfusion of trypan blue.

study, however, Ferguson and Woodbury (1969) have followed uptake of ^{14}C inulin and ^{14}C sucrose into both brain and CSF of developing rats and have discussed their results in terms of a steadily decreasing extracellular space, a variable sink action of the CSF and a variable blood–brain barrier to the solutes. There is little doubt that at the earliest stage studied, namely, 4 days before birth, the blood–CSF barrier is considerably reduced so that the concentration in the CSF nearly reaches the plasma concentration after about 24 hours. Such a situation might be expected were the CSF being formed as a simple filtrate of plasma at this early stage. In these animals the inulin space for brain was some 30%, and this doubtless corresponded with the extracellular space which is high in the fetal animal (Brizzee and Jacobs, 1959). With increasing age, both rate of equilibration and absolute steady-state level decreased, and the results are consistent with an increasing barrier leading to more effective sink-action by the CSF, associated with a real decrease in extracellular space until the adult value of 13.5% is reached (Woodward *et al.*, 1967).[26]

C. Chemical Composition of Cerebrospinal Fluid

We have seen that the cerebrospinal fluid is characteristically different from a dialysate of plasma, a difference that is attributable to active transport processes involved in the elaboration of the fluid. It is reasonable, because of the close relationships between brain extracellular fluid and CSF, to assume that ontogeny of the compositions of the CSF will parallel that of the blood–brain barrier since this latter is a reflexion of the active processes controlling the composition of the extracellular fluid.

1. *Cl⁻ and Urea*

Flexner (1938) selected as characteristic features of the CSF the chloride and urea concentrations, the one being larger than that required of a dialysate of plasma and the other less. In the pig, embryos of 3.5 to 5.5 cm length gave concentrations corresponding roughly with those in a plasma dialysate, but at 6 to 7 cm the value of R_{CSF} for Cl⁻ was 1.17 and for urea 0.85; at 10–15 cm the ratio for Cl⁻ had reached 1.29. We may note that Ames *et al.* (1964) found that the concentration of Cl⁻ in the

---

[26] Luciano (1968) showed that the water and sodium contents of newborn rat brain were 88.8% and 71 mEq/kg wt. compared with 78.8% and 47 mEq/kg wt. in the adult. The kinetics of uptake of ^{24}Na indicated a more rapid uptake by the newborn animal.

CSF freshly secreted by the choroid plexus was much lower than that obtained in bulk from the cisterna magna, suggesting that the high concentration is reached by virtue of exchanges with the extracellular fluid of the brain, i.e., that the brain is more responsible for the secretory process that causes the concentration to be high than the choroid plexuses. If this is true, then Flexner's results reflect on the ontogeny of the development of secretory activity in the parenchyma rather than the choroid plexuses.

2. Na^+, K^+, and Cl^-

Figure 44 shows the progressive changes in R_{CSF} for Cl^-, Na^+, and K^+ in the growing rat obtained by Ferguson and Woodbury (1969). Here the most striking change is that for the K^+ distribution ratio, which falls from the dialysis value of about 0.94 in the fetal animal to about 0.6 in the adult.

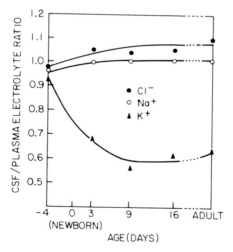

Fig. 44. Plot of CSF/plasma electrolyte concentration ratios at various ages. (Ferguson and Woodbury, 1969.)

3. K^+, Ca^{++}, and Mg^{++}

Bito and Myers (1970) studied the changes in concentration of K, Ca, and Mg in the CSF of the rhesus monkey from 50 days of intrauterine life to the adult. The study is especially valuable since they analyzed fluid from several loci, namely, the spinal subarachnoid space, the cisterna magna, the cortical subarachnoid space, and the lateral ventricles. As indicated earlier, the cortical subarachnoid fluid has a considerably lower concentration of K^+ than that from the other loci; with Mg the cortical fluid is greater in concentration than that in the cisternal. Thus, with both ions the secretory processes that cause the concentrations to be discrepant from those required for equilibrium have been more active by the time the fluid has reached the cortical subarachnoid space, and this reflects secretory activity on the part of the brain tissue, the fluid secreted by the choroid plexuses having, presumably, concentrations that are not so far removed from equilibrium. As the fluid passes through the cerebrospinal system exchanges with extracellular fluid take place leading to losses of K and gains of Mg. Figure 45 shows that the cisternal R_{CSF} for K decreases to reach its adult value of about 0.6 at some 360 days.

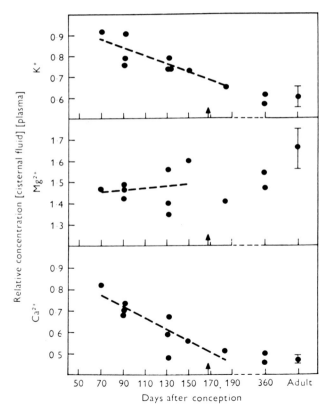

Fig. 45. Changes in the value of R_{CSF} for K^+, Mg^{++}, and Ca^{++} in the developing monkey. (Bito and Myers, 1970.)

The Mg ratio is already high at the earliest stage studied and increases less dramatically. The large changes in R_{CSF} for Ca may be related to the protein content of the fluid since a large fraction of the Ca is bound to protein. Of some interest is the development of the cortical/cisternal gradient of concentration, and this is shown in Fig. 46. During fetal life this gradient does not exist, and the large change occurs some time between 190 days, i.e., in the 3-week-old infant, and adulthood. By contrast,

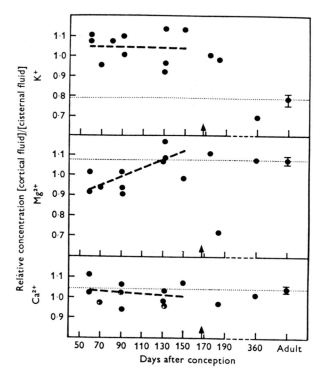

Fig. 46. Changes in the cisternal-cortical gradient of concentration of K+, Mg++, and Ca++ with development in the monkey. (Bito and Myers, 1970.)

the cortical/cisternal gradient for Mg shows a significant increase during the second trimester of gestation, reaching the adult value by the 120th day of fetal life.

To return to the situation with K+, we may note that the distribution ratio for the earliest fetuses studied, namely, 50 days after conception, is the same as for dialysis of adult plasma, and so at this stage there is no evidence for secretory activity. As Fig. 45 shows, the value of R_{CSF} for

K$^+$ does not reach its adult value until after birth; however, if the *absolute concentration* in CSF is considered, rather than the ratio R_{CSF}, it is found that the adult concentration is reached by about 130 days after conception, i.e., before birth. This is because the plasma K decreases with age, and the finding that the adult concentration in CSF is achieved early means that the homeostatic mechanism that ensures that the CSF concentration is largely independent of plasma concentration is operative at this early stage.

In general, this study of Bito and Myers establishes the earliness with which secretory activity occurs in the cerebrospinal system. Since such activity is inconceivable without a corresponding development of the blood–brain barrier, this work shows that, in primates at any rate, "barrier activity" occurs at an early embryonic stage.

D. Secretory Processes

A characteristic feature of the choroid plexus is its power of accumulating iodide against a concentration gradient *in vivo* or *in vitro*. Robinson *et al.* (1968b) have shown that this feature develops very early in fetal cats and rabbits. In the earliest fetuses studied (7–10 days preterm in rabbits and 1–2 days preterm in cats) *in vitro* accumulation of iodide was as great as in adult choroid plexuses; interestingly, higher tissue/medium ratios were found in late fetal plexuses than in adult ones. Sulphate is also accumulated by the isolated plexus, and significant accumulation of this anion developed later, at 1–3 days after birth.

Again, the rate of secretion may be expected to increase with development; Shaywitz *et al.* (1969) found that this increased from 3.3 μliters/minute in 20-day kittens to 11.3 at 8 weeks old and to 17.1 in adults. Associated with this development there was a large drop in efflux of ^{24}Na from the ventricles, presumably associated with a decrease in passive permeability of the choroid plexuses and brain capillaries to sodium.[27]

E. Morphology

The morphology of the developing rabbit and human choroid plexuses has been reviewed recently by Tennyson and Pappas (1968); the devel-

---

[27] Bures (1957) has shown that the dc potential between the surface of the rat's cortex and the sciatic nerve is only 1.3 mV at 5 days old but reaches its adult value of about 6 mV by 15 days.

opment in the chick has been described by Meller and Wechsler (1965). According to Kappers (1958), the development may be divided into three stages in man, and corresponding stages were described by Tennyson and Pappas, in the rabbit. In the first phase, at about 6 weeks, the choroid plexus is represented by a simple fold into the lateral ventricle consisting of pseudostratified epithelium; the stroma is filled with developing blood cells and strands of angioblasts forming capillaries. The second phase appears at about 8 weeks when the plexus becomes lobular and occupies almost the whole ventricle; at this stage the epithelium consists of a single layer of low columnar cells containing glycogen. The third period occurs when the fetus is in its fourth month; the choroid plexus decreases in volume in relation to the ventricle; most of the epithelial cells still contain glycogen, but some cuboidal cells resembling the mature epithelium have appeared. According to the electron-microscopical study of Tennyson and Pappas, stage 2 is accompanied by an increase in number of microvilli on the epithelial cells, as well as in the infoldings and interdigitations of the basal regions of adjacent cells. Stage III is associated with a reduction in the number of microvilli while the basal infoldings become less complex. Meller and Wechsler (1965), in their study of the chick, suggest that the early signs of development in the epithelial cells are related to the requirement for *absorption* from the primitive CSF. Only later does the secretion of fluid become important, and this is associated with the microvilli and lateral interdigitations. In this connection we may note that Smith *et al.* (1964) observed that early chick embryonic plexuses actively absorbed labeled proteins.

XXI. Special Regions of the Brain

Certain regions of the brain are stained by trypan blue after intravenous injection, namely, the posterior lobe of the hypophysis, the tuber cinereum, the area postrema, the epiphysis or pineal body, the paraphysis, the wall of the optic recess and the eminentia saccularis of the hypophyseal stem. In these localized regions the blood–brain barrier seems to be defective. They are highly specialized areas of tissue not sharing the functions of the rest of the parenchyma. The vascular pattern in these regions is markedly different from that in nervous tissue proper, the outstanding feature being the presence of numerous sinusoidal blood vessels, with no apparent perivascular glial sheath but surrounded by dense argyrophile connective tissue sheaths. More modern studies, in which such solutes as $^{32}PO_4$ (Bakay, 1951, 1952), ^{82}Br (Gruner *et al.*, 1951), sulpha-guanidine and *N*-acetyl-4-amino-antipyrine (Brodie *et al.*, 1960) were studied, have generally confirmed the more rapid rate of penetration into these specialized regions, but the morphological feature of the blood vessels or their glial linings that deprives them of their barrier action has only recently been demonstrated. Thus Luse (1962), on the basis of her electron microscope study of the brain, was unable to point to a distinguishing feature of the capillaries of the nonneural regions; the existence of connective tissue spaces round the vessels was thought to be significant but Bodenheimer and Brightman (1968) showed that the cerebral capillaries of the urodele have large collagen-containing spaces around them, similar to those in the area postrema of higher vertebrates, but they failed to allow horseradish peroxidase to pass out, so that the mere occurrence of a pericapillary space is not necessarily coincident with the absence of a blood–brain barrier.

A. Fenestrated Capillaries

Hashimoto (1966) and Rivera-Pomar (1966) have shown that the capillaries of the area postrema are, in fact, fundamentally different from those of the brain proper in so far as they are fenestrated, like those in the choroid plexuses and in many endocrine organs. Thus, as described by Hashimoto and Hama (1968), the endothelial cells are attenuated to give typical diaphragms or pores some 700–800 Å in diameter; intravenously injected horseradish peroxidase was said to exude through these pores as in the choroid plexus. As noted by others, the basement membranes of the capillary endothelial cells are separated from the basement membrane of the adjacent glial cells by quite large spaces to give a system of perivascular spaces not seen in brain tissue proper; the horseradish peroxidase was seen distributed throughout these spaces. The astrocytic end-feet surround the capillary of the area postrema as in the rest of the brain, but in the area postrema the end-feet rest on the outer layer of basement membrane so that there is the large perivascular space between the astroglial lining and the endothelium, by contrast with the situation in brain proper where the basement membranes of endothelial cell and astrocytic end-feet are in close apposition. According to Rivera-Pomar, gaps in the astroglial lining provide direct communication between the perivascular space and the neuropil.

B. Ependymal Specialization

It was observed by Woollard (1924) and Mandelstamm and Krylow (1928) that when trypan blue was introduced into the CSF the specialized areas failed to stain; this was attributed by Davson (1956) to the rapid removal by the capillaries here which would be able to do so precisely because they lacked a blood–brain barrier. An additional factor, however, may be the modification of the ependyma in these regions; thus, Reese and Brightman (1968) showed that the cells of the ependyma adjacent to the median eminence are connected laterally by tight junctions and thus restrict the movement of trypan blue—at any rate of horseradish peroxidase. The development of these junctions in these regions serves to maintain the insulation of the bulk of the parenchyma from unrestricted access of materials from the blood. Without this modification, substances could pass out of the blood in these regions without restraint; they would then pass into the CSF and so gain access to other regions.

XXII. Peripheral Nerve

Early experimenters[28] on isolated peripheral nerve observed that the effects of changing the medium on the electrical characteristics were not immediate; thus to cause conduction block by removal of Na^+ requires

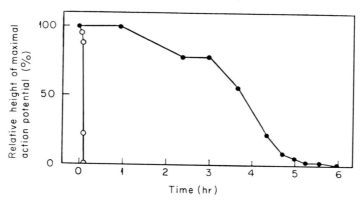

Fig. 47. Comparison of rate of loss of conduction in a frog sciatic nerve perfused with a Na-free, isotonic choline chloride solution, and in a control nerve placed in the same solution. ○—○, perfused nerve; ●—●, control nerve. (Krnjevic, 1954.)

---

[28] References to the classical literature on this point, dating from Bunzen in 1807, have been summarized by Krnjevic (1954).

hours (Fig. 47), although the time required for passive diffusion from the extracellular fluid would be of the order of minutes. This is presumably due to the presence of a low-permeability sheath separating the nerve fibers from the surrounding medium since Feng, for example, showed that the time required for blocking agents to exert their effects could be considerably reduced by slitting the sheath. Later studies of Feng and Liu (1949), Rashbass and Rushton (1949), Crescitelli (1951), Huxley and Stämpfli (1951), and Krnjevic (1954) have confirmed that the sheath of nerve constitutes a barrier to exchange with an outside medium, a barrier that may reduce the effective diffusion coefficient of K^+, for example, by a factor of 30 compared with that in free solution.

A. PERINEURIUM

The only matter of conjecture has been the anatomical identity of this barrier; thus, some investigators considered that the desheathed nerve was intact but for the removal of the connective-tissue epineurium, but Krnjevic showed that, in fact, the epineurium was also removed and he argued that it is this structure, rather than the epineurium, that is responsible for the barrier to diffusion of solutes from the intercellular spaces of the nerve fibers to the outside medium, i.e., the extracellular fluid of epineurium and adjacent tissue innervated by the nerve. As Shantha and Bourne (1968) have pointed out in Vol. I of this treatise, the terminology relating to the coverings of the individual fibers, and groups of fibers, constituting a peripheral nerve is confusing, but the important layer, histologically, seems to be the perineurium, namely, the epithelial layer surrounding a small bundle of fibers. As the bundle branches to produce smaller bundles with fewer and fewer fibers the perineurium divides, too, becoming thinner but remaining as an intact cellular covering to the fibers. By the time a single fiber is reached the perineurium appears as a single-celled layer while the endoneurium, beneath it, has largely disappeared. This ultimate sheath is often called the sheath of Henle[29] but is better described, in the motor fiber, as the bell mouth of Henle. The relations of epi-, peri-, and endoneurium are illustrated in Fig. 48. According to Shanthaveerappa and Bourne (1962), the perineurium is the direct continuation of the arachnoid membrane, which covers the nerve roots as they leave the cord and proceed peripherally, and as such it may be expected to constitute a barrier between the blood supply of

---

[29] The structure described as Henle's sheath is, in fact, the endoneurium and tends to disappear by the time the single fiber is reached.

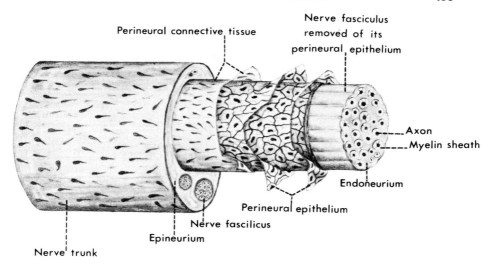

Fig. 48. Dissection of peripheral nerve showing relation of epi-, peri-, and endo-neurium. (Courtesy Dr. Shantha.)

the epineurium, which is analogous with the dura, and the fluid bathing the individual nerve fibers, which are embedded in endoneurium, in the same way that the arachnoid membrane may be regarded as a barrier between the blood vessels of the dura and the extracellular fluid bathing the central neurons.

B. Blood–Nerve Barrier

The restriction of passage of solutes from the medium to the nerve fibers will only have sense if there is a corresponding restraint on the passage from blood in the capillaries of the vasa nervorum that come into close relationship with the individual nerve fibers, namely, the capillaries that lie beneath the perineurium and are in the endoneurium; i.e., if there is a *blood–nerve barrier* analogous with the blood–brain barrier of the central nervous system. The blood supply to peripheral nerves has been described most recently by Lundborg and Brånemark (1968); essentially the epineurial blood vessels divide into ascending and descending branches which communicate by transverse vessels. These epineurial vessels are connected to the perineurial vessels, but there is no sharp demarcation between these two systems of the outer sheaths. In the perineurium itself there is a plexus of capillaries, arterioles, and venules, and at the entrance and exit of blood vessels to and from the endoneurium they acquire a perineurial sleeve which accompanies the vessel for a short distance into the endoneurium, as originally described by Key and Retzius (1876). Having penetrated into the endoneurium, the vessels branch in such a way as to form a meshwork whose strands run between the individual nerve fibers.

The study of Manery and Bale (1941) on the penetration of ^{24}Na into the various tissues of the body suggested the presence of a barrier between blood and an inner compartment of the nerve. Again, Krnjevic' study (1954), in which he compared the effects of perfusing the frog's limb with Na$^+$-free or K$^+$-rich solutions with corresponding effects on the isolated nerve, showed that there was a definite delay corresponding to some 15 minutes on average for the changed solutions to cause block of the nerve (Fig. 47). Krnjevic computed diffusion coefficients for Na$^+$ and K$^+$ under these conditions of $7.5.10^{-6}$ cm^2/second and $1.5.10^{-5}$ cm^2/second; these values compare with values of $7.8.10^{-4}$ and $9.1.10^{-4}$ cm^2/second for NaCl and KCl in pure water at 18°C and indicate a considerable restraint on passage out of the extracellular fluid, surrounding the fibers, to the blood. We may presume that this reflects restraint on passage into the vessels within the endoneurium (blood–nerve barrier) and restraint across the perineurium and into the blood vessels of the epineurium which, if comparable with those in the dura, exert no barrier action.

1. *Morphology*

That the vessels within the endoneurium are different from those in the epineurium was demonstrated by Olsson (1966), who labeled serum albumin with a fluorescent dye and observed the vessels and adjacent tissue in the fluorescence microscope. The blood vessels within the endoneurium, i.e., those supplying the nerve fibers, were sharply differentiated from those in the epineurium, in that the walls of the latter were strongly fluorescent and those of the former not at all. Furthermore, the tissue of the epineurium contained a large diffuse extravascular fluorescence, indicating escape of labeled protein, and, as Fig. 49 shows, this compares with the space within the endoneurium, where fluorescence can only be found within the lumen of the blood vessels.

2. *Tight Junctions*

A recent study of the capillaries of the endoneurium by Olsson and Reese (1971), using the peroxidase technique, has shown that, as in the central nervous system, the peroxidase was held up at tight junctions that

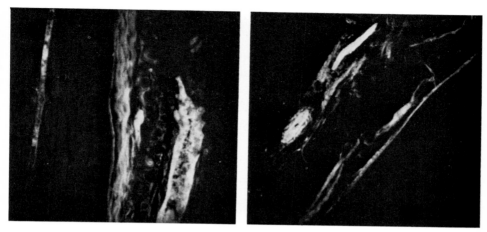

Fig. 49.   Illustrating the distribution of fluorescent albumin in peripheral nerve after intravenous injection. At the left a vast diffuse extravascular fluorescence can be seen in the surrounding connective tissue sheaths in contrast to the endoneurium, where fluorescence can only be found within the lumen of blood vessels. At the right it can be seen that the fluorescence extends to the innermost parts of the external nerve sheaths leaving the endoneurium uninvaded. The arrows mark the localization of the perineurial epithelium. (Olsson, 1966.)

block off the intercellular clefts of the capillary endothelium. By contrast, the epineurial capillaries allowed escape of peroxidase between their endothelial cells whose intercellular clefts were not occluded by tight junctions. The epithelial cells of the perineurium were sealed laterally by tight junctions at which peroxidase, applied to the sheath, was held up. Thus, both functionally and morphologically, the central and peripheral nervous systems seem to be essentially similar, passage from blood to the neuron, be it peripheral or central, being restrained by the tight junctions that seal the capillary endothelial clefts, while passage from dura or its analogue, the epineurium, to the underlying neuron is restrained by tight junctions that seal the clefts between arachnoidal or perineurial epithelial cells.

Appendix*

In the text the idea is developed that because the extracellular fluid bathes the capillaries and the cell membranes and is in turn open to the

* By K. Welch.

CSF which contacts choroid plexuses and arachnoid villi, processes at all these interfaces are coupled. Since the system is quite intractable to the kind of abstraction necessary for the analysis, this is carried out using a geometrically simplified model.

In this treatment consideration is given to a region, $0 < x < l$, bounded by parallel planes and consisting of a continuous and tortuous aqueous medium. At $x = 0$ the slab is backed by its mirror image so that at that plane there is no gradient. At $x = l$ the region is in contact with a fluid which is mixed and is continuously renewed. For that fluid the conservation equation is

$$V \frac{dC_{(l,t)}}{dt} + \frac{DA}{\varrho} \frac{\partial C}{\partial x}\bigg|_{l,t} + V\gamma C_{(l,t)} - V\gamma f C_{\text{Plasma}} = 0 \qquad (1)$$

in which V is the volume of fluid, C is the concentration in the fluid, and D is the coefficient of diffusion. A is the area of interface, ϱ is the tortuosity, $[\partial C/\partial x]_{l,t}$ is the gradient at the interface, γ is the rate constant for renewal of the fluid, C_{Plasma} is a forcing function which corresponds to concentration in circulating plasma and will be taken as a constant, and f is the fraction of C_{Plasma} at which new fluid is formed.

Within the bounded region there is a distributed source which contributes material to unit volume at the rate $\varkappa(C_{\text{Plasma}} - C_{(x,t)})$. Also within that region two states, c and s, are reversibly accessible to the material; c corresponds to extracellular material and is free to diffuse while s corresponds to intracellular material and is immobile. The two are related as follows:

$$\frac{\partial S}{\partial t} = K_i C - K_o S \qquad (2)$$

in which S and C are the amounts of material in the corresponding states, each referred to the volume of distribution of c. The K's are rate constants and include relative volumes of distribution.

The differential equation is

$$\frac{D}{\varrho^2} \frac{\partial^2 C}{\partial x^2} - \frac{\partial C}{\partial t} - \frac{\partial S}{\partial t} - \varkappa C = -\varkappa C_{\text{Plasma}} \qquad (3)$$

Initially, $C_{(x,o)} = 0$. The boundary conditions are $[\partial C/\partial X]_{o,t} = 0$, and at $x = l$ the boundary condition is given by Eq. (1).

The solution is

$$C_{(x,t)} = C_{\text{Plasma}} - \frac{[C_{\text{Plasma}} - fC_{\text{Plasma}}]h\gamma \cosh x\sqrt{\varkappa/D'}}{h\gamma \cosh l\sqrt{\varkappa/D'} + \sqrt{\varkappa/D'} \sinh l\sqrt{K/D'}}$$

$$- hC_{\text{Plasma}} \sum_{n=1}^{\infty} \frac{B_n\{\gamma f\lambda_n^2 + \varkappa/D'(P_n + \gamma)e^{P_n t}\} \cos x\,\lambda_n}{P_n\{\lambda_n^2(l - hB_n) + h(P_n + \gamma)(1 + hl)(P_n + \gamma)\} \cos l\lambda_n} \quad (4)$$

in which $h = V\varrho/DA$, $D/\varrho^2 = D'$ and

$$P_n = \tfrac{1}{2}\{- D'(\lambda_n^2 + \varkappa/D' + K_i/D' + K_0/D')$$
$$\pm [D'^2(\lambda_n^2 + \varkappa/D' + K_0/D' + K_i/D')^2 - 4D'K_0(\lambda_n^2 + K/D')]^{\frac{1}{2}}\}$$

$$B_n = -2D'/(1 + K_iK_0/(P_n + K_0)^2)$$

λ_n, $n = 1, 2, 3 \cdots$ are the roots of

$$\lambda_n \tan \lambda_n l = h(P_n + r) \quad (5)$$

There is thus an infinite series corresponding to each branch of λ_n, P_n, etc., and in connection with one or both there may be an imaginary root $i\lambda = \xi$. This appears when $-P_{n(\lambda=0)} > v$ and replaces the first branch of Eq. (5).

$S_{(x,t)}$ is obtained by multiplying the steady state terms in Eq. (4) by K_i/K_0 and the time-dependent terms by $K_i/(P_n + K_0)$. Average values for C and S are obtained from the appropriate definite integrals.

REFERENCES

Agnew, W. F., and Crone, C. (1967). *Acta Physiol. Scand.* **70**, 68–175.

Ahmed, N., and Van Harreveld, A. (1969). *J. Physiol. (London)* **204**, 31–50.

Ames, A., Sakanoue, M., and Endo, S. (1964). *J. Neurophysiol.* **27**, 672–681.

Ames, A., Higashi, K., and Nesbett, F. B. (1965a). *J. Physiol. (London)* **181**, 506–515.

Ames, A., Higashi, K., and Nesbett, F. B. (1965b). *J. Physiol. (London)* **181**, 516–524.

Ashcroft, G. W., Dow, R. C., and Moir, A. T. B. (1968). *J. Physiol. (London)* **199**, 397–425.

Atkinson, A. J., and Webb, M. F. (1969). *Amer. J. Physiol.* **216**, 1120–1126.

Bakay, L. (1951). *AMA Arch. Neurol. Psychiat.* **66**, 419–426.

Bakay, L. (1952). *AMA Arch. Neurol. Psychiat.* **68**, 629–640.

Bakay, L. (1953). *AMA Arch. Neurol. Psychiat.* **70**, 30–39.

Bakay, L. (1960). *Neurology* **10**, 564–571.

Bakay, L., and Lee, J. C. (1965). "Cerebral Edema." Thomas, Springfield, Illinois.

Bakay, L., Ballantine, H. T., and Bell, E. (1959). *Arch. Neurol. (Chicago)* **1**, 59–67.

Barlow, C. F., Domek, N. S., Goldberg, M. A., and Roth, L. J. (1961). *Arch. Neurol. (Chicago)* **5**, 102–110.

Becker, B. (1961). *Amer. J. Physiol.* **201**, 1149–1151.

Behnsen, G. (1926). *Muench. Med. Wochenschr.* **73**, 1143.

Behnsen, G. (1927). *Z. Zellforsch. Mikrosk. Anat.* **4**, 515–572.

Bekaert, J., and Demeester, G. (1951a). *Arch. Int. Physiol.* **59**, 262–264.

Bekaert, J., and Demeester, G. (1951b). *Arch. Int. Physiol.* **59**, 393–394.

Bekaert, J., and Demeester, G. (1952). *Arch. Int. Physiol.* **60**, 172–175.

Bennett, H. S., Luft, J. H., and Hampton, J. C. (1959). *Amer. J. Physiol.* **196**, 381–390.

Bering, E. A., and Sato, O. (1963). *J. Neurosurg.* **20**, 1050–1063.

Besson, J. M., Woody, C. D., Aleonard, P., Thompson, H. K., Albe-Fessard, D., and Marshall, W. H. (1970). *Amer. J. Physiol.* **218**, 284–291.

Bidder, T. G. (1968). *J. Neurochem.* **15**, 867–874.

Bito, L. Z. (1969). *Science* **165**, 81.

Bito, L. Z., and Davson, H. (1966). *Exp. Neurol.* **14**, 264–280.

Bito, L. Z., and Myers, R. E. (1970). *J. Physiol. (London)* **208**, 153–170.

Bito, L. Z., Bradbury, M. W. B., and Davson, H. (1966a). *J. Physiol. (London)* **185**, 323–354.

Bito, L. Z., Davson, H., Levin, E., Murray, M., and Snider, N. (1966b). *J. Neurochem.* **13**, 1057–1067.

Blahd, W. H., Goldberg, B., and Bauer, F. K. (1965). *In* "Nuclear Medicine" (W. H. Blahd, ed.), pp. 483–511 McGraw-Hill, New York.

Bodenheimer, T. S., and Brightman, M. W. (1968). *Amer. J. Anat.* **122**, 249–267.

Bowyer, F., and Widdas, W. F. (1958). *J. Physiol. (London)* **141**, 219.

Bradbury, M. W. B. (1971). Unpublished data.

Bradbury, M. W. B., and Davson, H. (1964). *J. Physiol. (London)* **170**, 195–211

Bradbury, M. W. B., and Davson, H. (1965). *J. Physiol. (London)* **181**, 151–174.

Bradbury, M. W. B., and Kleeman, C. R. (1967). *Amer. J. Physiol.* **213**, 519–528.

Bradbury, M. W. B., and Stubbs, J. D. (1963). *J. Physiol. (London)* **169**, 106–107.

Bradbury, M. W. B., and Štulcová, B. (1970). *J. Physiol. (London)* **208**, 415–430.

Bradbury, M. W. B., Stubbs, J., Hughes, I. E., and Parker, P. (1963). *Clin. Sci.* **25** 97–105.

Bradley, R. D., and Semple, S. J. G. (1962). *J. Physiol. (London)* **160**, 381–391.

Brightman, M. W. (1965a). *J. Cell Biol.* **26**, 99–123.

Brightman, M. W. (1965b). *Amer. J. Anat.* **117**, 193–220.

Brightman, M. W. (1967). *Progr. Brain Res.* **29**, 19–37.

Brightman, M. W., and Palay, S. L. (1963). *J. Cell Biol.* **19**, 415–439.

Brightman, M. W., and Reese, T. S. (1969). *J. Cell Biol.* **40**, 648–677.

Brizzee, K. R., and Jacobs, L. A. (1959). *Anat. Rec.* **134**, 97–105.

Brocklehurst, G. (1969). *J. Anat.* **105**, 467–475.

Brodie, B. B., Titus, E. O., and Wilson, C. W. M. (1960). *J. Physiol. (London)*, **152**, 20–22.

Broman, T. (1950). *Acta Psychiat. Neurol. Scand.* **25**, 19–31.

Bronstead, H. E. (1969). *Acta Physiol. Scand.* **76**, 32A.

Brooks, C. McC., Kao, F. F., and Lloyd, B. B., eds. (1965). "Cerebrospinal Fluid and the Regulation of Ventilation." Davis, Philadelphia, Pennsylvania.

Bruns, R. R., and Palade, G. E. (1968). *J. Cell Biol.* **37**, 244–276 and 277–299.

Bulat, M., and Supek, Z. (1968). *J. Neurophysiol.* **15**, 383–389.

Bures, J. (1957). *Electroencephalogr. Clin. Neurophysiol.* **9**, 121–130.

Burgess, A., and Segal, M. B. (1970). *J. Physiol. (London)* **208**, 88P–91P.

Caldwell, P. C. (1968). *Physiol. Rev.* **48**, 1–64.

Calhoun, A. M. C., Hurt, H. D., Eaton, H. D., Rousseau, J. E., and Hall, R. C. (1967a). *Amer. J. Dairy Sci.* **50**, 1486.

Calhoun, A. M. C., Hurt, H. D., Eaton, H. D., Rousseau, J. E., and Hall, R. C. (1967b). *Bull. Storrs Agr. Exp. Stat.* **401**, 22.

Cameron, I. R., and Kleeman, C. R. (1970). *J. Physiol. (London)* **207**, 68P–69P.

Cameron, I. R., Davson, H., and Segal, M. B. (1970). *Yale J. Biol. Med.* **42**, 241–247.

Carpenter, S. J. (1966). *J. Comp. Neurol.* **127**, 413–421.

Carver, M. J. (1965). *J. Neurochem.* **12**, 45–50.

Cestan, Sendrail, and Lassalle (1925). *C. R. Soc. Biol.* **93**, 475–478.

Chirigos, M. A., Greengard, P., and Udenfriend, S. (1960). *J. Biol. Chem.* **235**, 2075–2079.

Chutgow, J. G. (1968). *Proc. Soc. Exp. Biol. Med.* **128**, 555–558.

Clara, M. (1953). "Das Nervensystem des Menschen," 2nd ed. Barth, Leipzig.

Clemedson, C. J., Hartelius, H., and Holmberg, G. (1958). *Acta Pathol. Scand.* **42**, 137–149.

Clemente, C. D., and Holst, E. A. (1954). *AMA Arch. Neurol. Psychiat.* **71**, 66–79.

Coben, L. A., and Smith, K. R. (1969). *Exp. Neurol.* **23**, 76–90.

Cohen, H. (1927). *Quart. J. Med.* **20**, 173–186.

Cohen, H., and Davies, S. (1937). *J. Anat.* **72**, 23–52.

Cohen, H., and Davies, S. (1938). *J. Anat.* **72**, 430–455.

Cohen, M. W., Gerschenfeld, H. M., and Kuffler, S. W. (1968). *J. Physiol. (London)* **197**, 363–380.

Cooper, E. S., Lechner, E., and Bellet, S. (1955). *Amer. J. Med.* **18**, 613–621.

Courtice, F. C., and Simmonds, W. J. (1951). *Aust. J. Exp. Biol. Med. Sci.* **29**, 255–263.

Coxon, R. V., and Swanson, A. G. (1965). *J. Physiol. (London)* **181**, 712–727.

Crescitelli, F. (1951). *Amer. J. Physiol.* **166**, 229–240.

Crone, C. (1965). *J. Physiol. (London)* **181**, 103–113.

Csaky, T. Z., and Rigor, B. M. (1968). *Progr. Brain Res.* **29**, 147–158.

Cserr, H. (1965). *Amer. J. Physiol.* **209**, 1219–1226.

Cutler, R. W. P., and Barlow, C. F. (1966). *Arch. Neurol.* **14**, 54–63.

Cutler, R. W. P., Watters, G. V., Hammerstad, J. P., and Merler, E. (1967). *Arch. Neurol.* **17**, 620–628.

Cutler, R. W. P., Lorenzo, A. V., and Barlow, C. F. (1968a). *Arch. Neurol.* **18**, 316–323.

Cutler, R. W. P., Page, L., Gallicich, J., and Watters, G. V. (1968b). *Brain* **91**, 707–720.

Cutler, R. W. P., Robinson, R. J., and Lorenzo, A. V. (1968c). *Amer. J. Physiol.* **214**, 448–454.

Davson, H. (1955a). *J. Physiol. (London)* **129**, 111–133.

Davson, H. (1955b). *J. Physiol. (London)* **128**, 52–53.

Davson, H. (1956). "Physiology of the Ocular and Cerebrospinal Fluids." Churchill, London.

Davson, H. (1958). *Cerebrospinal Fluid; Prod., Circ., Absorption, Ciba Found. Symp.,* 1957, pp. 189–203.

Davson, H. (1963). *Ergeb. Physiol., Biol Chem. Exp. Pharmakol.* **52**, 20–73.

Davson, H. (1967). "Physiology of the Cerebrospinal Fluid." Churchill, London.

Davson, H., and Bradbury, M. B. (1965,a). *Symp. Soc. Exp. Biol.* **19**, 349–364.

Davson, H., and Bradbury, M. (1965b). *In* "Biology of Neuroglia" (E. D. P. De Robertis and R. Carrea eds.), pp. 124–134. Elsevier, Amsterdam.

Davson, H., and Bradbury, M. (1965c). *Progr. Brain Res.* **15**, 124–134.

Davson, H., and. Luck, C. P. (1957). *J. Physiol. (London)* **137**, 279–293.

Davson, H., and Pollay, M. (1963a). *J. Physiol. (London)* **167**, 239–246.

Davson, H., and Pollay, M. (1963b). *J. Physiol. (London)* **167**, 247–255.

Davson, H., and Segal, M. B. (1969). *Brain* **92**, 131–136.

Davson, H., and Segal, M. B. (1971). Unpublished data.

Davson, H., and Segal, M. B. (1971). *J. Physiol. (London)* **209**, 131–153.

Davson, H., and Spaziani, E. (1959). *J. Physiol. (London)* **149**, 135–143.

Davson, H., and Spaziani, E. (1962). *Exp. Neurol.* **6**, 118–128.

Davson, H., Kleeman, C. R., and Levin, E. (1961). *J. Physiol. (London)* **159**, 67–68.

Davson, H., Kleeman, C. R., and Levin, E. (1962). *J. Physiol. (London)* **161**, 126–142.

Davson, H., Kleeman, C. R., and Levin, E. (1963). *In* "Drugs and Membranes" (A. M. Hogben, and P. Lindgren, eds.), pp. 71–94. Pergamon, Oxford.

Davson, H., Hollingsworth, G., and Segal, M. B. (1971). *Brain* **93**, 665–678.

De Robertis, E. D. P. (1965). *Progr. Brain Res.* **15**, 1–11.

Dobbing, J. (1968). *Progr. Brain Res.* **29**, 417–425.

Domer, F. R. (1961). *J. Physiol. (London)* **158**, 366–373.

Domer, F. R. (1969a). *Exp. Neurol.* **24**, 54–64.

Domer, F. R. (1969b). *Exp. Neurol.* **24**, 65–75.

Edström, R. (1958). *Acta Psychiat. Neurol. Scand.* **33**, 403–416.

Ehrlich, P. (1887). *Ther. Monatsh.* **1**, 88–90.

Eidelberg, E., Fishman, J., and Hams, M. L. (1967). *J. Physiol. (London)* **191**, 47–57.

Esser, H., and Heinzler, F. (1952). *Deut. Med. Wochenschr.* **77**, 1329–1330.

Farquhar, M. G., and Palade, G. E. (1963). *J. Cell Biol.* **17**, 375–412.

Fencl, V., Miller, T. B., and Pappenheimer, J. R. (1966). *Amer. J. Physiol.* **210**, 459–472.

Feng, T. P., and Liu, Y. M. (1949). *J. Cell. Comp. Physiol.* **34**, 1–16.

Fenstermacher, J. D., and Johnson, J. A. (1966). *Amer. J. Physiol.* **211**, 341–346.

Ferguson, R. K., and Woodbury, D. M. (1969). *Exp. Brain Res.* **7**, 181–194.

Fishman, R. A. (1964). *Amer. J. Physiol.* **206**, 836–844.

Fleischhauer, K. (1957). *Z. Zellforsch. Mikrosk. Anat.* **46**, 729–767.

Fleischhauer, K. (1961). *In* "Regional Neurochemistry" (S. S. Kety and J. Elkes, eds.), pp. 279–283. Pergamon, Oxford.

Flexner, L. B. (1933). *Amer. J. Physiol.* **106**, 210–203.

Flexner, L. B. (1938). *Amer. J. Physiol.* **124**, 131–135.

Flexner, L. B., and Winters, H. (1932). *Amer. J. Physiol.* **101**, 697–710.

Frazier, C. H., and Peet, M. M. (1914). *Amer. J. Physiol.* **35**, 268–282.

Fremont-Smith, F., Dailey, M. E., Merritt, H. H., and Carroll, M. P. (1931). *Arch. Neurol. Psychiat.* **25**, 1290–1296.

Frick, E, and Scheid-Seydel, L. (1958,a). *Klin. Wochenschr.* **36**, 66–69.

Frick, E., and Scheid-Seydel, L. (1958b). *Klin. Wochenschr.* **36**, 857–863.

Frick, E., and. Scheid-Seydel, L. (1960). *Klin. Wochenschr.* **38**, 1240–1243.

Friedberg, F., and Greenberg, D. M. (1947). *J. Biol. Chem.* **168**, 411–413.

Geiger, A. Magnes, J., Taylor, R. M., and Veralli, M. (1954). *Amer. J. Physiol.* **177**, 138–149.

Gesell, R., and Hertzman, A. B. (1926). *Amer. J. Physiol.* **78**, 610–629.

Goldberg, M. A., Barlow, C. F., and Roth, L. J. (1963). *Arch. Neurol.* **9**, 498–507.

Goldmann, E. E. (1909). *Beitr. Klin. Chir.* **64**, 192–265.

Goldmann, E. E. (1913). *Abh. Preuss. Akad. Wiss., Phys.-Math. Kl.* No. 1. pp. 1–60.

Granholm, L., and Siesjo, B. K. (1969). *Acta Physiol. Scand.* **75**, 257–266.

Gray, E. G. (1961). *In* "Electronmicroscopy in Anatomy" (J. D. Boyd *et al.*, eds.), pp. 54–66, Arnold, London.

Grazier, F. M., and Clemente, C. D. (1957). *Proc. Soc. Exp. Biol. Med.* **94**, 758–760.

Greenberg, D. M., Aird, R. B., Boelter, M. D. D., Campbell, W. W., Cohn, W. E., and Murayama, M. M. (1943). *Amer. J. Physiol.* **140**, 47–64.

Gröntoft, O. (1954). *Acta Pathol. Microbiol. Scand.* Suppl. C, p. 109.

Gruner, J., Sung, S. S., Tubiana, M., and Segarra, J. (1951). *C. R. Soc. Biol.* **145**, 203–206.

Guroff, G. and Udenfriend, S. (1962). *J. Biol. Chem.* **237**, 803–806.

Hafferl, A. (1953). "Lehrbuch der Topographischen Anatomie." Springer-Verlag, Berlin and New York.

Harper, P. V., Lathrop, K. A., McCardle, R. J., and Andros, G. (1964). *Med. Radioisotope Scanning, Proc. Symp.*, pp. 33–45.

Hashimoto, P. H. (1966). *Acta Anat. Nippon.* **41**, 154–155.

Hashimoto, P. H., and Hama, K. (1968). *Med. J. Osaka Univ.* **18**, 331–346.

Heisey, S. R., Held, D. and Pappenheimer, J. R. (1962). *Amer. J. Physiol.* **203**, 775–781.

Held, D., Fencl, V., and Pappenheimer, J. R. (1964). *J. Neurophysiol.* **27**, 942–959.

Hill, N. C., McKenzie, B. F., McGuckin, W. F., Goldstein, N. P., and Svien, H. J. (1958). *Proc. Staff Meet. Mayo Clin.* **33**, 686–698.

Hill, N. C., Goldstein, N. P., McKenzie, B. F., McGuckin, W. F., and Svien, H. J. (1959). *Brain* **82**, 581–593.

Hochwald, G. M., and Wallenstein, M. C. (1967a). *Exp. Neurol.* **19**, 115–126.

Hochwald, G. M., and Wallenstein, M. C. (1967b). *Amer. J. Physiol.* **212**, 1199–1204.

Hochwald, G. M., Wallestein, M. C., and Matthews, E. S. (1969). *Amer. J. Physiol.* **217**, 348–353.

Hunter, G., and Smith, H. V. (1960). *Nature (London)* **186**, 161–162.

Hunter, G., Smith, H. V., and Taylor, L. M. (1954). *Biochem. J.* **56**, 588–597.

Huxley, A. F., and Stämpfli, R. (1951). *J. Physiol. (London)* **112**, 479–508.

Johnson, J. A. (1966). *Amer. J. Physiol.* **211**, 1261–1263.

Kamin, H., and Handler, P. (1951). *J. Biol. Chem.* **188**, 193–205.

Kappers, J. A. (1958). *Cerebrospinal Fluid ; Prod., Circ., Absorption, Ciba Fund. Symp.* 1957, pp. 3–25.

Karnovsky, M. J. (1967). *J. Cell Biol.*, **35**, 213–236.

Katzman, R., Graziani, L., Kaplan, R., and. Escriva, A. (1965). *Arch. Neurol.* **13**, 513–524.

Kemeny, A., Boldizsar, H., and Pethes, G. (1965). *Acta Physiol. Acad. Sci. Hung.* **27**, 111–117.

Key, G., and Retzius, A. (1876). "Anatomie des Nervensystems und des Bindegewebes." Stockholm.

Kjällquist, A., Messeter, K., and Siesjö, B. K. (1970). *Acta Physiol. Scand.* **78**, 94–102.

Kjällquist, A., Nardini, M., and Siesjö, B. K. (1969a). *Acta Physiol. Scand.* **76**, 485–494.

Kjällquist, A., Nardini, M., and Siesjö, B. K. (1969b). *Acta Physiol. Scand.* **77**, 241–251.

Klatzo, I., and Seitelberger, F. (Eds.) (1967). "Brain Edema." Springer, Vienna.

Kleeman, C. R., Davson, H., and Levin, E. (1962). *Amer. J. Physiol.* **203**, 739–747.

Klein, J. R., Hurwitz, R., and Olsen, N. S. (1946). *J. Biol. Chem.* **164**, 509–512.

Kral, A., Stary, Z., and Winternitz, R. (1929). *Z. Gesamte Neurol. Psychiat.* **122**, 308–316.

Krnjevic, K. (1954). *J. Physiol. (London)* **123**, 338–356.

Kuttner, R., Sims, J. A., and Gordon, M. W. (1961). *J. Neurochem.* **6**, 311–317.

Lajtha, A. (1957). *J. Neurochem.* **1**, 216–227.

Lajtha, A. (1958). *J. Neurochem.* **2**, 209–215.

Lajtha, A. (1968). *Progr. Brain Res.* **29**, 201–218.

Lajtha, A., and Toth, J. (1961). *J. Neurochem.* **8**, 216–225.

Lajtha, A., and Toth, J. (1963). *J. Neurochem.* **10**, 909–920.

Lajtha, A., Furst, S., Gerstein, A., and Warlsch, H. (1957). *J. Neurochem.* **1**, 289–300.

Le Fevre, P. G., and Peters, A. A. (1966). *J. Neurochem.* **13**, 35–46.

Leiderman, P. H., and Katzman, R. (1953). *Amer. J. Physiol.* **175**, 271–275.

Lemire, R. J., Shepherd, T. H., and Alvord, E. C. (1965) *Anat. Rec.* **152**, 9–16.

Leusen, I. (1950). *J. Physiol. (London)* **110**, 319–329.

Leusen, I. (1965). *In* "Cerebrospinal Fluid and the Regulation of Ventilation" (C. McC. Brooks, F. F. Kao, and B. B. Lloyd, eds.), pp. 55–89. Davis, Philadelphia, Pennsylvania.

Levin, E., Nogueira, G. J., and Argiz, C. A. G. (1966). *J. Neurochem.* **13**, 761–767.

Lewandowsky, M. (1900). *Z. Klin. Med.* **40**, 480–494.

Linder, G. C., and Carmichael, E. A. (1928)l *Biochem. J.* **22**, 46–50.

Ling, G. N., and Kromash, M. H. (1967). *J. Gen. Physiol.* **50**, 677–694.

Loeschke, H. H. (1956a). *Pfluegers Arch. Gesamte Physiol. Menschen Tiere* **262**, 517–531.

Loeschke, H. H. (1956b). *Pfluegers Arch. Gesamte Physiol. Menschen Tiere* **262**, 532–536.

Loeschke, H. H., and Sugioka, K. (1969). *Pfluegers Arch.* **312**, 161–188.

Lorenzo, A. V., and Cutler, R. W. P. (1969). *Amer. J. Physiol.* **216**, 353–358.

Lowenthal, A. (1954). *Acta Neurol. Psychiat. Belg.* **54**, 192–199.

Luciano, D. S. (1968). *Brain Res.* **9**, 334–350.

Luft, J. H. (1965). *In* "The Inflammatory Process" (B. W. Zweifach, L. Grant, and R. T. McCluskey, eds.), pp. 121–159. Academic Press, New York.

Lundborg, G., and Brånemark, P. I. (1968). *Advan. Microcirc.* **1**, 66–88.

Luse, S. (1962). *Res. Publ., Ass. Res. Nerv. Ment. Dis.* **40**, 1–26.

Luyendijk, W., ed. (1968). "Cerebral Circulation." Elsevier, Amsterdam.

Majno, G. (1965). *In* "Handbook of Physiology" (Amer. Soc. Physiol. J. Field, ed.), Sect. 2, Vol. III, pp. 2203–2375. Williams & Wilkins, Baltimore, Maryland.

Mandelstamm, M., and Krylow, L. (1928). *Z. Gesamte Exp. Med.* **60**, 63–85.

Manery, J. F., and Bale, W. F. (1941). *Amer. J. Physiol.* **132**, 215–231.

Maren, T. H. (1967). *Physiol. Rev.* **47**, 595–781.

Mark, J., Godin, Y., and Mandel, P. (1968). *J. Neurophysiol.* **15**, 141–143.

Maxwell, D. S., and Pease, D. C. (1956). *J. Biophys. Biochem. Cytol.* **2**, 467–474.

Mayer, S., Maickel, R. P., and Brodie, B. B. (1959). *J. Pharmacol.* **127**, 205–211.

Meller, K., and Wechsler, W. (1965). *Z. Zellforsch. Mikrosk. Anat.* **65**, 420–444.

Merritt, H. H. and Fremont-Smith, F. (1937). "The Cerebrospinal Fluid." Saunders, Philadelphia, Pennsylvania.

Mestrezat, W. (1911). Thesis, Montpelier.

Millen, J. W., and Hess, A. (1958). *Brain* **81**, 248–257.

Millen, J. W., and Woollam, D. H. M. (1961). *Brain* **84**, 514–520.

Millen, J. W., and Woollam, D. H. M. (1962). "The Anatomy of the Cerebrospinal Fluid." Oxford Univ. Press, London and New York.

Mitchell, R. A., Carman, C. T., Severinghaus, J. W., Richardson, B. W., Singer, M. M., and Shnider, S. (1965). *J. Appl. Physiol.* **20**, 443–452.

Mottschall, H. J., and Loeschke, H. H. (1963). *Pfluegers Arch. Gesamte Physiol. Menschen Tiere* **277**, 662–670.

Muir, A. R., and Peters, A. (1962). *J. Cell Biol.* **12**, 443–448.

Neame, K. D. (1968). *Progr. Brain Res.* **29**, 185–196.

Nelson, E., Blinzinger, K., and Hager, H. (1961). *Neurology* **11**, 285–295.

Nicholls, J. G., and Kuffler, S. W. (1964). *J. Neurophysiol.* **27**, 645–671.

Nobécourt, P., and Voisin, R. (1903). *Arch. Gen. Med.* **192**, 3018–3025.

Nyhan, W. L., and Tocci, P. (1966). *Annu. Rev. Med.* **17**, 133–160.

Oldendorf, W. H., and Davson, H. (1967). *Arch. Neurol.* **17**, 196–205.

Olsson, Y. (1966). *Acta Neuropathol.* **7**, 1–15.

Olsson, Y., and Reese, T. S. (1971). *J. Neuropathol. Exp. Neurol.* **30**, 105–119.

Oppelt, W. W., McIntyre, I., and Rall, D. P. (1963). *Amer. J. Physiol.* **205**, 959–962.

Oppelt, W. W., Patlak, C. S., and Rall, D. P. (1964). *Amer. J. Physiol.* **206**, 247–250.

Owman, C., and Rosengren, E. (1967). *J. Neurochem.* **14**, 547–550.

Pappenheimer, J. R. (1965–1966). *Harvey Lect.* **61**, 70–94.

Pappenheimer, J. R., Heisey, S. R., and Jordan, E. F. (1961). *Amer. J. Physiol.* **200**, 1–10.

Pappenheimer, J. R., Heisey, S. R., Jordan, E. F., and Downer, J. de C. (1962). *Amer. J. Physiol.* **203**, 763–774.

Park, C. R., Johnson, L. H., Wright, J. H., and Batsel, H. (1957). *Amer. J. Physiol.* **191**, 13–18.

Patten, B. M. (1953). *Amer. J. Anat.* **93**, 365–395.

Pitlyk, J. P., Tauxe, W. N., Kerr, F. W. L., Sedlack, R. E., and Svien, H. J. (1963). *Arch. Neurol.* **9**, 437–443.

Plum, F. M., and Posner, J. B. (1967). *Amer. J. Physiol.* **212**, 864–870.

Pollay, M. (1966). *Amer. J. Physiol.* **210**, 275–279.

Pollay, M., and Curl. F. (1967). *Amer. J. Physiol.* **213**, 1031–1038.

Pollay, M., and Davson, H. (1963). *Brain* **86**, 137–150.

Pollay, M., and Kaplan, R. J. (1970). *Brain Res.* **17**, 407–416.

Pontén, U. (1966). *Acta Physiol. Scand.* **68**, 152–163.

Posner, J. B., Swanson, A. G., and Plum, F. (1965), *Arch. Neurol.* **12**, 479–496.

Posner, J. B., Plum F., and Zee, D. (1969). *Arch. Neurol.* **20**, 664–667.

Prather, J. W., and Wright, E. M. (1970). *J. Membrane Biol.* **2**, 150–172.

Ragazzini, F. (1952). *Riv. Clin. Pediatr.* **50**, 381–388.

Rall, D. P., Oppelt, W. W., and Patlak, C. S. (1962). *Life Sci.* **2**, 43–48.

Rashbass, C., and Rushton, W. A. H. (1949). *J. Physiol. (London)* **110**, 110–135.

Reed, D. J., and Woodbury, D. M. (1963). *J. Physiol. (London)* **169**, 816–850.

Reed, D. J., Woodbury, D. M., Jacobs, L., and Squires, R. (1965). *Amer. J. Physiol.* **209**, 757–764.

Reese, T. S. (1971). Personal communication.

Reese, T. S., and Brightman, M. W. (1968). *Anat. Rec.* **160**, 414.

Reese, T. S., and Karnovsky, M. J. (1967). *J. Cell Biol.* **34**, 207–217.

Rhodin, J. A. G. (1962). *J. Ultrastruct. Res.* **6**, 171–185.

Riser (1929). "Le Liquide Céphalo-Rachidien." Masson, Paris.

Rivera-Pomar, J. M. (1966). *Z. Zellforsch. Mikrosk. Anat.* **75**, 542–554.

Roberts, R. B. (1968). *Progr. Brain Res.* **29**, 235–243.

Roberts, R. B., Flexner, J. B., and Flexner, L. B. (1959). *J. Neurochem.* **4**, 78–90.

Robin, E. D., Whaley, R. D., Crump, C. H., Bickelmann, A. G., and Travis, D. M. (1958) *J. Appl. Physiol.* **13**, 385–392.

Robinson, R. J., Cutler, R. W. P., Lorenzo, A. V., and Barlow, C. F. (1968a). *J. Neurochem.* **15**, 1169–1174.

Robinson, R. J., Cutler, R. W. P., Lorenzo, A. V., and. Barlow, C. F. (1968b). *J. Neurochem.* **15**, 455–458.

Rodriguez-Peralta, L. A. (1957). *J. Comp. Neurol.* **107**, 455–469.

Rothman, A. R., Freireich, E. J., Gaskins, J. R., Patlak, C. S., and Rall, D. P. (1961). *Amer. J. Physiol.* **201**, 1145–1148.

Royer, P. (1950). *Biol. Med.* (*Paris*) **39**, 237–269.

Rubin, R. C., Henderson, E. S., Ommaya, A. K., Walker, M. D., and Rall. D. P. (1966). *J. Neurosurg.* **25**, 430–436.

Sachs, J. R., and Welt, L. G. (1967). *J. Clin. Invest.* **46**, 65–76.

Sadler, K., and Welch, K. (1967). *Nature* (*London*), **215**, 884–885.

Sahar, A., Hochwald, G. M., Sadik, A. R., and Ransohoff, J. (1969a). *Arch. Neurol.* **21**, 638–644.

Sahar, A., Hochwald, G. M., and Ransohoff, J. (1969b). *Exp. Neurol.* **25**, 200–206.

Schaltenbrand, G., and Putnam, T. (1927). *Deut. Z. Nervenheilk* **96**, 123–132.

Schanker, L. S., Prockop, L. D., Schou, J., and Sisodia, P. (1962). *Life Sci.* **10**, 515–521.

Schultze, H. E. M., Schonenberger, M., and Schwick, G. (1956). *Biochem. Z.* **328**, 267–284.

Selverstone, B., and Moulton, M. J. (1957). *Brain* **80**, 362–375.

Severinghaus, J. W. (1964). *Fed. Proc. Fed. Amer. Soc. Exp. Biol.* **23**, 259.

Severinghaus, J. W. (1965). *In* "Cerebrospinal Fluid and the Regulation of Ventilation" (C. McC. Brooks, F. F. Kao, and B. B. Lloyd, eds.), pp. 277–279. Davis, Philadelphia, Pennsylvania.

Shabo, A. L., and Maxwell, D. S. (1968a). *J. Neurosurg.* **29**, 451–463.

Shabo, A. L., and Maxwell, D. S. (1968b). *J. Neurosurg.* **29**, 464–474.

Shantha, T. R., and Bourne, G. H. (1968). *In* "The Structure and Function of Nervous Tissue." (G. H. Bourne, ed.), Vol. 1, pp. 379–459. Academic Press, New York.

Shanthaveerappa, T. R., and Bourne, G. H. (1962). *J. Anat.* **96**, 527–537.

Shaywitz, B. A., Katzman, R., and Escriva, A. (1969). *Neurology* **19** 1159–1168.

Siesjö, B. K. (1965). *In* "Cerebrospinal Fluid and the Regulation of Ventilation" (C. McC. Brooks, F. F. Kao, and B. B. Lloyd, eds.), pp. 331–371. Davis, Philadelphia, Pennsylvania.

Smith, D. E., Streicher, E., Milkovic, K., and Klatzo, I. (1964). *Acta Neuropathol.* **3**, 372–386.

Spatz, H. (1934). *Arch. Psychiat. Nervenkr.* **101**, 267–358.

Spina-Franca, A. (1960). *Arch. Neuropsiquiat. S. Paulo* **18**, 19–28.

Steger, J. (1953). *Deut. Z. Nervenheilk.* **171**, 1–19.

Stern, L., and Gautier, R. (1921). *Arch. Int. Physiol.* **17**, 138–192.

Stern, L., and Gautier, R. (1922). *Arch. Int. Physiol.* **17**, 391–448.

Stern, L., and Peyrot, R. (1927). *C. R. Soc. Biol.* **96**, 1124–1126.

Stosseck, K., and Acker, H. (1969). *Pfluegers Arch.* **312**, R149.

Sweet, W. H., Selverstone, B., Solloway, S., and Stetten, D. (1950). "American College of Surgeons Surgical Forum," pp. 376–381. Saunders. Philadelphia, Pennsylvania.

Tennyson, V. M., and Pappas, G. D. (1961). *In* "Disorders of the Developing Nervous System" (W. S. Fields and M. M. Desmond, eds.), pp. 267-318. Thomas, Springfield, Illinois.

Tennyson, V. M., and Pappas, G. D. (1962). *Z. Zellforsch. Mikrosk. Anat.* **56**, 595–618.

Tennyson, V. M., and Pappas, G. D. (1968). *Progr. Brain. Res.* **29**, 63–85.

Tochino, Y., and Schanker, L. S. (1965). *Biochem. Pharmacol.* **14**, 1557–1566.

Tochino, Y., and Schanker, L. S. (1966). *Amer. J. Physiol.* **210**, 1229–1233.

Tschirgi, R. D., and Taylor, J. L. (1958). *Amer. J. Physiol.* **195**, 7–22.

Tschirgi, R. D., Frost, R. W., and Taylor, J. L. (1954). *Proc. Soc. Exp. Biol. Med.* **87**, 373–376.

Tubiana, M., Benda, P., and Constans, J. (1951). *Rev. Neurol.* **85**, 17–35.

Tveten, L. (1965). *Acta Neurol. Scand.* **41**, 80–91.

Van Harreveld, A., and Ahmed, N. (1968). *Brain Res.* **11**, 32–41.

Van Harreveld, A., Ahmed, N., and Tanner, D. J. (1966). *Amer. J. Physiol.* **210**, 777–780.

Van Vaerenbergh, P. J. J., Demeester, G., and Leusen, I. (1965). *Arch. Int. Physiol. Biochim.* **73**, 738–747.

Vernadakis, A., and Woodbury, D. M. (1962). *Amer. J. Physiol.* **203**, 748–752.

Vernadakis, A., and Woodbury, D. M. (1965). *Arch. Neurol.* **12**, 284–293.

Von Monakow, P. (1920). *Arch. Neurol. Psychiat.* **6**, 183–200.

Waggener, J. D., and Beggs, J. (1967). *J. Neurophatol.* **26**, 412–426.

Wallace, G. B., and Brodie, B. B. (1939). *J. Pharmacol. Exp. Ther.* **65**, 220–226.

Wallace, G. B., and Brodie, B. B. (1940). *J. Pharmacol. Exp. Ther.* **70**, 418–427.

Walter, K. (1925). *Z. Gesamte Neurol. Psychiat.* **95**, 522–540.

Wang, J. (1948). *J. Gen. Physiol.* **31**, 259–268.

Weed, L. H. (1914). *J. Med. Res.* **31**, 51–91.

Weed, L. H. (1917). *Contrib. Embryol. Carneg: Inst.* **5**, 3-116.

Welch, K. (1962). *Proc. Soc. Exp. Biol. Med.* **109**, 953–954.

Welch, K. (1965). *In* "Cerebrospinal Fluid and the Regulation of Ventilation" (C. McC., Brooks, F. F. Kao, and B. B. Lloyd, eds.), pp. 413–421. Blackwell, Oxford.

Welch, K. (1969). *Brain Res.* **16**, 453–468.

Welch, K., and. Friedman, V. (1960). *Brain.* **83**, 454–469.

Welch, K., and Pollay, M. (1961). *Amer. J. Physiol.* **201**, 651–654.

Welch, K., and Sadler, K. (1965). *J. Neurosurg.* **22**, 344–349.

Welch, K., and Sadler, K. (1966). *Amer. J. Physiol.* **210**, 652–660.

Welch, K., Sadler, K., and Hendee, R. (1969). *Brain Res.* **19**, 465–482.

Wiechert, P. (1963). *Acta Biol. Med. Ger.* **10**, 305–310.

Wislocki, B., and Ladman, A. J. (1958). *Cerebrospinal Fluid ; Prod. Circ., Absorption, Ciba Found. Symp., 1957* pp. 55–75.

Wolff, H. G. (1963). *Z. Zellforsch. Mikrosk. Anat.* **60**, 409–431.

Wolff, H. G., and Lennox, W. G. (1930). *Arch. Neurol. Psychiat.* **23**, 1097–1120.

Woodward, D. I., Reed, D. J., and Woodbury, D. M. (1967). *Amer. J. Physiol.* **212**, 367–370.

Woody, C. D., Marshall, W. H., Besson, J. M., Thompson, H. K., Aleonard, P., and Albe-Fessard, D. (1970). *Amer. J. Physiol.* **218**, 275–283.

Woollard, H. H. (1924). *J. Anat.* **58**, 89–100.

Wright, E. M., and Diamond, J. M. (1969). *Proc. Roy. Soc. Ser. B.* **172**, 203.

Wright, E. M., and Prather, J. W. (1970). *J. Membrane Biol.* **2**, 127–149.

Wright, S. L., Herr, E. P., and Paul, J. R. (1930). *J. Clin. Invest.* **9**, 443–461.

Zuckermann, E. C., and Glaser, G. H. (1968). *Exp. Neurol.* **20**, 87–110.

10

The Extracellular Space in the Vertebrate Central Nervous System

A. Van Harreveld

I. Space Determinations with Extracellular Markers 449
   A. Natural Extracellular Markers 449
   B. Artificial Extracellular Markers 451
   C. The Spaces Determined by Extracellular Markers and the Extra-
      cellular Space 458
   D. The Extracellular Space of the Brain during Fetal and Postnatal
      Development 462
II. Electrical Impedance of Central Nervous Tissue 463
   A. Extracellular Space Estimated from the Tissue Impedance . . . 463
   B. Impedance Changes in Central Nervous Tissue 468
III. Chloride and Water Movements in Central Nervous Tissue 474
   A. Methods for the Study of Chloride and Water Movements . . . 475
   B. Chloride and Water Movements Accompanying Major Impedance
      Changes 475
IV. Electron Microscopy of Central Nervous Tissue 479
   A. Micrographs Prepared with Conventional Fixation Methods . . 479
   B. The Spaces in Electron Micrographs and the Extracellular Space. 481
   C. The Use of Freeze Substitution for the Preservation of the Water
      Distribution 482
   D. Extracellular Space in Electron Micrographs Prepared by Freeze
      Substitution 484
   E. Changes in Extracellular Space during Fixation for Electron Mi-
      croscopy 489
   F. The Spaces in Electron Micrographs Prepared by Freeze Substi-
      tution and the Extracellular Space 493
   G. Abnormal Fluid Uptake by Cellular Elements during Asphyxiation,
      Spreading Depression, and Fixation 496
   H. Differences in the Extracellular Space in Deep and Superficial
      Layers of the Cerebral Cortex 497

V. Mechanisms Involved in the Electrolyte and Water Transport in Central Nervous Tissue 499

A. The Electrolyte and Water Transport 499

B. A Mechanism for the Increase of the Membrane Permeability for Sodium 501

References 506

The extracellular space (ECS) in the vertebrate central nervous system (CNS) has been a subject of controversy. Different methods of estimation gave values varying from a few percent of the tissue volume to 30% and more. Lately, it has been realized that central nervous tissue has features which make it impossible to apply methods for ECS determinations which are used routinely for other organs without modification to the brain. Furthermore, the ECS in the nervous system is not stable and can change markedly. Taking these special features of central nervous tissue into consideration, more recent determinations with different methods have yielded values for the ECS which are less divergent and which may approach a reasonable estimate of this entity in the central nervous system.

Three general principles have been used in investigations of the ECS. The method most frequently employed is based on the use of extra cellular markers, substances which readily pass the capillary wall allowing a rapid equalization of the concentrations of the marker in the ECS and in the blood plasma, without entering the intracellular compartment of the organ. When these conditions are satisfied, the extracellular space can be computed from the concentrations of the marker in plasma and in the organ, i.e.,

$$\frac{\text{concentration in organ}}{\text{concentration in plasma}} \times 100 = \% \text{ ECS}$$

A large number of compounds have been used as extracellular markers —some ionized, such as thiocyanate, thiosulfate, bromide, iodide, sulfate, and p-aminohippurate; others nonionized, like inulin, sucrose, mannitol, and raffinose. Certain complications have to be taken into consideration, such as the possible adsorption of the marker on the plasma proteins, the difference in water content of plasma and extracellular fluid, and the Donnan distribution of ionized compounds across the capillary wall. However, when the necessary corrections are applied a reliable estimate can be made of the ECS of body organs but not, as will be discussed, of the brain.

A second method is based on the fact that low-frequency alternating current passing through a tissue is carried mainly by extracellular ions. The impedance of the tissue can therefore be considered as a measure of the extracellular space. A great advantage of this method is that it can be used to detect rapid changes in the magintude of the ECS.

Finally, the extracellular space has been estimated from electron micrographs (EM) of central nervous tissue. The results obtained with these three approaches to the study of the ECS in the CNS will be discussed with respect to those special features of the brain which affect the determination of this entity.

The present review was restricted to the ECS in the vertebrate central nervous system, which is by far the most extensively investigated. Furthermore, vertebrate central nervous tissue exhibits a mechanism which can produce major changes in the magnitude of the ECS and which may be unique for this phylum. Studies on the ECS in the invertebrate CNS were recently reviewed by Treherne and Moreton (1970).

I. Space Determinations with Extracellular Markers

A. NATURAL EXTRACELLULAR MARKERS

The bulk of the sodium and chloride ions of a tissue is generally present in the ECS, and these ions have therefore been used as natural extracellular markers. Manery and Hastings (1939) found a chloride space of 25% in the rat brain and 35% in the rabbit brain on the assumption that the Cl^- concentration in the extracellular material is the same as in serum ultrafiltrate and that all the chloride is extracellular. The sodium space was 38% in rabbit brain. In the dog similar Cl^- and Na^+ spaces were determined (Eichelberger and Richter, 1944).

These spaces overestimate the ECS since part of the Cl^- and Na^+ are undoubtedly situated intracellularly. An estimate can be made for the intracellular Cl^- and Na^+ concentrations from the inhibitory and excitatory equilibrium potentials for these ions (Eccles, 1957). Also, the assumption by Manery and Hastings (1939) of an equality of the concentrations of these ions in serum and extracellular material is subject to doubt even after applying a correction for the difference in water content of plasma and CSF and for the Donnan distribution across the capillary wall. A relatively free exchange between the extracellular material in the tissue lining the ventricles and the CSF occurs. Even large molecules such as inulin pass relatively easily across the ependymal lining (Rall *et al.*, 1962). Davson (1958) suggested that due to this easy exchange the composition of the CSF during its passage through the ventricular system assumes the composition of extracellular material. The Cl^- concentration of the cisternal CSF of the rabbit is 1.21 times as high as that in the plasma water (Davson, 1956). Making corrections for the postulated higher Cl^- concentration in the extracellular material and for the chloride in the intracellular compartment, Davson's figure (1956) of 31.4% for the chloride space of this species is reduced to 21.4%; the Na space, from 34.6 to 24.2% (Van Harreveld, 1966). Ames and Nesbett (1966) came to a similar conclusion. The difference between the Cl^- and Na^+ spaces may be due to nonionized binding of intracellular sodium to acidic lipids such as phosphatidyl serine and diphosphoinositide (Katzman, 1961; Folch *et al.*, 1956).

Doubt remains, however, that the corrected chloride space represents the ECS. Especially the chloride and natrium contents of the glial elements are not known. Determinations of these ions in abnormal tissues consisting mainly of glia such as glial tumors (Katzman, 1961) or central nervous tissue in which the nervous elements had been made to degenerate (Koch *et al.*, 1962) showed a higher Cl^- and Na^+ content but may not supply reliable values for normal glia (Van Harreveld, 1966). Several investigators using intracellular techniques found unexcitable cells exhibiting a high membrane potential in central nervous tissue and which were considered to be glial cells (Coombs *et al.*, 1955; Phillips, 1956; Li, 1959; Krnjević and Schwartz, 1967). The high membrane potential suggests that the Cl^- and Na^+ concentration of these cells is similar to that of nerve cells.

Sulfate can also be used as a natural extracellular marker. Barlow *et al.* (1961) estimated a 4% space in cat brain from the distribution of intravenously administered labeled sulfate between brain and plasma. The sulfate concentration in the CSF is much lower than that in plasma, however. Richmond and Hastings (1960) found this ratio to be 0.15 for $^{35}SO_4^{--}$ in dogs. Van Harreveld *et al.* (1966) determined a ratio of 0.24 for the naturally occurring sulfate in cats. Assuming that the sulfate concentration of the extracellular material is similar to that of the CSF, the figure of the sulfate space of Barlow *et al.* (1961) can be reinterpreted to give an extracellular space of 16 to 24% (Ames and Nesbett, 1966; Van Harreveld *et al.*, 1966).

B. ARTIFICIAL EXTRACELLULAR MARKERS

The intravenous administration of extracellular markers which gives satisfactory results in the body organs leads to erroneous values when applied to the CNS because of the presence of the blood–brain barrier (BBB). In its original concept the brain would be separated from the blood by structures which impede the free diffusion of compounds between plasma and extracellular material. This simplistic concept has given way to the realization that the blood–brain barrier is a complicated mechanism in which restricted access from plasma to the ECS is complemented by mechanisms which transport compounds in and out of the brain. An equalization of the concentrations of an extracellular marker in plasma water and ECS can therefore, in general, not be achieved by the simple intravenous administration of the compound. There results, after some time, a steady state in which the concentration of the marker in the extracellular material may be considerably lower than that in the plasma water. These features deprive this method of ECS determination of one of its basic requirements. Extracellular markers can be used successfully for the CNS only when the exchange across the blood–brain barrier is taken into full consideration and appropriate methods are taken to insure an equal concentration of the marker in the plasma water and in the extracellular material of the brain.

1. The Blood–Brain Barrier

There is ample evidence that the access from plasma to the brain is restricted. It takes much longer for an intravenously administered compound to enter the CNS than most body organs. This was shown, for instance, for radioactive sodium (Manery and Bale, 1941) and chloride (Manery and Haege, 1941). Equilibrium between the sodium in plasma and muscle was reached within an hour; in the brain this took up to 12 hours. Compounds used as extracellular markers such as ^{14}C sucrose or ^{14}C inulin reach a constant concentration in muscle within a few hours; in the brain this takes 24 hours or more (Reed and Woodbury, 1963; Ferguson and Woodbury, 1969). Reese and Karnovsky (1967) and Brightman and Reese (1969) demonstrated "gap" junctions between the endothelial cells of brain capillaries which deny access of protein molecules (peroxidase) to the ECS. These gap junctions may retard the entrance of smaller molecules to the brain.

Once a compound has entered the brain ECS it can be removed again by a mechanism suggested by Davson (1963), which is called the sink

action of the CSF. This feature is based on the presence of active mechanisms which transport compounds from the CSF into the blood against
a concentration gradient. Such a transport was shown by Pappenheimer
et al. (1961) for phenolsulfonphtlalein and Diodrast and, later, for a number of compounds used as extracellular markers such as ^{131}I, thiocyanate,
p-aminohippurate, and sulfate (Davson *et al.*, 1962; Davson and Pollay,
1963; Pollay and Davson, 1963; Coben *et al.*, 1965; Pollay, 1966; Cutler
et al., 1968b; Hammerstad *et al.*, 1969). Since the isolated choroid plexuses accumulate ^{131}I, sulfate, and thiosulfate (Becker, 1961; Welch,
1962a,b; Kaplan and Pollay, 1968; Robinson *et al.*, 1968), it is generally
believed that these structures are involved in the transport from CSF

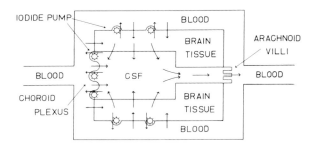

Fig. 1. Schematic representation of the central nervous system. The arrows indicate
the direction of iodide movements. Iodide moves from the blood through blood–brain
barrier into the brain extracellular space and from there through the brain–CSF barrier.
Also, iodide would pass from blood into the CSF through the choroid plexuses. Iodide
is removed with the CSF through the arachnoid villi (sink action) and by active transport
in the choroid plexuses from the CSF and across the lining of the brain capillaries from
the ECS into the blood. (From Ahmed and Van Harreveld, 1969.)

to blood. The concentration of such compounds in the CSF produced by
the choroid plexuses and the fluid formed by the brain tissue (Bering and
Sato, 1963; Bering, 1965; Pollay and Curl, 1967) and which passes over
these structures is, therefore, low. This CSF can take up markers from
the ECS of the brain tissue during its passage through the ventricular
system, finally leaving the brain case through the arachnoid villi. The
ependymal lining of the ventricles is quite permeable (Rall *et al.*, 1962),
which fact facilitates this mechanism. The sink action of the CSF can be
expected to keep the mean concentration of the marker in the ECS lower
than in the blood plasma. Figure 1, which is adopted from a figure of
Reed *et al.* (1965), shows a scheme of the sink action. Davson and Segal
(1969) demonstrated the sink action of the CSF by administering [14]C

sucrose intravenously and perfusing the ventricles with either an artificial CSF or low-viscosity silicone, which does not take up sugar. The sugar space of the silicone perfused brain was significantly larger than when artificial CSF was used.

Oldendorf and Davson (1967) proposed the perfusion of the ventricles with an artificial CSF containing the same marker concentration as present in the plasma as a method to prevent the sink action of the CSF. They found, indeed, that the perfusion of the ventricles in this way increased the sucrose space of the brain from 2.5%, when the marker was administered intravenously only, to 9%.

There may still be another mechanism which affects the concentration of markers in the ECS. As there is a mechanism in the choroid plexuses which removes compounds from the CSF, there could well be similar pumps which transport markers from the ECS to the blood through the lining of the brain capillaries (Fig. 1). Evidence for an active cation transport across this component of the BBB was presented by Bito and Davson (1966), Bito (1969) and by Ahmed and Van Harreveld (1969).

2. *The Iodide Space of the Brain*

Radioactive iodide (^{131}I) is a marker which has been investigated in detail (Reed *et al.*, 1965; Bito *et al.*, 1966; Cutler *et al.*, 1968a; Ahmed and Van Harreveld, 1969) and which exhibits all the transport mechanisms mentioned above. To demonstrate the large effect of these mechanisms on the iodide space some figures from the investigation of Ahmed and Van Harreveld (1969) follow.

It takes several hours for the iodide to attain a constant concentration in the central nervous tissue. It was therefore necessary to prevent the elimination of the marker by the kidneys. However, even after nephrectomy the level of the marker in the plasma could be kept constant only by repeated small injections. The iodide space reached a constant level 4 to 5 hours after the start of intravenous administration of the marker. For the entire rabbit brain this space had a value of about 2.5% after correction for the ^{131}I in the blood remaining in the vessels of the tissue. The concentration of the marker in the CSF was about 1% of that of the plasma. The difference between the iodide concentration in the tissue and in the CSF can be expected to result in the sink action especially when the distribution of the marker in the tissue is taken into consideration. Much of the ^{131}I will be confined to a relatively small ECS, making the iodide concentration gradient between the extracellular material and the CSF much larger than appears from the iodide space and the CSF concentration. Indeed, when the sink action was eliminated by perfusing the ventricle system with an artificial CSF containing the same concentration of the marker as the plasma, the iodide space rose to 10%.

The active transport of iodide can be inhibited by perchlorate (Wyngaarden *et al.*, 1953) or by supplying much more of the marker than can be handled by the transport mechanism, resulting in its saturation. If the iodide transport in the choroid plexuses which reduces the concentration of the marker in the CSF and thus makes the sink action possible were the only active transport mechanisms depressing the iodide level in the ECS of the brain, then the administration of perchlorate could not be expected to change the iodide space in a preparation in which the sink action was eliminated by ventricle perfusion. However, perchlorate administration enhanced, in such preparations, the iodide space to 17%. The administration of unlabeled iodide to a serum concentration of 30 mM which saturates the mechanisms for active transport, enhanced the iodide space in ventricle perfused preparations to 21%. There seems therefore to be present in the brain another active transport mechanism than that in the choroid plexuses, which tends to decrease the iodide concentration in the tissue by pumping iodide from the ECS directly into the blood. Coben (1969) suggested that if such a pump exists it should be located at the luminal side of the capillary endothelium.

In some experiments the concentration of labeled and unlabeled iodide in the perfusion fluid was so adjusted that the fluid neither gained nor lost iodide during its passage through the ventricles. This indicated that the perfusion fluid was in equilibrium with the extracellular material. In these experiments the iodide concentration of the perfusion fluid was therefore used for the computation of the iodide space, yielding a value of 22.5%. The I concentration in the perfusion fluid was, under these conditions, about 10% lower than that of plasma. The difference may be due to the binding of iodide to the plasma proteins. It can be computed from these figures that 15% of the iodide is bound to plasma proteins, a similar value as found by Bito *et al.* (1966) with a different method. The observations on the iodide space described above are in general agreement with those of the latter authors.

It is obvious that the iodide space can be affected markedly by eliminating mechanisms which tend to remove the marker from the brain tissue. For the equalization of the marker concentration in the plasma water and in the extracellular material it is necessary to consider the sink action of the CSF and the possibility of a transport mechanism across the lining of the brain capillaries. A correction for binding of the marker to the plasma proteins is, in general, necessary. For different markers each of these features may be of different importance. Determinations of spaces with markers carried out before the transport mechanisms were known and, thus, not taken into consideration, can be expected to have yielded erroneous values.

3. *Recent Space Determinations with Extracellular Markers*

In recent investigations some or all of the transport mechanisms which interfere with the equalization of the marker concentration in plasma water and extracellular material were eliminated. Streicher (1961) determined a 4% thiocyanate space in rat brain when the marker concentration in the plasma water was 2 to 2.5 mM. An increase of the plasma concentration to about 10 mM enhanced the thiocyanate space to 15%. An effect of the administered amount of this marker on the magnitude of the thiocyanate space had been earlier observed in chicken brain by Lajtha (1957). Saturation also enhanced the thiocyanate concentration of the CSF to about 80% of that of the plasma water at a plasma concentration of 8 mM (Streicher et al., 1964). The efficiency of the sink action of the CSF under the latter circumstances was probably not very high. Since both active transport across the brain capillaries and the sink action of the CSF can be expected to be impaired by high thiocyanate concentrations in the plasma, the marker concentration in plasma water and extracellular material may have been approximately equal. The maximum value of the thiocyanate space observed by Streicher (1961) may therefore approach a value obtained under conditions which satisfy one of the requirements for ECS determinations. Pollay (1966) performed similar experiments using ^{35}S-labeled thiocyanate. Saturation with the unlabeled marker or inhibition of the active transport with iodide administered intravenously or with dinitrophenol injected into the lateral ventricles resulted in a thiocyanate space of about 15%.

Woodward et al. (1967) injected ^{14}C-labeled inulin intravenously and perfused the ventricles for 6 hours with an artificial CSF containing a similar concentration of the marker as present in the plasma water. The value for the inulin space determined in the cerebral cortex was 14%.

Cutler et al. (1968a) determined the sulfate space in cats by intravenous administration of ^{35}S-sulfate and simultaneous ventriculo-cisternal perfusion. The sulfate concentration of the perfusate was about 80% of that of the plasma. Radioautograms indicated a higher concentration of the label in regions of the brain in close contact with the perfusion fluid, and accordingly, the sulfate space was higher in these areas. No attempts were made to arrest a possible transport of the marker across the capillary lining by saturation or inhibition. The authors estimated the overall sulfate space as 10 to 15%. These experiments demonstrate the difficulty of enhancing the marker concentration uniformly in the entire ECS which might have been accomplished by suppressing active transport.

Baethmann *et al.* (1970) administered ^{35}S-labeled thiosulfate in rats intravenously and by ventricular perfusion. The thiosulfate space of the whole brain after 2 hours equilibration was about 12%. Reulen *et al.* (1970) using the same mode of application in dogs determined a thiosulfate space of 9.3% in the cortex, 13.3% in the nucleus caudatus, 9.5% in the medulla, 11.9% in the cerebellum, and 8.5% in the white matter. Also, in these experiments no attempt was made to suppress a possible transport across the lining of the brain capillaries.

Reed *et al.* (1965) determined a ^{131}I space in rats of about 12% by saturation with 10 mM/kg unlabeled iodide and of 7% by perchlorate administration but without ventricular perfusion. Cutler *et al.* (1968a) who applied ventriculo-cisternal perfusion, but no saturation found regional differences in the iodide space ranging from 5 to 20%. Bito *et al.* (1966) administered ^{131}I intravenously, and prevented the sink action by ventricular perfusion and active transport with perchlorate. They determined an iodide space of 19%. As mentioned above, Ahmed and Van Harreveld (1969) found an iodide space of 17% with the procedure used by Bito and a space of about 22% when active transport was depressed by saturation.

4. *Local Application of Extracellular Markers*

Several investigators introduced markers into the brain not through the BBB but through the more permeable brain–CSF barrier. Davson *et al.* (1961) replaced the CSF surrounding the spinal cord repeatedly by fluids containing sucrose and *p*-aminohippurate and determined spaces for these markers of about 12%. In a more recent investigation Bito *et al.* (1966) perfused the spinal subarachnoidal space with marker solutions and determined an inulin space in the cord of 9% and an iodide space of about 25%.

Rall *et al.* (1962) perfused the ventricles of dogs with ^{14}C-labeled inulin and determined 3–5 hours later the concentration of the label in the tissue as a function of the distance from the ventricle. The 1 to 2 mm of caudate nucleus tissue nearest the ventricle contained an average of 10% of the inulin concentration in the perfusate. In the tissue farther way from the ventricle the inulin concentration fell rapidly. Extrapolating for the concentration in the tissue immediately adjoining the ventricle Rall (1964) suggested an inulin space of 13% in the caudal nucleus and of 12% in the pons. When using sucrose as the marker the spaces were larger, i.e., 17 and 19% for the same structure. In these experiments it was assumed that the ventricle ependyma is completely permeable for inulin. If this structure forms an impediment for inulin diffusion, as suggested by Ferguson and Woodbury (1969), a concentration gradient across the ependyma will be established and the extrapolated inulin space will be too low. Furthermore, the marker may diffuse through the lining of the brain capillaries into the blood (Pollay and Kaplan, 1970), which also will make the space smaller. The differences between the inulin and sucrose spaces observed may indicate that these features for sucrose are different than those for inulin.

Bourke et al. (1965) injected ^{14}C-labeled thiocyanate, sucrose, and inulin into the cisterna of a number of species and collected, 6 hours later, the subarachnoidal CSF and cortical tissue. The thiocyanate space computed from these samples was similar to the chloride space in the cortex. The sucrose and inulin spaces were similar and smaller and were found to increase with the brain weight of the species investigated: ranging from 19 and 22% in the guinea pig and rabbit, to 28% in the cat and 33% in the monkey. However, Fenstermacher and Bartlett (1967), applying sucrose by subarachnoidal perfusion, found in the rabbit much lower average values (about 10%) for the sucrose space of the cerebral and cerebellar cortex and even lower values (7 to 8%) for the brain stem and spinal cord. In some experiments much higher values were found and the authors considered the possibility that only in these instances the perfusion had been "truly good." In a more recent paper Fenstermacher et al. (1970) and Levin et al. (1970) combined subarachnoidal perfusion with the extrapolation technique of Rall (1964) mentioned above, and determined inulin and sucrose spaces of 17–20% in the cerebral cortices of rabbits, cats, dogs, and monkeys. Contrary to the observation of Bourke et al. (1965), no correlation between brain size and the magnitude of the extracellular space was found. Finally, Bradbury et al. (1968) superfused the rabbit cerebral cortex with an artificial CSF containing ^{35}S-labeled sulfate. The concentration of the marker extrapolated to the pial surface suggested an 18.3% sulfate space.

Several authors have used tissue slices for ECS determinations. Although it is possible to circumvent in this way the blood–brain and brain–CSF barriers, there are serious objections to such preparations. The mechanical damage to the cut surfaces of the slice creates a layer of tissue which is so abnormal that it takes up labeled protein (Pappius *et al.*, 1962). This effect is especially serious in thin slices. If thicker slices are used, the oxygenation of the central part of the slice may be impaired, which, as will be shown below, can cause a shift of extracellular material into the intracellular compartment.

Two preparations of isolated central nervous tissue have been used which are not subject to these objections. Bradbury *et al.* (1968) used the whole frog brain, which is small and has a low metabolism. Inulin, sucrose, and sulfate spaces of 19, 24, and 21.5% respectively were determined. Zadunaisky and Curran (1963) suggested a similar space based on the washout of ^{24}Na from preloaded frog brain. Ames and Hastings (1956) used the isolated rabbit retina as a sample of central nervous tissue. This preparation responded to light for hours (Ames and Gurian, 1960) and, thus, seemed to remain in a viable state. The retina is situated inside the blood–aqueous humor barrier and has, itself, apparently no structures which seriously impede the exchange of compounds with the surrounding solution. When bathed in an inulin solution the concentration of the marker in the retina reached a steady value in a few minutes. An average inulin space of 29% was found. This high value may be explained by the inclusion of the relatively large spaces between the light-sensitive elements, which strictly are not part of the tissue ECS (Van Harreveld and Khattab, 1968a), and of a canal system in the Müller cells, which communicate with the ECS (Lasansky and Wald, 1962).

C. The Spaces Determined by Extracellular Markers and the Extracellular Space

1. *The Marker Concentration in the Extracellular Space*

A better understanding of the mechanisms which determine the concentration of markers in the extracellular material and the CSF has made it possible to devise conditions under which equality of the marker concentration in the extracellular material and in plasma or the fluid in the ventricles can be approached. The necessity of eliminating the sink action of the CSF seems now well accepted. An active transport from the ECS into the blood across the lining of the brain capillaries must be considered as a distinct possibility, especially for small ions. For compounds with a relatively large molecular weight such as inulin (MW 5000) active transport seems less likely. Since diffusion of such compounds proceeds slowly (Pollay *et al.*, 1969), times of the order of 24 hours have to be allowed for equilibration (Ferguson and Woodbury, 1969). However, prolonging the equilibration time in ventricle perfused preparations beyond 6 hours, as practiced by Woodward *et al.* (1967), may seriously jeopardize the normal functional state of the brain. It will therefore be difficult to combine complete equalization with the elimination of the sink action when using inulin as an extracellular marker.

Not much attention has been paid to a feature of the CSF production which may impair the equalization of the marker concentration in the ECS and plasma water or ventricle perfusate. The CSF is not only produced by the choroid plexuses but is also released by the ependymal lining of the ventricles and in the arachnoidal space (Bering and Sato, 1963; Bering, 1965; Pollay and Curl, 1967). The origin of this CSF will be extracellular fluid produced in the brain tissue by the capillaries. Such a fluid may have a marker concentration which is materially lower than that of the plasma water from which it originates. The low inulin content of the CSF (1–3%, Reed *et al.*, 1965) after intravenous administration of the marker may be taken as an example. It is unlikely that this low concentration is due to an active transport of inulin from CSF to the blood but more likely the result of fluid production by secretion or molecular sieving (Pappenheimer, 1953). Another example is the ^{131}I concentration of the CSF, which did not exceed 30% of that of the plasma after active transport had been suppressed by perchlorate or saturation (Bito *et al.*, 1966; Ahmed and Van Harreveld, 1969). The release in the brain ECS of a fluid with a lower marker concentration than in the plasma water will establish a steady state even in ventricle perfused preparations which will prevent the equalization of the marker concentrations in the ECS, the plasma water, and the ventricle perfusate. This will lower the marker space, probably especially when compounds of a high molecular weight, such as inulin, are used.

The application of markers through the CSF–brain barrier circumvents some of the difficulties described above. The extrapolation of the marker concentration up to the ependymal lining seems a promising approach. It may be significant that the marker spaces determined in this way are among the largest reported. Even these figures may be too low due to the possibilities, mentioned above, that the CSF–brain barrier impedes the diffusion of the marker into the tissue and that the capillaries of the brain remove the marker from the ECS.

2. *The Penetration of the Marker into the Intracellular Compartment*

One of the conditions for the determination of the magnitude of the ECS is that the marker does not penetrate into the intracellular compartment. That relatively small ions such as iodide, thiocyanate, sulfate, or thiosulfate would remain restricted completely to the ECS seems unlikely. Indeed, there is evidence that they enter the intracellular compartment. P. F. Baker (1965) bathed crustacean nerve in 150 mM iodide solutions for as short a period as 10 seconds after removing the chloride by washing in a nitrate solution and, subsequently, precipitated the I⁻ with silver ions. Some of the silver iodide was observed within axons in electron micrographs of this material. It was mainly associated with mitochondria.

Also, markers of higher molecular weight seem to enter the intracellular compartment. Nicholls and Wolfe (1967) found in autoradiographs of the leech ventral nerve cord charged with ¹⁴C-labeled inulin (M.W. 5000–5500) and dextran (MW 15,000–17,000) clusters of silver grains especially over nerve cells but also over glial cells. It was suggested that these large molecules are taken up by pinocytosis. The intracellular inulin and dextran would account for the 5–10% of the total tracer content of the tissue which could not be removed by prolonged washing. Brown *et al.* (1969) measured the grain density in radioautographs of frozen dried sections of the superior cervical and the nodose ganglion of cats after administration of labeled methoxy-inulin, D-mannitol, and sulfate. Silver grains were observed over ganglion cells. Their density was 10–15% of that over the vessels which had a high density due to the blood they contained. Assuming that the marker was present mainly in the plasma, its activity was about twice that of blood and the density of the silver granules in the ganglion cells 5–7% of that in the plasma, a value close to that suggested by Nicholls and Wolfe (1967) for leech cells and the surrounding bathing fluid.

Cutler *et al.* (1968a) considered the possibility that inhibition or saturation of the transport mechanisms may impede not only the transport of a marker in the choroid plexus (and in the lining of brain capillaries) but also the mechanisms normally excluding these compounds from the cellular elements of the brain. Such a view was supported by an observation of French (1965), who found that the thiocyanate space of muscle and erythrocytes increases markedly with the concentration of the marker. On the other hand, Reed *et al.* (1965) and Ahmed and Van Harreveld (1969) found that the iodide space in muscle is independent of the plasma concentration of the marker and, also, is not affected by perchlorate which inhibits iodide transport. Furthermore, the iodide space of muscle determined by the latter authors was very similar to the inulin space (Creese *et al.*, 1955; Law and Phelps, 1966), making it unlikely that a significant part of the iodide moved intracellularly after suppression of active transport. One cannot be sure that brain cells behave like muscle fibers, but the observations on muscle suggest strongly that the increased iodide space caused by inhibition or saturation of the iodide transporting mechanism is not due to a penetration of the marker into the intracellular compartment but to an effect on the BBB. The latter observations support the postulate that the exclusion of markers from the cellular elements is not based on a transport mechanism but on special features of the marker molecule or ion. Bradbury *et al.* (1968), for instance, suggested that sulfate ions are almost completely excluded from cells because of the divalency of the sulfate ion and the large negative potential of both neurons and glial cells.

3. *The Extracellular Space of Central Nervous Tissue*

As has been pointed out, the two conditions necessary for a determination of the extracellular space cannot be completely satisfied. A better understanding of the mechanisms involved in the solute distribution in the brain has made it possible to devise methods which made it possible to circumvent some of the difficulties involved in the determination of meaningful marker spaces. The application of this knowledge has resulted in a substantial increase in the estimate of the marker spaces, which run in the more recent estimates from 12 to 20% and more. Some of the unresolved difficulties mentioned above suggest that some of these figures may underestimate the marker spaces. On the other hand, there is direct evidence that even markers of high molecular weight are not completely excluded from the intracellular compartment. These considerations make it impossible to suggest a definitive figure for the magnitude of the ECS.

As will be shown below, the magnitude of the ECS is quite variable under adverse conditions such as asphyxiation. Also, during spreading depression large changes occur in this entity. It seems quite likely that, also, more normal functional activities result in changes of the ECS. Furthermore, the extracellular space of the brain is not of uniform magnitude. Estimates of extracellular space in specific areas by local application of markers may therefore yield values which differ considerably from the overall figures determined for the whole brain or large parts thereof. However, a value of 15% or more of the volume of the whole brain may be an ultimate figure for this entity.

D. The Extracellular Space of the Brain during Fetal and Postnatal Development

A decrease of the chloride space during development was noted by L. B. Flexner and Flexner (1949) and J. B. Flexner and Flexner (1950) in the guinea pig. This value showed a maximum of 47% at the 41st day of gestation, declining to 31% at term, which is slightly larger than the chloride space of the adult. Lajtha (1957) extended these observations to chickens in which the chloride space fell from about 40% 1 week before hatching to the adult level of 23%. In rats 2 days after birth the chloride space was 38%, falling to 28% during the first 4 weeks of postnatal life. The thiocyanate space followed a similar course. Barlow *et al.* (1961) determined a sulfate space for the cerebral cortex in 3- to 7-day-old kittens of about 17% which decreased in 2 months to 4%. For cerebral white matter the figures were 33.5% and 6%. These results were corrected for the sulfate incorporated in the tissue, which can be expected to be much larger in the growing central nervous system than in the adult (Dobbing, 1961).

Vernadakis and Woodbury (1965), using ^{36}Cl, determined in 8-day-old rats a chloride space of 56% and an inulin space of 22%. The chloride space decreased to 30% in the adult, and the inulin space to 5% in 32-day-old rats. The ^{36}Cl uptake curves of 8- and 17-day-old rats could be resolved in two components, in older rats in three components. The inulin uptake curve of animals of all ages yielded only one component. The single component of the inulin curve and one of the components of the ^{36}Cl curves were assigned to the extracellular compartment. The other two chloride components were assigned to the neuronal and glial compartments.

In rats the BBB has not yet developed before birth (Ferguson and Woodbury, 1969). The CSF is an ultrafiltrate of the plasma so that no sink action is possible. In 4-day prenatal animals the brain/plasma and brain/CSF ratios for inulin and sucrose approached each other, indicating that the marker concentrations in plasma, CSF, and ECS were near equal. The inulin and sucrose spaces (40–50%) would reflect, at this age, the extracellular space. During maturation the brain/plasma ratio declines due to the development of the sink action of the CSF.

II. Electrical Impedance of Central Nervous Tissue

A. EXTRACELLULAR SPACE ESTIMATED FROM THE TISSUE IMPEDANCE

1. Theoretical Considerations

An independent method for the determination of extracellular space is based on the observations of Fricke (1924a,b, 1933) and of Cole and his co-workers (Cole, 1928, 1940; Cole and Spencer, 1938; Cole *et al.*, 1969) that the specific resistance of a cell suspension measured with low-frequency alternating current is a function of the ratio of the cell volume and that of the fluid in which the cells are suspended. This is due to the fact that the plasma membrane of cells impede ion movements and thus have a relatively high electrical resistance. Much of the current used in impedance measurements of tissues therefore flows through the extracellular space. The theoretical basis for this relationship is given by an equation derived about a century ago by Maxwell (1873) for the specific resistance of a suspension of spheres of certain specific resistance suspended in a medium of different resistivity.

$$\frac{1 - (r_1/r)}{2 + (r_1/r)} = \varrho \, \frac{1 - (r_1/r_2)}{2 + (r_1/r_2)}$$

In this equation r and r_1 are the specific resistances of the suspension and the medium respectively, r_2 the resistance of the spheres, and ϱ is the volume concentration of the spheres. If, as proved to be the case in cell suspensions, the resistance of the particles is very large compared with that of the medium, the equation can be simplified to

$$\frac{1 - (r_1/r)}{2 + (r_1/r)} = \frac{\varrho}{2}$$

The cell volume (ϱ) can in this way be computed from the specific resistances of the suspension and of the fluid in which the spheres are suspended. Cole and Spencer (1938) measured the resistance of suspensions of spherical sea urchin (*Arbacia punctulata*) eggs in seawater with alternating current of varying frequencies. The volume concentration computed from these values was compared with the volume of the eggs determined by the cell count and the mean diameter of the cells (Cole, 1940). In suspensions ranging from 30 to 70 vol % of eggs these determinations corresponded within the experimental error. Similar investigations were performed by Fricke (1924b, 1933) on suspensions of erythrocytes. A modification of Maxwell's equation was used, adapting it to the nonspherical shape of the red cells. Again, a comparison of the cell volume based on the impedance measurements of the suspension corresponded closely, over a wide range of concentrations, with the cell volume determined in other ways.

The specific impedance of the cells in the above investigations was considered to be infinite, making the simplification of Maxwell's equation possible. This may seem surprising since neither the cytoplasm nor the cell membrane have a very high resistance. The explanation is given by an equation for a spherical body of certain specific resitance surrounded by a thin shell of another resistance, derived by Cole (1928) from a more general equation by Maxwell (1873):

$$r_2 = r_3 + (r_4/a)$$

In this equation r_2 is the specific resistance of the particle, r_3 is that of the inner sphere, r_4 is the resistance of the outer shell (the plasma membrane) expressed in ohms per unit area, and a is the radius of the sphere. This equation shows that the specific resistance of a cell is not only determined by the resistance of its plasma membrane but is also a function of its size; the smaller the cell, the larger the resistance. For instance, the specific resistance of a sea urchin egg cell with a membrane resistance of 100 Ω cm^2 (Cole, 1941) and a mean radius of 36 μ (Shapiro, 1935) is about 28,000 Ω cm. Since the specific resistance of sea water is 20 Ω cm, the simplification of Maxwell's equation seems justified.

It would seem that the observations on cell suspensions can be applied to tissues. These also consist of cells surrounded by plasma membranes, which impede ion movements, suspended in extracellular material. The Maxwell equation was derived for dilute cell suspensions of spherical bodies, and objections have been made against its use for the much higher cell volumes found in tissues (Horstmann and Meves, 1959). However, the highest cell volumes (70 and 80%) computed by Cole (1940) and by Fricke (1924b, 1933) from the specific resistance of the suspensions corresponded well with the cell volumes determined in other ways. Additional justification for the use of Maxwell's equation for cell suspensions of high volume concentration was recently presented by Cole et al. (1969). Objections have been raised, furthermore, against the assumption that cells can be considered to have an infinite resistance. The resistance of plasma membrane of nerve cells was generally found to be high, e.g., for the motoneuron values of 500–1000 Ω cm² (Coombs *et al.*, 1955; Frank and Fuortes, 1956) were determined. However, because of the relatively high capacitance of the neuronal membrane, i.e., 6 μF/cm² (Eccles, 1957), the impedance is much lower, i.e., (about 28 Ω cm² at 1000 Hz. Hild and Tasaki (1962) computed a membrane resistance of 3–10 Ω cm² for glia cells in tissue culture. Since the glia processes were neglected in this calculation, this value may be too small. Furthermore, such low values of the membrane resistance seem not to be a general property of glia. Kuffler and Potter (1964) computed a membrane resistance of 1000 Ω cm² for glial cells of the leech, and Trachtenberg and Pollen (1970) determined a value of 200–500 Ω cm² for the membrane resistance of cortical glial cells. However, even with such low membrane resistances as reported by Hild and Tasaki, the small dimension of central nervous elements causes the specific resistance to be relatively high. A spherical cell of 10-μ diameter and with a membrane resistance of 3 Ω cm² would still have a specific resistance of 6000 Ω cm, which is large in comparison to that of the extracellular material (less than 100 Ω cm).

A more valid objection against the use of Maxwell's equation is that it was derived for particles of a definite and uniform geometrical shape whereas the cellular elements of nervous tissue are highly irregular. Furthermore, Ranck (1963b) pointed out that, although the dimensions of cells and the cross sections of fibers are small, fibers situated in the direction of the current lines may be the equivalents of rather large elements. The specific impedance of a fiber parallel with the current lines may therefore be materially lower than that of fibers at right angle with the current. This concept is supported by the finding that the specific impedance of white matter is much larger when determined at right angles with the fiber direction than measured in the direction of the fibers (Ranck and BeMent, 1965; Nicholson, 1965).

2. Determinations of the Specific Impedance of Central Nervous Tissue

The specific impedance of cerebral cortical tissue has been determined by several authors with different methods. Freygang and Landau (1955) constructed a pool of Ringer's solution on the cat's cortex. They applied current pulses through the pool and underlying tissue and measured the potential drop per unit distance in these media, which is proportional to the specific resistance. These experiments yielded a mean specific resistance for the cortex of 222 Ω cm. With electrodes placed on the cortical surface and in the lateral ventricle, Van Harreveld *et al.* (1963) established

in rabbits a uniform 1000 Hz alternating current field in a tissue slab consisting of the cerebral cortex and the underlying white matter. The mean
specific impedance of the slab was determined. Bennett (1969) found a
resistance of 50–100 Ω cm² for the arachnoidal membrane, which might
interfere with the determination of the mean impedance of the tissue slab.
However, this membrane has a capacitance of at least 30 μF/cm², which
would give it a very low impedance (about 0.5–1 Ω cm²) when measured
with a 1000 Hz current. The ratio of the specific impedance of the gray
and white matter in the tissue slab were determined by passing a probe
through the tissue and measuring the potential differences between the
probe and the electrode in the lateral ventricle as a function of its position
in the tissue. These data yielded a mean specific cortical impedance of
208 Ω cm. Corrected for the conductivity of the blood in the vessels, this
value became 234 Ω cm for the cortical tissue proper. Ranck (1963a)
measured the potential at various distances from an electrode placed on
the surface of the cortex and computed the specific resistance of the cortex from this value and the current distribution in the hemispherical field
surrounding the point electrode. A specific impedance of 256 Ω cm, corrected for the conductivity of the blood in the pial vessels, was measured
at a frequency of 5000 Hz. Finally, Li *et al.* (1968) and Fenstermacher
et al. (1970) determined the specific resistance of the cat's cerebral cortex
with current pulses using a method similar to that of Ranck. The electrodes were placed in the cortical tissue instead of on the surface, however.
The results were at variance with the earlier findings; a value of about
555 Ω cm was found for the specific cortical resistance. As will be shown
below, the impedance of gray matter is a labile entity which tends to
increase markedly under unfavorable conditions of the cortex. The placement of electrodes in the cortex, which cannot but disturb the tissue
in the surrounding of the electrodes, may explain the higher values observed by these authors.

The impedance of white matter measured at right angles with the fiber
direction is appreciably larger than that of gray matter. Van Harreveld
et al. (1963) found the subcortical white matter impedance determined
normal to the fiber direction four to five times as large as that of the cortex (800 to 1000 Ω cm). Nicholson (1965), Ranck and BeMent (1965),
and Li *et al.* (1968) observed similar values in the corpus callosum, the
dorsal column, and the subcortical white matter. When measured in the
length direction a much smaller impedance (90–200 Ω cm) was determined by Nicholson (1965) and by Ranck and BeMent (1965); Li *et al.*
(1968) found a value of 580 Ω cm.

3. *Tissue Resistance and Extracellular Space*

A computation of the extracellular space with the Maxwell equation from Freygang and Landau's figure (1955) for the specific impedance of the cortex and the specific resistance of CSF (Crile *et al.*, 1922) as a model for the extracellular material yielded a value of about 30% (Van Harreveld and Schadé, 1960). Fenstermacher *et al.* (1970) applied Maxwell's equation to the larger cortical impedance determined with the method of Li *et al.* (1968) and suggested a 15–20% extracellular space. As mentioned above, the figure for the ECS computed by Van Harreveld and Schadé (1960) is probably too high since glial and neuronal fibers situated in the direction of the current lines may not have the high specific resistance required for the application of the simplified Maxwell equation. Ranck (1963b) took the low resistance of fibers in the direction of the current lines into consideration and assumed a low membrane resistance of the glial plasma membrane (Hild and Tasaki, 1962), resulting in his assumption that $\frac{1}{3}$ of the glial volume is the electrical equivalent of interstitial space. He considered his figure for the cortical specific resistance (256 Ω cm) to be consistent with an ECS of 2–15% of the tissue volume. It would seem, however, that the glial membrane resistance cannot be neglected. Krnjevic and Schwartz (1967) measured a higher resistance across the plasma membrane of unresponsive (glia) cells than of neurons. Trachtenberg and Pollen (1970) estimated a value of 200–500 Ω cm^2 for the resistance of the cortical glial plasma membrane. Also, the specific resistance of the glial cytoplasm is undoubtedly larger than that of the CSF used in the above models for the extracellular material. Nicholson (1965) computed an ECS of the white matter of 10% if the membrane resistance of the oligodendrocytes is not lower than 8 Ω cm^2.

The determination of the magnitude of the ECS from the specific tissue resistance, although in theory promising, has met practical difficulties mainly due to the structure of the tissue and to the uncertainty of the glial membrane resistance. Although these difficulties make it impossible to give a definitive figure for the ECS, the low specific impedance of gray matter determined by several investigators suggests an appreciable ECS. The figure may be larger than that suggested by Ranck (1963b) and certainly smaller than that computed by Van Harreveld and Schadé (1960). The value of 15% or more suggested above from the use of extracellular markers would seem consistent with the specific impedances determined.

B. Impedance Changes in Central Nervous Tissue

Large impedance changes of the gray matter have been observed during asphyxiation, spreading depression, and perfusion fixation. The relation between tissue impedance and the extracellular space suggests that these are an indication of changes in the magnitude of this entity.

1. *Asphyxial Impedance Changes*

Leão and Ferreira (1953) were the first to mention an impedance increase of the cerebral cortex during asphyxiation. This observation was confirmed by Freygang and Landau (1955) and by Van Harreveld and Ochs (1956). Figure 2 shows the asphyxial impedance changes of the rabbit cerebral cortex caused by circulatory arrest. During the first 3 minutes there is a slight increase in impedance which can be ascribed to the draining of blood, which has a lower impedance than the nervous tissue, from the vessels. After about 3.5 minutes there develops a rapid rise of the impedance, during which this value almost doubles, followed by an increase at a diminishing rate. Simultaneous with the rapid rise in impedance a surface negativity (asphyxial slow potential change) develops. Collewijn and Schadé (1964a) found a longer latency of the asphyxial impedance rise in cooled preparations (28°C).

A similar asphyxial impedance increase, be it with a somewhat different time course, was recorded in the cerebellum (Van Harreveld, 1961). In the spinal gray matter the impedance change had a much shorter (10–15 seconds) latency than that in cerebral cortex (Van Harreveld and Biersteker, 1964). The spinal cord can be asphyxiated by clamping the

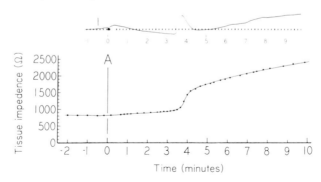

Fig. 2. Asphyxial potential (upper trace) and resistance changes (lower graph) of rabbit cerebral cortex after circulatory arrest at A. The calibration line in the upper record indicates 5-mV deflection for the asphyxial potential. (From Van Harreveld and Ochs, 1956.)

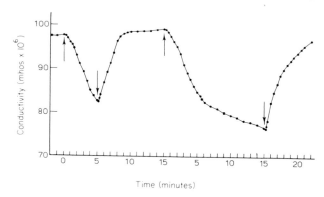

Fig. 3. Conductivity changes of spinal gray matter caused by clamping the thoracic aorta for 5 and 15 minutes. At the arrows pointing up the aorta was clamped, at the arrows pointing down the clamp was released. (From Van Harreveld and Biersteker, 1964.)

thoracic aorta and reoxygenated by reestablishing the circulation. Figure 3 shows the conductivity (reciprocal of the impedance) loss of the spinal gray matter during 5 and 15 minutes of asphyxiation and the prompt recovery during reoxygenation. A similar return to the preasphyxial level of the tissue impedance was observed in the reoxygenated cerebral cortex (Van Harreveld and Tachibana, 1962). The impedance changes are caused by the oxygen lack and not by the accumulation of CO_2 or other metabolites. Figure 4 shows a similar conductivity drop of the spinal gray matter during ventilation of the preparation with nitrogen as during arrest of the circulation (Van Harreveld and Biersteker, 1964).

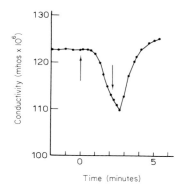

Fig. 4. Changes in the conductivity of spinal gray matter by ventilating the preparation with nitrogen. During the period between the arrows nitrogen was fed into the apparatus for artificial respiration. (From Van Harreveld and Biersteker, 1964.)

2. *Impedance Changes during Spreading Depression*

Spreading depression (SD) was first described by Leão (1944) as a depression of the electrocorticogram which spreads slowly (2–4 mm/minute) from a stimulated area in a more or less concentric fashion over the cerebral cortex. The depression of the corticogram is accompanied by a slow potential change consisting of a surface negativity of the cortex followed by a positivity (Leão, 1947, 1951) and by an increase in the cortical impedance (Leão and Ferreira, 1953; Freygang and Landau, 1955; Van Harreveld and Ochs, 1957; Ranck, 1964; Rosenblueth and Garcia Ramos, 1966; Wong, 1969). Figure 5 shows the depression of the corticogram during SD in the rabbit, accompanied by a slow potential change

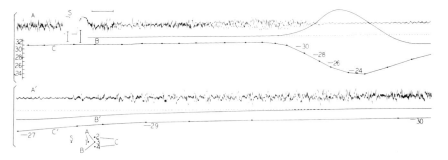

Fig. 5. Electrocorticogram (A, A'), slow potential change record (B, B') and conductivity change in mhos $\times$ 10^5 (C, C') during spreading depression. S indicates stimulation with 4 V dc. In the insert are shown the position of the stimulating electrode (s), the electrodes leading off the electrocorticogram (1 and 3) and the slow potential change (3), and of the electrodes for the resistance measurement (2 and 4). The first vertical calibration line indicates 1 mV for the electrocorticogram, the second 5 mV for the slow potential change. The horizontal calibration line indicates 10 seconds. (From Van Harreveld and Ochs, 1957.)

and a transient conductivity loss of the tissue. The loss in conductivity is smaller than during asphyxiation (of the order of 15%). Freygang and Landau (1955) noted simultaneously with the cortical impedance rise during spreading depression an about 5% drop in the resistance of the underlying white matter. Rosenblueth and Garcia Ramos (1966) and Wong (1969) made similar observations.

3. *Impedance Changes during the Perfusion of the Cortex with Fixatives*

The electron micrographs of brain tissue fixed by submersion or perfusion with the usual fixatives show, in general, a paucity of extracellular space which is not in accord with the more recent determination of the ECS with extracellular markers and with the low specific resistance of gray matter. An investigation of the impedance during the fixation procedure as a measure of possible changes in extracellular space seemed therefore indicated. The perfusion of the cerebral cortex with Bodian and Taylor's fixative (1963), which contains the Ringer's salts, 20% formalin, and 0.1% chloral hydrate, caused in the course of a few minutes a decrease in cortical conductivity comparable in magnitude with the asphyxial drop (Van Harreveld, 1966). Nevis and Collins (1967) measured the cortical resistance during perfusion with a number of fixatives in combination with various buffers and additives. Glutaraldehyde in a veronal acetate buffer (pH 7.4) caused a large and sustained impedance increase. The impedance changes caused by osmium tetroxide varied from a sustained increase to an initial increase followed by a decline, depending on the additives used. Van Harreveld and Khattab (1968c) recorded a sustained conductivity decrease of similar magnitude as the asphyxial drop, during cortical perfusion with a 5% glutaraldehyde solution in a $1/15$ M phosphate buffer at pH 7.4 to which sodium chloride had been added to give the perfusion fluid a similar conductivity as plasma (Fig. 6A). The conductivity drop started after a shorter latency than the asphyxial loss, indicating that the impedance change was caused by the perfusion and not by the arrest of the oxygen supply. Glutaraldehyde perfusion had no significant effect on the tissue conductivity after the cortex had sustained an asphyxial conductivity drop (Fig. 6B). This indicates that the conductivity drops caused by O_2 deprivation and by perfusion fixation are due to the same cause, presumably a loss of extracellular electrolytes. Perfusion with an osmium tetroxide solution in $1/15$ M phosphate buffer caused an initial drop in conductivity followed by a rise to, and sometimes above, the preinfusion level (Fig. 6C) as was also observed in some of Nevis and Collins' experiments (1967). Perfusion of the cortex with osmium tetroxide after asphyxiation and after glutaraldehyde fixation enhanced the conductivity of the tissue (Fig. 6D and E). Perfusion with hydroxyadipaldehyde, a fixative proposed by Torack (1965), caused a biphasic change of the tissue conductivity (Fig. 7A), i. e., an initial drop followed by a rise as observed during OsO_4 fixation (Van Harreveld and Khattab, 1969). After the cortex had sustained an asphyxial loss in conductivity, perfusion with hydroxyadipaldehyde enhanced the conductivity again (Fig. 7B).

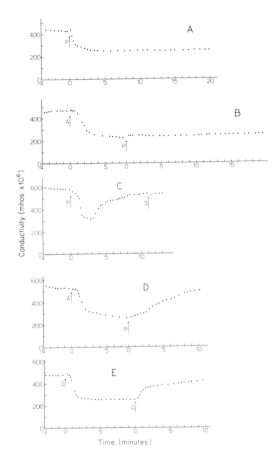

Fig. 6. Mouse cerebral cortex conductivity during fixation and asphyxiation. A. At the arrow (P) the front part of the animal is perfused with Ringer's solution for 10 seconds immediately after circulatory arrest, then with 5% glutaraldehyde in a phosphate buffer. B. At the first arrow (A) the circulation is arrested; at the second arrow (P) the brain is perfused with the glutaraldehyde solution after 10 seconds of perfusion with Ringer's solution. C. At the first arrow (P) the front part of the mouse is perfused for 10 seconds with Ringer's solution, then with 1% osmium tetroxide in the buffer solution. At the second arrow (S) the perfusion is stopped. D. At the first arrow (A) the circulation is arrested; at the second arrow (P) the brain is perfused first with Ringer's for 10 seconds then with the OsO$_4$ solution. E. At the first arrow (G) the front part of the animal is perfused with the glutaraldehyde solution, at the second arrow (O) the brain is perfused with OsO$_4$. (From Van Harreveld and Khattab, 1968c.)

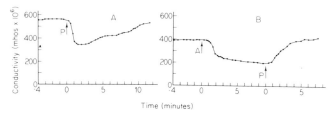

Fig. 7. A. Change in conductivity of mouse cerebral cortex during perfusion with hydroxyadipaldehyde (4.5%) in a Na-cacodylate buffer. The perfusion starts at the arrow (P). B. At the arrow (A) the circulation is arrested, at the arrow (P) the brain is perfused with the hydroxyadipaldehyde solution. (From Van Harreveld and Khattab, 1969.)

4. Impedance Changes Produced in Other Ways

Collewijn and Schadé (1962) observed a decrease of the cortical conductivity of 23% when the cortex was cooled from 37° to 28°C. They explained this impedance change by the effect of temperature on the conductivity of the various media transmitting the measuring current. Fenstermacher et al. (1970) made similar observations and, taking the physical effect of temperature on the resistivity into account, concluded that this impedance increase does not signify a contraction of the ECS.

Several investigators noted that cortical activity changes the tissue impedance. Freygang and Landau (1955) found during the direct cortical response an about 3% decrease in impedance which reached its maximum 5 msec after the stimulus was applied. A similar impedance drop followed by a rise was observed by Klivington and Galambos (1967) during cortical responses evoked by auditory and photic stimulation. Convulsive activity and transcallosal stimulation caused relatively small (less than 5%) increases of the cortical impedance (Efron, 1961; Van Harreveld and Schadé, 1962). Morlock et al. (1964) observed a 0.1–0.3% impedance rise in the geniculate body during photic stimulation. Adey et al. (1962) recorded with a coaxial electrode, chronically implanted in the hippocampus, both increases and decreases of the tissue impedance during enhanced activity. Also, effects were observed on the tissue impedance of alerting, orienting, and discriminative performance, especially in the hippocampus (Adey et al., 1966). Ranck (1966, 1970) recorded in rats during paradoxical sleep a 25% impedance increase in the subiculum and smaller increases in other areas of the brain. Finally, Wang and Adey (1969) observed a marked drop in the resistance of the periventricular tissue after the injection of calcium solutions in the lateral ventricle. A similar drop in the cortical impedance was found after superfusion with Ca solutions (Van Harreveld et al., 1971).

5. *Impedance Changes and the Extracellular Space*

From the above discussion on tissue resistance it can be concluded that large increases in tissue resistance can be explained most readily by contraction of the ECS. An increase in membrane resistance cannot be expected to have much effect since the tissue elements, because of their small dimensions, have already a relatively high specific resistance even if their membrane resistance is not very large. Only in the unlikely case that an appreciable percentage of the tissue elements would feature a very low resistance, much lower than the $3-10 \, \Omega$ cm² estimated by Hild and Tasaki (1962) for glia in tissue cultures, could this explanation account for the large impedance rises observed. A marked increase in tissue impedance therefore indicates, almost with certainty, a contraction of the ECS.

A drop in tissue impedance may be due to an expansion of the ECS but could also be caused by a greatly increased permeability of the cell membranes. Smaller changes may in addition to changes in the magnitude of the ECS be due to changes in conductivity of the extracellular material, variations in the filling of blood vessels, and physiological variations of the membrane resistance. It is sometimes possible to distinguish between these alternatives because of the time course of the phenomenon. It would seem that the small and rapid (measured in milliseconds) drop in tissue resistance during direct cortical responses (Freygang and Landau, 1955) and evoked responses (Klivington and Galambos, 1967) could well be due to excitatory changes in membrane resistances. More gradually developing impedance changes of longer duration are more likely to be of vascular origin, due to changes in the magnitude of the ECS or to changes in conductivity of the extracellular material. For instance, the small impedance decrease of the subcortical white matter during spreading depression observed by Freygang and Landau (1955), Rosenblueth and Garcia Ramos (1966), and Wong (1969) might well be caused by an increased filling of the vessels with blood, which has a much higher conductivity than the white matter.

III. Chloride and Water Movements in Central Nervous Tissue

As discussed above, it seems likely that a marked enhancement of the tissue resistance is due to a loss of extracellular electrolytes. It seems unlikely that these ions move out of the central nervous system through the BBB, leaving the alternate possibility that they are taken up by the intracellular compartment where they are surrounded by cell membranes and cannot freely participate any more in the transport of the measuring current. A movement of extracellular ions, mainly sodium and chloride accompanied by water to maintain osmotic equilibrium into cells and fibers of the tissue, can therefore be expected during asphyxiation, spreading depression and perfusion with some of the fixatives for electron microscopy. Independent evidence has been obtained for this postulate.

A. METHODS FOR THE STUDY OF CHLORIDE AND WATER MOVEMENTS

Chloride and water movements were studied in freeze substituted material. To this end the water and electrolyte distribution in the tissue was fixed by rapid freezing with isopentane cooled to its fusion point. The ice in the tissue was then substituted at low temperature (—20°C) by ethanol. The tissue was embedded and sectioned after staining with one of Cajal's silver impregnation methods. It can be expected that preparations made in this way reflect the water distribution at the moment of freezing (Van Harreveld, 1957). A similar method was used to study the position of chloride in the tissue. To accomplish this the substitution was carried out in 90% ethanol saturated with silver nitrate. As the chloride ions were freed at the plane of substitution they were precipitated by the silver ions as silverchloride, which in the histological preparations made subsequently from this material could be made visible by reduction to a brown or yellow subhalide. The substitution fluid was acidified with nitric acid to prevent the precipitation of anions other than chloride by the silver ions. The low temperature at which the substitution was carried out prevented a reaction between silver nitrate and the proteins of the tissue which is responsible for the well-known methods of silver staining in use for central nervous tissue (Van Harreveld and Potter, 1961).

B. CHLORIDE AND WATER MOVEMENTS ACCOMPANYING MAJOR IMPEDANCE CHANGES

1. *Asphyxial Chloride and Water Transport*

Cerebral and cerebellar cortices frozen while the circulation was intact were compared with material frozen after 6–8 minutes of asphyxiation when the large impedance increase had occurred. Preparations of nonasphyxiated material treated with the histochemical method for chloride showed a rather uniform distribution of the brown and yellow silver subhalide. Only the pia mater and the vessels filled with blood showed a concentration of colored material (Fig. 8A). In the asphyxiated cortices the distribution was different. In the cerebral cortex (Fig. 8B) an accumulation of chloride had occurred in the apical dendrites which stood out as darkened structures on a light background (Van Harreveld and Schadé, 1959). Collewijn and Schadé (1964b) observed this asphyxial chloride shift not only at the normal temperature of the cortex but also at 28° and 20°C.

In the asphyxiated cerebellar cortex chloride had accumulated in the dendrites and often in the somas of the Purkinje cells. Chloride was also present in the fibers of Bergmann, glial structures which run in a radial direction through the molecular layer. They originate from cells situated in the layer of Purkinje cells and form endfeet on the surface, which together constitute a glial membrane. This observation shows that the chloride accumulation can occur both in neural and in glial tissue elements (Van Harreveld, 1961).

A comparison of the diameter of apical dendrites measured at the same distance from the surface in cerebral cortices frozen while the circulation was intact and after 8 minutes of asphyxiation showed statistically significant differences. The apical dendrites in asphyxiated cortex were about 30% thicker than those in the nonasphyxiated control material, indicating that the volume of these structures had increased by 70% (Van Harreveld, 1957). Collewijn and Schadé (1964b) observed a similar asphyxial water uptake at 37°C and at 28°C. At 20°C the apical dendrites in nonasphyxiated cortex were enlarged and did not increase in volume after circulatory arrest. The chloride and water uptake by apical dendrites can be reversed by reoxygenation of the cortex even after relatively long periods of asphyxiation (Van Harreveld and Tachibana, 1962). The diameter of the Bergmann fibers in the cerebellum increased during asphyxiation about 70% in diameter, which corresponds with a volume increase of almost 200% (Van Harreveld, 1961).

2. *Chloride and Water Transport during Spreading Depression*

Rabbit's cerebral cortex, frozen when the impedance increase caused by spreading depression was at a maximum, showed a similar accumulation of chloride in apical dendrites as observed in asphyxiated cortex. In the rabbit the retrospleneal area of the cortex is, under normal circumstances, not invaded by SD (Leão, 1944). In preparations of cortices frozen during SD the chloride accumulation can be seen to stop rather sharply

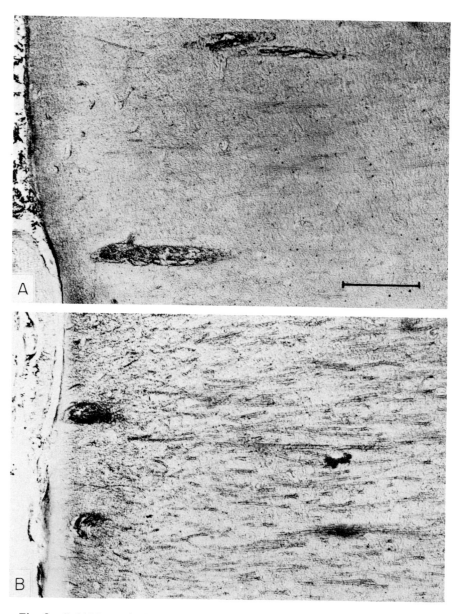

Fig. 8. Rabbit's cerebral cortex treated with a histochemical method for chloride. (A) A section of cortex is shown frozen while the circulation was intact. The pia mater and the blood vessels have a high chloride content. The outlines of apical dendrites are just discernible. (B) A section of cortex which was frozen after the asphyxial impedance change had taken place. The apical dendrites stand out as dark fibers. The tissue in between the apical dendrites is lighter in B than in A. The calibration line indicates 200 μ. (From Van Harreveld, 1966.)

at the parasaggital sulcus, which forms the lateral boundary of the retro-spleneal area (Van Harreveld and Schadé, 1959).

An about 15% increase in the diameter of the apical dendrites was found during spreading depression. This is demonstrated in an experiment in which SD was elicited in the cortex of one hemisphere while the other served as control. Both cortices were frozen when the impedance increase measured between two electrodes placed on the experimental side was at a maximum (Fig. 9). After freeze substitution the cortices were cut in strips and the mean diameter of the apical dendrites was determined in each of these. The figure shows that the diameters of the

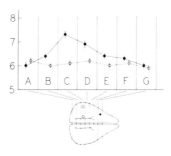

Fig. 9. The figure of the brain shows the locations of the stimulating electrode (closed circle) and resistance electrodes (open circles). The lines indicate the slices cut from the experimental and control cortices after freeze substitution. In the graph is plotted on the ordinate the mean diameter of the apical dendrites in each of the slices (expressed in an arbitrary unit) on the control side (open circles) and the experimental side (closed circles). The vertical lines through the circles and points indicate the standard error of each determination. (From Van Harreveld, 1958.)

apical dendrites in the control cortex did not differ more than can be expected from the standard error of each determination. In the experimental cortex the apical dendrites were significantly larger in the strip where the enhanced impedance indicated the presence of a fully developed SD. The diameters in the adjoining strips are also larger, diminishing with the distance from the strip in which the impedance was measured. This demonstrates the changes in dendritic diameter during the development and recovery from SD (Van Harreveld, 1958).

3. *Chloride Movements during Glutaraldehyde Fixation*

Mouse cerebral cortices frozen after 5 minutes perfusion with a 5% glutaraldehyde solution in a 1/15 *M* phosphate buffer (pH 7.4) were subjected to the histochemical method for chloride. The resulting preparations showed an accumulation of chloride in apical dendrites, which was quite comparable with the asphyxial uptake. The cerebellar cortex perfused for 5 minutes with the glutaraldehyde solution exhibited a movement of chloride into fibers of Bergmann and in some instances into the dendrites of the Purkinje cells as observed during asphyxiation (Van Harreveld and Khattab, 1968b).

4. *The Transport of Electrolytes and Water and the Impedance Changes*

The observed chloride transport during asphyxiation, spreading depression, and glutaraldehyde perfusion of central nervous tissue supports the explanation that the loss of tissue conductivity observed under these conditions is due to a loss of extracellular material. It is assumed that the chloride is accompanied by cations, mainly Na^+, and that the swelling is due to a water uptake to maintain osmotic equilibrium. The postulated Na^+ transport into cellular elements may account for the observation of Hartmann (1966), who found in electron micrographs of material fixed by immersion in an OsO_4 solution and then treated with a histochemical method for Na^+ a high concentration of sodium in astrocytes.

It is possible that during asphyxiation additional mechanisms, such as the hydrolysis of large molecules, enhance the osmoconcentration of the cytoplasm and cause in this way swelling of tissue elements. The hydrolysis of organic phosphates and the increase of the lactic acid concentration developing after arrest of the oxygen supply (Schneider, 1956) could have such an effect. Collewijn and Schadé (1964b) explained in this way the swelling of apical dendrites in a non-asphyxiated cortex at 18°C body temperature which was not accompanied by an accumulation of chloride in these structures. It seems likely, however, that it is mainly the transport of sodium chloride into cellular elements which causes the volume increase of cellular elements during asphyxiation and spreading depression.

IV. Electron Microscopy of Central Nervous Tissue

A. MICROGRAPHS PREPARED WITH CONVENTIONAL FIXATION METHODS

Wyckoff and Young (1956), studying the motoneuron surface in spinal gray matter fixed by perfusion with osmium tetroxide solutions, seem to have been the first to emphasize the absence of an appreciable extracellular space in electron micrographs of such material. This paucity of extracellular space is a striking feature in electron micrographs prepared by chemical fixation methods published before (Pease and Baker, 1951; Dempsey and Wislocki, 1955; Luse, 1956) and in numerous papers after the paper of Wyckoff and Young appeared (e.g., Palay *et al.*, 1962). Improvement of the technique made it possible to estimate the slits between the tissue elements as from 100 to 200 Å wide. These slits are so uniform that Horstmann and Meves (1959) estimated the extracellular space in the optic tectum of the dog fish (*Scylliorhinus canicula*) from the mean diameter of the cellular elements on the assumption that these are separated by 200 Å wide spaces. The amount of extracellular space determined in this way varied with the size of the cellular elements from an appreciable value in the neuropil to very low figures at regions where large structures such as somas were present. The mean ECS of the gray matter was estimated as 5%. More recently, Karlsson and Schultz (1965) and Schultz and Karlsson (1965) observed in EM's of tissue fixed by perfusion with formaldehyde or glutaraldehyde and postfixed with OsO_4 even less extracellular space. They concluded that the plasma membranes are closely apposed (tight junctions) and that the extracellular space consists only of small triangular spaces where three cellular elements meet. González-Aguilar (1969) observed in gray matter of the rat fixed by perfusion with 12 *M* formaldehyde and postfixed with OsO_4 areas featuring 150–200 Å extracellular slits in addition to regions in which the cell membranes were closely approximated. An extracellular space of less than 5% was estimated for the gray matter.

An exception to the almost unanimous findings of a small ECS in EM's prepared with conventional fixation methods was the observation of Torack (1965), who fixed the tissue by perfusion with hydroxyadipaldehyde and postfixed with OsO_4. The resulting EM's exhibited a much larger ECS which was mainly distributed in bundles of small profiles, probably unmyelinated axons. At places where neuronal and glial structures came in contact, slits of the usual dimensions were seen between the tissue elements.

The estimate of an ECS of 5% or less from EM's prepared with conventional fixation procedures was readily accepted because this figure agreed with the spaces determined by the simple intravenous administration of extracellular markers such as inulin or sulfate. The postulated absence of an appreciable ECS posed a question about the way in which metabolites and the products of metabolism would be transported between the brain capillaries and the cells. It was suggested that the glial components of the tissue would substitute for the ECS of the body organs as a pathway for these compounds (Schultz *et al.*, 1957; Farquhar and Hartmann, 1957; Luse, 1960a,b, 1962; Bondareff, 1965). Although it is now quite likely that the ECS in the gray matter is larger than suggested by these early papers, the intimate relationship of certain glial and nervous elements may well be the expression of a metabolic interaction of these tissue components.

B. THE SPACES IN ELECTRON MICROGRAPHS AND THE EXTRACELLULAR SPACE

Before a tissue can be viewed under the electron microscope it has to be subjected to a long series of processes, each of which can, and probably does, cause changes in the relative magnitude of cellular structures and spaces. The tissue has to be fixed which in the past was usually carried out by treatment with osmium tetroxide alone but, presently, mostly by perfusion with glutaraldehyde or formaldehyde followed by post-fixation with OsO_4. The aldehyde solutions used were in general highly hyperosmotic (e.g., Karlsson and Schultz, 1965; González-Aguilar, 1969).

When fixation is performed by immersion of the tissue a period of asphyxiation can be expected to precede the action of the fixative because of the time involved in the diffusion of the fixative into the material. The increase in tissue impedance and the transport of chloride and water into cellular elements suggested that during asphyxiation a contraction of the ECS occurs. During immersion fixation the antecedent asphyxiation thus may cause a reduction of the ECS before the fixative has time to diffuse into the material.

It has been suggested that the asphyxial contraction of the extracellular space can be prevented by perfusion fixation which was believed to fix the tissue before oxygen deficiency develops. However, perfusion with formaldehyde (Van Harreveld, 1966) and glutaraldehyde produced impedance increases of the same magnitude as asphyxiation (Nevis and Collins, 1967; Van Harreveld and Khattab, 1968c). The observation that after the asphyxial impedance increase had been elicited, perfusion with glutaraldehyde was without effect on the tissue resistance (Van Harreveld and Khattab, 1968c) suggested that both these impedance rises are due to identical causes, i.e., to a contraction of the ECS. This conclusion was supported by the observation that during glutaraldehyde perfusion chloride accumulates in the same tissue elements as during asphyxiation. A transport of extracellular material into the intracellular compartment is obviously not accompanied by any externally observable change in tissue volume.

After fixation the tissue is dehydrated usually with acetone or ethanol which then is replaced with a compound such as propylene oxide miscible with these solvents and with the embedding material. After this, the material is impregnated with plastics such as methacrylate, Maraglass, or Epon, which finally are polymerized to yield a block suitable for thin sectioning. Nevis and Collins (1967) showed that dehydration results in a volume decrease of the tissue but that embedding in Epon causes little if any additional shrinking.

The shrinkage of the tissue caused by dehydration and embedding may affect both the extra- and intracellular compartments resulting in changes in the absolute magnitude of these entities but probably has only a small effect on the ratio of the compartments. The change in space distribution suggested by the impedance increase during glutaraldehyde perfusion, however, is specifically an alteration of the ratio of the extra- and intracellular spaces causing a much more severe distortion of the ECS than dehydration.

In view of these considerations the assurances given by proponents of particular fixatives that they do not affect the space distribution in the tissue cannot be accepted on face value. In order to investigate the magnitude of extracellular space in central nervous tissue special methods are needed which circumvent the mechanism that causes the contraction of the ECS during conventional fixation procedures.

C. THE USE OF FREEZE SUBSTITUTION FOR THE PRESERVATION OF THE WATER DISTRIBUTION

As will be discussed below it is postulated that the transport of extracellular ions into the intracellular compartment is caused by an increase in the sodium permeability of the plasma membrane. This disturbs the double Donnan equilibrium which maintains the normal distribution of electrolytes between the extra- and intracellular compartments. The permeability change results in a movement of extracellular sodium chloride into the affected cellular elements, accompanied by water to maintain osmotic equilibrium. As pointed out by Van Harreveld *et al.* (1965), freeze substitution can be expected to hamper this process for the following reasons. The material is after freezing placed in 100% acetone or ethanol at low temperature. The solvents proceed to dissolve ice to the maximum water concentration they can contain at the temperature of substitution. Acetone at —85°C, the temperature at which the substitution was routinely carried out (Van Harreveld and Crowell, 1964), can contain maximally 2% water. The water diffuses into the surrounding acetone or ethanol and the plane of substitution moves in this way slowly deeper into the tissue. Since the water concentration cannot rise above 2%, the ice in the tissue is replaced directly by 98% acetone. The solubility of NaCl in acetone saturated with water at this temperature is very low, i.e., 0.0018% (Van Harreveld et al., 1965). The mechanism of the transport from extra- in to the intracellular compartment which depends on the solubility of NaCl may therefore be greatly retarded and perhaps prevented. Furthermore, the possibility will be discussed below that the increased sodium permeability of the membrane is due to glutamate released from the extracellular compartment into the ECS. Nothing is known about the effect of low temperatures either on the release of this amino acid nor on its ability to alter the Na permeability of the plasma membrane. It seems likely, however, that these processes will be greatly depressed at —85°C and in the abnormal millieu of 98% acetone. Freeze-drying was used as an alternate method of tissue preparation for the electron microscope. A transport of electrolytes from the extra- into the intracellular compartment seems even less likely with this method.

Although freeze substitution and freeze-drying can be expected to prevent the transport of extracellular material into the intracellular compartment during fixation, the replacement of the water of the tissue by acetone or ethanol and the subsequent embedding in plastic may introduce more or less serious distortion of the space distribution.

Freezing followed by freeze substitution for electron microscopy poses problems since extensive ice crystal formation tends to mask the fine structure of the tissue. The material is usually frozen by immersion in liquid propane, Freon or isopentane cooled close to their fusion points, and substituted in solvents such as acetone or ethanol. The results of attempts to freeze substitute in this way relatively large tissue specimen without the use of protective additives such as glycerol or dimethyl sulfoxide have in general not been encouraging (Rebhun, 1965; Bondareff and Pysh, 1968). Pease (1967a,b) reported satisfactory results from freezing in Freon and on cold metal and substitution in ethylene- or propyleneglycol. It seems likely, however, that the latter compounds do not fix the material and, therefore, do not preserve the ice crystal ghosts in the tissue as acetone and ethanol do. Fernandez-Morán (1960) and Bullivant (1960) used helium II for freezing, which in addition to its low temperature, has the advantage of being superconductive for heat.

This promises an extremely rapid heat transport from the surface of the object.

In a less demanding technique the tissue was brought in contact with a polished and carefully cleaned cold metal surface (Van Harreveld and Crowell, 1964). Silver was used for this purpose because of its good heat-conducting properties. The metal surface, situated at the bottom of a deep well, was cooled to about —207°C by liquid nitrogen under reduced pressure. Condensation of water, carbon dioxide, and oxygen on the surface was prevented by a stream of cooled helium which filled the well. The tissue fell at a controlled speed through the well on the cold metal surface. It is possible that the firm contact which in this way is established between tissue and cooling surface is a factor in the success of this method, in addition to the good heat conduction of the metal. The rate of freezing with this method is high (Van Harreveld and Crowell, 1964) which tends to preserve the water distribution in the tissue (Mazur, 1970). The material was freeze substituted for 2 days at —85°C in 100% acetone or ethanol in which 2% OsO_4 had been dissolved. Neither the solvent (J. R. Baker, 1958) nor the OsO_4 seem to affect the tissue at this low temperature. When the material was brought to room temperature, the OsO_4 which had diffused into the tissue caused the usual blackening. Finally, the tissue was embedded in a plastic in the usual fashion. This method yielded in a fair percentage of the trials EM's in which the superficial 10–15 μ did not show ice formation. In the deeper layers the fine structure was always seriously disturbed by ice crystals.

D. Extracellular Space in Electron Micrographs Prepared by Freeze Substitution

1. *Extracellular Space in the Cerebellar Cortex*

Asphyxiation and mechanical disturbances have been found to cause an impedance rise in central nervous tissue, suggesting a loss of extracellular material. The cerebellar cortex was therefore frozen shortly (within 30 seconds) after circulatory arrest (by decapitation), before an asphyxial impedance increase can be expected. Furthermore, to avoid mechanical disturbance the tissue was not taken from the brain case. After removal of the occipital bone the isolated head was fixed on a carrier in such a way that the exposed vermis was parallel with the silver freezing surface. Then the whole head was lowered into the well. This necessitated the use of a small animal such as the mouse which has been used exclusively in these investigations. Furthermore, the pia is thin in these animals, which is an advantage since in larger species this membrane would form an appreciable part of the superficial 10–15 μ layer of tissue suitable for electron microscopy.

A comparison was made between EM's of cerebellar cortex prepared in the way described above with those of material frozen 6–8 minutes after decapitation, sufficiently long to elicit the asphyxial impedance rise (Van Harreveld et al., 1965; Van Harreveld and Steiner, 1970a). The EM's of the surface of the cerebellar cortex frozen shortly after circulatory arrest and cut at right angles with the folia of the vermis show numerous cross sections of nonmyelinated parallel fibers, dendrites of Purkinje cells and their spines, and length sections of Bergmann fibers forming endfeet on the surface (Figs. 10–12). The glia between the nervous elements consists mostly of processes of the latter fibers. Numerous synapses are generally found in this tissue. All the cellular elements have a more or less uniform electron density. Electron micrographs of this material exhibit, in general, an appreciable extracellular space which is particularly prominent in the fields of parallel fibers. These fibers have a rounded contour and lack the polygonal shape forced on them by the close packing of the fibers in EM's prepared by conventional fixation methods. The spaces between glia and pre- and post-synaptic structures consist of 150–250 Å wide slits. The synaptic cleft was 200 to 300 Å wide, which is not different from the dimension observed in conventionally fixed preparations.

The EM's of cerebellar cortex treated in the same way but for an interval of 6–8 minutes between decapitation and freezing, exhibited a very different appearance (Figs. 13–15). The fibers of Bergmann, their endfeet, and their processes between the neural elements were considerably enlarged and had a lower electron density than the profiles of the parallel fibers. Also the dendrites and dendritic spines appeared swollen and electron transparent. The parallel fibers never exhibited swelling. The most striking difference with EM's of nonasphyxiated tissue was the paucity of ECS between the profiles of the parallel fibers most of which were polygonal and were closely approximated, often forming five-layered junctions. Also, the slits between the glia and the pre- and post-synaptic structures were narrower than in the nonasphyxiated material. The synaptic gap had the usual dimension of about 250 Å.

Similar EM's were obtained from asphyxiated and nonasphyziated cerebellar cortex prepared by freeze drying instead of freeze substitution (Van Harreveld and Malhotra, 1966).

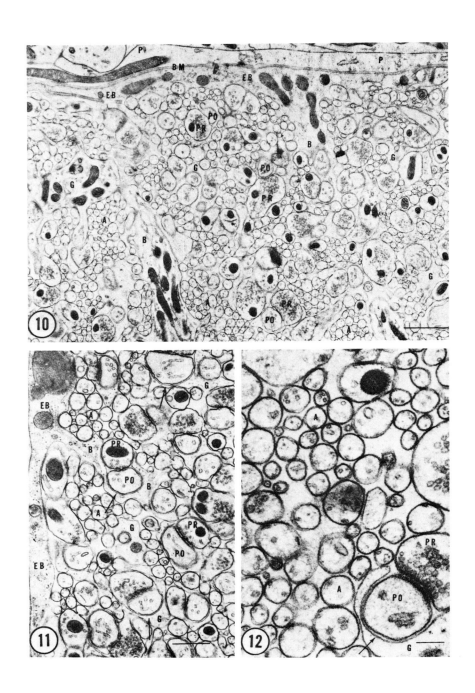

2. *Extracellular Space in the Cerebral Cortex*

Cerebral cortex was frozen in the same way as the cerebellar cortex by positioning its surface parallel to the silver freezing surface. Although the molecular layer exhibits less regularity in its structure than the cerebellar cortex, the same elements can be distinguished. Again, EM's of tissue frozen shortly after circulatory arrest were compared with those of asphyxiated cortex (Van Harreveld and Malhotra, 1967; Van Harreveld and Steiner, 1970a). In nonasphyxiated cortex the profiles of nonmyelinated axons were rounded and an appreciable ECS was present between these fibers. The electron density of the various tissue elements was again rather uniform. In asphyxiated cortex the space betwen the profiles of small axons which had become more polygonal had disappeared. Their plasma membranes were closely approximated, often forming five-layered junctions. No swelling of these fibers was ever observed. However, there were present in the asphyxiated cortex large electron transparent, apparently swollen, elements some of which could be identified as dendritic elements by synaptic contacts whereas others may have been of a glial nature.

Bondareff and Pysh (1968) froze rat cerebral cortex in liquid propane and prepared EM's from this material by substitution in acetone. Although marred by ice crystals, the EM's exhibited an appreciable extracellular space located mainly in bundles of nonmyelinated axons. They observed a larger extracellular space in immature animals than in adults. Less ECS was observed by Bondareff (1967) in freeze-dried cerebral cortex.

Since spreading depression causes a smaller but in all other aspects similar impedance increase of cerebral cortex as asphyxiation, EM's of cortex frozen during spreading depression elicited by electrical stimulation or by placing a small square of filter paper moistened with a KCl

---

Figs. 10, 11, and **12.** Electron micrographs of the molecular layer of the cerebellar cortex. The cerebellum was frozen within 30 seconds of circulatory arrest. There is an appreciable extracellular space between the bundles of nonmyelinated axons. Between the glia and pre- and post-synaptic structures are 100 to 200 Å wide slits (arrows). The electron density of the tissue elements (including the glia) is quite uniform. The letter A in this and subsequent electron micrographs stands for a field of axons, B for a fiber of Bergmann, BM for basement membrane, D for dendrite, EB for endfoot of a Bergmann fiber, M for mitochondrium, G for glia, P for pia, PO for a post-synaptic structure, and PR represents a pre-synaptic terminal. The calibration line in Fig. 10 indicates 1 μ. In Figs. 11 and 12 the lines represent 0.5 and 0.2 μ respectively. (From Van Harreveld and Steiner, 1970a.)

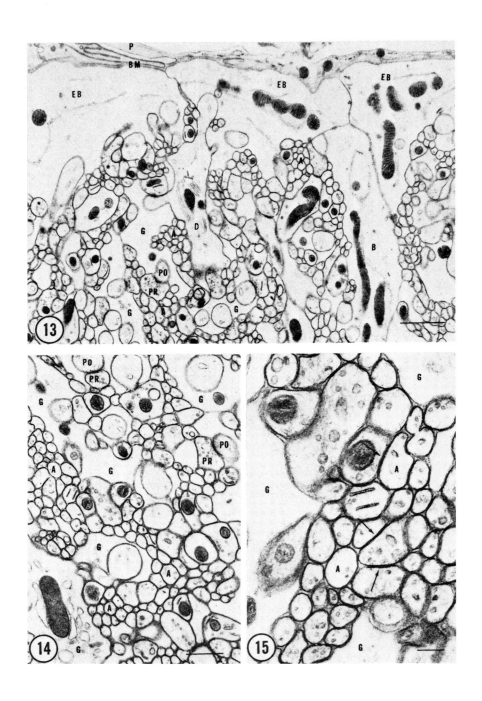

solution on the cortex were compared with those of tissue not invaded by this phenomenon (Van Harreveld and Khattab, 1967). A loss of extracellular space and the presence of swollen electron transparent structures was found in EM's of cortices frozen during spreading depression. Many of the swollen structures could be identified as dendrites or dendritic spines. No swelling of the thin axons was observed. These experiments are of interest since they made possible the comparison of tissues of the same cortex prepared in exactly the same way but under different physiological conditions.

Treatment of the cerebral cortex with an isotonic $CaCl_2$ solution caused a marked drop in tissue resistance. In EM's of this material prepared by freeze substitution, an enlarged extracellular space was found (Van Harreveld et al., 1971).

3. Extracellular Space in White Matter

The white matter at the dorsal surface of the medulla was frozen in a way similar to that described for the cerebellar vermis (Malhotra and Van Harreveld, 1966). The specific resistance of white matter is considerably larger than that of gray, suggesting a smaller ECS. Indeed the myelinated fibers and the oligodendrocytes associated with them form a compact tissue exhibiting very little ECS. However, an appreciable amount of extracellular material was present in bundles of nonmyelinated fibers.

E. CHANGES IN EXTRACELLULAR SPACE DURING FIXATION FOR ELECTRON MICROSCOPY

1. Glutaraldehyde Perfusion

The impedance rise of gray matter and the transport of chloride into cellular elements of the cerebellar and cerebral cortices during glutaral-

---

Figs. 13, 14, and 15. Electron micrographs of the molecular layer of the cerebellar cortex frozen 8 minutes after circulatory arrest, after the asphyxial impedance increase had developed. The Bergmann fibers and their endfeet are swollen and electron transparent. Also, the glia in the neuropil is swollen, as are dendritic structures. Much of the extracellular material present in nonasphyxiated cortex has disappeared. The nerve fibers in the axon fields are so closely approximated that at many places five-layered junctions are formed by their plasma membranes (arrows in Fig. 15). Also the slits between glia and pre- and post-synaptic structures are narrower than in nonasphyxiated material. The calibration line in Fig. 13 indicates 1 μ; in Figs. 14 and 15, 0.5, and 0.2 μ respectively. (From Van Harreveld and Steiner, 1970a.)

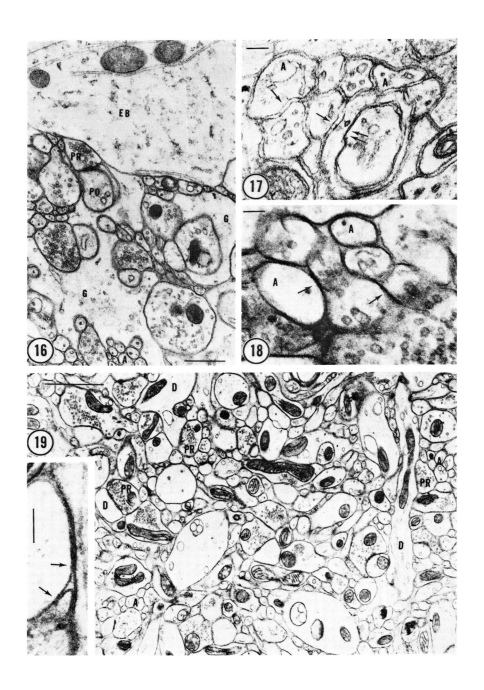

dehyde perfusion suggested a similar loss of extracellular material to the intracellular compartment as observed during asphyxiation. Since the impedance rise started with a shorter latency than the asphyxial increase, it was concluded that the transport of extracellular material is due to the action of the fixative rather than to O_2 deficiency. Electron micrographs of the cerebral and cerebellar cortices freeze substituted after 10–15 minutes of perfusion with 2.5 and 5% glutaraldehyde solutions in a 1/15 M phosphate buffer at pH 7.4 (Figs. 16, 18, 19) resembled similar EM's of asphyxiated tissue (Van Harreveld and Khattab, 1968c; Van Harreveld and Steiner, 1970a). They showed a paucity of extracellular space between the small axons although this was not always as pronounced as in asphyxiated material. Still, the plasma membranes of these fibers were often so closely approximated that five layered junctions resulted. In the cerebellar cortex the fibers of Bergmann and the Purkinje cell dendrites were enlarged and electron transparent; in the cerebral cortex the swollen structures were often of a dendritic nature. The thin, non-myelinated axons never participated in the swelling.

2. *The Effect of Osmium Tetroxide Postfixation*

The glutaraldehyde perfused and freeze substituted material yielded EMS which differed from those usually obtained by more conventional fixation by glutaraldehyde perfusion and osmium tetroxide postfixation. In the former there is less extracellular space which is mainly restricted to triangular spaces where three tissue elements meet. At many places

---

Fig. 16. Molecular layer of the cerebellar cortex, freeze substituted after 10 minutes of glutaraldehyde perfusion. The endfoot of the Bergmann fiber and the glia in the neuropil are swollen. The extracellular space in the bundles of small nerve fibers has disappeared. This EM resembles that of asphyxiated cerebellum (Fig. 13). The calibration line indicates 0.5 μ. (From Van Harreveld and Steiner, 1970a.)

Fig. 17. Cerebral cortex, perfused with glutaraldehyde and afterward postfixed for 2 hours with osmium tetroxide, frozen, and substituted. An axon field is shown exhibiting uniform slits between the tissue elements (arrows). At one spot the membranes are more closely approximated (double arrows). Calibration line indicates 0.1 μ. (From Van Harreveld and Khattab, 1968c.)

Figs. 18 and 19. Cerebral cortex perfused with glutaraldehyde, frozen, and subjected to freeze substitution. Some of the electron transparent, swollen elements can be identified as dendritic by synaptic contacts. The extracellular space is often reduced to triangular spaces where three cellular elements meet. At many places the cell membranes show five-layered junctions (arrows in the insert of Fig. 19 and in Fig. 18). Calibration line indicates 1 μ in Fig. 19; in the insert of Fig. 19 and in Fig. 18 it is 0.1 μ. (From Van Harreveld and Khattab, 1968c.)

the plasma membranes, especially of the small nonmyelinated fibers, are closely approximated. In OsO_4 treated material the extracellular space is characteristically present in the form of the uniformly wide slits between the cellular elements which enabled Horstmann and Meves (1959) to estimate the extracellular space from the magnitude of the tissue elements. Perfusion of the cerebral cortex with an OsO_4 solution after perfusion with glutaraldehyde reduced the tissue impedance which was greatly enhanced during the application of glutaraldehyde (Fig. 6E). As mentioned above, this impedance change can be interpreted in several ways, one of them being an increase of the extracellular material. The impedance drop during OsO_4 perfusion of glutaraldehyde fixed cortex may therefore be the expression of the change of a tissue with very little space after glutaraldehyde perfusion to a tissue with the larger spaces of uniform width after OsO_4 postfixation. Indeed, EM's of material perfused with glutaraldehyde, postfixed with OsO_4, and then freeze substituted showed the typical uniform slits of tissue prepared in the same way but not subjected to freeze substitution (Fig. 17).

Perfusion with osmium tetroxide solution caused an impedance rise followed by a drop to, or below, the preinfusion figure (Fig. 6C). It seems likely that this signifies a contraction of the ECS as during glutaraldehyde perfusion followed by the formation of the uniform slits typical for OsO_4 treated material. One can speculate on the mechanism involved in the creation of uniform tissue slits by OsO_4. It could be surmised that the application of this compound results in the formation of an electrical charge on the membranes. The repulsion by charges of equal sign on opposing membranes then could explain the uniformity of the slits.

The course of events during glutaraldehyde fixation and OsO_4 postfixation can now be pictured as follows. During the glutaraldehyde fixation the extracellular material is taken up by specific cellular elements which swell and become electron transparent. The postfixation then creates a new space consisting of the uniform slits. This leads to the familiar picture of central nervous tissue treated in this way in which one may find structures (dendrites, glia) that are swollen and electron transparent as compared with the same structures in EM's of freeze substituted nonasphyxiated tissue and that exhibits the typical uniform slits between the tissue elements.

3. *Extracellular Space during Hydroxyadipaldehyde Fixation*

Torack (1965) observed in hydroxyadipaldehyde perfused, OsO_4 postfixed cortex an appreciable extracellular space mainly between nonmyelinated fibers, similar to that found in nonasphyxiated freeze substituted material. The cortical impedance during perfusion with this fixative showed an increase during the first minutes of perfusion followed by a decrease often to below the preperfusion level (Fig. 7A). This could be the expression of a contraction followed by an expansion of the ECS. Indeed cerebral cortices frozen and substituted at the height of the initial impedance rise yielded EM's exhibiting a paucity of ECS between the small axons, five-layered junctions between these fibers, and the presence of swollen structures some of which could be identified by synaptic contacts as dendrites (Fig. 20). Eletron micrographs of cortex frozen after 15–20 minutes of perfusion with hydroxyadipaldehyde when the impedance had decreased again exhibited an abnormally large ECS between the small tissue elements which showed rounded profiles. Enlarged tissue elements were still present which often contained grossly swollen mitochondria (Fig. 21). When this tissue was postfixed with OsO_4 and then frozen, EM's were obtained which resembled those published by Torack showing a substantial extracellular space between the small tissue elements although less than in the non-postfixed material (Van Harreveld and Khattab, 1969).

The observation of Torack (1966) that the extracellular space of rat cortex is accessible to Thorotrast in tissue perfused with hydroxyadipaldehyde but not in glutaraldehyde perfused material is in accord with the differences in ECS produced by these fixatives.

F. The Spaces in Electron Micrographs Prepared by Freeze Substitution and the Extracellular Space

Reasons for the postulate that freeze substitution preserves the space distribution in central nervous tissue more faithfully than conventional fixation methods were mentioned above. Although one cannot be sure that the spaces observed in the EM's correspond exactly with those present in the tissue at the moment of freezing, the differences in ECS observed under various conditions which are in good agreement with the predictions made from the impedance changes and the movements of chloride and water strongly suggest that EM's prepared by freeze substitution at least reflect the magnitude of the extracellular space. The conclusion to be drawn from this then is that in the normal living gray matter there is an appreciable extracellular space. This space contracts during asphyxiation and spreading depression by a movement of extracellular material into specific cellular elements which become swollen and electron transpar-

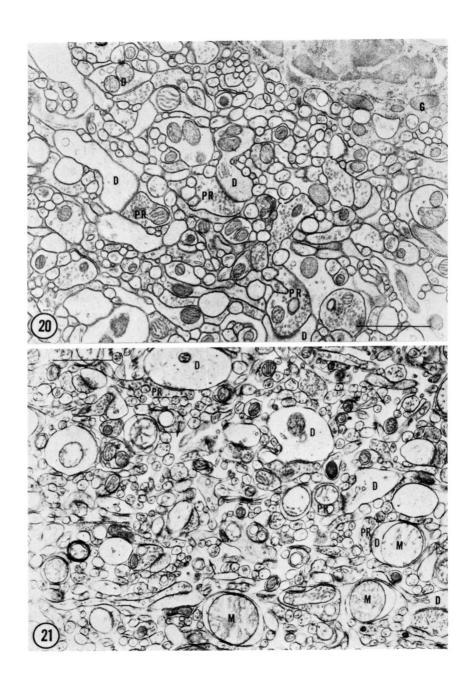

ent. Treatment with fixatives causes more complicated contractions and expansions of the ECS. In the cases investigated the first effect of these chemicals was a severe contraction of the space which could be followed by an expansion. The expansion was especially marked during prolonged hydroxyadipaldehyde perfusion. A special feature of OsO_4 application was the tendency to form uniform clefts between the tissue elements.

The determination of the magnitude of the ECS from EM's of freeze substituted material is hazardous. In addition to the doubt whether these EM's represent exactly the space in the living tissue there is the difficulty that an electron micrograph represents only a very small part of the tissue. Most of the extracellular space is found in bundles of small non-myelinated axons. In regions where many large elements such as somas are present the extracellular space will be small. Van Harreveld et al. (1965) determined with the Chalkley method an ECS of 18–25.5% with a mean of 23.5% in EM's prepared by freeze substitution of the surface neuropil of the cerebellar cortex. Since there are no large tissue elements in these regions, this figure may be larger than the overall extracellular space in the nervous system which includes white matter and regions with numerous nerve cell bodies in which there is less ECS. Bondareff and Pysh (1968) measured an extracellular space of 21.5% in EM's of cerebral cortex of adult rats prepared by freeze substitution.

The conclusion that an appreciable extracellular space exists in the central nervous system in supported by the observation of movements of relatively large particles in the spaces between tissue elements. This was shown for ferritin by Brightman (1965a,b), for saccharated iron oxide by Pappas and Purpura (1966), and by Villegas and Fernandez (1966) for thorium dioxide.

It is of interest that the EM's of central nervous tissue of immature animals prepared by conventional fixation methods exhibit a materially larger ECS than those of adult material (Karlsson, 1967; Sumi, 1969;

Fig. 20. Cerebral cortex frozen after 2 minutes of hydroxyadipaldehyde perfusion and then subjected to freeze substitution. Some of the swollen, electron transparent structures can be identified as dendritic in nature by synaptic contacts. The tissue is characterized by a paucity of extracellular material. The plasma membranes are closely approximated. Calibration line indicates 1 μ. (From Van Harreveld and Khattab, 1969.)

Fig. 21. The same tissue perfused with hydroxyadipaldehyde for 20 minutes and then subjected to freeze substitution. Enlarged dendrites are present, some of the mitochondria are enormously swollen. An abundant extracellular space is found (arrows) between the unmyelinated axons which have a rounded profile. The calibration line indicates 1 μ. (From Van Harreveld and Khattab, 1969.)

Pysh, 1969; Caley and Maxwell, 1968a,b, 1970). This is in agreement with the reduction of the ECS determined with extracellular markers during maturation (see above). Caley and Maxwell (1970) considered the possibility that the larger extracellular spaces in immature animals may be better preserved because the process which causes a transport of extracellular material into the intracellular compartment during fixation has not yet developed.

G. Abnormal Fluid Uptake by Cellular Elements during Asphyxiation, Spreading Depression, and Fixation

In general the bone and dura over the cerebral cortex cannot be removed without mechanical disturbance of the tissue which may elicit spreading depression. Even if this is not produced, the mechanical stimulation may cause transient changes in the space distribution in the cortex. To give the cortex time to recover it was superfused for some time after its exposure with a physiological salt solution warmed to body temperature. When in these experiments the cortex was frozen shortly after circulatory arrest, the space distribution of the resulting EM's was not different from micrographs of material which was frozen without superfusion. However, when such cortices were asphyxiated while being superfused they yielded EM's which showed grossly swollen structures. These could sometimes be identified as dendrites or dendritic spines by synaptic contacts (Van Harreveld and Malhotra, 1967). Similar observations were made on cortices in which spreading depression was elicited by flooding the cortical surface with an isotonic KCl solution. The swelling of dendritic elements was so large that they could be seen with the light microscope as transparent spots, often containing small dark structures which probably were mitochondria. The swelling due to SD in superfused cortex was to a large degree reversible (Van Harreveld and Khattab, 1967). Perfusion with glutaraldehyde of cortices superfused with a physiological salt solution also led to enormous swelling of tissue elements, some of which could be identified as dendrites. The swelling was often so large that the plasma membranes ruptured (Fig. 22). Also these swollen tissue elements could be observed with the light microscope (Figs. 23 and 24) as transparent spots (Van Harreveld and Khattab, 1968c).

The enormous swelling of these cellular elements cannot possibly be explained by the uptake of extracellular material. It would seem, therefore, that the superfusion fluid which is present in near unlimited quantity is available to these structures. This explanation is supported by the observation that the swollen elements viewed with the light microscope are present only in the upper $\frac{1}{3}$ of the molecular layer (Figs. 23 and 24). The gross swelling of dendritic elements of superfused cortex during asphyxiation, spreading depression and glutaraldehyde fixation is an indication of the avidity with which these structures take up fluid from their surrounding under these circumstances. It is of interest that the perfusion fluid used for fixation does not seem to be available to cortical dendrites since in the not superfused cortex these tissue elements seem to take up only the extracellular material, swelling to about the same degree as in asphyxiated nonsuperfused freeze substituted cortex. It is possible that the hypertonicity of the glutaraldehyde solutions used (800 mosmols) prevented its uptake by the cellular elements.

H. DIFFERENCES IN THE EXTRACELLULAR SPACE IN DEEP AND SUPERFICIAL LAYERS OF THE CEREBRAL CORTEX

Karlsson and Schultz (1965), Johnston and Roots (1967), and González-Aguilar (1969) observed more extracellular space in superficial than in deep regions of central nervous tissue prepared by aldehyde perfusion and OsO_4 postfixation. The superficial layer is in a special position since it has access to fluid on the surface of the cortex. Even when the cortex is not intentionally flooded as in the above experiments, the superficial cortical tissue has access to the thin layer of CSF in the subarachnoidal space which will be taken up during the perfusion with glutaraldehyde by the same elements that accumulate the extracellular material. A more pronounced swelling of these structures can therefore be expected in the superficial layers of the cortex than in the deeper regions where only the extracellular material is available for transport into the intracellular compartment. A comparison of EM's of superficial and deep regions of the cortex fixed with glutaraldehyde and OsO_4 showed, ideed, a more pronounced swelling of dendritic structures in the superficial regions than in the deep ones (Van Harreveld and Steiner, 1970b).

During the OsO_4 postfixation a redistribution of water occurs in the tissue which results in the more or less uniformly wide slits between the tissue elements, typical for OsO_4 treated material. In the cerebellum this was accompanied by a shrinking of the fibers of Bergmann which had taken up extracellular material during glutaraldehyde perfusion (Van Harreveld and Steiner, 1970a) suggesting that these structures give up material to form the OsO_4 slits. It would seem possible that the magnitude

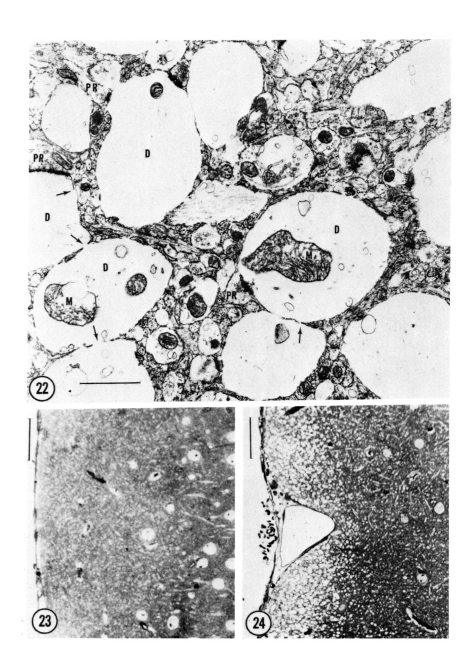

of these slits is in this way related to the dendritic swelling which would explain the difference in the ECS in superficial and deep tissue fixed by glutaraldehyde and OsO_4.

To test the postulated effect of dendritic swelling on the width of the slits between the tissue elements, the swelling was greatly enhanced by perfusing the cortex with glutaraldehyde while it was superfused with a physiological salt solution. After OsO_4 postfixation EM's of this material featured spaces between the tissue elements which at places were more than 500 Å wide, supporting the concept that the width of the tissue spaces formed by OsO_4 postfixation are affected by material available in the dendritic elements, swollen during glutaraldehyde perfusion. This seems to be another instance of the complexity of the processes involved in the fixation of nervous tissue which have to be known for an understanding of the resulting space distribution.

V. Mechanisms Involved in the Electrolyte and Water Transport in Central Nervous Tissue

A. The Electrolyte and Water Transport

The distribution of water and electrolytes in the central nervous system has been found to be a labile one, which can be altered profoundly by asphyxiation, spreading depression and by the chemical stimulation provided by the treatment of the tissue with fixatives. It seems likely that the mechanism which causes the observed transport of extracellular material into cellular elements of the tissue is the same in all these in-

---

Fig. 22.   Cerebral cortex perfused with glutaraldehyde shortly after circulatory arrest while being flooded with a salt solution, then postfixed with osmium tetroxide. Enormously swollen elements are present some of which can be identified as dendritic by synaptic contacts. Some of these structures contain swollen mitochondria and endoplasmic reticulum. The plasma membranes of the swollen structures show frequent breaks (arrows). Calibration line indicates 1 μ. (From Van Harreveld and Khattab, 1968c.)

Figs. 23 and **24.**   Photomicrographs of the cerebral cortex perfused immediately after circulatory arrest with glutaraldehyde, stained with methylene blue and azure II. The cortex shown in Fig. 23 was not flooded with a salt solution, the tissue yielding Fig. 24 was flooded during the perfusion. The latter photomicrograph shows swollen structure which correspond with those in the electron micrograph of Fig. 22. The swelling is present only in the surface layer. The nonflooded cortex has a granular appearance. The calibration line indicates 50 μ. (From Van Harreveld and Khattab, 1968c.)

stances. A change in the ion permeability of the plasma membrane of the structures involved has been postulated as the basic cause of this transport (Van Harreveld and Ochs, 1956; Van Harreveld, 1966). Such a change disturbs the mechanism by which the differences in ionic composition of the extra- and intracellular compartment are maintained. The main ions in the extracellular compartment are sodium and chloride; the main intracellular cation is potassium. The intracellular anions have not been defined in the vertebrates, but may consist of proteins, amino acid, phosphate, etc. An investigation of the axoplasm of giant fibers of the squid showed it to be mainly a specific amino acid (isethionic acid). In crustaceans other amino acids, aspartic acid, and to a smaller extent, glutamic acid, alanine, and taurine form the bulk of the organic anions. The differences in intra- and extracellular ion composition are maintained by membrane properties and ion pumps which establish a steady state sometimes called the "double Donnan equilibrium." It is assumed that the plasma membrane is impermeable for the large intracellular anions, preventing the exchange of these ions for extracellular Cl^- which can pass the membrane without much restriction. The membrane is also supposed to be impermeable for Na^+ even though experiments with labeled Na^+ have shown that this is by no means true for the plasma membrane of nervous elements. The membrane restricts the movements of sodium, however, and an active mechanism (ion pump) transports sodium which leaked into the cellular structures back into the extracellular space, establishing a functional impermeability of the membrane for this ion. This prevents an exchange of intracellular K^+, which can readily pass the membrane, for extracellular Na^+. When the Na^+ permeability is markedly increased a situation is created studied by Gibbs and Donnan in which a membrane separates two compartments, one containing a salt of which both the anions and cations can pass the membrane. The membrane is impermeable for one of the ion species present in the other compartment. Under these conditions the solutes distribute themselves between the two compartments in such a way that the product of the concentrations of the ions in each compartment for which the membrane is permeable are equal (Donnan, 1924). This results in a net gain of ions in the compartment containing the ion species for which the membrane is impassable. The resulting increase in osmotic pressure has to be balanced by hydrostatic pressure or if this is impossible as in cellular elements, which do not have the mechanical strength to withstand such pressures, water will accompany the moving salt.

An increase in Na^+ permeability of susceptible structures in the brain tissue would thus cause a transport of extracellular sodium chloride and water into the intracellular compartment, resulting in the observed impedance increase, chloride accumulation in certain tissue elements, and the loss of ECS and swelling of cellular elements observed in the EM's of freeze substituted tissue. An increase in Na^+ permeability is not an unusual occurrence in central nervous tissue. It is the basic membrane change underlying excitation in electrically excitable structures. In chemically excitable regions the increase in the ion permeability is a more general one (Eccles, 1957). This results in depolarization of the tissue elements which has been recorded with intracellular methods during spreading depression and asphyxiation (Collewijn and Van Harreveld, 1966; Brožek, 1966; Karahashi and Goldring, 1966). The depolarization may account for the slow potential changes which accompany O_2 deficiency and spreading depression.

Since no swelling of nonmyelinated axons was found in EM's of tissue subjected to asphyxiation, spreading depression or fixation, it would seem that the mechanism involved in the Na permeability changes of the plasma membranes in electrically excitable tissue plays no part in the water and electrolyte transport observed. Dendrites tend to swell which suggests other properties for their plasma membranes. Indeed, the chemical excitability of the sub-synaptic areas of these structures distinguishes their plasma membrane from that of axons. Certain glial components of the tissue such as the Bergmann fibers of the cerebellum take up extracellular material during asphyxiation and fixation. The plasma membrane of these structures thus seem to react to these stimuli in the same way as the dendritic cell membrane. It would seem that a single permeability change, an increase of the Na permeability of the plasma membrane of specific cellular structures in the gray matter, can account for the various concomitants of asphyxiation, spreading depression and fixation.

B. A MECHANISM FOR THE INCREASE OF THE MEMBRANE PERMEABILITY FOR SODIUM

1. *The Arrest of Active Ion Transport*

The mechanism which causes the postulated increase in Na^+ permeability can now be considered. Asphyxiation will affect the functional impermeability of the plasma membrane for Na^+ by the arrest of the ion pumps because of lack of oxidative energy. This could lead to an inflow of sodium chloride and water. An uptake of NaCl from the medium by tissue slices of the kidney and other body organs by interference with the metabolism was explained in this way (Conway and Geoghegan, 1955; Leaf, 1956). Such a mechanism may also account for the impedance rise and loss of extracellular material in body organs such as kidney, liver and salivary glands after arrest of the circulation. This is a rather slow process which takes 10–60 minutes to develop (Van Harreveld and Biber, 1962). It seems unlikely, however, that this mechanism underlies the asphyxial electrolyte and water transport in central nervous tissue. The arrest of the ion pumps and the accumulation of NaCl in the cellular elements can be expected to develop gradually, whereas the asphyxial impedance increase and the accompanying slow potential change appear rather suddenly often after a considerable latency. Furthermore, although the arrest of the ion pump and the resulting inflow of sodium chloride and water can be expected to involve all cellular elements, the asphyxial swelling was observed selectively in certain constituents of the tissue and not in others. Finally this explanation does not fit the impedance and slow potential changes accompanying spreading depression, which is not accompanied by a marked oxygen deficiency (Van Harreveld and Ochs, 1957; Marshall, 1959). It would seem, therefore, that an alternate mechanism such as the release of a compound able to cause the increase in Na^+ permeability has to be postulated especially in the case of spreading depression.

2. The Nature of Spreading Depression

Before the importance of an increase in ion permeability of the plasma membrane for the explanation of the concomitants of spreading depression was realized, Grafstein (1956) proposed an ingeneous mechanism for the slow propagation of this phenomenon. She postulated that during SD potassium is released from cellular structures, depolarizing adjacent elements, which discharge and in doing so release more potassium, etc. This postulate was supported by the demonstration of unit discharges at the start of SD (Grafstein, 1956; Morlock et al., 1964; Collewijn and Van Harreveld, 1966) and by the release during this phenomenon of ^{42}K from cortices charged with radioactive potassium (Křivánek and Bureš, 1960; Brinley et al., 1960). The depolarization of cellular elements which is a feature of spreading depression (Collewijn and Van Harreveld, 1966; Brožek, 1966; Karahashi and Goldring, 1966) would be a direct consequence of this mechanism. In Grafstein's postulate the depolarization is caused by an equalization of the K^+ concentration in the intra- and extracellular compartments which cannot readily explain the transport of extracellular material into susceptible structures whereas an increase in sodium permeability can account both for the depolarization and for the transport. Such an increase in ion permeability could be produced by a release of glutamate from the intra- into the extracellular compartment. Glutamate is present in the brain in a concentration of 10 mM/kg (Schwerin *et al.*, 1950; Berl and Waelsch, 1958). It depolarizes virtually all nerve cells when deposited iontophoretically in their neighborhood (Curtis *et al.*, 1960; Krnjević and Phillis, 1963), which is accomplished by an increase in ion permeability of the plasma membrane (Bradford and McIlwain, 1966). By replacing a release of potassium in Graftstein's explanation by a release of glutamate the slow propagation of SD with all its concomitants can be accounted for including the unit discharge at the beginning of this phenomenon which would be caused by glutamate induced depolarization. The release of labeled potassium from the cortex which is the central feature of Grafstein's postulate can also be expected when the membrane depolarization is induced by a glutamate release. The increased Na$^+$ permeability will result in an outflow of K$^+$ from the structures involved, which then can diffuse into a salt solution superfusing the cortex (Brinley *et al.*, 1960; Křivánek and Bureš, 1960). The potassium release may arrest the conduction in axons which are not directly involved in the electrolyte and water transport during spreading depression. Such an effect was observed on white matter situated in close proximity of tissue exhibiting spreading depression (Fifková and Bureš, 1966; Bureš *et al.*, 1967; Ichijo and Ochs, 1967, 1970; Bureš and Fifková, 1968).

3. Glutamate, Spreading Depression, and Asphyxiation

The concept that a release of glutamate is the primary cause of the complex of phenomena observed during spreading depression and perhaps also during asphyxiation is supported by the following observations. If glutamate is involved in spreading depression it should be possible to elicit this phenomenon by applying the amino acid to the tissue. Indeed, SD can be elicited by topical application of glutamate to the cerebral cortex. The threshold concentration is quite low (about 15 mM), much lower than that of potassium chloride, i.e., 110 mM (Van Harreveld, 1959). In chickens the BBB develops a few days after hatching. When glutamate is administered intravenously before that time, it causes impedance increases and slow potential changes in the corpus striatum which closely resemble those recorded during asphyxiation and spreading depression (Fifkova and Van Harreveld, 1970).

Glutamate, deposited iontophoretically in the rat cerebral cortex, produces a region characterized by enormously swollen structures and shrunken nerve cells. An examination of this spot with the electron microscope revealed that some of the swollen structures were dendrites as shown by synaptic contacts, others were pre-synaptic terminals containing synaptic vesicles. The glia in this area is difficult to identify, but some of the swollen structures may have been derived from this tissue element. Grossly swollen perivascular glia was observed. It is of interest that the small nonmyelinated fibers do not participate under these circumstances, in the uptake of material (Van Harreveld and Fifkova, 1971). These observations show that glutamate is able to cause a gross swelling of the same tissue elements as occurs during SD and after asphyxiation.

Ames (1956, 1958) found that the rabbit retina bathed in a medium containing *l*-glutamate took up Na^+, Cl^-, and water, as certain cellular elements do during asphyxiation and SD. A large swelling of elements in the inner plexiform layer was observed in EM's of the turtle retina treated with glutamate by Wald and de Robertis (1961). Van Harreveld and Khattab (1968a) also found in mouse retinas bathed in a medium containing glutamate swelling of dendritic elements in this layer. No swelling was observed of the nonmyelinated axons, nerve cells, and Müller cells.

If glutamate is released during spreading depression and asphyxiation, it should be possible to demonstrate the amino acid in a salt solution superfusing the cerebral cortex. In attempts to show this, a continuous marked release of amino acids was found in a similar proportion as present in the blood plasma. These amino acids, probably derived from the pial vessels, masked any release which might have been due to SD (Van Harreveld and Kooiman, 1965). Recently, the isolated chicken retina, which can exhibit SD characterized by a change in transparency of the tissue (Martins-Ferreira and de Oliveira Castro, 1966), was found to be a more favorable object for the demonstration of an amino acid release during this phenomenon (Van Harreveld and Fifkova, 1970). The retina was charged with ^{14}C-labeled glutamate and superfused with a physiological salt solution. One-minute portions of the superfusion fluid were collected, subjected to electrophoresis, and passed through a strip counter which made a record of the labeled compounds. When not stimulated the retina released mainly glutamine, metabolized from the label, but very little glutamate. Stimulation with direct current or superfusion with a KCl solution caused an increase in transparency of the tissue indicating that SD had been elicited. The samples of the superfusion fluid collected during this period contained in addition to glutamine an appreciable amount of labeled glutamate. Also the superfusion with unlabeled glutamate (0.2–1 mM) caused a transparency increase and a marked release of the radioactive amino acid (Fig. 25). The release of intracellular labeled by unlabeled glutamate suggests the presence of a process with positive feedback. The release of some glutamate in the extracellular space may increase the permeability of the plasma membrane of susceptible structures for this amino acid. More glutamate will flow out which enhances the permeability even more until a maximum release is established. Such a mechanism may account for the all-or-none character of spreading depression.

It can be postulated that a glutamate release which seems to account for the concomitants of SD also causes the asphyxial changes. As a pos-

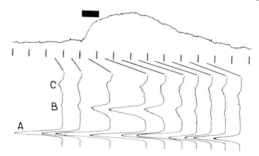

Fig. 25. The upper record shows the transparency change in the isolated chicken retina, charged with ^{14}C glutamate and superfused with a salt solution, caused by stimulation with unlabeled glutamate in a concentration of 5 mM for 1 minute (indicated by the bar). The time signal indicates minutes. In the lower part of the figure records of the radioactivity in 1-minute portions of the superfusion fluid are shown. The peak A is caused by glutamine, B by glutamate, and C by aspartate and nonaminated metabolites of glutamate.

sible mechanism it is suggested that glutamate leaks out of the tissue elements continually but normally is actively transported back into the intracellular compartment. When the O_2 supply is arrested and the available energy reserves have been used up the active glutamate transport becomes impossible. Glutamate would now accumulate in the extracellular space and when a sufficient concentration is reached, set in motion the process with positive feedback which results in a maximum release of the amino acid. Such a mechanism explains the rather sudden onset of the asphyxial impedance and slow potential changes after a latency often as long as several minutes.

Some evidence was obtained for the possibility that the electrolyte and water transport observed during glutaraldehyde fixation is also caused by a glutamate release. During superfusion of the isolated retina with a glutaraldehyde solution a transparency increase and a release of amino acids were observed. There is evidence that one of the amino acids released is glutamate. This release may be responsible for the uptake of extracellular material by the intracellular compartment during the fixation process by an increase of the membrane permeability for Na^+. It is also possible, however, that the ion permeability is affected more directly by the fixative (Van Harreveld and Fifkova, 1972).

The release of glutamate as a mechanism for the transport of extracellular material into the intracellular compartment seems to be specific for central nervous tissue. There is no evidence for a comparable mechanism in the body organs. The glutamate effect may be an abnormal activity of a more normal function of this amino acid, which for the time being is unknown. This mechanism may not be present in the CNS of other phyla than the vertebrates, which may react to asphyxiation and chemical stimulation in other ways.

REFERENCES

Adey, W. R., Kado, R. T., and Didio, J. (1962). *Exp. Neurol.* **5**, 47.

Adey, W. R., Kado, R. T., McIlwain, J. T., and Walter, D. O. (1966). *Exp. Neurol.* **15**, 490.

Ahmed, N., and Van Harreveld, A. (1969). *J. Physiol. (London)* **204**, 31.

Ames, A. (1956). *J. Neurophysiol.* **19**, 213.

Ames, A. (1958). *Neurology* **8**, 64.

Ames, A., and Gurian, B. S. (1960). *J. Neurophysiol.* **23**, 676.

Ames, A., and Hastings, A. B. (1956). *J. Neurophysiol.* **19**, 201.

Ames, A., and Nesbett, F. B. (1966). *J. Physiol. (London)* **184**, 215.

Baethmann, A., Steude, U., Horsch, S., and Brendel, W. (1970). *Eur. J. Physiol.* **316**, 51.

Baker, J. R. (1958). "Principles of Biological Microtechnique." Methuen, London.

Baker, P. F. (1965). *J. Physiol. (London)* **180**, 439.

Barlow, C. F., Domek, N. S., Goldberg, M. A., and Roth. L. J. (1961). *Arch. Neurol.* **5**, 102.

Becker, B. (1961). *Amer. J. Physiol.* **201**, 1149.

Bennett, M. V. L. (1969). *Brain Res.* **15**, 584.

Bering, E. A. (1965). In "Cerebrospinal Fluid and the Regulation of Ventilation" (C. McC. Brooks, F. Kao, and B. B. Lloyd, eds.), pp. 395-412. Davis, Philadelphia, Pennsylvania.

Bering, E. A., and Sato, O. (1963). *J. Neurosurg.* **20**, 1050.

Berl, S., and Waelsch, H. (1958). *J. Neurochem.* **3**, 161.

Bito, L. Z. (1969). *Science* **165**, 81.

Bito, L. Z., and Davson, H. (1966). *Exp. Neurol.* **14**, 269.

Bito, L. Z., Bradbury, M. W. B., and Davson, H. (1966). *J. Physiol. (London)* **185**, 323.

Bodian, D., and Taylor, N. (1963). *Science* **139**, 330.

Bondareff, W. (1965). *Anat. Rec.* **152**, 119.

Bondareff, W. (1967). *Z. Zellforsch. Mikrosk. Anat.* **81**, 366.

Bondareff, W., and Pysh, J. J. (1968). *Anat. Rec.* **160**, 773.

Bourke, R. S., Greenberg, E. S., and Tower, D. B. (1965). *Amer. J. Physiol.* **208**, 682.

Bradbury, M. W. B., Villamil, M., and Kleeman, C. R. (1968). *Amer. J. Physiol.* **214**, 643.

Bradford, H. F., and McIlwain, H. (1966). *J. Neurochem.* **13**, 1163.

Brightman, M. W. (1965a). *J. Cell Biol.* **26**, 99.

Brightman, M. W. (1965b). *Amer. J. Anat.* **117**, 193.

Brightman, M. W., and Reese, T. S. (1969). *J. Cell Biol.* **40**, 648.

Brinley, F. J., Kandel, E. R., and Marshall, W. H. (1960). *J. Neurophysiol.* **23**, 246.

Brown, D. A., Stumpf, W. E., and Roth, L. J. (1969). *J. Cell Sci.* **4**, 265.

Brožek, G. (1966). *Physiol. Bohemoslov.* **15**, 98.

Bullivant, S. (1960). *J. Biophys. Biochem. Cytol.* **8**, 639.

Bureš, J., and Fifková, E. (1968). *Physiol. Bohemoslov.* **17**, 405.

Bureš, J., Hartmann, G., and Lukyanova, L. D. (1967). *Exp. Neurol.* **18**, 404.

Caley, D. W., and Maxwell, D. S. (1968a). *J. Comp. Neurol.* **133**, 17.

Caley, D. W., and Maxwell, D. S. (1968b). *J. Comp. Neurol.* **133**, 45.

Caley, D. W., and Maxwell, D. S. (1970). *J. Comp. Neurol.* **138**, 31.

Coben, L. A. (1969). *Amer. J. Physiol.* **217**, 89.

Coben, L. A., Gottesman, L., and Jacobs, M. (1965). *Neurology* **15**, 951.

Cole, K. S. (1928). *J. Gen. Physiol.* **12**, 29.

Cole, K. S. (1940). *Cold Spring Harbor Symp. Quant. Biol.* **8**, 110.

Cole, K. S. (1941). *Tabulae Biol.* **19**, 24.

Cole, K. S., and Spencer, J. M. (1938). *J. Gen. Physiol.* **21**, 583.

Cole, K. S., Li, C.-L., and Bak, A. F. (1969). *Exp. Neurol.* **24**, 459.

Collewijn, H., and Schadé, J. P. (1962). *Arch. Int. Physiol. Biochim.* **70**, 200.

Collewijn, H., and Schadé, J. P. (1964a). *Arch. Int. Physiol. Biochim.* **72**, 181.

Collewijn, H., and Schadé, J. P. (1964b). *Arch. Int. Physiol. Biochim.* **72**, 194.

Collewijn, H., and Van Harreveld, A. (1966). *Exp, Neurol.* **15**, 425.

Conway, E. J., and Geoghegan, H. (1955). *J. Physiol. (London)* **130**, 438.

Coombs, J. S., Eccles, J. C., and Fatt, P. (1955). *J. Physiol. (London)* **130**, 291.

Creese, R., d'Silva, J. L. and Hashish, S. E. E. (1955). *J. Physiol. (London)* **127**, 525.

Crile, G. W., Hosmer, H. R., and Rowland, A. F. (1922). *Amer. J. Physiol.* **60**, 59.

Curtis, D. R., Phillis, J. W., and Watkins, J. C. (1960). *J. Physiol. (London)* **150**, 656.

Cutler, R. W. P., Lorenzo, A. V., and Barlow, C. F. (1968a). *Arch. Neurol.* **18**, 316.

Cutler, R. W. P., Robinson, R. J., and Lorenzo, A. V. (1968b). *Amer. J. Physiol.* **214**, 448.

Davson, H. (1956). "Physiology of the Ocular and Cerebrospinal Fluid." Churchill, London.

Davson, H. (1958). *Cerebrospinal Fluid ; Prod., Circ., Absorption, Ciba Found. Symp.,* 1957, pp. 189-208.

Davson, H. (1963). *Ergeb. Physiol. Biol. Chem. Exp. Pharmakol.* **52**, 20.

Davson, H., and Pollay, M. (1963). *J. Physiol. (London)* **167**, 239.

Davson, H., and Segal, M. B. (1969). *Brain* **92**, 131.

Davson, H., Kleeman, C. R., and Levine, E. (1961). *J. Physiol. (London)* **159**, 67P.
Davson, H., Kleeman, C. R., and Levine, E. (1962). *J. Physiol. (London)* **161**, 126.
Dempsey, E. W., and Wislocki, G. B. (1955). *J. Biophys. Biochem. Cytol.* **1**, 245.
Dobbing, J. (1961). *Physiol. Rev.* **41**, 130.
Donnan, F. G. (1924). *Chem. Rev.* **1**, 73.
Eccles, J. C. (1957). "The Physiology of Nerve Cells." Johns Hopkins Press, Baltimore, Maryland.
Efron, R. (1961). *In* "Transactions of the 5th Research Conference Chemotherapy in Psychiatry," Vol. 5, p. 11. U. S. Veterans Admin., Washington, D. C.
Eichelberger, L., and Richter, R. B. (1944). *J. Biol. Chem.* **154**, 21.
Farquhar, M. G., and Hartmann, J. F. (1957). *J. Neuropathol. Exp. Neurol.* **16**, 18.
Fenstermacher, J. D., and Bartlett, M. O. (1967). *Amer. J. Physiol.* **212**, 1268.
Fenstermacher, J. D., Li, C.-L., and Levin, V. A. (1970). *Exp. Neurol.* **27**, 101.
Ferguson, R. K., and Woodbury, D. M. (1969). *Exp. Brain Res.,* **7**, 181.
Fernandez-Morán, H. (1960). *Ann. N. Y. Acad. Sci.* **85**, 689.
Fifková, E., and Bureš, J. (1966). *Physiol. Bohemoslov.* **15**, 344.
Fifkova, E., and Van Harreveld, A. (1970). *Exp. Neurol.* **28**, 286.
Flexner, J. B., and Flexner, L. B. (1950). *Anat. Rec.* **106**, 413.
Flexner, L. B., and Flexner, J. B. (1949). *J. Cell. Comp. Physiol.* **34**, 115.
Folch, J., Lees, M., and Sloane-Stanley, G. H. (1956). *In* "Metabolism of the Nervous System" (D. Richter, ed.), pp. 174-181. Pergamon, Oxford.
Frank, K., and Fuortes, M. G. F. (1956). *J. Physiol. (London)* **134**, 451.
French, C. M. (1965). *J. Physiol. (London)* **178**, 55P.
Freygang, W. H., and Landau, W. M. (1955). *J. Cell. Comp. Physiol.* **45**, 377.
Fricke, H. (1924a). *Phys. Rev.* **24**, 575.
Fricke, H. (1924b). *J. Gen. Physiol.* **6**, 741.
Fricke, H. (1933). *Cold Spring Harbor Symp. Quant. Biol.* **1**, 117.
González-Aguilar, F. (1969). *J. Ultrastruct. Res.* **29**, 76.
Grafstein, B. (1956). *J. Neurophysiol.* **19**, 154.
Hammerstad, J. P., Lorenzo, A. V., and Cutler, R. W. P. (1969). *Amer. J. Physiol.* **216**, 353.
Hartmann, J. F. (1966). *Arch. Neurol.* **15**, 633.
Hild, W., and Tasaki, I. (1962). *J. Neurophysiol.* **25**, 277.
Horstmann, E., and Meves, E. (1959). *Z. Zellforsch. Mikrosk. Anat.* **49**, 569.
Ichijo, M., and Ochs, S. (1967). *Physiologist* **10**, 209.
Ichijo, M., and Ochs, S. (1970). *Brain Res.* **23**, 41.
Johnston, P. V., and Roots, B. I. (1967). *J. Cell Sci.* **2**, 377.
Kaplan, R. J., and Pollay, M. (1968). *Proc. Soc. Exp. Biol. Med.* **129**, 133.
Karahashi, Y., and Goldring, S. (1966). *Electroencephalogr. Clin. Neurophysiol.* **20**, 600.
Karlsson, U. (1967). *J. Ultrastruct. Res.* **17**, 158.
Karlsson, U., and Schultz, R. L. (1965). *J. Ultrastruct. Res.* **12**, 160.
Katzman, R. (1961). *Neurology* **11**, 27.
Klivington, K. A., and Galambos, R. (1967). *Science* **157**, 211.
Koch, A., Ranck, J. B., and Newman, B. L. (1962). *Exp. Neurol.* **6**, 186.
Křivánek, J., and Bureš, J. (1960). *Physiol. Bohemoslov.* **9**, 494.
Krnjević, K., and Phillis, J. W. (1963). *J. Physiol. (London)* **165**, 274.
Krnjević, K., and Schwartz, S. (1967). *Exp. Brain, Res.* **3**, 306.
Kuffler, S. W., and Potter, D. D. (1964). *J. Neurophysiol.* **27**, 290.

Lajtha, A. (1957). *J. Neurochem.* **1**, 216.

Lasansky, A., and Wald, F. (1962). *J. Cell Biol.* **15**, 463.

Law, R. O., and Phelps, C. F. (1966). *J. Physiol. (London)* **186**, 547.

Leaf, A. (1956). *Biochem. J.* **62**, 241.

Leão, A. A. P. (1944). *J. Neurophysiol.* **7**, 359.

Leão, A. A. P. (1947). *J. Neurophysiol.* **10**, 409.

Leão, A. A. P. (1951). *Electroencephalogr. Clin. Neurophysiol.* **3**, 315.

Leão, A. A. P., and Ferreira, H. M. (1953). *An. Acad. Brasil. Cienc.* **25**, 259.

Levin, V. A., Fenstermacher, J. D., and Patlak, C. S. (1970). *Amer. J. Physiol.* **219**, 1528.

Li, C.-L. (1959). *J. Neurophysiol.* **22**, 436.

Li, C.-L., Bak, A. F., and Parker, L. O. (1968). *Exp. Neurol.* **20**, 544.

Luse, S. A. (1956). *J. Biophys. Biochem. Cytol.* **2**, 531.

Luse, S. A., (1960a). *Anat. Rec.* **138**, 461.

Luse, S. A. (1960b). *J. Histochem. Cytochem.* **8**, 398.

Luse, S. A. (1962). *Res. Publ., Ass. Res. Nerv. Ment. Dis.* **40**, 1.

Malhotra, S. K., and Van Harreveld, A. (1966). *J. Anat.* **100**, 99.

Manery, J. F., and Bale, W. F. (1941). *Amer. J. Physiol.* **132**, 215.

Manery, J. F., and Haege, L. F. (1941). *Amer. J. Physiol.* **134**, 83.

Manery, J. F., and Hastings, A. B. (1939). *J. Biol. Chem.* **127**, 657.

Marshall, W. H. (1959). *Physiol. Rev.* **39**, 239.

Martins-Ferreira, H., and de Oliveira Castro, G. (1966). *J. Neurophysiol.* **29**, 715.

Maxwell, J. C. (1873). "A Treatise on Electricity and Magnetism." 3d Ed. Clarendon Press, Oxford. (Dover, London and New York, 1954).

Mazur, P. (1970). *Science* **168**, 939.

Morlock, N. L., Mori, K., and Ward, A. A. (1964). *J. Neurophysiol.* **27**, 1192.

Nevis, A. H., and Collins, G. H. (1967). *Brain Res.* **5**, 57.

Nicholls, J. G., and Wolfe, D. E. (1967). *J. Neurophysiol.* **30**, 1574.

Nicholson, P. W. (1965). *Exp. Neurol.* **13**, 386.

Oldendorf, W. H., and Davson, H. (1967). *Arch. Neurol.* **17**, 196.

Palay, S. L., McGee-Russell, S. M., Gordon, S., and Grillo, M. A. (1962). *J. Cell Biol.* **12**, 385.

Pappas, G. D., and Purpura, D. P. (1966). *Nature (London)* **210**, 1391.

Pappenheimer, J. R. (1953). *Physiol. Rev.* **33**, 387.

Pappenheimer, J. R., Heisey, S. R., and Jordan, E. F. (1961). *Amer. J. Physiol.* **200**, 1.

Pappius, H. M., Klatzo, I., and Elliott, K. A. C. (1962). *Can. J. Biochem. Physiol.* **40**, 885.

Pease, D. C. (1967a), *J. Ultrastruct. Res.* **21**, 75.

Pease, D. C. (1967b). *J. Ultrastruct. Res.* **21**, 98.

Pease, D. C., and Baker, R. F. (1951). *Anat. Rec.* **110**, 505.

Phillips, C. G., (1956). *Quart. J. Exp. Physiol.* **41**, 58.

Pollay, M. (1966). *Amer. J. Physiol.* **210**, 275.

Pollay, M., and Curl, F. (1967). *Amer. J. Physiol.* **213**, 1031.

Pollay, M., and Davson, H. (1963). *Brain* **86**, 137.

Pollay, M., and Kaplan, R. J. (1970). *Brain Res.* **17**, 407.

Pollay, M., Stevens, A., and Kaplan, R. (1969). *Anal. Biochem.* **27**, 381.

Pysh, J. J. (1969). *Amer. J. Anat.* **124**, 411.

Rall, D. P. (1964). *In* "The Cellular Functions of Membrane Transport" (J. F. Hoffman, ed.), pp. 269-282. Prentice-Hall, Engelwood Cliffs, New Jersey.

Rall, D. P., Oppelt, W. W., and Patlak, C. S. (1962). *Life Sci.* **1**, 43.

Ranck, J. B. (1963a). *Exp. Neurol.* **7**, 144.

Ranck, J. B. (1963b). *Exp. Neurol.* **7**, 153.

Ranck, J. B. (1964). *Exp. Neurol.* **9**, 1.

Ranck, J. B. (1966). *Exp. Neurol.* **16**, 416.

Ranck, J. B. (1970). *Exp. Neurol.* **27**, 454.

Ranck, J. B., and BeMent, S. L. (1965). *Exp. Neurol.* **11**, 451.

Rebhun, L. I. (1965). *Fed. Proc., Fed. Amer. Soc. Exp. Biol.* **24**, S217.

Reed, D. J., and Woodbury, D. M. (1963). *J. Physiol. (London)* **169**, 816.

Reed, D. J., Woodbury, D. M., Jacobs, L., and Squires, R. (1965). *Amer. J. Physiol.* **209**, 757.

Reese, T. S., and Karnovsky, M. J. (1967). *J. Cell Biol.* **34**, 207.

Reulen, H. J., Hase, U., Fenske, A., Samii, M., and Schürmann, K. (1970). *Acta Neurochir.* **22**, 305.

Richmond, J. E., and Hastings, A. B. (1960). *Amer. J. Physiol.* **199**, 814.

Robinson, R. J., Cutler, R. W. P., Lorenzo, A. V., and Barlow, C. F. (1968). *J. Neurochem.* **15**, 1169.

Rosenblueth, A., and Garcia Ramos, J. (1966). *Acta Physiol. Lat. Amer.* **16**, 141.

Schneider, M. (1956). *In* "Metabolism of the Nervous System" (D. Richter, ed.), pp. 238-244. Pergamon, Oxford.

Schultz, R. L., and Karlsson, U. (1965). *J. Ultrastruct. Res.* **12**, 187.

Schultz, R. L., Maynard, E. A., and Pease, D. C. (1957). *Amer. J. Anat.* **100**, 369.

Schwerin, P., Bessman, S. P., and Waelsch, H. (1950). *J. Biol. Chem.* **184**, 37.

Shapiro, H. (1935). *Biol. Bull.* **68**, 363.

Streicher, E. (1961). *Amer. J. Physiol.* **201**, 334.

Streicher, E., Rall, D. P., and Gaskins, J. R. (1964). *Amer. J. Physiol.* **206**, 251.

Sumi, S. M. (1969). *J. Ultrastruct. Res.* **29**, 398.

Torack, R. M. (1965). *Z. Zellforsch. Mikrosk. Anat.* **66**, 352.

Torack, R. M. (1966). *J. Ultrastruct. Res.* **14**, 590.

Trachtenberg, M. C., and Pollen, D. A. (1970). *Science* **167**, 1248.

Treherne, J. E., and Moreton, R. B. (1970). *Int. Rev. Cytol.* **28**, 45.

Van Harreveld, A. (1957). *Amer. J. Physiol.* **191**, 233.

Van Harreveld, A. (1958). *Amer. J. Physiol.* **192**, 457.

Van Harreveld, A. (1959). *J. Neurochem.* **3**, 300.

Van Harreveld, A. (1961). *J. Cell. Comp. Physiol.* **57**, 101.

Van Harreveld, A. (1966). "Brain Tissue Electrolytes" Molecular Biology and Medicine Series (E. Bittar, ed.). Butterworth, London.

Van Harreveld, A., and Biber, M. P. (1962). *Amer. J. Physiol.* **203**, 609.

Van Harreveld, A., and Biersteker, P. A. (1964). *Amer. J. Physiol.* **206**, 8.

Van Harreveld, A., and Crowell, J. (1964). *Anat. Rec.* **149**, 381.

Van Harreveld, A., and Fifkova, E. (1970). *J. Neurobiol.* **2**, 13.

Van Harreveld, A., and Fifkova, E. (1971). *Exp. Mol. Pathol.* **15**, 61.

Van Harreveld, A., and Fifkova, E. (1972). *J. Neurochem.* **19**, 237.

Van Harreveld, A., and Khattab, F. I. (1967). *J. Neurophysiol.* **30**, 911.

Van Harreveld, A., and Khattab, F. I. (1968a). *Anat. Rec.* **161**, 125.

Van Harreveld, A., and Khattab, F. I. (1968b). *Anat. Rec.* **162**, 467.

Van Harreveld, A., and Khattab, F. I. (1968c). *J. Cell Sci.* **3**, 579.

Van Harreveld, A., and Khattab, F. I. (1969). *J. Cell Sci.* **4**, 437.

Van Harreveld, A., and Kooiman, M. (1965). *J. Neurochem.* **21**, 431.

Van Harreveld, A., and Malhotra, S. K. (1966). *J. Cell Sci.* **1**, 223.

Van Harreveld, A., and Malhotra, S. K. (1967). *J. Anat.* **101**, 197.

Van Harreveld, A., and Ochs, S. (1956). *Amer. J. Physiol.* **187**, 180.

Van Harreveld, A., and Ochs, S. (1957). *Amer. J. Physiol.* **189**, 159.

Van Harreveld, A., and Potter, R. L. (1961). *Stain Technol.* **36**, 185.

Van Harreveld, A., and Schadé, J. P. (1959). *J. Cell. Comp. Physiol.* **54**, 65.

Van Harreveld, A., Schadé, J. P. (1960). *Struct. Funct. Cereb. Cortex, Proc. 2nd Int. Meet. Neurobiol.*, 1959, pp. 239-254.

Van Harreveld, A., and Schadé, J. P. (1962). *Exp. Neurol.* **5**, 383.

Van Harreveld, A., and Steiner, J. (1970a). *Anat. Rec.* **166**, 117.

Van Harreveld, A., and Steiner, J. (1970b). *J. Cell Sci.* **6**, 793.

Van Harreveld, A., and Tachibana, S. (1962). *Amer. J. Physiol.* **202**, 59.

Van Harreveld, A., Murphy, T., and Nobel, K. W. (1963). *Amer. J. Physiol.* **205**, 203.

Van Harreveld, A., Crowell, J., and Malhotra, S. K. (1965). *J. Cell Biol.* **25**, 117.

Van Harreveld, A., Ahmed, N., and Tanner, D. J. (1966). *Amer. J. Physiol.* **210**, 777.

Van Harreveld, A., Daffny, N., and Khattab, F. I. (1971). *Exp. Neurol.* **31**, 358.

Vernadakis, A., and Woodbury, D. M. (1965). *Arch. Neurol.* **12**, 284.

Villegas, G. M., and Fernandez, J. (1966). *Exp. Neurol.* **15**, 18.

Wald, F., and de Robertis, E. (1961). *Z. Zellforsch. Mikrosk. Anat.* **55**, 649.

Wang, H. H., and Adey, W. R. (1969). *Exp. Neurol.* **25**, 70.

Welch, K. (1962a). *Amer. J. Physiol.* **202**, 757.

Welch, K. (1962b). *Proc. Soc. Exp. Biol. Med.* **109**, 953.

Wong, E. K. (1969). *Acta Physiol. Lat. Amer.* **19**, 71.

Woodward, D. L., Reed, D. J., and Dixon, D. H. (1967). *Amer. J. Physiol.* **212**, 367.

Wyckoff, R. W. G., and Young, J. Z. (1956). *Proc. Roy. Soc., Ser. B* **144**, 440.

Wyngaarden, J. B., Stanbury, J. B., and Rapp, B. (1953). *Endocrinology* **52**, 568.

Zadunaisky, J. A., and Curran, P. F. (1963). *Amer. J. Physiol.* **205**, 949.

Author Index

Numbers in italics refer to the pages on which the complete references are listed.

A

Acker, A., 365, *444*
Ádám, G., 222, 230, *243*, *244*
Adams, D. H., 190, *211*
Adams, R. D., 142, *170*
Adey, W. R., 232, *243*, 473, *506*, *511*
Adrian, E. D., 232, *243*, 309, *317*
Aghajanian, G. K., 24, 33, *55*, 234, *243*
Agnew, W. F., 401, *431*
Agranoff, B. W., 218, 219, 220, *243*, *244*
Ahmed, N., 360, 364, 365, 368, 413, *437*, *445*, 450, 452, 453, 456, 459, 460, *506*, *511*
Aird, R. B., 341, *441*
Aitken, J. T., 39, *55*
Akert, K., 32, *56*, 85, *101*, 208, *212*
Akiyama, T., 267, *289*
Albe-Fessard, D., 389, 390, *438*, *445*
Albers, R. W., 272, 274, 275, *283*, *287*, *288*
Aldridge, V. J., 293, 314, 315, *320*
Alemán, V., 194, 195, 196, *214*
Aleonard, P., 389, 390, *438*, *445*
Alkon, D. L., 122, *127*
Alksne, J. F., 61, 68, *101*
Allen, K. W., 117, *127*
Allegranza, A., 151, 152, *170*
Alpert, M., 158, *177*
Altman, J., 43, 47, *55*
Alvord, E. C., 118, *120*, 420, *442*
Alzheimer, A., 159, 165, *170*
Amaldi, P., 209, *211*

Amano, M., 191, 192, 193, *213*
Amaro, J., 117, 120, *127*
Ames, A., 382, 385, 386, 416, 424, *437*, 450, 458, 504, *506*
Andersen, P., 12, 13, *55*, 305, *317*
Anderson, N. G., 117, *127*
Anderson, W., 156, 160, *171*
Andersson, E., 182, 183, 184, 186 (19), *211*
Andersson, S. A., 303, 305, *317*
Andres, K. H., 205, *211*
Andrews, J. M., 136, 139, *170*, *173*
Andros, G., 414, *441*
Angeletti, P. U., 206, 207, *213*, *214*
Ansell, G. B., 109, *122*
Anthoni, J. F., 226, *247*
April, R. S., 38, *55*
Aprison, M. H., 239, *243*, 275, 279, 280, 281, 282, 283, 284, 285, *289*
Argiz, C. A. G., 406, *442*
Armstrong, J., 41, *55*
Armstrong-James, M. A., 24, *55*
Arnaiz, J. R. de L., 115, *127*
Asada, Y., 268, *283*
Aserinsky, E., 25, *55*, *317*
Ash, A. S. F., 264, *283*
Ashcroft, G. W., 369, *437*
Atkinson, A. J., 399, *437*
Atwood, H. L., 266, *283*, *287*
Austin, G. M., 35, *58*, 96, *102*
Austin, J., 151, 152, 153, *174*, *177*
Austin, L., 183, 209, *211*, *214*
Awapara, J., 250, *283*
Axelrod, J., 66, *104*

B

Babich, F. R., 221, 222, 223, 230, *243*
Baethmann, A., 456, *506*
Bain, J. A., 275, *286*
Bak, A. F., 463, 464, 466, 467, *507*, *509*
Bakay, L., 362, 414, 415, 421, 422, 430, *437*
Baker, C. P., 53, *59*
Baker, J. R., 484, *506*
Baker, P. F., 125, *127*, 460, *506*
Baker, R. E., 27, *58*
Baker, R. F., 480, *509*
Balázs, R., 47, *55*, 183, 194, *211*, 274, 276, *283*
Bale, W. F., 434, *442*, 451, *509*
Ball, M. J., 146, 157, 167, *174*
Ballantine, H. T., 414, *437*
Banna, W. R., 273, *283*
Barden, H., 155, 158, *170*
Barer, R., 66, *101*
Barker, L. A., 117, 120, *127*
Barker, L. F., 179, 180, 208, *211*
Barlow, C. F., 360, 361, 367, 415, 428, *438*, *439*, *440*, *444*, 450, 452, 453, 455, 456, 460, 462, *506*, *507*, *510*
Barlow, J. S., 306, 310, *317*, *318*
Barondes, S. H., 218, 219, 220, *243*, *244*
Barr, M. L., 35, *56*
Barradough, C. A., 48, *55*
Barron, K. D., 28, *55*, 96, *101*, 140, *170*, *171*
Bartlett, M. O., 451, *508*
Bateson, P. P. G., 218, *243*
Batini, C., 299, *317*
Batsel, H., 401, *443*
Bauer, F. K., 414, *438*
Baxter, C. F., 264, 274, *283*
Baxter, D. W., 136, 143, 158, *171*, *177*
Baylor, D. A., 15, *55*
Bazelon, M., 157, 158, *170*, *171*
Bazemore, A., 250, 251, 266, *283*
Beach, G., 218, *243*
Beaver, D. L., 158, *174*
Beck, A., 293, 301, 306, *317*
Becker, B., 366, *438*, 452, *506*
Beggs, J., *445*
Beheim-Schwarzbach, D., 148, 150, *170*
Behnsen, G., 421, *438*

Bekaert, J., 339, *438*
Bell, E., 414, *437*
Bellet, S., 339, *439*
Be Ment, S. L., 465, 466, *510*
Benitez, H. A., 136, 139, *173*
Bennett, E. L., 42, *59*, 223, *244*
Bennett, H. S., *438*
Bennett, M. V. L., 466, *506*
Bensch, K. G., 160, 165, *170*, *173*
Beránek, R., 116, *128*, 278, *283*
Beresford, W. A., 96, *101*
Bergamasco, B., 313, *317*
Bergamini, L., 313, *317*
Berger, B. D., 223, *244*
Berger, H., 292, 293, 297, *317*
Bering, E. A., 363, 364, 416, *438*, 452, 459, 466, *506*
Berl, S., 503, *506*
Berlin, L., 159, *170*
Berneis, K. H., *128*
Bernhard, W., 136, *171*
Bernsohn, J., 96, *101*, 190, *211*
Bernstein, J., 155, *171*
Bernstein, J. J., 27, *57*, 96, *101*, *102*
Bernstein, M. E., 96, *101*
Berry, R. W., 46, *55*, 203, *211*
Bertrand, I., 157, 159, *170*, *176*
Bessman, S. P., 250, 275, *283*, 503, *510*
Besson, J. M., 389, 390, *438*, *445*
Best, R. M., 239, *243*
Beswick, F. B., 11, *55*
Bethlem, J., 148, 150, *170*, *171*
Betz, W. J., 9, *55*
Biber, M. P., 502, *510*
Bickford, R. G., 296, 313, *317*, *318*
Bidder, T. G., 399, *438*
Biederman, M. A., 251, 252, *285*
Biersteker, P. A., 468, 469, *520*
Bignami, A., 74, *101*
Bindman, L. J., 6, *55*
Biondi, G., 142, *170*
Birks, R., 106, 107, 108, 113, 115, 119, 120, 122, 123, 124, *127*
Bito, L. Z., 338, 361, 366, 367, 368, 379, 380, 381, 383, 403, 425, 426, 427, *438*, 453, 454, 456, 459, *506*, *507*
Bittner, G. D., 255, *286*
Björklund, A., 66, 97, *101*, *103*

Black, R. G., 32, *60*
Blackstad, T. W., 61, 68, 93, *101*
Blahd, W. H., 414, *438*
Blanchard, C. L., 312, *317*
Bleier, R., 29, *55*
Bligh, J., 108, *122*
Blinzinger, K., 28, *56*, 365, *443*
Blioch, Z. L., 10, *56*
Bliss, T. V. P., 4, 5, 6, 7, 54, *56*
Bloom, F. E., 24, 33, *55*, 234, *243*
Blum, N. R., 160, *172*
Blumenthal, H., 159, *170*
Bodenheimer, T. S., 430, *438*
Bodian, D., 24, 28, *56*, 133, 139, *170*, 182, *211*, 471, *507*
Boelter, M. D. D., 341, *441*
Boeris, W., 13, *59*
Bogacz, J., 313, *317*
Bagoch, S., 218, *243*
Boisacq-Schepens, N., 6, 7, *55*, *56*
Boistel, J., 251, 257, 258, *283*
Boldizsar, H., 339, *441*
Bondareff, W., 33, *56*, 155, *170*, 483, 487, 495, *507*
Bondy, S. C., 46, *56*, 181, 192, 197, 198, 199, *211*, *214*
Booth, D. A., 218, 238, *243*
Bornstein, M. B., 40, *56*, 164, *174*
Borsanyi, S. J., 312, *317*
Bosanquet, F. D., 148, 150, 159, *171*
Boullin, D. J., 263, *283*
Bourke, R. S., 451, *507*
Bourne, G. H., 139, *175*, 432, *444*
Bouteille, M., 136, *170*
Bowman, R. E., 217, *243*
Bowman, W. C., 122, 123, *127*
Bownds, M. D., 253, 265, 272, 277, 278, *285*, *286*
Bowyer, F., 400, *438*
Boycott, B. B., 14, *56*
Bozsik, G., 133, *170*
Bradbury, M., 360, *440*
Bradbury, M. W. B., 337, 338, 339, 340, 349, 356, 360, 361, 363, 364, 366, 367, 368, 377, 383, 385, 386, 399, 403, 412, *438*, *440*, 453, 454, 456, 457, 458, 459, 461, *507*
Bradford, H. F., 503, *507*

Bradley, K., 32, *58*
Bradley, R. D., 391, *438*
Brady, R. O., 272, 275, *283*
Brånemark, P. I., 433, *442*
Brattgàrd, S.-O., 186 (10, 12), 192, 205, 206, *211*
Braud, W. G., 221, *243*
Bray, J. J., 209, *211*, *214*
Brazier, M. A. B., 293, 294, 296, 297, 298, 301, 304, 306, 308, 309, 310, 311, 313, 314, *318*
Breese, G. R., 124, *128*
Bregoff, H. M., 250, 275, *288*
Breinin, G. M., 85, *101*
Bremer, F., 300, 313, *318*
Brenda, P., 382, *445*
Brendel, W., 456, *506*
Briggs, H. M., 236, *243*
Brightman, M. W., 333, 372, 373, 374, 375, 376, 430, 431, *438*, *443*, 451, 495, *507*
Brindley, G. S., 2, 13, 55, *56*
Brink, J. J., 219, *243*
Brinley, F. J., 502, 503, *507*
Brizzee, K. R., 424, *438*
Brock, L. G., 32, *58*
Brocklehurst, G., 420, *438*
Brodal, P., 79, *102*
Brodie, B. B., 337, 350, 352, 353, 366, 430, *438*, *442*, *445*
Brody, A., 25, *56*, 158, *170*
Broman, T., 423, *438*
Bronstead, T., 401, *438*
Brooks, C. McC., 396, *438*
Brooks, V. B., 121, 123, *127*
Brown, D. A., 460, *507*
Brown, G. L., 29, *56*
Brown, T. S., 305, *319*
Brown, W. J., 139, *170*
Browning, E. T., 110, *127*
Brožek, G., 501, 502, *507*
Brückner, G., 92, *103*
Bruggencate, G. T., 269, 273, 279, 282, *283*
Bruner, J., 314, *318*
Bruns, R. R., 371, *438*
Bubash, S., 221, 222, 223, 230, *243*
Buck, C., 223, *245*

Budd, G. C., 124, *127*
Budtz, P. E., 92, *101*
Budtz-Olsen, O. E., 43, *60*
Bulat, M., 369, *438*
Bullivant, S., 483, *507*
Bullock, T. H., 4, *56*, 231, 234, *246*
Bunge, M. B., 164, *170*
Burge, R. P., 164, *170*
Bunina, T. L., 143, *170*
Burdman, J., 164, *172*
Burdman, J. A., 164, *170*
Bureš, J., 428, *438*, 502, 503, *507*, *508*
Burgen, A. S. V., 252, 267, *185*
Burgess, A., 335, 336, *439*
Burke, W., 38, 39, 44, *56*
Burns, B. D., 4, 5, 6, 7, 54, *56*
Busca, G., 209, *211*
Byrne, W. L., 222, 223, *244*

C

Caldwell, P. C., 396, *439*
Caley, D. W., 496, *507*
Calhoun, A. M.C., 420, *439*
Cameron, I. R., 388, 391, 415, *439*
Campbell, W. W., 341, *441*
Canevini, P., 151, 152, *170*
Caputto, R., 43, *57*
Carey, F. M., 223, *245*
Carlson, P. L., 223, *244*
Carman, C. T., 393, 394, 395, *442*
Carmichael, E. A., 411, *442*
Carpenter, S., 162, *170*
Carpenter, S. J., 333, *439*
Carroll, M. P., 411, *440*
Carta, F., 44, *58*
Carver, M. J., 404, *439*
Casby, J. U., 306, 313, *318*
Casola, L., 218, 219, *243*
Caspersson, T., 180, *213*
Caton, R., 292, 306, *318*
Cegrell, L., 66, *101*
Cerf, J. A., 45, *56*
Cestan, 392, *439*
Chacko, L. W., 45, *56*
Chakrin, L. W., 109, 119, *127*
Chambers, W. W., 35, *58*, 96, *102*
Chandel, R. L., 139, *170*

Chandler, K. A., 160, *171*
Chandler, R. L., 139, *170*
Chapman, D. D., 252, *285*
Chapouthier, G., 222, 227, 228, *244*, *247*
Chargaff, E., 180, *211*
Chatrian, G. E., 312, 313, *318*
Cheng-Minoda, K., 85, *101*
Chiang, T. Y., 28, *55*
Chiappetta, L., 223, *244*
Chirigos, M. A., 405, *439*
Chopra, S. P., 45, *59*, 218, *246*
Chornock, F. W., 235, *245*
Chorover, S. L., 223, *244*
Chou, S. M., 146, 159, 162, *170*, 208, *211*
Chow, K. L., 43, *56*, *59*
Christensen, B. N., 122, *127*
Chutgow, J. G., 338, *439*
Cigánek, L., 310, *318*
Clara, M., 334, *439*
Clark, A. W., 18, *56*
Clark, H. J., 155, *174*
Clark, R. H., 222, 223, 225, *247*
Clemedson, C. J., 414, *439*
Clemente, C. D., 62, *101*, 298, 299, *318*, 371, 423, *439*, *441*
Clendinnen, B. G., 47, 49, *56*
Clouet, D., 182, *211*
Cobb, W. A., 309, *318*
Coben, L. A., 368, *439*, 452, 454, *507*
Cocks, W. A., 47, *55*, 183, 194, *211*
Cody, T. R., 313, *317*
Cohen, E. B., 73, *101*
Cohen, H., 411, 420, *439*
Cohen, H. D., 219, 220, *243*, *244*
Cohen, M. W., 337, 384, *439*
Cohn, W. E., 341, *441*
Cole, K. S., 463, 464, *507*
Cole, M., 96, *101*, *103*
Coleman, P. D., 44, *56*
Collewijn, H., 468, 473, 476, 479, 501, 502, *507*
Collier, B., 106, 107, 109, 115, 116, 117, 119, 122, 124, *127*
Collins, G. H., 37, *58*, 151, 152, 153, *170*, *172*, 471, 481, 482, *509*
Colmant, H. J., 151, 152, *175*
Colonnier, M., 64, 83, 84, *101*

Colvin, R. B., 275, *285*
Conroy, R. T. W. L., 11, *55*
Constans, J., 382, *445*
Converse, W. K., 37, *58*
Conway, E. J., 502, *507*
Cook, W. H., 35, *56*
Coombs, J. S., 450, 465, *507*
Cooper, E. S., 339, *439*
Cooper, J. R., 114, *128*
Cooper, R., 293, 306, 314, 315, *318, 320*
Corbin, H. P. F., 296, *318*
Cori, G. T., 153, *172*
Corning, W. C., 221, *244*
Cornwell, A. C., 17, *56*
Corsellis, J. A. N., 159, *170*
Corson, J. A., 223, *244*
Côté, L. J., 275, *285*
Cotman, C., 117, *127*
Courtice, F. C., 330, *439*
Cowan, S., *286*
Cowan, W. M., 34, *58*
Cowden, R. R., 151, 152, 153, *170*
Cowen, D., 155, *176*
Cowdry, E. V., 132, *170*
Coxon, R. V., 392, *439*
Cragg, B. G., 6, 15, 17, 22, 24, 25, 26, 34, 37, 41, 43, 44, 47, 52, 54, *56*, 233, 235, *244*
Craighead, J. E., 133, *176*
Craik, K. J. W., 242, *244*
Crain, S. M., 40, *56*
Creese, R., 461, *507*
Crescitelli, F., 432, *439*
Creutzfeldt, O. D., 300, 305, 316, 317, *318, 319*
Crile, G. W., 467, *507*
Crone, C., 350, 399, 401, *437, 439*
Crough, D. G., 222, *244*
Crow, H. J., 306, *318*
Crowell, J., 482, 483, 484, 485, 495, *570, 511*
Crump, C. H., 392, *443*
Csaky, T. Z., 369, *439*
Cserr, H., 385, *439*
Cuénod, M., 32, *56*, 85, *101*
Cummins, R. A., 43, *60*
Curl, F., 364, 416, *443*, 452, 459, *509*
Curran, P. F., 458, *511*

Curtis, D. R., 251, 268, 273, 274, 277, 279, 280, *284*, 503, *507*
Cutler, R. W. P., 344, 361, 367, 368, 409, 415, 416, 418, 428, *439*, 442, *444*, 452, 453, 455, 456, 460, *507, 508, 510*

D

Daffny, N., 473, 489, *571*
Daft, F. S., 158, *173*
Daginawala, H. F., 205, *214*
Dahl, D., 276, *283*
Dahl, E., 136, 139, *170*
Dahl, N. A., 8, *56*
Dahlstrom, A., 15, *56*, 116, *127*, 255, *284*
Dailey, M. E., 411, *440*
Dale, H. H., 259, *284*
Daliers, J., 222, *244*
Daneholt, B., 186 (12), 192, *211*
Daniels, A. C., 28, *55*
D'Anzi, F. A., 22, *56*
Da Prada, M., 118, *128*
Darnell, J., 195, *214*
Darnell, J. E., 193, *212*
David-Ferreira, J. F., 146, *171*
David-Ferreira, K. L., 146, *171*
Davidoff, R. A., 279, 280, 281, 282, *283, 284, 289*
Davidson, N., 274, *284*
Davies, S., 420, *439*
Davis, C. J. F., 40, *56*
Davis, H., 297, 308, *319*
Davis, P. A., 297, *319*
Davis, R. E., 218, 219, 220, *243, 244*
Davson, H., 324, 329, 330, 332, 337, 338, 342, 343, 345, 346, 349, 351, 355, 357, 359, 360, 361, 363, 364, 365, 366, 367, 368, 377, 379, 380, 381, 383, 391, 396, 399, 403, 406, 415, 416, 417, 418, 423, *438, 439, 440, 441, 443*, 450, 451, 452, 454, 456, 459, 483, *507, 508, 509*
Dawson, G. D., 308, 309, *318, 319*
Deanin, G. G., 223, *245*
Deeke, L., 315, *319*
de Jager, A., 152, *176*
de la Haba, G., 219, *244*
Delarue, J., 136, *170*
Del Castillo, J., 10, *56*

Dellmann, H.-D., 92, *101*
Dembitzer, H. M., 145, 146, 148, 157, 160, *172*
Demeester, G., 339, 392, *438*, *445*
Dement, W., 299, *319*
Dempsey, E. W., *319*, 480, *508*
den Hartog Jager, W. A., 148, 150, *170*, *171*
de Oliveira Castro, G., 504, *509*
Derbyshire, A. J., 298, *319*
de Ribaupierre, F., 66, *103*
de Robertis, E., 15, 22, *56*, 84, 90, 92, *101*, *104*, 115, *127*, 276, *288*, 370, *440*, 504, *511*
Desiderio, D. M., 231, *247*
de Thé, G., 136, *171*
Deutsch, J. A., 236, *244*
Dewar, A. J., 46, *56*
Diamond, I., 106, 107, *122*
Diamond, J., 64, *101*, 268, 280, *284*, *288*
Diamond, J. M., 357, *445*
Diamond, M. C., 42, 48, 49, *56*, *59*
Didio, J., *506*
Dierks, R. E., 135, *171*
Dingman, C. W., 193, 194, *211*
Dingman, W., 216, 218, *244*
Dixon, D. H., 455, 459, *511*
Dixon, J. S., 136, 139, *171*
D'Monte, B., 45, *59*, 218, *246*
Dobbing, J., 422, *440*, 462, *508*
Dodge, F. A., Jr., 121, *127*
Dolivo, M., 66, *103*
Domagk, G. F., 221, 222, 228, 230, *247*
Domek, N. S., 360, *438*, 450, 462, *506*
Domer, F. R., 385, 417, 418, *440*
Donahue, S., 146, 158, *171*, *177*
Donnan, F. G., 500, *508*
Doolin, P. F., 140, *170*, *171*
Dore, E., 207, *214*
Doty, W., 34, *59*
Dow, R. C., 369, *437*
Dowe, G., 118, *128*
Dowling, J. E., 14, 15, *56*, *60*
Downer, J. de C., 343, *443*
Dreifuss, J. J., 272, *284*
Dreyfus-Brisac, C., 296, *319*
Droz, B., 235, *244*
d'Silva, J. L., 461, *507*

Dubois, D., 152, *176*
Dubois-Dalcq, M., 151, 152, *171*
Dubrovsky, B., 7, *58*
Duchen, L. W., 26, *56*
Duchett, S., 155, *174*
Dudel, J., 251, 252, 259, 260, *284*
Duffy, P. E., 150, 158, *171*
Duggan, A. W., 274, 277, 279, 280, *284*
Duginawala, H. F., 218, *246*
Duke, L., 314, *319*
Dunant, Y., 66, *103*
Duncan, D., 140, 155, *171*, *174*
Dupont, J. R., 134, *171*
Dutcher, J. D., 223, *244*
Dutta, C. R., 139, *176*
Dyal, J. A., 222, *244*
Dylcen, P., 158, *177*
Dziewiatkouski, D., *211*

E

Eakin, R. M., 43, *57*
Earle, K. M., 134, 143, 146, 148, 152, 153, 159, 162, 164, 165, 169, *171*, *172*, *173*, *175*
Eaton, H. D., 420, *439*
Eayrs, J. T., 41, 47, 48, 49, *55*, *56*, *57*
Eccles, J. C., 32, 35, 36, 37, 39, *57*, 64, *101*, *102*, 233, *244*, 250, 251, 268, 269, 273, 274, 280, 281, *284*, 449, 450, 465, 501, *507*, *508*
Eccles, R. M., 35, 36, 39, *57*
Edgar, G. W. F., 152, *171*
Edds, M. V., 35, *52*, 95, *102*
Edström, A., 182, 183, 184, 186 (1920), 209, 210, *211*, *212*, *213*
Edström, J.-E., 180, 182, 183, 186 (7, 9, 10, 11, 17, 18, 20, 22), 187, 202, 203, 205, 206, 208, 209, 210, *211*, *212*, *214*
Edström, R., 323, *440*
Edwards, C., 251, 264, 266, 267, 280, *285*, 287
Efron, R., 473, *508*
Egyházi, E., 186 (3, 4, 23), 197, 201, 205, 208, *212*
Ehrlich, P., 323, 326, *440*
Eichelberger, L., 449, *508*

Eichner, D., 182, 186 (17, 20, 22), 187, 202, *211*, *212*
Eidelberg, E., 272, 275, *288*, *399*, *440*
Einarson, L., 158, *171*
Elfvin, L.-G., 145, *171*
Eliot, C. R., 252, *285*
Elizan, T. S., 145, 146, 148, 157, 159, *172*
Ellingson, R. J., 296, 309, *319*
Elliott, K. A. C., 250, 251, 266, 267, 273, 274, 276, 277, *283*, *285*, *286*, 452, 458, *509*
Elliott, L., 223, *245*
Ellis, C. H., 251, *285*
Elmqvist, D., 10, *51*, 116, 120, 123, *127*
Elul, R., 233, *244*
Emmens, M., 218, *243*
Endo, M., 10, *59*
Endo, S., 382, 424, *437*
Engberg, I., 269, 273, 279, 282, *283*, *284*
Engel, J. P., 13, 52, *57*, *59*
Enger, P. E. S., 267, *285*
Enesco, H. E., 223, *244*
Epstein, L., 222, 226, 230, *244*
Escriva, A., 385, 417, 428, *441*, *444*
Esser, H., 337, *440*
Essner, E., 155, *171*
Eterovic, V. A., 43, *57*
Evangelista, I., 35, *57*, 156, 160, *171*
Evans, C. A. N., 253, *285*
Evans, C. C., 311, *319*
Evarts, E. V., 38, *58*
Eyerman, G. S., 275, *287*
Eyzaguirre, C., 267, *287*

F

Fahn, S., 275, *285*
Faiszt, J., 222, 230, *243*, *244*
Falck, B., 66, *101*
Farquhar, M. G., 335, *440*, 481, *508*
Farrow, J. T., 222, 230, *246*
Fatt, P., 250, 251, 257, 258, *283*, *284*, *285*, 450, 465, *507*
Feher, O., 23, *59*
Feldman, R. G., 160, *171*, *173*
Felix, D., 274, *284*
Fenc, V., 337, 338, *440*, *441*
Feng, T. P., 432, *440*

Fenichel, G. M., 157, 158, *170*, *171*
Fenichel, R. L., 223, *244*
Fenske, A., 456, *570*
Fenstermacher, J. D., 350, *440*, 457, 464, 467, 473, *508*, *509*
Fényes, I., 148, 159, *171*
Ferchmin, P. A., 43, *57*
Ferguson, R. K., 424, 425, *440*, 451, 457, 459, 462, *508*
Feria-Valasco, A., 134, 135, *171*
Fernandez, J., 495, *511*
Fernandez-Morán, H., 483, *508*
Ferreira, H. M., 468, 470, *509*
Few, A., 155, *171*
Fickenscher, L., 64, *102*
Field, E. J., 139, 146, *171*, *174*
Field, P. M., 99, *102*
Fifkova, E., 44, *57*, 503, 504, *508*, *570*
Fifková, E., 503, *507*
Filias, N., 279, *286*
Fish, I., 48, *57*
Fisher, M. A., 275, *285*
Fishman, J., *399*, *440*
Fishman, R. A., 399, *440*
Fjerdingstad, E. J., 220, 221, 222, 228, 230, *244*, *246*, *247*
Fleischhauer, K., 373, *440*
Flexner, J. B., 219, 220, *244*, 422, *443*, 462, *508*
Flexner, L. B., 209, *212*, 219, 220, 234, *244*, *246*, 341, 342, 422, 424, *440*, *443*, 462, *508*
Florey, E., 250, 251, 252, 266, 267, *283*, *285*, *286*
Folch, J., 450, *508*
Foley, J. M., 143, 158, *171*
Fonnum, F., 112, *127*, 272, 276, *286*
Forbes, A., 298, *319*
Forno, L. S., 142, 148, 150, 159, *171*
Foroglou-Karameus, C., 66, *103*
Foulkes, D., 299, *319*
Fox, C. A., 139, *176*
Franguelli, R., 44, *58*
Frank, B., 224, *244*
Frank, K., 465, *508*
Frankel, S., 250, *288*
Fraser, H., 135, 145, *171*
Frazier, C. H., 341, *440*

Freeman, A. F., 278, *288*
Fremont-Smith, F., 338, 411, *440, 442*
French, C. M., 460, *508*
Freygang, W. H., 465, 467, 468, 470, 473, 474, *508*
Freireich, E. J., 342, *444*
Frick, E., 409, *440*
Fricke, H., 463, 464, *508*
Friedberg, F., 404, *440*
Friede, R. L., 155, 158, *171*
Friedman, R. M., 202, *213*
Friedman, V., 331, *445*
Friesen, A. J. D., 109, *127*
Frommes, S. P., 136, *176*
Frost, R. W., 416, *445*
Fuerst, R., 250, *283*
Fujisawa, T., 195, *213*
Fukuda, J., 273, *286*
Fukuya, M., 268, *285*
Fuortes, M. G. F., 15, *55*, 465, *508*
Furshpun, E. J., 251, 267, *285*
Furst, S., 405, *442*

G

Gage, P. W., 10, *57*
Gaito, J., 205, *212*, 240, *245*
Gajdusek, D. C., 169, *173*
Galambos, R., 223, *244*, 308, *319*, 473, 474, *508*
Galindo, A., 273, 279, *285*
Gallicich, J., 344, 416, 418, *439*
Galvan, L., 222, 223, 225, 228, *247*
Gambetti, P., 139, *171*, 219, *244*
Gandini, D. A., 207, *214*
Ganote, C. E., 158, *174*
Garcia-Austt, E., 313, *317*
Garcia Ramos, J., 470, 474, *510*
Gardiner, M. F., 312, *319*
Gardner, R., 223, *244*
Gardner-Medwin, A. R., 2, 3, 13, 55, *57*
Garel, J. P., 194, 195, 198, *212*
Gartside, I. B., 6, 7, 9, 55, *57*
Gaskins, J. R., 342, *444*, 455, *510*
Gastaut, Y., 311, *319*
Gautier, R., 327, *444*
Gautron, J., 115, 117, *127*
Gay, A. J., 140, *176*

Gay, R., 222, 226, 230, *244*
Gaze, R. M., 62, 99, *102*
Geel, B. K., 218, *246*
Geiger, A., 399, *440*
Gelfan, S., 52, 53, *57*
Geoghegan, H., 502, *507*
Gerschenfeld, H. M., 337, 384, *439*
Gerstein, A., 405, *442*
Gesell, R., 392, *440*
Getty, R., 155, *171*
Gibbs, C. J., Jr., 146, 169, *171, 173*
Gibbs, C. L., 11, *57*
Gibby, R. G., 222, *244*
Girard, M., 193, *212*
Girardier, L., 258, *288*
Giuditta, A., 194, 195, 197, 198, *214*
Giurgea, C., 222, *244*
Glagoleva, I. M., 10, *56*
Glaser, G. H., 160, *171*, 384, *445*
Glassman, E., 217, 218, 219, 233, *244*
Globus, A., 41, 45, 46, *57, 58*
Glover, V. A. S., 107, 108, 109, 111, 112, *127, 128*
Glück, B., 148, 150, *173*
Goddard, G. V., 7, *57*
Godfraind, J. M., 274, *285*
Godin, Y., 402, *442*
Goel, B. K., 45, *59*
Goldberg, A. L., 34, *57*
Goldberg, B., 414, *438*
Goldberg, L. H., 207, *214*
Goldberg, M. A., 360, 415, *438, 440*, 450, 462, *506*
Goldberg, S., 94, *102*
Goldfischer, S., 155, *171*
Goldman, E. E., 323, 326, 327, *440*
Goldring, S., 501, 502, *508*
Goldstein, N. P., 337, 407, 408, *441*
Golub, A. M., 222, 223, 226, 230, *244*
Gomez, C. J., 155, *171*
Gonatas, N. K., 35, *57*, 139, 155, 156, 160, *171, 176*, 219, *244*
González-Aguilar, F., 480, 481, 497, *508*
González-Angulo, A., 134, 135, *171*
Goodchild, M., 274, *285*
Goodman, D. C., 35, *57*, 97, *102*
Goodman, H. M., 34, *57*
Goodman, L., 43, *57*

Gordon, J. E., 48, *59*
Gordon, H. W., 223, *245*, 422, *442*
Gordon, S., 480, *509*
Gorski, R. A., 48, *55*
Grafstein, B., 502, *508*
Grahm, A., 195, *214*
Graham, D. G., 135, *174*
Graham, L. T., 275, 279, 280, 281, *284*, *285*
Grahn, B., 194, 200, *213*
Grampp, W., 182, 186 (18), 202, 203, *211*, *212*
Gray, E. G., 41, *57*, 61, 64, 83, *101*, 102, 371, *441*
Gray, E. W., 145, *171*
Graziani, L., 385, *441*
Grözier, F. M., 423, *441*
Green, J. P., 122, *127*
Greenberg, D. M., 341, 404, *440*, *441*
Greenberg, E. S., 451, *507*
Greenfield, J. G., 143, 148, 150, 159, *171*
Greengard, P., 405, *439*
Grenell, R. G., 180, *213*, 234, *245*
Griffith, J. F., 135, *174*
Griffith, J. S., 237, *245*
Grillo, M. A., 480, *509*
Gröntoft, O., 423, *441*
Grofova, I., 73, 79, *102*
Gross, C. R., 223, *245*
Grossfeld, R. M., 277, 278, *286*
Grossman, R. G., 73, *104*
Grundfest, H., 251, 258, 259, 260, 266, 267, 278, *285*, *289*, *288*
Gruner, J., 430, *441*
Grunholm, L., 397, *441*
Gryder, R., 252, 260, *284*
Guillery, R. W., 41, *57*, 61, 64, 81, 83, 84, *101*, *102*
Gurian, B. S., 458, *506*
Guroff, G., 191, *212*, 405, *441*
Guth, L., 27, *57*, 95, 96, *102*
Guth, P. S., 117, 118, 120, *127*
Gutmann, E., 95, *104*
Gutmann, L., 95, *104*
Gutrecht, J. A., 146, 162, *170*
Gwynn, R. H., 223, *245*
Gyllensten, L., 43, 44, *57*

H

Habel, R. E., 135, 139, *176*
Haber, B., 269, 274, 275, *285*, *287*, *288*
Haberland, C., 157, 159, *171*
Hadjiolov, A. A., 194, 195, *214*
Haën, C., 207, *214*
Haege, F. F., 451, *509*
Häggendal, J., 116, 126, *127*
Hafferl, A., 330, *441*
Hageman-Bal, M., 151, 152, 153, *176*
Hagen, D. Q., 275, *285*
Hager, H., 365, *443*
Hagiwara, S., 251, 266, 267, *285*
Halász, B., 92, *103*
Halkerston, I. D. K., 237, *245*
Hall, R. C., 420, *439*
Hall, Z. W., 252, 253, 255, 260, 261, 262, 263, 264, 265, 266, 272, 278, *285*, *286*, *287*
Hall-Craggs, E. C. B., 39, *57*
Hallén, O., 202, *212*
Hallervorden, J., 148, 159, *172*
Halstead, W. C., 216, 238, *245*
Hama, K., 430, *441*
Hamberger, A., 202, *212*
Hamlyn, L. H., 83, *102*
Hammerstad, J. P., 409, *439*, 452, *508*
Hammond, B. J., 274, *283*
Hámori, J., 28, *57*, 70, 73, 83, 84, 85, 87, 90, 92, 97, *102*, *103*
Hampton, J. C., *438*
Hams, M. L., 399, *440*
Handler, P., 313, *317*, 404, *441*
Hanzlikova, V., 37, 39, *59*
Hardman, J. M., 146, 148, 159, 162, *175*
Harper, P. V., 414, *441*
Harriman, D. G. F., 151, 152, *172*
Harris, A. B., 140, *176*
Harris, G. W., 48, *57*
Harrison, A. K., 135, *171*
Hartelias, H., 414, *439*
Harter, M. R., 311, *319*
Harth-Edel, S., 180, 181, 189, 190, *213*
Hartmann, G., 503, *507*
Hartmann, H. A., 167, *170*, 186 (7, 8), 208, *211*, *212*, *214*
Hartmann, J. F., 479, 481, *508*

Hartroft, W. S., 155, 158, *174*
Harvey, A. M., 264, *285*
Harvey, E. N., 297, *319*
Harwood, J. R., 276, *283*
Hase, U., 456, *570*
Hashida, Y., 133, *172*
Hashimoto, P. H., 430, *441*
Hashish, S. E. E., 461, *507*
Hassler, R., 44, *57*, 148, *172*
Hassoun, J., 152, *176*
Hastings, A. B., 449, 450, 458, *506, 509 510*
Hata, F., 117, *128*
Hayashi, T., 250, *285*
Hayhow, W. R., 38, 39, 44, *56*
Haymaker, W., 159, *173*
Hebb, C. O., 112, *127*, 281, *285*
Hebb, D. O., 233, 237, *245*
Hechter, O., 237, *245*
Heding, A., 205, *214*
Heiner, L., 32, *57*, 63, 68, 81, *102*
Heinzler, F., 337, *440*
Heisey, S. R., 343, 363, 366, 419, *441, 443, 509*
Held, D., 363, 388, 419, *441*
Hellauer, H., 281, *287*
Heller, H., 66, *101*
Hemsworth, B. A., 122, 123, *127*
Hendee, R., 399, *445*
Henderson, E. S., 344, 416, *444*
Hendrickson, A., 94, *102*
Herblin, W. F., 222, *246*
Herdklotz, J. H., 117, *127*
Herman, M. M., 140, 158, *172*
Herndon, R. M., 135, *172*
Herr, E. P., 411, *445*
Herrington, R. M., 310, *319*
Hertzman, A. B., 392, *440*
Herzog, E., 148, 150, *172*
Hespe, W., 275, *285*
Hess, A., 423, *442*
Heuser, J., 34, *57*
Hiatt, H. H., 207, *214*
Hidaka, T., 267, *285*
Higashi, K., 385, 386, 416, *437*
Highstein, S. M., 273, *286, 287*
Hild, W., 465, 467, 474, *508*
Hill, D. K., 17, *58*

Hill, N. C., 337, 407, 408, *441*
Hinds, P. L., 74, *103*
Hirano, A., 143, 145, 146, 148, 157, 159, 160, 162, 164, 165, 169, *172, 173, 177*
Hirano, S., 276, *288*
Hirsch, H. E., 253, *285*
Hishio, A., 117, *128*
Hobart, G., 297, *319*
Hochstein, P., 207, *213*
Hochwald, G. M., 332, 348, 364, 407, 409, 419, *441, 444*
Hodgkin, A. L., 106, 108, *127*
Hökfelt, T., 209, 210, *211*, 272, *285*
Hoffman, J., 158, *177*
Hogans, A. F., 191, *212*
Hogenhuis, L. A. H., 191, 192, *212*
Holland, J., 223, *245*
Holland, J. M., 151, *172*
Holländer, H., 68, 79, *102*
Hollander, J., 155, *174*
Hollingsworth, G., 332, *440*
Holloway, R. L., 43, *58*
Holmberg, G., 414, *439*
Holmgren, E., 139, *172*
Holst, E. H., 371, *439*
Holt, C. E., III, 223, *244*
Honig, G. R., 207, *212*
Hopkin, J. M., 280, *285*
Horányi, B., 133, *170*
Horel, J. A., 35, *57*, 97, *102*
Horfat, J., 242, *245*
Horn, G., 48, *57*, 218, *243*
Horovitz, Z. P., 223, *244*
Horsch, S., 456, *506*
Horstmann, D. M., 133, 139, *170*
Horstmann, E., 464, 480, 492, *508*
Hösli, L., 279, 280, *284, 286*
Hosmer, H. R., 467, *507*
Howard, E., 48, *58*
Hoy, R. R., 255, *286*
Hsü, C. S., 194, 198, *214*
Hsu, D., 165, *173*
Hubbard, J. I., 10, 18, *57, 58*, 116, *127*
Hubel, D. H., 28, 43, 55, *58, 60*
Hughes, A., 209, *212*
Hughes, I. E., 412, *438*
Hughes, J. R., 38, *58*
Huikuri, K., 85, *103*

Hull, R. C., 310, *320*
Hunt, C. C., 85, *102*
Hunter, G., 337, 338, 366, 413, *441*
Hurlbut, W. P., 18, *56*
Hurst, E. W., 134, 139, *172*
Hurt, H. D., 420, *439*
Hurwitz, R., 401, *441*
Hutt, L. D., 223, *245*
Huxley, A. F., 432, *441*
Hydén, H., 180, 183, 186 (2, 3, 4, 5, 10, 16, 23, 24), 190, 197, 201, 202, 204, 205, 206, 208, *211, 212*, 216, 217, 218, 219, 230, 237, *245*

I

Ichijo, M., 503, *508*
Iizuka, R., 155, 158, *174*
Illingworth, B., 153, *172*
Ingham, C., 49, *56*
Innes, J. R. M., 135, 140, *172*
Iraldi, A. P., 115, *127*
Iravani, J., 260, *286*
Irwin, L. N., 217, 222, 228, 236, *247*
Ishii, T., 159, *172*
Ishikawa, H., 136, *172*
Israël, M., 115, 117, 126, *127, 128*
Issidorides, M., 155, *172*
Ito, M., 64, *102*, 268, 269, 371, 273, 276, 281, *284, 286, 287*
Ito, Y., 267, *285*
Itoh, T., 191, 201, *212*
Iversen, L. L., 260, 261, 262, 263, 264, 266, 273, 276, 277, 278, *286, 287*
Iwasaki, S., 267, *286*

J

Jabbur, S. J., 273, *283*
Jacob, H., 151, 152, *175*
Jacob, M., 194, 195, 196, 197, 198, *212, 214*
Jacobs, L., 367, 368, *443*, 452, 456, 459, 460, *570*
Jacobs, L. A., 424, *438*
Jacobson, A., 221, 222, 223, 230, *243*
Jacobson, A. L., 221, 222, 223, 230, *243*
Jacobson, J. L., 313, *317*

Jacobson, M., 27, *58*, 233, 234, *245*
Jacobson, S., 207, *213*
Jakoby, W. B., 253, 261, 270, *286*
James, W., 216, *245*
Janeway, R., 151, 152, *172, 174*
Janković, B. D., 242, *245*
Jansen, J., 268, 270, *289*
Järlfors, U., 116, *128*
Jarlstedt, J., 182, 183, 184, 186 (13, 14, 19), 202, *211, 212*
Jarvik, M. E., 218, 223, *243, 244*
Jasper, H. H., 273, 274, *285, 286*
Jenis, E. H., 152, 153, *172*
Jervis, G. A., 159, *172*
Jobsis, F. F., 11, *58*
John, E. R., 232, 233, 237, *245*, 310, *319*
Johnson, A. B., 160, *172*
Johnson, E. A., 11, *57*
Johnson, F. R., 24, *55*
Johnson, J. A., 350, 359, *440, 441*
Johnson, L. H., 401, *443*
Johnson, R. E., 49, *56*
Johnson, T., 223, *245*
Johnston, G. A. R., 274, 277, 279, 280, *284*
Johnston, I. H., 279, 280, *284*
Johnston, P. V., 234, *245*, 497, *508*
Johnstone, J. R., 96, *102*
Jones, A., 266, *283*
Jones, E. G., 32, *58*
Jones, S. F., 18, 19, *58*, 116, 118, 120, 122, 124, *127*, 265, 266, *286*
Jones, W. H., 45, *58*
Jonsson, G., 277, *283*
Jordan, E. F., 343, 366, *443, 509*
Joseph, B. S., 94, *102*
Journey, L. J., 164, *172*
Jouvet, M., 300, *319*
Judes, C., 194, 197, *212*
Julian, T., 274, *283*
Jund, R., 194, 197, *212*

K

Kado, R. T., *506*
Kadota, K., 116, *127*

Kahn, R. T., 273, *286*

Kaji, A., 252, 260, *284, 285*

Kakefuda, T., 276, 282, *287, 289*

Kalifat, S. R., 136, *170*

Kalyuzhnaya, P. I., 222 ,230, *245*

Kamin, H., 404, *441*

Kanaseki, T., 116, *127*

Kandel, E. R., 4, 37, *58,* 231, 233, *245,* 502, 503, *507*

Kao, F. F., 396, *438*

Kaplan, R. J., 362, 385, *441, 443,* 452, 457, 459, *508, 509*

Kappers, J. A., 139, *175,* 429, *441*

Karahashi, Y., 501, 502, *508*

Karczewski, W., 162, *177*

Karlsson, U., 24, *58,* 480, 481, 495, 497, *508, 510*

Karnovsky, M. J., 371, 372, *441, 443,* 451, *510*

Katchalsky, A., 237, *245*

Katz, B., 10, 11, *56, 58,* 120, 122, *127,* 251, 257, 263, 265, *285, 286*

Katz, J. J., 216, 238, *245*

Katzman, R., 385, 417, 428, *441, 442, 444,* 450, *508*

Kawai, N., 269, 271, 282, *286*

Kawakita, Y., 188, *214*

Keefe, J. R., 154, 155, *175*

Kellerth, J.-O., 273, *286*

Kelley, D. E., 195, *214*

Kelley, J. S., 272, *284*

Kelly, D. E., 234, *245*

Kelly, J. S., 11, *58*

Kemeny, A., 339, *441*

Kennedy, D., 255, *286*

Kennedy, E. P., 106, 107, *122*

Kerkut, G. A., *286*

Kernell, D., 203, 204, *212, 214*

Kerr, F. W. L., 414, *443*

Kerrigan, J. A., 133, *175*

Key, G., 434, *441*

Khattab, F. I., 458, 471, 472, 473, 479, 481, 489, 491, 493, 495, 496, 499, 504, *510, 511*

Kibrick, S., 133, *175*

Kidd, M., 160, *172*

Killam, K. F., 275, *286*

Kim, S. U., 136, 139, *173*

Kimberlin, R. H., 188, 192, 194, *212*

Kimble, D. P., 218, 223, *243, 245*

Kimble, R. J., 223, *245*

King, P. B., 273, *288*

Kingsley, J. R., 37, *58*

Kirkland, J. A., 115, 117, *128*

Kishida, K., 274, *286*

Kitto, G. B., 236, *243*

Kjallquist, A., 396, 416, *441*

Klatzo, I., 162, *173, 175,* 415, 429, *441, 444,* 452, 458, *509*

Kleeman, C. R., 339, 340, 342, 349, 351, 356, 357, 381, 385, 388, *438, 439, 440, 441,* 456, 457, 458, 461, *507, 508*

Klein, J. R., 401, *441*

Kleitman, N., *317*

Klintworth, G. K., 135, *174*

Klivington, K. A., 473, 474, *508*

Klopp, C. T., 26, *59*

Koch, A., 450, *508*

Koelle, G. B., 182, *213*

Koenig, E., 182, 183, 184, 186 (1, 25), 200, 208, 209, 210, *212, 213*

Koenig, H., 187, 191, 192, 207, *213*

Koffas, D., 159, *170*

Konishi, S., 279, *286*

Konrad, K. W., 7, *58*

Kooiman, M., 504, *511*

Kopin, I. J., 124, *128*

Korey, S. R., 155, *171*

Kornhüber, H. H., 315, *319*

Korr, I. M., 235, *245*

Kotani, M., 94, *102*

Kotetsu, K., 250, *284*

Kotorii, K., 139, *170*

Kovacs, S., 47, *55*

Koval, G. J., 274, *283*

Kozak, W., 37, *57, 58*

Kral, A., 412, *441*

Krauss, K. R., 124, *128*

Kravitz, E. A., 252, 253, 255, 256, 260, 261, 262, 263, 264, 265, 266, 272, 274, 277, 278, 281, *184, 285, 286, 287*

Krech, D., 42, *56*

Kreutzberg, G., 15, 28, 46, *56, 58*

Krigman, M. R., 160, *173*

Krishan, A., 165, *173*

Křivánek, J., 502, 503, *508*

Krnjević, K., 11, 37, *57*, *58*, 112, 122, 123, *127*, *128*, 272, 276, 279, *284*, *285*, *287*, 431, 432, 433, *441*, 450, 467, 503, 508
Kromash, M. H., 359, 387, *442*
Krücke, W., 159, *173*
Kruger, L., 53, *59*, 73, *102*, 150, 151, *173*
Krylov, O. A., 222, 239, *245*
Krylow, L., 431, *442*
Kuffler, S. W., 251, 252, 259, 260, 264, 266, 267, 268, 278, 280, 281, *284*, *285*, *286*, *287*, 337, 384, *439*, *443*, 465, *508*
Kuhlman, R. E., 45, *58*
Kuno, M., 250, 253, *287*
Kupfer, C., 44, *58*
Kuriyama, H., 267, *285*
Kuriyama, K., 269, 274, 275, 276, *285*, *287*, *288*, 289
Kurland, L. T., 143, 145, 146, 148, 157, 159, 160, *172*, *173*
Kusano, K., 251, 266, 267, *285*
Kuttner, R., 422, *442*
Kwak, S., 140, *171*
Kwanbunbumpen, S., 18, 19, 33, *58*, 116, 118, 120, 122, 124, *127*, 265, 266, *286*

L

Ladewig, P. P., 146, 148, 159, 162, *175*
Ladman, A. J., 333, *445*
Lafora, G. R., 148, 150, 151, *173*
Lajtha, A., 236, *245*, 403, 405, 406, 422, *442*, 455, 462, *509*
Lalich, J. J., 208, *212*
Lamarche, J. B., 159, *176*
Lambert, E. F., 298, *319*
Lampert, P. W., 143, 146, 148, 153, 157, 162, 164, 165, 167, 169, *173*, *175*
Landau, E. M., 19, 33, *58*
Landau, W. M., 465, 467, 468, 470, 473, 474, *508*
Landauer, T. K., 237, *245*
Landström, H., 180, *213*
Landua, A. J., 250, *283*
Láng, E., 85, 87, 90, *102*
Lange, P. W., 186 (16), 205, *212*, 217, 218, *245*
Larramendi, L. M. H., 64, *102*

Larson, M. D., 280, *287*
Larson, S. J., 22, *59*
Lasansky, A., 458, *509*
Lasek, R. J., 94, *102*, 182, *213*
Lashley, K. S., 237, 238, *245*
Lassalle, 392, *439*
Laszlo, J., 207, *213*
Latham, H., 193, *212*
Lathrop, K. A., 414, *441*
Law, R. O., 461, *509*
Lawrence, C. A., 39, *57*
Layne, E. C., 250, 275, *283*
Lazarte, J. A., 312, 313, *318*
Leaf, A., 502, *509*
Leaf, G., 278, *288*
Leaf, R. C., 223, *244*
Leake, L. D., *286*
Leão, A. A. P., 468, 470, 476, 502, *509*
Leblond, C. P., 191, 192, 193, *213*
Lechner, E., 339, *439*
Lee, J. C., 415, *437*
Lederis, K., 66, *101*
Leech, C. K., 7, *57*
Lees, M., 450, *508*
Leestma, J. E., 136, *173*
LeFevre, P. G., 399, 401, *442*
Leiderman, P. H., 385, *442*
Lemire, R. J., 420, *442*
Lemkey-Johnston, N., 64, *102*
Lennox, W. G., 415, *445*
Leonhardt, H. L., 223, *245*
Lesbats, B., 115, 117, *127*
Leusen, I., 342, 343, 392, 393, *442*, *445*
Levi-Montalcini, R., 206, 207, *213*, *214*
Levin, E., 342, 357, 361, 381, 406, *440*, *441*, *442*
Levin, V. A., 451, 466, 467, 473, *508*, *509*
Levine, E., 452, 456, *508*
Levine, S., 48, *57*
Levy, L. L., 160, *171*
Lewandowsky, M., 323, 326, *442*
Lewy, F. H., 148, *173*
Li, C.-L., 450, 457, 463, 464, 466, 467, 474, *507*, *508*, *509*
Liberman, E. A., 10, *56*
Libet, B., 66, *102*
Libert, B., 32, *57*

Lickey, M., 218, *243*
Lillie, R. D., 143, 155, 158, *173*
Lim, R., 218, 219, *243*
Lin, J., 186 (8), 208, *212*
Lindell, J.-O., 106, *128*
Lindenberg, R., 146, 157, 167, *175*
Linder, B., 42, *56*
Linder, G. C., 44, *442*
Lindsley, D. B., 296, *319*
Lindström, B., 182, *213*
Ling, G. N., 109, *127*, 359, 387, *442*
Lipkin, L. E., 143, 148, 150, *173*
Lipmann, F., 198, *213*
Lippold, O. C. J., 6, *55*, *57*
Liu, C. N., 35, *58*, 96, *102*, *103*
Liu, C. Y., 35, *58*, 96, *102*
Liu, Y. M., 432, *440*
Ljungdahl, Å., 277, *285*
Lloyd, B. B., 306, *438*
Lloyd, D. P. C., 3, 11, 12, 55, *58*
Lømo, T., 6, 12, 13, *55*, *56*
Loening, U. E., 193, 195, *213*, *214*
Loeschke, H. H., 337, 339, 387, 389, 395, *442*, *443*
Løvtrup-Rein, H., 194, 195, 200, *213*
Loewenstein, W. R., 234, 235, *245*, *246*
Loewi, O., 220, *245*, 265, 281, *287*
Logan, J. E., 180, *213*
Longenecker, H. E., 18, *56*
Loomis, A. L., 297, *319*
Lorenzo, A. V., 361, 367, 368, 428, *439*, *442*, *444*, 452, 453, 455, 456, 460, *507*, *508*, *510*
Lorey, R. A., 237, *246*
Love, R., 133, *173*
Lowe, I. P., 275, *287*
Lowenthal, A., 412, *442*
Lowry, O. H., 45, *58*, 270, *387*
Lu, C. Y., 207, *213*
Luciano, D. S., 424, *442*
Luck, C. P., 416, *440*
Luft, J. H., 371, *438*, *442*
Lukyanova, L. D., 503, *507*
Lund, J. S., 73, *102*
Lund, R. D., 73, 81, 83, *102*
Lundborg, G., 433, *442*
Luse, S. A., 160, *173*, 430, *442*, 480, 481, *509*

Luttges, M., 223, *245*
Lux, H. D., 46, *58*, 300, 316, *319*
Luyendijk, W., 396, *442*

M

McCallum, W. C., 293, 314, 315, *320*
McCance, R. A., 48, *58*
McCardle, R. J., 414, *441*
McCarty, K. S., 207, *213*
McCombs, R. M., 135, *173*
McConnell, J. V., 216, 221, 222, 223, 226, 230, 235, 237, *244*, *245*
McCormick, W. F., 136, 143, 153, 158, 160, *175*, *177*
McCouch, G. P., 35, *58*, 96, *102*
McGaugh, J., 220, 223, 236, *245*
McGavran, M. H., 135, *173*
McGeer, E. G., 267, *187*
McGeer, P. L., 267, *187*
McGee-Russell, S. M., 480, *509*
McGuckin, W. F., 337, 407, 408, *441*
Machili, P., 278, *288*
Machiyama, Y., 274, *283*
Machlus, B., 240, *245*
McIlwain, H., 503, *506*, *507*
MacIntosh, F. C., 106, 107, 108, 109, 113, 115, 119, 120, 122, 123, 124, *127*, 264, *285*
McIntyre, A. K., 13, 32, 37, *57*, *58*
McIntyre, D. C., 7, *57*
McIntyre, I., 340, *443*
McKenzie, B. F., 337, 407, 408, *441*
Mackey, E. A., 205, *213*
McKhann, G. M., 274, *287*
McKhawn, G. M., 158, *172*
McLennan, H., 267, 272, 274, *287*
McManan, U. J., 61, 84, *102*
McMenemey, W. H., 157, 159, *173*
Maekawa, K., 302, *319*
Magalhães, M. M., 139, *173*
Magnes, J., 399, *440*
Magoun, H. W., 301, *319*
Mahler, H. K., 117, *127*, 187, 188, 192, 193, 194, *213*, *214*, 237, *245*
Maikel, R. P., 350, 352, 353, *442*
Majno, G., 335, 369, *442*

Malamud, N., 143, 145, 146, 148, 157, 159, 160, *172, 173*
Malawista, S. E., 165, *170*
Maletta, G. J., 44, *58*
Malhotra, S. K., 482, 483, 485, 487, 489, 495, 496, *509, 511*
Malis, L. I., 53, *59*
Mallart, A., 8, *58*
Malmfors, T., 43, 44, *57*, 126, *127*
Mandel, P., 180, 181, 189, 190 ,194, 195, 196, 197, 198, *212, 213, 214*, 402, *442*
Mandelstamm, M., 431, *442*
Manery, J. F., 434, *442*, 449, 451, *509*
Mangan, J. L., 276, *287*
Mannell, W. A., 180, *213*
Manocha, S. L., 139, *175*
Mann, G., 139, *173*
Maraini, G., 44, *58*
Marantz, R., 165, *173*
Marchbanks, R. M., 106, 107, 115, 117, 118, 119, 126, *128*
Marco, L. A., 305, *319*
Mardell, R., 180, 181, 189, 190, *213*
Maren, T. H., 416, *442*
Margolis, F. L., 46, 48, *56, 60*
Margolis, G., 157, 159, *173*
Margules, D. L., 223, *244*
Marinesco, G., 135, 143, *173*
Marin-Padilla, M., 25, *58*
Mark, J., 402, *442*
Mark, R. F., 26, 27, 37, 55, *58*, 96, *102*
Markesbery, W. R., 142, *173*
Marotte, L. R., 26, *58*, 96, *102*
Márquiz-Monter, H., 134, 135, *171*
Marrone, R. L., 222, *244*
Marsden, C. D., 158, *173*
Marshall, W. H., 38, *58*, 389, 390, 438, *445*, 502, 503, *507, 509*
Martin, A. R., 8, *58*
Martin, J. D., 142, 162, *170*
Martin, K., 106, 107, 108, *127, 128*
Martin, R., 122, *127*
Martins-Ferreira, H., 504, *509*
Masiarz, F. R., 222, 223, *244*
Masurovsky, E. B., 136, 139, *173*
Mathews, J. D., 146, *171*
Matthews, E. S., 407, 409, *441*

Matthews, M. R., 34, 45, *58*, 64, 85, 91, *102, 103*
Matsuda, T., 113, *128*
Matsumoto, S., 134, *174*
Mauro, A., 18, *56*
Maxwell, D. S., *173*, 332, 333, *442, 444*, 496, *507*
Maxwell, J. C., 464, *509*
May, L., 180, *213*
Maynard, E. A., 481, *570*
Mazur, P., 484, *509*
Meller, K., 429, *442*
Melnick, J. L., 133, 135, *173, 174*
Mendell, J., 142, *173*
Mendelson, M., 277, *289*
Melzaek, R., 7, *58*
Mercier, C., 153, *173*
Merler, E., 409, *439*
Merritt, H. H., 338, *440, 442*
Messeter, K., 416, *441*
Mestrezat, W., 411, *442*
Meves, E., 464, 480, 492, *508*
Meyer, D. D., 96, *103*
Meyers, J. P., 155, *176*
Michaelson, I. A., 115, 117, *128*
Mickelsen, O., 274, *287*
Mikovic, K., 429, *444*
Miledi, R., 10, 11, 34, 37, *57, 58*, 71, 85, 93, *103*, 121, 122, *127*, 234, *245*
Millar, J. H. D., 151, 152, *172*
Millen, J. W., 325, 373, 423, *442*
Miller, C., 159, *170*
Miller, D. S., 207, *213*
Miller, P. L., 278, *283*
Miller, R. G., 222, *246*
Miller, T. B., 337, *440*
Mirra, S. S., 147, *171*
Mitchell, J. F., 122, 123, *128*, 273, *286, 287*
Mitchell, R. A., 393, 394, 395, *442*
Miyasishi, T., 155, 158, *174*
Miyamoto, K., 134, *174*
Miyata, Y., 269, 270, 271, 273, 275, 281, 282, 283, *287*
Mobelli, A. M., 313, *317*
Moir, A. T. B., 369, *437*
Molenaar, P. C., 124, *128*
Molinoff, P. B., 252, 253, 255, 264, 265, 266, 272, 278, *286, 287*

Monné, L., 216, *245*
Monod, N., 296, *319*
Montgomery, A., 40, *56*
Moossy, J., 142, 157, *174, 177*
Moore, G. P., 231, *245*
Moore, R. Y., 97, *103*
Moore, W. J., 187, 188, 192, 193, 194, *213, 214*
Morales, R., 140, 143, 155, *171, 174*
Morecki, R., 134, *174*
Morel, F., 159, *174*
Moreton, R. B., 449, *510*
Morgan, I. G., 183, *211*
Mori, K., 473, 502, *509*
Morin, W. A., 266, *287*
Morison, R. S., *319*
Morlock, H. C., 312, *320*
Morlock, N. L., 38, *58*, 423, 502, *509*
Morrell, F., 4, 13, 52, *57, 59, 60*, 230, *246*
Morris, D., 114, *128*
Morris, J. A., 146, *171*
Moruzzi, G., 299, 301, *317, 319*
Moscona, A. A., 234, *246*
Moscona, M. H., 234, *246*
Moses, H. L., 158, *174*
Mosley, J., 49, *60*
Motokizawa, F., 258, *287*
Mottschall, H. J., 387, *443*
Moulton, M. J., 414, *444*
Mountford, S., 15, *59*
Mouravieff, F., 222, *244*
Mugnaini, E., 64, 83, 84, *103, 104*
Muir, A. R., 371, *443*
Mullinges, A. M., 15, *59*
Muramatsu, M., 195, *213*
Murayama, M. M., 341, *441*
Murphy, F. A., 135, *171*
Murphy, T., 466, *571*
Murray, J. G., 27, *59*
Murray, M. R., 136, 139, *173*
Murthy, M. R. V., 191, 194, 197, *213*
Musgrave, F. S., 300, 301, *320*
Myers, R. E., 372, 425, 426, 427, *438*

N

Nagai, K., 250, *285*
Nagai, M., 109, *122*

Nagata, Y., 276, *288*
Nagayama, M., 276, *287*
Nahmias, A. J., 133, *175*
Naka, K.-I., 274, *286*
Naka, S., 188, *214*
Nakamura, R., 276, *287*
Nakamura, T., 191, 192, *214*
Nall, D., 155, *171*
Namba, M., 152, 153, *174*
Nardini, M., 396, 416, *441*
Narkiewicz, O., 162, *177*
Nauta, W. J. H., 35, *59*, 96, *101*
Nayyar, R., 207, *213*
Neal, M. J., 273, 274, 276, 277, 280, *285, 286, 287*
Neame, K. D., 403, *443*
Nelson, E., 365, *443*
Nelson, P. G., 38, *59*, 85, *107*
Nenashev, N. A., 10, *56*
Nesbett, F. B., 385, 386, 416, *437*, 450, *506*
Nevis, A. H., 151, 152, 153, *170*, 471, 481, 482, *509*
Newman, B. L., 450, *508*
Nicander, L., 136, *174*
Nicholls, J. H., 384, *443*, 460, *509*
Nicholson, P. W., 465, 466, 467, *509*
Nicholson, V. J., 124, *128*
Nickel, E., 85, 90, 91, *103*, 116, 117, 119, 126, *128*
Nishi, S., 66, *103*
Nishioka, N., 158, *174*
Nissen, T., 221, 222, 228, 230, *244, 246*
Nobécourt, P., 411, *443*
Nobel, K. W., 466, *511*
Noble, A., 181, *214*
Nogueira, G. J., 406, *442*
Nonomura, Y., 10, *59*
Norgello, H., 190, *211*
Norman, R. M., 159, *174*
Norrlin, M. L., 44, *57*
Norrlin-Grettve, M. L., 43, 44, *57*
Novikoff, A. B., 155, *171*
Noyan, B., 159, *174*
Nurnberger, J. A., 182, *213*
Nyhan, W. L., 405, *443*

O

Obara, S., 267, *289*
Obata, K., 268, 269, 270, 271, 272, 273, 275, 276, 279, 281, 282, 283, *286*, *287*
Oceguera-Navarro, C., 221, 222, 230, *247*
Ochi, R., 268, 269, 276, 281, *287*
Ochs, S., 468, 470, 500, 502, 503, *508*, *571*
O'Connor, M. J., 11, *58*
Odor, D. L., 151, 152, *172, 174*
Oester, Y. T., 34, *59*
Oldendorf, W. H., 361, *443*, 483, *509*
Oldershaw, J. B., 96, *101*, 140, *170*
O'Leary, J. L., 140, *176*
Olsen, N. S., 401, *445*
Olsson, Y., 434, 435, *441*
Olszewski, J., 151, 159, *176*
Ommaya, A. K., 344, 416, *449*
Onari, K., 167, *174*
Oplatka, A., 237, *245*
Oppelt, W. W., 340, 361, 362, 416, *443*, 450, 452, 456, *570*
Ordy, J. M., 154, 155, *175*
Orkand, P. M., 266, *287*
Orrego, F., 191, 198, 201, *213*
Orton, S. T., 139, *177*
Ota, T., 152, 153, *174*
Otsuka, M., 10, *59*, 253, 255, 256, 260, 261, 262, 263, 269, 270, 271, 273, 275, 278, 279, 281, 282, 283, *286, 287*
Overton, R. K., 236, *246*
Owman, C., 406, *443*
Owsley, P. A., 92, *101*
Ozawa, T., 85, *101*
Ozeki, M., 278, *288*

P

Page, L., 344, 416, 418, *439*
Pagni, C. S., 309, *319*
Palade, G. E., 182, 192, *213*, 335, 371, *438*, *440*
Palay, S. L., 66, *104*, 139, 140, 162, *174, 176*, 182, *213*, 372, 373, *438*, 480, *509*
Palestini, M., 299, *317*
Pallis, C. A., 155, *174*

Palmer, P., 44, *58*
Pannese, E., 205, *213*
Papp, M., 133, *170*
Pappas, G. D., 24, *60*, 73, *101*, 235, *247*, 333, 334, 373, 428, *444, 445*, 495, *509*
Pappenheimer, A. M., 158, *174*
Pappenheimer, J. R., 337, 343, 363, 366, 388, 396, 419, *440, 441, 443*, 452, 458, 459, *509*
Pappius, H. M., 452, 458, *509*
Parducz, A., 23, *54*
Park, C. R., 401, *443*
Parker, J. C., Jr., 135, *174*
Parker, L. O., 466, 467, *509*
Parker, P., 412, *438*
Parr, W., 231, *247*
Pascoe, J. E., 29, *56*
Pasqualini, E., 32, *59*, 73, 83, *103*
Passonneau, J. V., 270, *287*
Pastan, I., 207, *213*
Patlak, C. S., 342, 361, 362, 416, *443*, 444, 450, 452, 456, 457, *509*, *570*
Patten, B. M., 420, *443*
Paul, J. R., 411, *445*
Peacock, A. C., 193, 194, *211*
Pearce, L. A., 151, 152, *172, 174*
Pearlman, A. L., 38, *58*
Pearse, A. G. E., 155, *174*
Pease, D. C., 74, *103*, 333, *442*, 480, 481, 483, *509, 510*
Pecci-Saavedra, J., 32, *59*
Peet, M. M., 341, *440*
Pelc, S., 133, 136, 139, *174*
Penman, S., 193, 195, *212, 213, 214*
Peña, C., 162, *176*
Penn, R. D., 234, *246*
Penny, J. E., 43, *60*
Périer, O., 133, 136, 139, 148, 150, *174*, *176*
Perkel, D. H., 231, 232, *245, 246*
Perry, R. P., 193, 195, *213, 214*
Perry, W. L. M., 251, *288*
Perwein, J., 274, *288*
Peters, A., 73, 81, *102, 103*, 140, *174*, 271, *443*
Peters, A. A., 399, 401, *442*
Peters, G., 140, 142, *174*
Petersen, M. C., 312, 313, *318*

Peterson, E. R., 40, *56*, 164, *174*
Peterson, J. A., 209, *214*
Peterson, R. P., 194, 199, 203, 204, *212*, *214*
Pethes, G., 339, *441*
Petrinovitch, L., 236, *245*
Petsche, H., 295, *319*
Pevzner, L. Z., 186 (21), 187, 201, *214*
Peyrot, R., 421, *444*
Phelps, C. F., 461, *509*
Phillips, C. G., 450, *509*
Phillis, J. W., 251, 268, 279, *284*, *287*, 503, *507*, *508*
Pickles, H. G., 280, *287*
Pigon, A., 186 (24), 202, 204, *212*
Pinching, A. J., 32, 33, *59*
Pinkerton, H., 132, 159, *173*, *174*
Pitlyk, J. P., 414, *443*
Pletscher, A., 118, *128*
Plum, F., 391, 398, *443*
Polak, R. L., 124, *128*
Pollay, M., 331, 338, 355, 362, 363, 364, 366, 367, 368, 416, *440*, *443*, *445*, 452, 455, 457, 459, *507*, *508*, *509*
Pollen, D. A., 295, *319*, 465, 467, *510*
Pontén, U., 396, *443*
Popoff, N., 136, 139, *174*
Porta, E. A., 155, 158, *174*
Posner, J. B., 391, 398, *443*
Potter, D. D., 251, 252, 253, 255, 256, 260, 266, 267, 278, 280, 281, *284*, *285*, *286*, *287*, 288, 465, *508*
Potter, L. T., 11, *59*, 66, *104*, 106, 107, 108, 109, 112, 113, 115, 116, 117, 118, 119, 120, 121, 122, 123, 124, *128*
Potter, R. L., 475, *511*
Powell, T. P. S., 32, 34, 45, *58*
Prather, J. W., 357, 400, *443*, *445*
Pravdich-Neminsky, V. V., 307, *319*
Prenant, A., 139, *174*
Prieur, D. J., 151, *172*
Prins, H., 275, *285*
Prockop, L. D., 368, *444*
Pumain, R., 274, *285*
Purpura, D. P., 24, *60*, 296, 300, 301, 302, 303, *319*, *320*, 495, *509*
Putnam, T., 364, *444*
Pysh, J. J., 483, 487, 495, 496, *507*, *509*

Q

Quastel, D. M. J., 10, *57*, 116, 120, 123, *127*
Quastel, J. H., 191, 201, *212*
Quilliam, J. P., 19, *59*

R

Rabinovitz, M., 207, *210*
Rady-Reimer, P., 154, 155, *175*
Ragazzini, F., 413, *443*
Rahamimoff, R., 121, *127*
Rahmann, H., 218, *246*
Raine, C. S., 139, 146, *171*, *174*
Raisman, G., 36, *59*, 66, 81, 92, 97, *102*, *103*
Rake, A., 195, *214*
Rakić, L., 242, *245*
Rall, D. P., 340, 342, 344, 361, 362, 416, *443*, *444*, 450, 452, 455, 456, 457, *509*, *510*
Rall, D. R., 457, *509*
Ralston, H. J., 74, 81, 83, *101*, *102*, *103*, 140, *172*
Ramón y Cajal, S., 139, *174*, *233*, *246*
Ramsey, H. J., 146, 148, *174*
Ranck, J. B., 450, 465, 466, 467, 470, 473, *508*, *510*
Randall, J., 157, *170*
Ransohoff, J., 332, 364, *444*
Raphelson, A., 222, 226, 230, *244*
Rapisarda, A. F., 53, *57*
Rapp, B., 454, *511*
Rappelsberger, P., 245, *319*
Rappoport, D. A., 205, *214*, 218, *246*
Rasch, E., 43, *59*
Rashbass, C., 432, *443*
Rasmussen, G. L., 41, *59*
Ravens, J. R., 151, 152, *172*, *174*
Raymond, A., 42, *56*
Reader, T. A., 32, *59*, 73, 84, *103*
Reading, H. W., 46, *56*
Rebhun, L. I., 483, *570*
Redfearn, J. W. T., 6, *55*
Reed, D. J., 348, 360, 361, 367, 368, 416, 424, *443*, *445*, 451, 452, 455, 456, 459, 460, *510*, *511*

Reese, T. S., 333, 366, 371, 372, 373, 374, 375, 376, 431, 434, *438*, *443*, 451, *507*, *510*
Rehmet, R., 140, *174*
Reich, E., 207, *214*
Reichel, W., 155, *174*
Rein, H., 180, 181, 189, 190. *213*
Reinis, S., 221, *246*
Rémond, A., 295, *320*
Rempel, B., 298, *319*
Rensch, B., 218, *246*
Ressig, M., 133, *174*
Réthehyi, M., 92, 95, *103*
Retzius, A., 434, *441*
Reuben, J. P., 251, 258, 259, 260, 266, *285*, *287*, *288*
Reulen, H. J., 456, *570*
Revel, J.-P., 207, *214*
Revel, M., 207, *214*
Revzin, A. M., 46, *59*
Rewcastle, N. B., 146, 157, 167, *174*
Reynolds, E. S., 133, *176*
Rhine, S., 222, 230, *246*
Rhodin, J. A. G., 335, *443*
Ribot, T. A., 216, *246*
Riccio, D., 221, *244*
Richardson, B. W., 393, 394, 395, *442*
Richardson, E. P., 148, 159, *174*
Richardson, J. C., 157, 159, *176*
Richardson, K. C., 41, *55*, 66, 85, *103*, *104*
Richmond, J. E., 450, *510*
Richter, D., 274, *283*
Richter, R. B., 449, *508*
Rickelmann, A. G., 392, *443*
Rickles, W. H., 251, 259, *285*
Riehl, J.-L., 139, *170*
Riesen, A. H., 43, 44, *56*, *59*
Rigor, B. M., 369, *439*
Ringborg, U., 186 (15), 190, *214*
Rinvik, E., 64, 73, 79, *102*, *103*
Riser, 341, *443*
Ritzén, M., 66, *101*
Rivera-Pomar, J. M., 430, *443*
Rivière, M., 136, *171*
Rizzoli, A. A., 279, *288*
Robbins, J., 259, 260, 277, 278, 279, *288*
Robbins, N., 38, *59*

Robert, E. D., 34, *59*
Roberts, E., 231, *246*, 250, 264, 267, 269, 272, 274, 275, 276, 277, 282, *283*, *285*, *287*, *288*, *289*
Roberts, R. B., 219, 234, *244*, *246*, 405, 406, 422, *443*
Roberts, S., 197, 198, *211*, *214*
Robin, E. D., 392, *443*
Robins, E., 253, 275, *285*, *287*
Robinson, C. E., 237, *246*
Robinson, R. J., 367, 428, *439*, *444*, 452, *507*, *510*
Rock, M. K., 270, *287*
Rodieck, R. W., 39, *59*
Rodriguez, E. M., 92, *101*
Rodriguez-Peralta, L. A., 365, *444*
Røigaard-Petersen, H. H., 221, 222, 228, 230, *244*, *246*
Roncoroni, L., 139, *175*
Roots, B. I., 234, *245*, 497, *508*
Roper, S., 268, 280, *288*
Rosan, R. C., 133, *175*
Rose, J. E., 53, *59*
Rose, S. P. R., 46, *59*, 218, *243*, *246*
Rosen, J., 224, *244*
Rosenblatt, F., 222, 225, 227, 228, 230, 239, 242, *246*
Rosenblueth, A., 26, *59*, 470, 474, *510*
Rosenbluth, J., 90, *103*
Rosengren, E., 66, *101*, 406, *443*
Rosenthal, E., 221, *246*
Rosenzweig, M. R., 42, *56*, *59*, 223, *244*
Rossen, J., 250, 275, *283*
Rossi, G. F., 299, *317*
Rossiter, R. J., 180, *213*
Roth, C. D., 85, *103*
Roth, L. J., 360, 415, *438*, *440*, 450, 460, 462, *506*, *507*
Rothman, A. R., 342, *444*
Rouiller, C., 66, *103*
Rousseau, J. E., 420, *439*
Rowland, A. F., 467, *507*
Roy, S., 150, *175*
Royer, P., 342, *444*
Rubenstein, L. J., 135, 158, *172*
Rubin, R. C., 344, 416, *444*
Rubinstein, M. K., 276, *289*
Rudomin, P., 250, 253, *287*

Rushtop, W. A. H., 432, *443*
Ryall, R. W., 273, *284*

S

Saavedra, J. P., 73, 83, *103*
Saborio, J. L., 194, 195, 196, *214*
Sachs, E., 236, *246*
Sachs, J. R., 386, *444*
Sadik, A. R., 332, *444*
Sadler, K., 356, 357, 383, 388, 399, *444*, *445*
Saelens, J. K., 109, 112, *128*
Saffran, E., 42, *59*
Sahar, A., 332, 364, *444*
Saito, S., 251, 266, 267, *285*
Sakai, M., 151, 152, 153, *175*, *177*
Sakakura, H., 34, *59*
Sakanoue, M., 382, 424, *437*
Salganicoff, L., 115, *127*, *276*, *288*
Salive, H., 222, *245*
Salpeter, M. M., 124, *127*
Salvador, R. A., 275, *288*
Samec, J., 194, 195, 196, 197, 198, *212*, *214*
Samii, M., 456, *510*
Samli, M. H., 198, *214*
Samorajski, T., 154, 155, *175*
Samson, F. E., 33, *59*, 217, *246*
Samuel, D., 223, *244*
Sances, A., 22, *59*
Sandri, C., 32, *56*, 85, *101*
Sanghavi, P., 207, *213*
Santori, M., 44, *58*
Sass, R. L., 117, *127*
Sato, N., 268, 269, 276, 281, *287*
Sato, O., 363, 364, 416, *438*, 452, 459, *506*
Saunders, L. Z., 135, 140, *172*
Saunders, N. R., 112, 123, *128*, 253, *285*
Sayre, G. P., *172*
Schadé, J. P., 467, 468, 473, 476, 478, 479, 485, 487, 489, 491, 497, *507*, *511*
Schaffer, K., 159, *175*, 182, 195, *214*
Schaltenbrand, G., 364, *444*
Schanter, L. S., 368, 369, *444*, *445*
Scheibel, A. B., 41, 45, *57*, 93, *103*
Scheibel, M. E., 93, *103*
Scheid-Seydel, L., 409, *440*

Schiaffino, S., 37, 39, *59*
Schiller, P. H., 223, *244*
Schmidt, D. E., 122, *127*
Schmidt, R. F., 273, 274, *284*, *288*
Schmitt, F. O., 33, *59*, 217, 237, *246*
Schnabel, R., 151, 152, *175*
Schneider, G. E., 35, *59*
Schneider, M., 479, *510*
Schochet, S. S., Jr., 136, 143, 146, 148, 152, 153, 157, 158, 159, 160, 162, 164, 165, 167, *172*, *175*, *177*
Schonenberger, M., 337, *444*
Schor, N., 186 (17), 202, *211*
Schou, J., 368, *444*
Scrimshaw, N. S., 48, *59*
Schubert, P., 46, *58*
Schuberth, J., 106, 107, *128*
Schuffman, S. S., 158, *174*
Schuller, E., 49, *60*
Schulman, M. P., 110, *127*
Schultze, H. E. M., 337, *444*
Schulz, D. W., 270, *287*
Schultz, R. L., 480, 481, 497, *508*, *510*
Schürmann, K., 456, *510*
Schwartz, S., 272, 276, 279, *285*, *287*, 450, 467, *508*
Schwarz, G. A., 151, 152, *175*, *177*
Schwerin, P., 503, *510*
Schwick, G., 337, *444*
Scott, D., Jr., 96, *103*
Scott, E. M., 253, 261, 270, *286*
Scott, I. H., 180, *214*
Scotto, J., 118, *128*
Seale, B., 250, *283*
Sebrell, W. H., Jr., 158, *173*
Sedlack, R. E., 414, *443*
Seeman, P., 252, *285*
Segal, M. B., 332, 335, 336, 361, 365, 391, 415, 417, 418, *438*, *439*, *440*, 452, *507*
Segarra, J., 430, *441*
Segundo, J. P., 231, *245*
Seil, F. J., 162, 164, *175*
Seïto, R., 136, 139, 145, *175*
Seitelberger, F., 151, 152, 157, 159, *175*, 415, *441*
Sekhon, S. S., 139, *170*
Selverstone, B., 342, 414, *444*

Semon, R., 216, *246*
Semple, S. J. G., 391, *438*
Sendrail, 392, *439*
Setton, A., 39, *59*
Severinghaus, J. W., 385, 393, 394, 395, *442, 444*
Shabo, A. L., 332, *444*
Shank, R. P., 275, 279, 280, 281, *283, 284, 285*
Shanklin, W., M., 155, *172*
Shannon, C. W., 293, *320*
Shantha, T. R., 139, *175*, 432, *444*
Shanthaveerappa, T. R., 432, *444*
Shapira, A., *286*
Shapiro, H., 464, *510*
Sharman, M., 39, *55*
Sharpless, S. K., 4, 17, *54, 56*
Shashoua, V. E., 218, *246*
Shaywitz, B. A., 417, 428, *444*
Shealy, C. N., 35, 36, 39, *57*
Shelanski, M. L., 164, 165, *173, 175, 176, 177*
Shelby, J. M., 221, *145*
Shende, M. C., 273, *288*
Shepherd, T. H., 420, *442*
Sheridan, M. N., 117, *128*
Sherrington, C. S., 232, *246*
Shigehisa, T., 222, *245*
Shimada, M., 191, 192, *214*
Shinder, S., 393, 394, 395, *442*
Shinozaki, H., 269, 273, 279, 282, *286, 287*
Shiraki, H., 133, *176*
Shively, M. C., 186 (8), 208, *212*
Shofer, R. J., 300, 301, 302, 303, *320*
Sholl, D. A., 6, *59*
Siegesmund, K. A., 22, *59*, 139, *176*
Siegrist, G., 66, *103*
Siesjö, B. K., 392, 396, 397, 416, *441, 444*
Silver, A., 112, 122, *127, 128*
Simeone, F. A., 26, *59*
Simmonds, W. J., 330, *439*
Simon, L., 85, 87, 90, *102*
Sims, J. A., 422, *442*
Singer, M. M., 393, 394, 395, *442*
Sisken, B., 267, 269, 274, 277, *287, 288*
Sisodia, P., 368, *444*

Sjöstrand, J., 33, *56*, 205, *214*
Skoff, R. P., 74, *103*
Slagel, D. E., 186 (7), 208, *214*
Slagle, R. W., 42, *59*
Slater, C. R., 71, 85, 93, *103*, 121, *128*, 234, *245*, 277, 278, *286*
Sloane-Stanley, G. H., 450, *508*
Sluga, E., 152, *176*
Smith, C. E., 236, *246*
Smith, D. E., 429, *444*
Smith, D. S., 116, *128*
Smith, H. V., 337, 338, 366, 413, *441*
Smith, J. M., 140, *176*
Smith, K. R., 160, *173*, 368, *439*
Smith, M. G., 135, *173*
Smith, M. V., 366, *441*
Smith, P. S., 39, *59*
Smith, W., 145, *171*
Sörbo, B., 106, 110, 111, *128*
Sokoloff, L., 274, *287*
Sokolov, E. N., 293, *320*
Solitare, G. B., 159, *176*
Sollenberg, J., 111, *128*
Solloway, S., 342, *444*
Somjen, G., 11, *58*
Sotelo, G., 85, 90, *103*, 139, 162, *176*
Southwick, C. A. P., 274, *284*
Spanner, S., 109, *127*
Sparbes, S. B., 221, *246*
Sparf, B., 107, *128*
Spatz, H., 167, *174*, 365, 421, *444*
Spaulding, S. W., 191, 192, *212*
Spaziani, E., 359, 360, 363, 416, *440*
Spehlman, R., 310, *320*
Spencer, J. M., 463, *507*
Spencer, W. A., 4, 37, 38, *55, 58*, 231, 233, *245*
Sperry, R. W., 234, 235, *246*
Spina-Franca, A., 337, *444*
Spiro, D., 205, *213*
Sporn, M. B., 216, 218, *244*
Squires, R., 367, 368, *443*, 452, 456, 459, 460, *510*
Srinivasan, V., 273, *286, 287*
Srivanij, P., 158, *176*
Stämpfli, R., 432, *441*
Stanbury, J. B., 454, *511*
Standlan, E. M., 155, *176*

Stanford, A. L., Jr., 237, *246*
Stary, Z., 412, *441*
Stavraky, G. W., 52, *59*
Steele, J. C., 157, 159, *176*
Steger, J., 337, *444*
Streicher, E., 455, *510*
Stein, A., 155, *171*
Stein, D. G., 224, *244*
Stein, L., 223, *244*
Steiner, J., 485, 487, 489, 491, 497, *511*
Stell, W. K., 93, *103*
Stenevi, U., 97, *103*
Sterba, G., 92, *103*
Sterc, J., 295, *319*
Stern, L., 327, *421*, *444*
Sternon, J. E., 148, 150, *176*
Stetten, D., 342, *444*
Steude, U., 456, *506*
Stévenin, J., 194, 195, 196, 197, 198, *212*, *214*
Stevens, A., 459, *509*
Stevens, W. F., 226, *247*
Stewart, S., 136, 139, *174*
Stockinger, L., 152, *176*
Stone, S., 49, *56*
Storm-Mathisen, J., 272, *285*
Stosseck, K., 365, *444*
Strada, G. P., 151, 152, *170*
Straschill, M., 274, *288*
Straughan, D. W., 122, *128*
Strehler, B. L., 155, *174*, *176*
Streicher, E., 162, *173*, 429, *444*
Strobel, D. A., 217, *243*
Stromblad, B. C. R., 26, *59*
Stubbs, J. D., 361, 412, *438*
Štulcová, B., 385, 386, *438*
Stumpf, W. E., 460, *507*
Sugioka, K., 395, *442*
Sulkin, D. F., 155, *176*
Sulkin, N. M., 155, 158, *176*
Sumi, S. M., 495, *510*
Sundwall, A., 106, 107, *128*
Sung, J. H., 155, *176*
Sung, S. S., 430, *441*
Supek, Z., 369, *438*
Sutton, S., 310, *319*
Susz, J. P., 274, *288*
Suzuki, K., 151, 152, *172*

Suzuki, Y., 194, 198, *214*
Svien, H. J., 337, 407, 408, 414, *441*, *443*
Swanson, A. G., 391, 392, *439*, *443*
Swanson, J. L., 133, *176*
Sweet, W. H., 342, *444*
Swift, H., 43, *59*
Szentágothai, J., 64, 70, 83, 84, 92, 95, 102, *103*, 269, *284*
Szilagyi, P. I. A., 122, *127*
Szilard, L., 238, *246*
Szlachta, H. L., 135, 139, *176*
Szumski, A. J., 273, *286*

T

Tachibana, S., 469, 476, *511*
Takahashi, K., 277, 278, *286*
Takahashi, Y., 194, 198, *214*
Takayata, N., 155, 158, *174*
Takeda, K., 269, 272, 273, 279, 282, *287*
Takei, Y., 147, *176*
Takeuchi, A., 257, 258, 259, 260, 264, 266, 277, 278, *288*
Takeuchi, N., 257, 258, 259, 260, 264, 266, 277, 278, *288*
Takeno, K., 117, *128*
Talwar, G. P., 45, *59*
Tamarind, D. L., 19, *59*
Tanaka, Y., 269, 270, 271, 273, 275, 281, 282, 283, *287*
Tanner, D. J., 360, 364, 365, *445*, 450, *511*
Tarlov, I. M., 52, *57*
Tasaki, I., 465, 467, 474, *508*
Tashiro, N., 267, *285*
Tauc, L., 314, *318*
Tauxe, W. N., 414, *443*
Taxi, J., 85, *103*
Taylor, E. W., 165, *175*
Taylor, J. L., 388, 416, *445*
Taylor, L. M., 366, *441*
Taylor, N., 471, *507*
Taylor, R. M., 399, *440*
Taylor, S. H., 47, *57*
Tebécis, A. K., 279, *286*
Teichgraber, P., 47, *55*
Telwar, G. P., 218, *246*
Teneheva, Z. S., 194, 195, *214*

Tennyson, V. M., 150, *158, 171,* 333, 334, 373, 428, *444, 445*
Teravainen, H., 85, *103*
Terry, R. D., 146, 155, 160, 162, 164, 169, *171, 176, 177*
Thesleff, S., 26, 33, *59*
Thienes, C. H., 251, *285*
Thies, R. E., 121, 123, *127*
Thios, S. J., 222, *244*
Thomas, D. B., 45, *58*
Thompson, H. G., 142, 159, 162, *170*
Thompson, H. K., 389, 390, *438, 445*
Thompson, J. W., 27, *59*
Thompson, R. J., 187, 188, *213*
Tille, J., 11, *57*
Timiras, P. S., 44, *58*
Titus, E. O., 430, *438*
Tocci, P., 405, *443*
Tochino, Y., 369, *445*
Toga, M., 152, *176*
Tömböl, T., 70, 83, 84, *103*
Tongur, V. S., 222, 230, *245*
Torack, R. M., 471, 480, 492, 493, *510*
Torvik, A., 205, *214*
Toschi, G., 207, *214*
Toth, J., 406, *442*
Tower, D. B., 274, *287,* 457, *507*
Toyne, M. J., 94, *102*
Trachtenberg, M. C., 465, 467, *510*
Travis, D. M., 392, *443*
Treherne, J. E., 449, *510*
Trétiakoff, C., 148, *176*
Trueb, L., 151, 152, 153, *175*
Tsanev, R. G., 193, *214*
Tschirgi, R. D., 388, 416, *445*
Tsuchiya, T., 273, *286*
Tsukada, Y., 276, *288*
Tuazon, R., 157, 159, 165, *171*
Tubiana, M., 382, 430, *441, 445*
Tuček, S., 110, *128*
Tucker, J. F., 264, *283*
Tuncbay, T. O., 96, *101*
Tveten, L., 407, *445*

U

Ubell, E., 252, *285*
Uchizono, K., 64, *103,* 266, 271, *288*

Udenfriend, S., 191, *212,* 250, *288,* 405, *439, 441*
Udo, M., 269, 271, *286*
Ungar, G., 217, 221, 222, 223, 225, 226, 227, 228, 230, 231, 236, 239, *246, 247*
Ungerer, A., 228, *244*
Usenik, E., 136, *176*
Usherwood, P. N. R., 267, 278, *288*
Uttal, W. R., 231, 232, *241*
Uttley, A. M., 4, 5, 6, 7, 54, 55, *56, 60*

V

Vaaland, J. L., 68, *102*
Vaccarezza, O. L., 32, *59,* 73, 83, *103*
Valverde, F., 45, *60*
van Bogaert, L., 142, 157, 159, *170, 176*
Van Buren, J. M., 29, *60*
Vander Eecken, H., 142, *170*
Vanderhaeghen, J.-J., 133, 136, 139, 148, 150, 153, *174, 176*
Van der Kloot, W. G., 259, *288*
van Gelder, N. M., 275, 276, 277, *285, 288, 289*
Van Harreveld, A., 42, 52, *60,* 277, 278, 279, *289,* 360, 364, 365, 368, 413, *437, 445,* 450, 452, 453, 456, 458, 459, 460, 466, 467, 468, 469, 470, 471, 472, 473, 475, 476, 477, 478, 479, 481, 482, 483, 484, 485, 487, 489, 491, 493, 495, 496, 499, 500, 501, 502, 503, 504, *506, 507, 508, 509, 510, 511*
van Heycop ten Ham, M. W., 151, 152, *176*
van Hoof, F., 151, 152, 153, *176*
Van Marthens, E., 48, 49, *60*
Van Vaerenbergh, P. J. J., 392, *445*
Vanzulli, A., 313, *317*
Vaughan, H. G., 319, *320*
Varon, S., 276, *289*
Vaughn, J. E., 74, *103*
Vaz Ferreira, A., 22, *56*
Veralli, M., 399, *440*
Vernadakis, A., 422, *445,* 462, *511*
Vesco, C., 194, 195, 197, 198, *214*
Veskov, R., 242, *245*
Victor, J., 158, *174*
Villamil, M., 451, 458, 461, *507*

Villars, T., 222, 223, *244*
Villegas, G. M., 495, *511*
Voisin, R., 411, *443*
von Braunmühl, A., 148, 159, *176*
Voeller, K., 24, *60*
von Euler, U. S., 281, *289*
von Foerster, H., 216, *247*
von Hungen, K., 192, 193, 194, *214*
Von Monakow, P., 327, *445*

W

Waggener, J. D., 365, *445*
Wagner, A. R., 223, *244*
Waelach, H., 199, *211*
Waelsch, H., 182, *211*, 503, *506*, *510*
Waksman, A., 274, 276, *289*
Walberg, F., 61, 64, 68, 74, 79, 83, 84, *101*, *102*, *103*, *104*, 268, 270, 272, *285*, *286*
Wald, F., 458, 504, *509*, *511*
Wallace, G. B., 337, 366, *445*
Wallenstein, M. C., 348, 407, 409, 419, *441*
Walker, J. H., 35, *56*
Walker, M. D., 344, 416, *444*
Walker, R. J., *286*
Wall, P. D., 32, *57*
Walsh, G. O., 35, *57*
Walsh, R. N., 43, *60*
Walter, D. O., 312, *319*, *506*
Walter, K., 413, *445*
Walter, W. G., 293, 306, 309, 314, 315, *318*, *320*
Walter, W. J., 309, *320*
Wang, H. H., 473, *571*
Wang, J., 341, *445*
Ward, A., 52, *60*
Ward, A. A., 473, 502, *509*
Warlsch, H., 405, *442*
Waser, P. G., 85, 90, 91, *103*
Wasserman, E., 223, *244*
Watanabe, A., 267, *289*
Watanabe, I., 158, *171*
Watanabe, S., 300, 316, *319*
Watkins, J. C., 251, 268, 279, *284*, 503, *507*
Watson, W. E., 96, *104*, 199, 202, 205, 206, *214*
Watters, G. V., 344, 409, 416, 418, *439*

Waxman, S. G., 235, *247*
Webb, M. F., 399, *437*
Weber, A., 136, *176*
Weber, A. F., 136, *176*
Wechsler, W., 429, *442*
Weddell, G., 95, *104*
Weed, L. H., 330, 420, *445*
Weinberg, R. A., 195, *214*
Weiner, N., 12, *60*
Weinmann, R. L., 159, *176*
Weinstein, H., 276, 282, *289*
Weise, V. K., 124, *128*
Weiss, M., 160, *176*
Weiss, P., 234, 243, *247*
Welch, K., 331, 332, 353, 356, 357, 364, 366, 383, 399, 419, *444*, *445*, 452, *511*
Welt, L. G., 386, *444*
Werblin, F. S., 15, *60*
Werman, R., 239, *243*, 275, 279, 280, 281, 282, *283*, *284*, *285*, *289*
Westerman, R. A., 37, *57*, *58*
Westman, J., 79, *104*
Westrum, L. E., 32, 45, 52, *60*, 99, *104*
Whaley, A., 164, *172*
Whaley, R. D., 392, *443*
Whelan, W. J., 153, *173*
Whipp, S., 136, *176*
White, C. T., 311, *319*
White, J. G., 165, *177*
White, L., 52, *60*
White, L. E., 45, *60*, 61, 68, *101*
Whitlock, D. G., 94, *102*
Whittaker, V. P., 109, 115, 116, 117, 118, 119, *127*, *128*, 276, *287*, *289*
Widdas, W. F., 400, *438*
Widdowson, E. M., 48, *58*
Wiechert, P., 403, *445*
Wiersma, C. A. G., 251, *285*
Wiener, J., 205, *213*
Wiesel, T. N., 28, 43, 55, *58*, *60*
Wieskrantz, L., 43, *60*
Wilder, B. J., 52, *60*
Wildi, E., 159, *174*
Wildy, P., 133, *173*
Wilkinson, P. N., 235, *245*
Wilkinson, R. T., 312, *320*
Willems, M., 195, *214*
Williams, H. W., 165, 167, *177*

Williams, J. D., 114, *128*
Williams, T. H., 66, *104*
Williams, V., 73, *104*
Willis, J. S., 125, *127*
Willis, R., 139, *170*
Willis, W. D., 273, 274, *284*
Wilson, C. W. M., 430, *438*
Wilson, M. E., 94, *102*
Windle, W. F., 95, *102*
Winick, M., 48, *57*, 181, *214*
Winkler, R., 155, *171*
Winsburg, G. R., 43, *60*
Winternitz, R., 412, *441*
Winter, A. L., 293, 306, 314, 315, *318, 320*
Winters, H., 341, *440*
Wislocki, B., 333, *445*
Wislocki, G. B., 480, *508*
Wisniewska, K., 162, *177*
Wisniewski, H., 146, 160, 162, 164, 169, *173, 176, 177*
Wisotzkey, H. M., 142, *177*
Witmer, F., 151, 152, 153, *174, 177*
Wolf, A., 139, 155, *176, 177*
Wolfart, G., 180, *213*
Wolfe, D. E., 66, *104*, 460, *509*
Wolff, H. G., 370, 415, *445*
Wolman, L., 150, *175*
Wolthuis, O. L., 222, 226, *247*
Wong, E. K., 470, 474, *511*
Woodard, J. S., 150, 157, *177*
Woodbury, D. M., 361, 367, 368, 422, 424, 425, *440, 443, 445*, 451, 452, 456, 457, 459, 460, 462, *508, 570, 571*
Woodsbury, W. A. H., 432, *443*
Woodward, D. I., 361, 424, *445*
Woodward, D. L., 455, 459, *511*
Woody, C. D., 389, 390, *438, 445*
Woollam, D. H. M., 325, *442*
Woollard, H. H., 431, *445*
Wright, E. M., 351, 400, *443, 445*
Wright, J. H., 401, *443*

Wright, S. L., 411, *445*
Wu, S. Y., 42, *59*
Wyatt, R. B., 136, 143, 158, 160, *175, 177*
Wykoff, R. W. G., 479, *571*
Wyngaarden, J. B., 454, *571*

Y

Yamada, H., 143, 158, *173*
Yamagami, S., 188, *214*
Yamamoto, C., 282, *286*
Yamamoto, T., 133, *176*
Yanagiya, I., 117, *128*
Yanoff, M., 151, 152, *175, 177*
Yasargil, G. M., 64, *101*
Yokoi, S., 151, 152, *177*
Yoshida, H., 122, *128*
Yoshida, M., 268, 269, 271, *286*
Young, J. Z., 39, 41, *55*, 479, *511*
Young, R. R., 32, *57*
Yuen, P., 136, *177*
Yunis, E. J., 133, *172*

Z

Zadunaisky, J. A., 458, *511*
Zambrano, D., 92, *104*
Zamenhof, S., 48, 49, *60*, 180, *211*
Zanchetti, A., 299, *317*
Zavala, B. J., 134, 135, *171*
Zee, D., 398, *443*
Zelená, J., 115, *128*
Zelleveger, H., 153, *175*
Zeman, W., 146, 158, *171, 177*
Zetterstrom, B., 17, *60*
Zieher, L., 115, *127*
Zimmerman, H. M., 134, 143, 145, 146, 148, 157, 159, 160, 165, *172, 174*
Zippel, H. P., 221, 222, 228, 230, *247*
Zomzely, C. E., 198, *214*
Zuchermann, E. C., 384, *445*

Subject Index

A

Acetazoleamide, reduction of CSF secretion, 416–417
Acetylcholine, 105–126
  assay, 122
    quantal, 120–122
  quantum content of, 122
  release of, 113, 120–126
    mechanisms for, 124–126
    rate of, 122–124
  resynthesis after hydrolysis, 109–110
  in synaptic vesicles, 115–118
    release of, 125–126
  synthesis, 106–114
  turnover in nerve terminals, 119
    in vesicles, 119–120
  storage, 114–120
    site, 114–115
Acetylcoenzyme A
  in acetylcholine synthesis, 110–111
  source of, 110–111
Acidophilic granules, 143, 145
Acoustic stimuli, EEG response, 311–312
Actinomycin D, 107
  effects on nervous system, 207
    on RNA, 207
Alpha-blocking. 301-302
Alpha rhythm, 294–295
  definition, 294
Alzheimer's neurofibrillary tangles, 159
Amino acids
  blood-brain exchange, 404–405
  in blood plasma, 402–406
  brain-blood exchange, 406
  in cerebrospinal fluid, 402–406

in dog plasma, 402–403
passage from blood to cerebrospinal fluid, 403–404
γ-Aminobutyric acid (GABA), 249–283
  amino acids related to, 277–280
  distribution in crustacean nervous system, 251–256
    in Deiters cells, 269–272
  enzymes in pathway of metabolism, 274–275
  metabolism in mammalian central nervous system, 274–277
  as neurotransmitter, 280–283
  release
    from inhibitory nerves, 260–264
    in Purkinje axon terminals, 272
  storage and uptake in crustacean tissue, 265–266
  subcellular distribution, 275–276
  uptake in mammalian central nervous system, 276–277
γ-Aminobutyric acid (GABA)-glutamate transaminase in mammalian central nervous system, 275
Antipyrine, penetration of, into brain, 352
Apical dendrites, size change in spreading depression, 478
Aqueduct of Sylvius, drainage of cerebrospinal fluid, 341–342
Arachnoid villi
  role in cerebrospinal fluid drainage, 330–332
  valvular action, 331
Asphyxiation
  abnormal fluid uptake by cellular elements and, 496–497

causing impedance change, 468–469
Astrocytes, 73–79
Atrophy, trans-synaptic, effect on axon terminal, 34–35
Axon, ribonucleic acid content, 182–184
Axon-cytolysomes, 87
Axon terminals, 22–23, 28–32
    degeneration, 28–29
    density in tissue, 41–42
    presynaptic, GABA inhibition in crayfish, 259
    trans-synaptic atrophy effect, 34–35
Axonal sprouting, 35–36, 96–99
Axotomy, effect on ribonucleic acid, 205–206

B

Beta rhythm, definition, 294
Bicarbonate
    in blood-brain barrier, 392
    in blood-cerebrospinal fluid barrier, 392
Bicuculline as GABA antagonist, 274
Bioassays for molecular code, 220–231
    chemical aspects, 230–231
    importance of variables, 224–227
    method specificity, 227–229
    optimal conditions, 222–223
    reliability, 222–227
    types, 221–222
Biological assays, see Bioassays
Blood, pH, 392–395
Blood-brain barrier, 323–437
    active transport, 378
    capillary exchanges, 325
    choroidal exchanges, 324–325
    definition, 328
    effect on RNA metabolism, 191–192
    historical aspects, 326–329
    loci of exchange, 328–329
    modifications, 410–420
        inorganic ions in disease, 411–413
        protein concentration in disease, 410
    morphology, 323–329, 369–376
    ontogeny, 420–429
    peripheral nerve and, 431–435
    significance, 376–384
    trans-meningeal exchanges, 325–326
Blood-brain direct exchange, 414–415

Blood-brain flow of materials, 347–349
Blood-brain uptake and maturity, 421–424
Blood-cerebrospinal fluid
    kinetics of, passage of materials, 345–347
    passage of infused material from, 344–350
    slowly equilibrating substances, 347, 358
Blood-nerve barrier, 433–435
    morphology, 434
Brain
    active transport
        of hydrogen ion, 396
        outward from, 366–369
    capillaries in, morphology, 369–372
    chemical analysis relating to information processing, 217–218
    development
        perinatal factors, 47
        postnatal factors, 47–52
    drainage route, 420–421
    effect of novelty in information storage, 313
    electrical activity, 292–317
        computer techniques in detection, 306
        peripheral stimulation effect, 3ù6–316
    extracellular fluid, 379,391
    extracellular space, 358–361
        in fetal and postnatal development, 462
        influence of volume on uptake of ions, 422
        measurement by infusion-perfusion, 361
            by silicone perfusion, 361
            by ventricular perfusion, 360–361
    growth
        effects of hormones, 47–52
        of starvation, 48, 49
    habituation to sensory stimulation, 312–314
    lactate concentration, 396–398
    penetration by substances from blood, 350–356
    pH, 395–398
    potentials, 387–391
        surface, 388
    pyruvate concentration, 396–398

ribonucleic acid in tissue, 180–181, 188, 190
of vertebrates (table), 181
sucrose space, 359
transport out of, 367–368
uptake of phosphate, 422
Brain–cerebrospinal fluid equilibriation of
mathematical analysis, 353–354
exchanges, 362–365
transapial, 364–365
transependymal, 362–363
Bunina bodies, 141, 143

C

Calcium
effect on acetylcholine release, 121, 124–125
in central nervous system, 11
increase in transmitter release in muscle, 10–11
Capillaries, fenestrated, and blood-brain barrier, 430
Cell firing, poststimulus histogram, 13
Cell suspensions, for impedance measurement, 463–465
Cell types, RNA synthesis in, 199–200
Central nervous system
cellular elements in abnormal fluid uptake, 496–497
degeneration, 73–84
regeneration, 62, 96–97
Central nervous tissue
anions, 499–501
electrical impedance of, 463–474
changes caused by, 468–474
affecting electrolyte transport, 479
affecting water transport, 479
effect of temperature, 473
increase and contraction of extracellular space, 474
relation to extracellular space, 467
electrolyte transport mechanisms, 499–506
electron microscopy of, 479–499
freezing with cold metal surface, 484
water distribution, preservation of by freeze substitution, 482–484

extracellular space, 461–462
variation in magnitude, 461–462
micrographs of, 479–481
determination of extracellular space, 480–481
extracellular space affected by freeze substitution, 484–486
fixation methods and extracellular space, 493–496
freeze substitution preserving extracellular space, 493–496
water movement in, 474–479
water transport mechanisms, 499–506
Cerebellar cortex, extracellular space, 484–486
micrographs, 484–485
Cerebral blood flow, effect of brain potential, 389–391
Cerebral cortex
extracellular space, 487–489
differences in deep and superficial layers, 497–499
micrographs, 487–489
GABA as inhibitory transmitter, 272
Cerebral cortical tissue, electrical impedance, 465–466
Cerebrospinal fluid
acid-base parameters, 391–398
brain potentials and, 387–391
calcium content, 425
chemistry, 336–341
chloride content, 424–425
clearance of injected substances, 342–344
composition, 337–341, 424–428
drainage, 330–332
subarachnoid, 341
electrochemical potential, 339
as equivalent of lymphatic system, 332
freshly secreted, 382–383
glucose concentration, 383–384
potassium content, 383–384
magnesium content, 425–427
passage of material from blood into, 344–350
pH changes, 392
potassium content, 425–428

protein in, 337

rate of secretion, 341–344

  development and, 428

  inhibitors of, 417–418

  pressure affecting, 419–420

  in various species, 344

secretion, 332–336

  modified by inhibitors, 415–420

sink action, 360, 451–453

  effect of maturity, 423–424

urea content, 424

variations in concentration of solutes, 378–382

Cerebrospinal fluid-brain exchange, 377–378

Cerebrospinal fluid-brain flow of materials, 349

Chloride

  in asphyxiated cerebral cortex, 475–476

  movement

    in central nervous tissue, 474–479

    during glutaraldehyde fixation, 478–479

  space during development, 462

Choline

  in acetylcholine synthesis, 106–110

  central nervous system tissue content, 109–110

  nerve terminal uptake, 106–108

  peripheral nervous tissue content, 106–109

Choline acetyltransferase, 111–113

  in acetylcholine synthesis, 113–114

  distribution, 112–113

Cholinergic terminals, choline content, 107–108

Choroid plexus

  anatomy, 333–334

  capillaries, 373

  morphology, 428–429

  permeability, 356–357

  permeability constants for substances, 357

  potential, 388–389

  role in formation of cerebrospinal fluid, 332–333

Chronic survival experiments in terminal degeneration, 94–95

Clarke's columns, 37–38

Colloid inclusions, 140–142

Color preference training, 228–229

Conductivity, cortical, effect of stimulation, 4–6

Cortex, human, EEG response to peripheral stimulation, 307–308

Cortex perfusion with fixatives, impedance change during, 470–471

Cortical activity causing impedance change, 473

Crustacean muscle, effect of L-glutamate, 277–278

Crustacean neuromuscular junction, 251–265

Crustacean stretch receptor, GABA inhibition, 266–267

CSF, *see* Cerebrospinal Fluid

Cycloheximide as inhibitor of protein synthesis, 219

Cytoplasmic bodies laminated, 139–141

Cytoplasmic inclusions, 134

  nonviral, 139–158

D

Dark-avoidance training, 228, 230, 231

Darkness, *see also* Light

  dark-rearing

    neurons in monkeys and, 43

    optical nerve in mice and, 43–44

    synapses in rats and, 43, 45

Degeneration, *see also* specific types

  autoradiographic study of, 94

  electron dense, 73–74, 81

  limitation of methods, 93–95

  synaptic, *see* Synaptic degeneration

  terminal, electron microscopy of, 70–92

Deiters nucleus, inhibitory synapses, 268–272

Denervation, partial, of neurons, 52–53

Depression, *see* Spreading depression

Dreaming and REM, 299

Dura in brain-cerebrospinal fluid exchanges, 365

Dural mesothelium as barrier to diffusion, 365

E

Electrical activity of brain, *see* Brain
Electrical stimulation and RNA synthesis, 201
Electroencephalograph
neuronal mechanisms, 300–305, 316–317
normal human adult, 293–296
metabolic disease and, 297
normal human child, 296
sleep spindles, 304–305
thalamic stimulation patterns, 302–304
Electron micrographs, *see* Micrographs
Endplate potentials, miniature, 18, 120–121
Environment and synaptic structure, 42–43
Eosinophilic bodies, 135
Ependyma
blood-brain barrier and, 431
morphology, 373
Ependymal permeability, 362–363
Epileptic foci, 7, 52
Extracellular space
estimated from tissue impedance, 463–467
relation to increase in tissue resistance, 474
in vertebrate CNS, 447–551
determination, with markers, 449–462
Extracellular space markers, 449–462
artificial, 451–458
blood-brain barrier effect, 451–453
effect of CSF production, 459
high molecular weight, 460
marker concentration, 458–459
natural, 449–450
penetration into intracellular compartment, 460–461
role of transport mechanisms, 460–461

F

Fibrillary aggregates, 162–165
Fibrous protein neuronal inclusions, 159–169

Fixation
for electron microscopy
abnormal fluid uptake by cellular elements, 496–497
changes in extracellular space during, 489–493
of information, 220
Fluids in brain-cerebrospinal exchanges, 364
Freeze substitution in electron microscopy, 482–484
Functional activity
RNA metabolism and, 203–204
RNA synthesis and, 200–205
Functional validation, 233

G

Gap-junctions in central nervous system, 373–376
Glia
relationship with neurons, 204
ribonucleic acid relationship, 204
Glial end-feet in blood-brain barrier, 370–371
Glutamate, in spreading depression and asphyxiation, 503–506
L-Glutamate, 277–279
as neurotransmitter, 280–281
release in lobster tissue, 278
in vertebrate central synapses, 278–279
Glutamate decarboxylase
distribution in Deiters cells, 269–272
in mammalian central nervous system, 275
Glutaraldehyde fixation of cortex affecting chloride movement, 478–479
Glutaraldehyde perfusion fixation, 489, 491
Glycine, 279–282
distribution in nervous system, 280
as postsynaptic inhibitory transmitter, 279–280
Goldmann-Stern hypothesis of blood-brain exchange, 327
Golgi technique, 92–93
Growth hormone, effect on brain growth, 49

H

Halogen anions in brain-blood relationship, 366
Halogen ions as extracellular markers, 449–450
Hirano bodies, 145–148
    ultrastructure, 146–148
Homeostasis
    in brain, 384–387
        carrier mechanism, 384–387
    in cerebrospinal fluid, 339–341
Hormones and synaptic growth, 47–52
Horseradish peroxidase penetration of capillaries, 371–372
Hydroxyadipaldehyde fixation for micrographs, effect on extracellular space, 492–493
Hypercapnia and direct blood-brain exchange, 414–415

I

Impedance measurement of tissues, 463–466
    theory, 463–465
Information coding,
    labeled lines in, 232
Information processing, 215–243
    chemical correlates, 217–220
    connector hypothesis, 239–241
    connectors in, 239–241
    effect of metabolic inhibitors, 218–220
    electrical field theory, 237
    molecular hypotheses, 235–241
    nonneurological hypotheses, 236–237
    RNA composition change, 217–218
    RNA synthesis increase, 217–218
Inhibitory synapses, 266–274
    invertebrate, 266–267
    vertebrate, 266–267, 272–274
Intercellular clefts
    in capillaries, 371–372
    tight junction sealing of, 372
Intranuclear filamentous inclusions, 139
Internuclear inclusions, 132–134
Inulin as extracellular space marker, 455, 456–457

Iodide as extracellular space marker, 453–456
Iodide space of brain, 453–456
Ions, flow into cerebrospinal fluid, 347

K

K complex in sleep, 297
Kernicterus and blood-brain barrier, 421

L

Lafora bodies, 150–154
    analysis, 152
    distribution, 151–152
    ultrastructure, 152–153
Lambda wave, 311
Lateral geniculate nucleus
    cat, 35, 38–39
    monkey, 34, 43
    rat, 44–45
Lattice-work inclusions, 143, 145
Learning, 233
Lewy bodies, 148–150
Light
    encephalographic response, 309–311
    synapses density and, 15–17, 43–46
Light microscopy of synapses, 40–42, 63, 66–69
Lipid solubility of brain penetrants, 350
Lipofuscin
    derivatives of, 157–158
    neuronal, 154–157
        histochemical reactions, 155
        ultrastructure, 155
Lobster
    abdominal ganglion, 253–256
        GABA content, 253–256
    axons, 252–253
        GABA content, 252–253
    nerve-muscle preparation, GABA release, 260–263
        uptake, 266
    nervous tissue, GABA metabolism in, 264–265
Lyssa bodies, 134

M

Marinesco bodies, 135–137

Maxwell's equation for specific resistance, applied to tissue impedance, 463–465

Medulla white matter extracellular space, 489

Memory, effect of metabolic inhibitors, 219–220

Meningitis
effect on blood-CSF and blood-brain barrier, 410–413
on ion concentration in cerebrospinal fluid, 411–413

Metabolic inhibitors as indicators of RNA role in information processing, 218–220

Micrograph spaces and extracellular space, 481–482
effects of fixation techniques, 481–482

Molecular code, bioassays for, *see* Bioassays for molecular code

Muscle membrane, crustacean postsynaptic GABA effect, 257–259

Muscles
innervated antigravity, 39
stretch receptors, 37–39

N

Negri bodies, 134–135

Nerve growth factor, 206–207
definition, 206
effect or RNA, 207

Nerve stimulation and acetylcholine release, 123–124

Nerve terminal degeneration, 70

Nervous system as chemical computer, 242–243

Nervous tissue cells, ribonucleic acid content of, 185–186

Neural coding
electrical phenomena, 232–233
molecular basis, 231–243

Neural pathways, labeled, 234–235
molecular code, 238–241

Neurofibrillary tangles, 148, 159–165
filamentous composition, 162–165
topographic distribution, 159

twisted tubule composition, 159–161

Neurofilamentous degeneration, 81–84

Neurofilamentous hypertrophy, 81, 83–84

Neurohypophysial degeneration, 92

Neuromelanin, 157–158

Neuromuscular junction, 8–12
endplates, 18–19
pharmacology of inhibition in crayfish, 259–260
structural studies, 18–23

Neuronal firing, 52
anesthesia effect, 6–7
polarization and, 6–8

Neuronal inclusions, 129–169
classification, 130
characteristic of viral infections, 132–133
Cowdry type A, 132–133
Cowdry type B, 133–134
definition, 129
pathological significance, 130
topographic distribution, 131

Neurons
chromatolytic, 28–32
overactive, 52
pigmented, 143, 145
resting potentials of central, 384

Neuropil, 40–41, 44
growth in starvation, 48–49
ultrastructure, 70, 78

Nissl substance, 179–180

Nitriles
effect on cellular RNA, 208
neurotoxicity, 208

Nuclear bodies, 136–139

Nutrition and brain growth, 48, 49

O

Optic nerve terminals
electrical stimulation, 38
long-term darkness and, 38–39

Organic bases, removal from cerebrospinal fluid, 368–369

Osmium tetroxide postfixation for micrographs
as cause of impedance change, 492
effect on extracellular space, 491–492

P

Parkinsonism, 148–150
Pattern stimulation, electroencephalographic response, 310–311
Peptides, role in neural coding, 230–231
Perineurium, 432–433
    tight junctions, 434–435
Peripheral nervous system
    degeneration, 84–91
    regeneration, 62, 95–96
Physiological stimulation as cause of RNA synthesis, 201–202
Pia-glia, morphology, 373
Pick bodies, 165, 167–169
    ultrastructure, 167
Picrotoxin
    as CNS stimulant, 259–260
    as synapses inhibitor, 272–274
Planerian worm experiments, 221
Postsynaptic membrane, GABA effect, 257–260, 268–269
Post-tetanic potentiation
    central nervous system, 11–13
    at neuromuscular junction, 8-12
    spinal cord, 37
Potassium
    in cerebrospinal fluid, 339–340, 380
        homeostasis, 385–387
    equilibration between blood and brain, 356
Preganglionic terminals, degeneration, 85–90
Proteins
    in central nervous systems fluids, 407–410
    labeled molecule turnover, 409–410
    synthesis in lumbar fluid, 407–409
        accompanying visual experience, 45–46
        information processing and, 218–220, 236
Purkinje cells
    GABA content, 269–272
    relation with Deiters cells, 269–272
Puromycin and inhibition of metabolism, 219–220

Q

Quaternary ammonium compounds, elimination from cerebrospinal fluid, 368–369

R

Recruiting response, 300–302
Reflexion coefficients relating to brain penetrants, 350
Respiratory acidosis and alkalosis, 392–395
Retina
    role of GABA, 274
    structural studies, 14–17
Retinal axons in cat, 35–36
Retinal receptors, 14–15
    light effect, 15–17, 43
Ribonucleic acid, 179–211
    age relationship, 189–191
    analysis, 193–194, 199–200
    axonal
        origin, 208–209
        synthesis, 209–210
    brain tissue, 180–181
    cellular, 182–188
        analysis by cell types, 199–200
    electrophysiological activity and, 201–205
    messenger, synthesis, 197–199
    metabolism, 191–200
        uptake of precursors, 191–193
    nerve cell tissue, 182, 185
    neuronal, 183–187
    ribosomal, 187, 196
        synthesis, 195
    separation into classes, 193–194
    transfer, synthesis, 195
Rodlet of Ronconi, 138, 139

S

Salicylic acid, penetration of brain, 352
Scotophobin, 231
Sleep
    alpha rhythm during, 297
    electroencephalograph during, 297–300, 304–305

rapid eye movement in, 298–300
spindling stage, 297
Sodium
in brain-cerebrospinal fluid exchange, 363
in central nervous tissue
mechanism for increase of membrane permeability, 501–502
permeability, 500–501
equilibration between blood and brain, 355
inhibition of penetration from blood into brain, 418–419
Somato-sensory stimulation, electroencephalographic response, 307
Spinal cord synapses, 37
Spreading depression, 502–505
abnormal fluid nptake by cellular elements, 496–497
behavior of chloride in cortex, 476–478
impedance change during, 470
role of glutamate, 503–505
of potassium, 502–503
water transport in cortex during, 476–478
Starvation and brain growth, 48, 49
Stimulus specificity, 228–229
Stretch stimulation, RNA synthesis resulting in, 203
Substance I, 251–252
Sugar transport
from blood into brain, 401
into cerebrospinal fluid, 398–399
carrier mediation, 398–402
in frog plexus, 401
Sulfate
as extracellular marker, 450, 455,–456
outflux in blood-brain relationship, 367
Synapses
degeneration, 32, 63–95
orthograde, 61–95
detonator, 13
development of new, 35–36, 233–235
electron microscopy of, 63–69
excitatory, 13
functional studies
long-term, 37–40
short-term, 4–14

hormones and growth, 47
inhibitory, 12–13
tetanic stimulation, 12–13
inoperative, 23–28, 34
experimental evidence, 25–28
intensifying, 13
nutrition and growth, 47
regeneration, 62, 95–99
in central nervous system, 96–97
in peripheral nervous system, 95–96
structural studies
long-term, 40–53
short-term, 14–23
trophic influence, 24–25
Synaptic cleft, 33–34
postsynaptic change, 33
Synaptic connections, new, 233–235
Synaptic degeneration, electron microscopy of, 63–64, 92–93
Synaptic efficacy, 2
Synaptic mitochondria, neuromuscular junctions, 18–22
Synaptic modification
anesthetic dependency, 6–7
mechanisms, 8–14
stimulation frequency effect, 5–7
time effect, 4–7
Synaptic plasticity, 2–55
Synaptic transmitter, 10–12
Synaptic vesicles, 79–81
acetylcholine
acquisition, 117–118
content, 116–117
release, 125–126
storage, 115–118
age and number, 24–25
change in number, 18–23
in size, 18–19
neuromuscular junctions, 18–23
retinal, 17
source, 115–116

T

Testosterone and brain growth, 48
Thalamus, human, EEG response to peripheral stimulation, 307–308

Thiocyanate as extracellular space marker, 455, 457
Thyroxin and brain growth, 47–48
Transprinting, 239
Trans-synaptic atrophy, 34–35

U

Urea in cerebrospinal fluid, 381–382
Ventriculo-cisternal perfusion of cerebro-spinal fluid, 342–344

V

Vertebrate(s)
  brain tissue, ribonucleic acid content, 181

nonmammalian, GABA inhibitory action, 268
Vestibular stimulation and RNA synthesis, 202
Viral infections, neuronal inclusions, 132–133
Visual experience and protein synthesis, 45–46
Visual stimulation, electroencephalographic response, 310
Visual system structure and visual experience, 43–46

W

Wallerian degeneration, 63